Molecular Features Distinguishing Gastric Cancer Subtypes

Molecular Features Distinguishing Gastric Cancer Subtypes

Special Issue Editor

Valli De Re

MDPI • Basel • Beijing • Wuhan • Barcelona • Belgrade

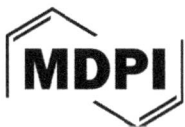

MDPI

Special Issue Editor
Valli De Re
Immunopathology and cancer biomarkers/Bio-proteomics facility,
Centro di Riferimento Oncologico, IRCCS
Italy

Editorial Office
MDPI
St. Alban-Anlage 66
4052 Basel, Switzerland

This is a reprint of articles from the Special Issue published online in the open access journal *International Journal of Molecular Sciences* (ISSN 1422-0067) from 2017 to 2018 (available at: https://www.mdpi.com/journal/ijms/special_issues/gastric_cancer_subtypes)

For citation purposes, cite each article independently as indicated on the article page online and as indicated below:

LastName, A.A.; LastName, B.B.; LastName, C.C. Article Title. *Journal Name* **Year**, *Article Number*, Page Range.

ISBN 978-3-03897-404-8 (Pbk)
ISBN 978-3-03897-405-5 (PDF)

Cover image courtesy of Vincenzo Canzonieri and Mara Fornasarig.

Contents

About the Special Issue Editor

Valli De Re, PhD, Biomedical Technologies Italy.   Birth: 10/06/1959, Belgium.   Project Manager/Bio-Proteomic facility Translational Researcher with expertise in Biomedical and Molecular Technologies.   Authorization of 2nd class professor class 06/A2 general and clinical pathology. Master in cytopathology assistance. Experience in the characterization of immunogenic and proteins involved in preneoplastic and neoplastic diseases, and in particular lymphoproliferative disorders and tumours of the gastrointestinal tract.   Research is focused on lymphomagenesis and gastric carcinoma in patients with a concomitant viral and/or bacterial infection (e.g., EBV, HCV, HIV, H. Pylori) and/or autoimmune disease (e.g., mixed cryoglobulinemia type II, celiac disease). Author/co-author of a patent: 009/016456 Idiotypic vaccine- PCT (n.85127032) WO2009016456 A2, 183 papers in PubMed, and 11 book chapters.

International Journal of
Molecular Sciences

MDPI

Editorial

Molecular Features Distinguish Gastric Cancer Subtypes

Valli De Re

Immunopathology and Cancer Biomarkers/Bio-Proteomics Facility, Centro di Riferimento Oncologico, IRCCS, 33081 Aviano, Italy; vdere@cro.it; Tel.: +39-0434-659-672; Fax: +39-0434-659-659

Received: 8 October 2018; Accepted: 10 October 2018; Published: 11 October 2018

Gastric cancer (GC) is a leading cause of cancer deaths. However, analysis of its molecular and clinical characteristics has been complicated by histological and etiological heterogeneity. Adenocarcinoma can be subdivided into histological Lauren and World Health Organization (WHO) classifications, however, this information has not led to the development of histologic subtype-specific treatment options. One way to potentially improve treatment for GCs is to better understand the molecular pathogenesis of the disease as well as the contribution of *Helicobacter pylori* infection and host immune responses leading to the development of an integrated histological and molecular classification schemes for GC.

Over the last several years, two major and comprehensive studies have been published focusing on a molecular classification of GC, the Cancer Genome Atlas (TCGA) and the Asian Cancer Research Group (ACRG) networks. Both Alessandrini [1] and Tirino [2], assessed the most common molecular GC classifications reported over the last years and found the main targetable molecular drivers highlighted by these studies. Indeed, only trastuzumab (anti-HER2 monoclonal antibody) and ramucirumab (anti-VEGFR monoclonal antibody) have proven to be successful in treating advanced or metastatic GC and they are currently used as a standard of care, but new drugs, e.g., nivolumab (PD-1 immune check-point inhibitor) showed activity against MSH-high locally advanced GC. Although the patient's condition improved by using these drugs, clinically, the practical use of the results remain is limited. Thus, GC remains one the most lethal diseases in the world with systemic chemotherapy still necessary to support its advanced stages. The hope is that combining histological and molecular classification will help identify more specific and limited in number biomarkers that consent to categorized patients who will really benefit from such therapies. With this aim Machlowska et al. [3], highlights the current status of prognostic molecular biomarkers that can be used in GC with a particular attention to those impacting on peritoneal spreading and neo-vascularization of the tumor, two of the most important mechanism by which tumors become more aggressive. In respect of the discovery of predictive tumor response markers in specific GC subset, Caggiari et al. [4], report that the characterization of a CDH1 haplotype is associated with improved survival in metastatic GC targeted by HER2 therapy. Indeed, the positivity for the HER2 status (by IHC or by fluorescence in situ hybridization) is a prerequisite for trastuzumab (anti-HER2 monoclonal antibody), which is the treatment currently used as a standard of care in advanced and metastatic GC. However, due to the heterogeneity of the tumor, the identification of the targeted HER2 molecules the treatment is not sufficient to predict drug response. In the present study, the authors also proposed a functional role of E-cadherin, the protein codified by the CDH1 gene in the HER2 pathway, which may be involved in better response to treatment. Although, the role of the CDH1 mutations in this context requires elucidation through further studies, the study is of interest for its novelty and for its potential utility in selecting patients who may benefit from new anti-HER2 agents. Hyperfibrinogenemia is also an important risk factor known to influence GC development and outcome, but the exact fragment of fibrinogens preferentially produced in the tumor environment is less known. A study reported by Repetto et al. [5], provides evidence of an increase in region D of the fibrinogen B chain fragments, as well as the entire fibrinogen chain production, in the tumor biopsies of patients with GC compared to the equivalent biopsies at least 5 cm from the tumor lesion of the same patients. Furthermore, they found a relationship between the increase in the load of fibrinogen fragments in tumor mass with an increase of the platelets number with a higher GC stage and the stomach corpus localization. Their results, thus, sustain the potential role of fibrinogen and platelets in the progression of tumor cell growth and aggressiveness of the tumor. Their data support the usefulness of plasma fibrinogen/fibrinolysis evaluation and platelet count in GC to evaluate the treatment response and patients' prognosis. Data have also helped to further characterize the interconnections between GC and platelet/coagulation pathways.

Part of the issue was focused on the characterization of specific GC subtypes to reinforce the TCGA classification. In this context Gullo et al. [6], investigate the transcriptomic landscape showed by EBV+ and the MSI-High subtypes identified in the TCGA classification. Their results strengthen the value for molecular segregation of these two subtypes and underline their relation with difference in clinical presentation. In particular, they confirm the importance of immunogenicity of EBV+ tumors and the mitotic signature of MSHI-high+ tumors, and reinforce the robustness of the Nanostring CodeSet proposed by TCGA classification. Notably, they highlighted a difference in the distribution of important checkpoint molecules, e.g., PD-1/PD-L1 molecules between EBV+ and MSHI-High subtypes, underling the best predictive value of protein expression rather than PD-L1 expression by immunohistochemistry to select GC patients eligible for anti-PD-1 immunotherapy. Their study offers a biological rationale to explain the unexpected positive response observed in patients harboring PD-L1-negative tumors, treated with anti-PD-1 therapy and a reasonable use of multiple immune targeted therapies in the specific EBV+ GC subtype, although further studies are necessary to sustain this proposal. The review reported by Dolcetti et al. [7], highlighted the observations of more recent advances in immunotherapeutic approaches overall of the GC subtypes. Indeed, immunotherapeutic approaches are still in the early phases but rapidly evolving in clinic. They discuss more important clinical trials reported by scientific communities, highlighting salient critical factors and possible solutions when they can be hypothesized. They also bring attention to the developments of more promising immunotherapies using adoptive cell and/or engineered cell; immune checkpoint inhibitors, immune modulator pathways, agonistic antibodies for co-stimulatory receptors, and cancer vaccines, thereby highlighting that for good clinical trials, the evaluation are also required to predict which patients will be responsive to particular treatments. Aldinucci et al. [8], focus on a particular immune axis: The interactions of chemokine CCL5, also known as RANTES, with its receptor CCR5, which regulates the immune and inflammatory responses by inducing lymphocytes and monocytes migration. Some researchers have demonstrated that cancer cells subvert the normal chemokine role, transforming them into a fundamental constituent of the immunosuppressive tumor microenvironment with tumor-promoting effects. The authors discuss the potential role of CCL5 leading to GC cell proliferation and metastasis and its proangiogenic effect in GC, although the exact functions of CCL5 in GC biology are not completely know. Moreover, CCR5 is not only a chemokine but also a co-receptor for HIV cell entry and a target of several drug researches, including GC treatment in pre-clinical and clinical trials as discussed by the authors. Notably, *H. pylori* increases the CCL5 secretion and interfere with the interaction between tumor cells and tumor microenvironment. Moreover, it was demonstrated that an increase in the CCL5 serum level and/or immunohistochemical staining is associated with more advanced GC stages and risk for peritoneal metastatization. Different algorithms include a CCL5 factor in order to predict treatment response, prognosis, and survival outcomes in GC. Thus, based on current knowledge, the CCL5/CCR5 axis may be considered a therapeutic target in GC.

Other landmark approaches to analytically photograph GC at molecular level are the modern mass spectrometry molecular imaging (MALDI-MSI) and flow cytometry. By using the first technique some pathologically significant molecules have already showed promise in the study of GC, providing greater insights into the molecular aspects of the disease and aiding in the identification of candidate biomarkers. Smith et al. [9] provided an overview of the MALDI-MSI innovative methodologies and summarize how the technique has been used to advance GC research for biomarker detection and for monitoring treatment response. Examples of MALDI-MSI applications in GC are the fasudil drug and its metabolites and inhibitors of the ROCK protein kinases, that can reach cancer cells in mice non-selectively. The proteomic differences may highlight a phenotypic tumor heterogeneity, which cannot be uncovered by using traditional histology; the identification is then successfully validated by immunohistochemistry of prognostic factors able to distinguish patients between stage I GC from those at the other stages; the identification of a protein profile predicting the HER+ GC tumor status with an accuracy of about 88–90%; the importance of difference in the distribution of lipids, metabolites and glicosilated fragments between the tumoral lesion and the non-neoplastic mucosa of a same patient. The second approach, the flow cytometry, has been used by Bockerstett [10], to analyze individually viable epithelial cells from gastric mucosa, which usually is limited due to difficulties in tissue processing. They develop and herein report an effective method for processing stomach tissue by enzymatic digestion and then analyze, via flow cytometry gastric epithelial cell, changes at single cell level from a large cell number of viable gastric cells in a model of inflammation induced gastric atrophy in mice. This approach results particularly useful for studying the inflammatory changes in surface markers on gastric epithelial cells during chronic disease. Their method confirms the up-regulation of MHC-II molecules on the epithelial cells caused by H-pylori-mediated inflammation. It is also possible that in the near future, a similar flow cytometric non-invasive diagnostic approach will be used to identify specific GC biomarker subtypes in circulating tumor cells.

The second part is in relation to environments and genetic factors that are known to increase the risk for GC development and how these factors may be useful to identify particular subjects that could be included in specific GC subtypes or at high risk for GC development.

H. pylori is the most abundant bacterium in the gastric epithelium and its presence was clearly associated with the risk of developing GC. In the last 100 years, infections have gradually declined due to new technologies, although other bacteria have been now identified in the stomach. Li and Perez. [11] discussed the potential role of the human gastric microbiota change in the presence or absence of *H. pylori* and moreover, they discuss which factors contribute to the increasing risk of GC. In particular, they confirm that the increased risk for GC is associated with the presence of highly virulent *H. pylori* strains (e.g., CagA+ and VacA+), and simultaneously by host genetic polymorphisms in the pro-inflammatory cytokine genes. However, it is now evident that during the progression of disease from *H. pylori* infection to GC, the stomach increases its pH thereby reducing the presence of *H. pylori*. In the same way, other bacteria increase with the possibility that the phenomena could be at patch trough the overall the stomach and with a different clinical outcome. Indeed, the change in the microbiota composition may also change the chronic inflammatory status in the stomach and a "point of no return" was reported in the cascade of events that lead to GC, which is associated with patients having intestinal metaplasia and dysplasia and is independent of *H. pylori* status. An elegant model to sustain gastric microbiota in the development of GC was in fact shown using the transgenic insulin-gastrin mouse model, but this could not be sufficient to demonstrate a direct role of microbiota in carcinogenesis. Nonetheless, the authors emphasize that in some regions, despite the decline of *H. pylori* infections, an increased incidence of GC was especially found in young adults (<40 years), GC diffuse type, and with no difference in the sex frequency. For the authors these new epidemiological data are particularly important since they could imply that changes in the gastric microbiota associated with new standards of living may be implicated in the specific increase in the GC development showed. On the other hand, the increase of GC incidence may be associated with the increase of another disease, like autoimmune gastritis that was found similarly to GC increase in the same population. Thus, a direct role for microbiota in GC development need further studies before being clearly accepted as a model of GC carcinogenesis. Kidane [12], discusses current molecular mechanisms that lead to DNA single and double-strand breaks and that reduce the capacity of DNA repair caused by *H. pylori* infection. The model discussed highlights the necessity for *H. pylori*-gastric cell contact and the infiltration of immune cells into the tumor microenvironment. The production of RONS, reactive oxygen species and nitrogen species, which cause DNA base damage and activation of the NF-κB factors that induces the cleavage of promoter gene regions and double strand breaks are the major consequence of *H. pylori* infection, although *H. pylori* itself may result directly from mechanisms not yet fully known through epigenetic alterations and overall a host genome instability. Excision DNA repair are complex and may be resumed in three major pathways that use different enzymes and recognition process: The base excision repair (BER) that use specific glycosylases and preferentially recognize small damages, the nucleotide excision repair (NER) involved also in bulky DNA reparation, and the DNA mismatch repair (MMR). BER, repairs during the cell cycle the majority of break damages resulting from oxidation and alkylation and it is the primary repair pathway occurring during *H. pylori* infection. Authors discuss how *H. pylori* is involved in BER and NER processes and the effect known today in enzyme alterations involved in these processes, including gene mutations occurring in the host and associated with the process of DNA repair. Authors also evidence that *H. pylori* infection enhances the transcription factor NF-κB pathway in immune and epithelial cells, thus resulting of the modulation of many DNA repair genes and the production of the inducible inflammatory mediator nitric oxide synthase (iNOS), which through the production of nitric oxide, contribute to enhanced inactivation of DNA repair enzymes and DNA double strand breaks. Thus, we can conclude that host genetic variants involved in DNA repair could modify the process of carcinogenesis in *H. pylori* infected hosts in any way, but that specific association among them require further studies. Indeed, the molecular mechanisms of DNA break formation, how these breaks are repaired and the interference of *H. pylori* in these processes remain largely to be clarified. Reprimo is a family of gene downstream effectors of p53-induced cell cycle arrest at G2/M checkpoint. Epigenetic silencing of RPRM, mainly by DNA methylation of its promoter region or P53 pathway, occurs at early stages and is a common event in GC. Amigo et al. [13], emphasize the role of this poorly studied gene in GC carcinogenesis. Of particular interest, previously authors demonstrated that methylation of the reprimo promoter region was associated with the infection of *H. pylori* and in particular with the more virulent cytotoxin-associated gene A (CagA) positive strains and that DNA methylation of reprimo may predict the progression of gastric lesions with a high sensitivity and specificity. Authors propose that reprimo methylation of cell-free DNA could be a marker for non-invasive discovery of GC in the next future.

While intestinal GC is more associated to *H. pylori* infection, the diffuse type composed by non-cohesive cells is more observable in a hereditary form. Ansari et al. [14], focus their review on the pathogenicity of this specific diffuse-GC type and report the most current understanding of the host factors, as well as the bacterial *H. pylori* factors that have been specifically involved. Although the pathogenicity of DGC has not yet been clarified in detail, authors indicate the central role of E-cadherin and cell-signaling pathways in the maintenance of cell integrity and function in particular in this subtype of GC. Melo et al. [15], highlight the state of art regarding the best methodologies, including the evaluation of migration dynamics of cells carrying E-cadherin variants in a transgene drosophila melanogaster model, to categorize the missense mutations in the CDH1, the gene codifying for the E-cadherin protein. Indeed, in the hereditary form of GC 155 different mutations have been reported to date but in about 17% of these cases the mutation remains with a function not predictable. The definition of how these alterations could perturb the expression and function of E-cadherin, as well as related signaling and cellular mechanisms, are fundamental to help clinicians and genetic counsellors in the management of the patients with GC and their familiars. Moreover, some mutations in the CDH1 gene may result in a slight down regulation rather than a complete abolition/function of the E-cadherin, and these alterations may be present also in other than hereditary form of GC. In that context, Melo and Seruca's group is considered a worldwide reference center to study the predictable function of CDH1 mutations. Their studies are also relevant to gain further understanding of the GC pathogenesis. In that context, the study of Caggiari et al. [4], highlight the possibility that CDH1 gene mutations can also be used as a potential prognostic factor for GC survival.

Bizzaro [16] noted that autoimmune diseases may also predispose individuals to malignancies. A link between chronic autoimmune gastritis and GC development has been known from some

Int. J. Mol. Sci. **2018**, *19*, 3121

time. Bizzaro et al. describes autoimmune gastritis and review its association with GC, in particular of the intestinal type and type I gastric carcinoid. The show particular attention to autoantibodies produced during autoimmune gastritis as markers for monitoring patient's response to treatment and during follow-up. The low sensitivity of autoantibodies has limited their application in clinical practice for an early detection of patient at risk for GC, but in the next future, the availability of new multiplex technology for the simultaneous detection of many autoantibodies could to overcome these limitations. Another important autoimmune disease associated with the development of GC and lymphoproliferative disorders is the common variable immunodeficiency disorder (CVID), a hypogammaglobulinemia, highly variable and heterogeneous in clinical manifestations, although frequently expresses severe, recurrent, and chronic bacterial infections of the respiratory and gastrointestinal tracts. The exact molecular pathways underlying the relationships between CVID and GC remain poorly understood. Leone et al. [17] assessed the most frequent genetic abnormalities resulting in CIVD discovered today, although they account for less than 15% of the overall cases. They also provided a hypothetical mechanism of GC development based on the peculiar features of the tumor occurring in these patients. Accordingly, they propose a protocol to screening patients with CVID at risk for GC by using three easy and non-invasive tests based on the evidence of a megaloblastic or macrocytic anemia, a deficiency in serum vitamin B12 and iron, and a positive urea breath test for *H. pylori* infection. Another hereditable predisposition for GC is the Lynch syndrome (LS) and familial adenomatous polyposis (FAP), two autosomal dominant genetic conditions leading to the development of colorectal cancer, but also to other tumors. Fornasig et al. [18] reported detailed clinical and molecular features of GC occurring in these patients since characteristics of GC associated with these diseases are still not well known. There information's added an important contribution to the recognition of patients at higher risk for GC development, which could be direct for the endoscopic surveillance. Family history of GC is a generic but a well-recognized risk factor for developing GC. Serum metabolic profiles including 188 serum metabolites were used by Corona et al. [19], to differentiate GC patients from first-degree relatives of patients with GC in two separate and independent series. The best discriminators they found belonged to phospholipids and acylcarnitines classes, and the discrimination increased in power when the C16 and M(OH)22:1 metabolites were integrated with serum pepsinogen-II value and with the age of the individual tested. The results of the study also provided new insights into the metabolism of GC. The increased acylcarnitines probably reflects alterations in the mitochondrial respiratory complex activities arising in GC that further increase *H. pylori* infection and the major age of patient with GC; while the decrease of some phosphatidylcholine lipid derivatives may be a consequence of a predisposition of tumor cells for a phospholipid storage. Authors propose that the effect of this storage may alter the cell lipid raft known to be involved in several tumor processes and at the same it may reflect the increase in tumor nerve growth observed in GC.

Funding: This research received no external funding.

Conflicts of Interest: The authors declare no conflict of interest.

References

1. Alessandrini, L.; Manchi, M.; De Re, V.; Dolcetti, R.; Canzonieri, V. Proposed Molecular and miRNA Classification of Gastric Cancer. *Int. J. Mol. Sci.* **2018**, *19*, 1683. [CrossRef] [PubMed]
2. Tirino, G.; Pompella, L.; Petrillo, A.; Laterza, M.M.; Pappalardo, A.; Caterino, M.; Orditura, M.; Ciardiello, F.; Galizia, G.; De Vita, F. What's New in Gastric Cancer: The Therapeutic Implications of Molecular Classifications and Future Perspectives. *Int. J. Mol. Sci.* **2018**, *19*, 2659. [CrossRef] [PubMed]
3. Machlowska, J.; Maciejewski, R.; Sitarz, R. The Pattern of Signatures in Gastric Cancer Prognosis. *Int. J. Mol. Sci.* **2018**, *19*, 1658. [CrossRef] [PubMed]

4. Caggiari, L.; Miolo, G.; Buonadonna, A.; Basile, D.; Santeufemia, D.A.; Cossu, A.; Palmieri, G.; De Zorzi, M.; Fornasarig, M.; Alessandrini, L.; et al. Characterizing Metastatic HER2-Positive Gastric Cancer at the CDH1 Haplotype. *Int. J. Mol. Sci.* **2017**, *19*, 47. [CrossRef] [PubMed]

5. Repetto, O.; Maiero, S.; Magris, R.; Miolo, G.; Cozzi, M.R.; Steffan, A.; Canzonieri, V.; Cannizzaro, R.; De Re, V. Quantitative Proteomic Approach Targeted to Fibrinogen beta Chain in Tissue Gastric Carcinoma. *Int. J. Mol. Sci.* **2018**, *19*, 759. [CrossRef] [PubMed]

6. Gullo, I.; Carvalho, J.; Martins, D.; Lemos, D.; Monteiro, A.R.; Ferreira, M.; Das, K.; Tan, P.; Oliveira, C.; Carneiro, F.; et al. The Transcriptomic Landscape of Gastric Cancer: Insights into Epstein-Barr Virus Infected and Microsatellite Unstable Tumors. *Int. J. Mol. Sci.* **2018**, *19*, 2079. [CrossRef] [PubMed]

7. Dolcetti, R.; De Re, V.; Canzonieri, V. Immunotherapy for Gastric Cancer: Time for a Personalized Approach? *Int. J. Mol. Sci.* **2018**, *19*, 1602. [CrossRef] [PubMed]

8. Aldinucci, D.; Casagrande, N. Inhibition of the CCL5/CCR5 Axis against the Progression of Gastric Cancer. *Int. J. Mol. Sci.* **2018**, *19*, 1477. [CrossRef] [PubMed]

9. Smith, A.; Piga, I.; Galli, M.; Stella, M.; Denti, V.; Del, P.M.; Magni, F. Matrix-Assisted Laser Desorption/Ionisation Mass Spectrometry Imaging in the Study of Gastric Cancer: A Mini Review. *Int. J. Mol. Sci.* **2017**, *18*, 2588. [CrossRef] [PubMed]

10. Bockerstett, K.A.; Wong, C.F.; Koehm, S.; Ford, E.L.; DiPaolo, R.J. Molecular Characterization of Gastric Epithelial Cells Using Flow Cytometry. *Int. J. Mol. Sci.* **2018**, *19*, 1096. [CrossRef] [PubMed]

11. Li, J.; Perez Perez, G.I. Is There a Role for the Non-Helicobacter pylori Bacteria in the Risk of Developing Gastric Cancer? *Int. J. Mol. Sci.* **2018**, *19*, 1353. [CrossRef] [PubMed]

12. Kidane, D. Molecular Mechanisms of *H. pylori*-Induced DNA Double-Strand Breaks. *Int. J. Mol. Sci.* **2018**, *19*, 2891. [CrossRef] [PubMed]

13. Amigo, J.D.; Opazo, J.C.; Jorquera, R.; Wichmann, I.A.; Garcia-Bloj, B.A.; Alarcon, M.A.; Owen, G.I.; Corvalan, A.H. The Reprimo Gene Family: A Novel Gene Lineage in Gastric Cancer with Tumor Suppressive Properties. *Int. J. Mol. Sci.* **2018**, *19*, 1862. [CrossRef] [PubMed]

14. Ansari, S.; Gantuya, B.; Tuan, V.P.; Yamaoka, Y. Diffuse Gastric Cancer: A Summary of Analogous Contributing Factors for Its Molecular Pathogenicity. *Int. J. Mol. Sci.* **2018**, *19*, 2424. [CrossRef] [PubMed]

15. Melo, S.; Figueiredo, J.; Fernandes, M.S.; Goncalves, M.; Morais-de-Sa, E.; Sanches, J.M.; Seruca, R. Predicting the Functional Impact of CDH1 Missense Mutations in Hereditary Diffuse Gastric Cancer. *Int. J. Mol. Sci.* **2017**, *18*, 2687. [CrossRef] [PubMed]

16. Bizzaro, N.; Antico, A.; Villalta, D. Autoimmunity and Gastric Cancer. *Int. J. Mol. Sci.* **2018**, *19*, 377. [CrossRef] [PubMed]

17. Leone, P.; Vacca, A.; Dammacco, F.; Racanelli, V. Common Variable Immunodeficiency and Gastric Malignancies. *Int. J. Mol. Sci.* **2018**, *19*, 451. [CrossRef] [PubMed]

18. Fornasarig, M.; Magris, R.; De Re, V.; Bidoli, E.; Canzonieri, V.; Maiero, S.; Viel, A.; Cannizzaro, R. Molecular and Pathological Features of Gastric Cancer in Lynch Syndrome and Familial Adenomatous Polyposis. *Int. J. Mol. Sci.* **2018**, *19*, 1682. [CrossRef] [PubMed]

19. Corona, G.; Cannizzaro, R.; Miolo, G.; Caggiari, L.; De Zorzi, M.; Repetto, O.; Steffan, A.; De Re, V. Use of Metabolomics as a Complementary Omic Approach to Implement Risk Criteria for First-Degree Relatives of Gastric Cancer Patients. *Int. J. Mol. Sci.* **2018**, *19*, 750. [CrossRef] [PubMed]

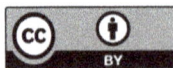

International Journal of
Molecular Sciences

MDPI

Review

Proposed Molecular and miRNA Classification of Gastric Cancer

Lara Alessandrini [1], Melissa Manchi [1], Valli De Re [2,*], Riccardo Dolcetti [3] and
Vincenzo Canzonieri [1,*]

[1] Pathology, IRCCS CRO National Cancer Institute, 33081 Aviano, Italy; lara.alessandrini@cro.it (L.A.);
manchi.melissa@gmail.com (M.M.)
[2] Immunopathology and Cancer Biomarkers, IRCCS CRO National Cancer Institute, 33081 Aviano, Italy
[3] The University of Queensland Diamantina Institute, Translational Research Institute, Woolloongabba,
QLD 4102, Australia; r.dolcetti@uq.edu.au
* Correspondence: vdere@cro.it (V.D.R.); vcanzonieri@cro.it (V.C.);
Tel.: +39-0434-659-672 (V.D.R.); +39-0434-659-618 (V.C.)

Received: 2 May 2018; Accepted: 1 June 2018; Published: 6 June 2018

Abstract: Gastric cancer (GC) is a common malignant neoplasm worldwide and one of the main cause of cancer-related deaths. Despite some advances in therapies, long-term survival of patients with advanced disease remains poor. Different types of classification have been used to stratify patients with GC for shaping prognosis and treatment planning. Based on new knowledge of molecular pathways associated with different aspect of GC, new pathogenetic classifications for GC have been and continue to be proposed. These novel classifications create a new paradigm in the definition of cancer biology and allow the identification of relevant GC genomic subsets by using different techniques such as genomic screenings, functional studies and molecular or epigenetic characterization. An improved prognostic classification for GC is essential for the development of a proper therapy for a proper patient population. The aim of this review is to discuss the state-of-the-art on combining histological and molecular classifications of GC to give an overview of the emerging therapeutic possibilities connected to the latest discoveries regarding GC.

Keywords: gastric cancer; gene expression profile; gene mutation; molecular gastric cancer subtype; EBV infection; microsatellite; preclinical models; miRNA

1. Introduction

Gastric cancer (GC) is the fifth malignant neoplasm worldwide and the third cause of cancer-related deaths [1]. Despite some advances in therapies for GC, long-term survival of patients with advanced disease is poor. GC is a multifactorial disease in which both genetic and environmental factors are involved. Historically, different types of classification have been used to shape prognosis and plan treatment [2–6]. Proposed in 1965, the Laurén system was widely used in GC classification for half a century, which was very useful in evaluating the natural history of GC carcinogenesis. Based on pathological morphology, the Laurén system divides GC into intestinal (G-INT), diffuse (G-DIF) and mixed GC (G-Mix). An improved prognostic classification for GC is essential for the development of a proper therapy for patients. Therefore, based on new knowledge of molecular pathways, new pathogenetic classifications for GC have been proposed. The aim of this review is to update molecular classifications of GC to give an overview of the emerging therapeutic possibilities

2. Histological and Molecular Classifications of GC

Based on the gene expression profile for GC cell lines and patients' tissue, Tan et al. [7] classified GC into two intrinsic genomic subtypes that overlapped with the histological Lauren's classification.

The G-INT subtype and the G-DIF are related to intestinal and diffuse histology, respectively. The two intrinsic subtypes have distinct patterns of gene expression.

In the G-INT subtype, genes associated with the carbohydrate and protein metabolism (FUT2) and cell adhesion (LGALS4, CDH17) are upregulated. The FUT2 gene codes for the galactoside 2-alpha-L-fucosyltransferase 2 enzyme affecting the Lewis blood group involved in *Helicobacter pylori* (*H. pylori*) infection; the LGALS4 gene codes the galectin 4 implicated in the modulation of the interaction between cell-cell and cell-matrix and the peptide transporter cadherin-17 coded by the CDH17 gene.

Instead, in the G-DIF subtype, genes related to cell proliferation (AURKB) and fatty acid metabolism (ELOVL5) are upregulated. The AURKB gene codes for the Aurora B kinase that functions in the attachment of the mitotic spindle to the centromere, and the ELOVL5 gene encodes the elongation of the very long chain fatty acids protein. The prognosis of G-DIF tumour type is poor, and the response to chemotherapy is reduced compared to those of the G-INT type. In vitro, G-INT cell lines are more sensitive to 5-FU and oxaliplatin than G-DIF lines, which result in being more sensitive to cisplatin [7,8]. There were many more other molecular studies based on the Laurén classification [9–12].

A molecular classification for GC, independent of the histological Laurent classification, was made in 2013 by Singapore Researchers. They categorized GC into three main types: [13] a proliferative profile associated with a high genomic instability and *TP53* gene mutation, a metabolic profile associated with a higher anaerobic glycolysis and resulting in tumour cells more sensitive to 5-FU therapy and a mesenchymal stem cell profile with a high capacity for self-renewal, immunomodulation and tissue regeneration showing a sensitivity to PIK3CA-mTOR pathway inhibitors.

Soon after, The Cancer Genome Atlas (TCGA) research group categorized GC into four main groups by introducing new technologies of large-scale genome sequencing analyses [14]: Epstein-Barr virus (EBV)-positive cancers (9% of all GC) characterized by DNA hypermethylation, a high frequency of PIK3CA mutations and PDL1/PDL2 overexpression, microsatellite instable (MSI, 22%) tumours, showing a very high number of mutations and DNA methylation sites and chromosome instable tumours (CIN, 50%) mainly coding for alteration in tyrosine kinase receptors and genome stable tumours (GS, 20%).

In 2015, by using similar multi-platform molecular approaches, the Asian Cancer Research Group (ACRG) developed a novel molecular classification for GC based on a pre-defined set of genetic pathways relevant to the biology of GC, including epithelial-mesenchymal transition (EMT), microsatellite instability, cytokine signaling and P53 activity [15]. The ACRG classification included four subtypes [16]: an MSI subtype (22.7%), a mesenchymal group microsatellite stable (MSS)/EMT (15.3%) based on the evidence of epithelial-to-mesenchymal transition, a microsatellite stable TP53-positive subtype MSS/TP53+ (26.3%) and a microsatellite stable TP53-negative subtype MSS/TP53− (35.7%), according to the presence/absence of P53 mutations. By using this approach, the MSI subtype had the best prognosis, while the MSS/EMT subtype had the worst one. The former occurred predominantly at an early stage in the distal part of the stomach and showed mainly an intestinal histology (according to Lauren's classification); the latter occurred at an advanced stage, at a younger age and with a diffuse histology (>80%) including a large set of signet ring cell carcinomas seeding in the peritonea with malignant ascites (64.1% vs. 15–24% in the other subtypes) and showed loss of CDH1 expression. Given the earlier stage of diagnosis, MSI and MSS/TP53− patients also had the best overall survival and when recurrence occurs, this was generally limited to liver metastasis (about 20%). EBV infection was more frequent in the MSS/TP53 active group.

In ACRG, the correlation between molecular classification and prognosis was validated using the TCGA [14] and the Gastric Cancer Project '08 Singapore datasets [16]. As shown in Table 1, the ACRG subtypes show a significant overlap with the TCGA subtypes, and this confirms the association between better survival and the MSI subtype [17]. However, the overlap is only partial and probably due to the differences in the patient population (Korea in ACRG and USA and Western Europe in

TCGA), tumour sampling and technical platforms used. Nonetheless, these novel classifications created a new paradigm in the definition of GC, although some limitations persist:

i. these classifications are based on a highly complex methodology, which is not always available in every laboratory;
ii. they lack a prospective validation on a large scale;
iii. they have striking differences in epidemiology, underlying molecular mechanisms and prognosis;
iv. their prognostic power is decreased by limited follow-up of patients;
v. none of them takes into account the active, non-malignant stromal cells

Table 1. Key characteristics of The Cancer Genome Atlas (TCGA) and the Asian Cancer Research Group (ACRG) molecular classifications of gastric cancer (GC). MSI, microsatellite instable; CIN, chromosome instable; GS, genome stable; EGJ, esophagogastric junction; MSS, microsatellite stable.

TCGA	EBV	MSI	CIN	GS
- Males >>> Females - Intestinal-type histology - Frequently located at fundus and body - JAK2 amplification - PIK3CA mutation (80% subtype) inactivating in the kinase domain (exon 20) - ARID1A (55%) mutations - Immune cell signaling enrichment	- >>>Females - Intestinal-type histology - An older age at diagnosis - Mutation in one of several different DNA mismatch repair genes (i.e., MLH1 or MSH2) - Lacks targetable amplifications		- Males >>> Females - Intestinal-type histology - Frequently located at EGJ - RTK-RAS amplifications (EGFR, ERRB2, ERRB3, VEGFA, FGFR2, MET, NRAS/KRAS, JAK2 and PIK3CA) - Amplification of cell cycle genes - TP53 mutations	- Males = Females - Distal location - Diffuse-type histology - An early age at diagnosis - Recurrent CDH1 inactivation, RHOA mutation, ARID1A mutation
ACGR	**MSS/TP53+**	**MSI**	**MSS/TP53-**	**MSS/EMT**
	- Frequently EBV-positive - Intermediate prognosis - Mutations in ARID1A, APC, KRAS, PIK3CQA and SMAD4	- Distal stomach - Intestinal-type histology - Early stage diagnosis - Favourable prognosis - Hypermutation	- TP53 mutation - Amplification of RTKs - Intermediate prognosis	- Diagnosed at younger age - Diffuse-type histology - Worse prognosis - Low number of mutations

3. Integrated Molecular Signatures to Discriminate Intestinal and Diffuse Histological GC Subtypes

Previous findings indicated that diffuse and intestinal GC might be two distinct diseases with different molecular bases, aetiologies, epidemiologies and, thus, response to therapies. A recent study based on a population of 300 GC identified 40 genes specifically expressed in diffuse or intestinal GC [12] and three genes associated with the patients' prognosis, namely EFEMP1 and FRZB in G-DIF and KRT23 in G-INT. The products of the former are an extracellular matrix glycoprotein and a secreted protein regulating bone development and influencing the Wnt/beta-catenin pathway. The latter encodes for a member of the keratin family, which regulates epithelial cell structures.

In the last year, a nine-gene signature, including two negative impact factors (NR1I2 and LGALSL) and seven positive ones (C1ORF198, CST2, LAMP5, FOXS1, CES1P1, MMP7 and COL8A1), was proposed to predict the outcome of GC, and the model was able to predict patients' outcome in terms of survival and recurrence, clustering GC cases into low-risk and high-risk groups [18].

Although molecular characterizations have identified the gene signature for prognosis in GC, today, signatures are still inadequate for accurate patient therapy. Identifying new tumour markers or constructing gene models is still the focus of many research works and studies.

4. TCGA Classification of GC and Related Signaling Pathways

4.1. EBV-Related GC

EBV-positive GC is one of the four subtypes of GC, as defined by TCGA, found in 9% of GC and characterised by high EBV burden [13]. EBV-positive tumours were more frequent in men (81% of the cases) and mainly occurred in the upper part of the stomach. In addition, EBV-positive GC was more prevalent in younger patients compared to older subjects (Figure 1). The histology of EBV-related GC is moderately- to poorly-differentiated adenocarcinoma, often accompanied by dense lymphocytic infiltration [19–22]. In this subtype were identified pathways related to the elevated expression of programmed death ligands 1 and 2 (PD-L1 and PD-L2), phosphatidylinositol-4,5-bisphosphate 3-kinase, the catalytic subunit α (PIK3CA) mutation and Janus kinase 2 (JAK2) amplification.

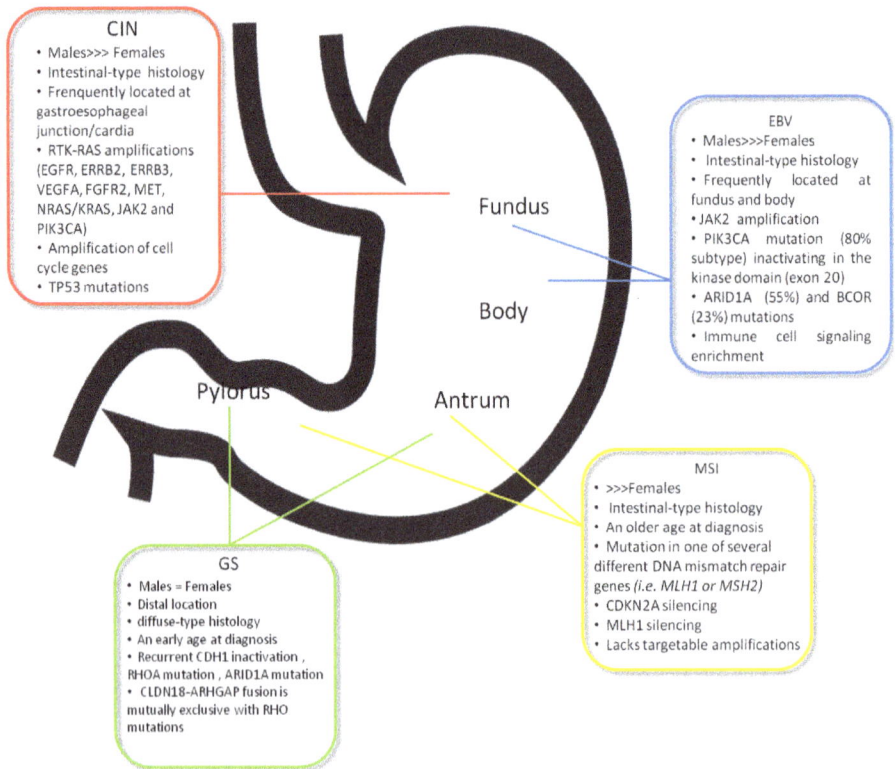

CIN
- Males>>> Females
- Intestinal-type histology
- Frenquently located at gastroesophageal junction/cardia
- RTK-RAS amplifications (EGFR, ERRB2, ERRB3, VEGFA, FGFR2, MET, NRAS/KRAS, JAK2 and PIK3CA)
- Amplification of cell cycle genes
- TP53 mutations

EBV
- Males>>>Females
- Intestinal-type histology
- Frequently located at fundus and body
- JAK2 amplification
- PIK3CA mutation (80% subtype) inactivating in the kinase domain (exon 20)
- ARID1A (55%) and BCOR (23%) mutations
- Immune cell signaling enrichment

Fundus

Body

Pylorus

Antrum

MSI
- >>>Females
- Intestinal-type histology
- An older age at diagnosis
- Mutation in one of several different DNA mismatch repair genes (*i.e. MLH1 or MSH2*)
- CDKN2A silencing
- MLH1 silencing
- Lacks targetable amplifications

GS
- Males = Females
- Distal location
- diffuse-type histology
- An early age at diagnosis
- Recurrent CDH1 inactivation , RHOA mutation , ARID1A mutation
- CLDN18-ARHGAP fusion is mutually exclusive with RHO mutations

Figure 1. The most relevant clinic-pathological and molecular features of TCGA subtypes.

PD-L1 helps neoplastic cells to escape from antitumoral immune response, by binding to PD-1, which is expressed on cytotoxic T-cells [23–25]. In the literature PD-L1, expressed on cancer cells or tumour infiltrating immune cells, has emerged as a prognostic factor in GC, but its specific role in EBV-related GC has not yet been described [26–30]. In a recent study [31] focusing on EBV-related GC, the expression of PD-1/PDL-1 on immune and neoplastic cells, respectively, was directly related to diffuse histology (according to Lauren's classification) and depth of tumour invasion. Therefore, targeted immune therapy against the PD-L1/PD-1 axis could be effective in this subtype. Pembrolizumab, a highly specific monoclonal antibody targeting the PD-1 receptor, showed an overall response rate of 22% in a cohort of patients previously treated with chemotherapy [32]. Subsequently,

PD-L1 expression in at least 1% of neoplastic cells from paraffin-embedded tissue was significantly related to response to this drug [33]. Another anti-immune strategy, already employed in melanoma, targeting both the PD-1/PD-L1 and the CTLA/B7 axis, is under evaluation in several clinical trials [34].

The PI3K family of intracellular kinases is involved in cell survival, proliferation, differentiation and migration [35]. In GC, the PI3K/AKT/mTOR pathway is frequently activated and associated with nodal metastasis: in 35–80% of GC cases, *PI3KCA* is overexpressed [27–29], and in 40–82% of GC cases, phosphorylation of AKT is described [36–40]. The EBV and MSI molecular subtypes of GC show alterations in PIK3CA, in 80% and 42% of cases, respectively [14]. However, molecular mechanisms responsible for sensitivity to PI3K inhibitors are not clearly defined, and the potential use of this drug category in advanced GC is still in the preclinical stage. [41]. In GC, the PIK3CA mutation could be predictive of response to everolimus and AKT inhibitors [42,43]. It is hypothesised that AKT affects the BCL2 protein and the NF-κB pathway. PI3K may also induce upregulation of the chemo-resistance proteins, MDR1/Pgp, BCL2 and XIAP, and downregulation of the expression of BAX and caspase 3. In vitro, in tumour tissues of GC patients, AKT activation and *PTEN* loss were associated with increased resistance to multiple chemotherapeutic agents (5-FU, doxorubicin, mitomycin C and cisplatin) [44]. Similarly, in GC cell lines, a combination of PI3K and AKT inhibitors with chemotherapy agents has successfully attenuated chemotherapeutic resistance [45,46].

The JAK/STAT signaling pathway has been identified in several types of tumours, including GC, and especially in the EBV-subtype [47,48]. The phosphorylation and subsequent activation of JAK2 lead to STAT activation by phosphorylation and activation of downstream gene expression involved in cell proliferation and apoptosis arrest [49]. Therefore, JAK2 inhibitors may also represent a potential therapeutic treatment for solid tumours, such as GC, despite them being primarily studied in inflammatory and myeloproliferative disorders [50]. Ruxolitinib, a JAK1 and JAK2 inhibitor, in combination with capecitabine has demonstrated preliminary efficacy in pancreatic cancer and, in combination with regorafenib, and is currently under evaluation in colorectal cancer (ClinicalTrials.gov identifier: NCI02119676) [51]. However, there are no trials ongoing in GC.

4.2. GC with MSI

Microsatellite instability (MSI) is the hallmark of the MSI subtype according to TGCA classification. MSI represents 15–30% of all GCs, is more frequently associated with intestinal histology and usually arises in the mucosa of the antrum, mainly in females at an older age [14,52,53] (Figure 1). MSI is a change that occurs in the DNA of certain cells (such as tumour cells) in which the number of repeats of microsatellites (short, repeated sequences of DNA) is different than the number of repeats in the DNA when it was inherited. The cause of MSI may be a defect in the ability to repair mistakes made when DNA is copied in the cell, determined by mutations in one of several different DNA mismatch repair genes (i.e., *MLH1* or *MSH2*) [54]. The principal mechanism causing MMR deficiency in this GC subtype relies on different *MMR* genes probably involved in MSI-high (MSI-H) sporadic GC without *MLH1* hypermethylation [55,56]. Zhu et al. in a meta-analysis showed a significant reduction of mortality in patients with MSI-H compared with MSI-L (low) or microsatellite stable (MSS) cases [57]. In the MRC MAGIC trial, the relationship between MMRd, MSI and survival in patients with resectable GC randomised to surgery alone or perioperative chemotherapy has been examined. MSI status and *MLH1* deficiency had a positive prognostic role in patients treated with surgery alone, while a negative prognostic effect was established in patients treated with chemotherapy [55]. In contrast to MSI in colorectal cancer, in MSI GC, alterations in *PIK3CA, ERBB3, ERB22* and *EGFR* genes, along with major histocompatibility complex I are known [14,53], whereas *BRAF* V600E mutations have never been found [14]. In MSI-positive colorectal cancer, pembrolizumab has shown objective response and progression-free survival rates of 40% and 78%, respectively [58]. Both MSI and EBV subtypes have been associated with a more favourable prognosis and are, therefore, detected in lower percentage in the metastatic setting, with subsequent difficult case finding in clinical trial design [59,60].

4.3. GC with CIN

The largest group, CIN subtype, accounts for approximately 50% of GCs, and its most frequent location is in the esophagogastric junction (EGJ)/cardia, as established by the TCGA study [14] (Figure 1). CIN GC with an intestinal type histology is associated with copy number gains of chromosomes 8q, 17q and 20q, whereas gains at 12q and 13q are more related to diffuse histology [61,62]. The effect of these alterations is the loss or gain of function of oncogenes and tumour suppressor genes [63]. In the CIN subtype, some specific mutations are frequently found, i.e., in the TP53 gene and receptor tyrosine kinases (RTKs), as well as amplifications of cell cycle genes (cyclin E1, cyclin D1 and cyclin-dependent kinase 6) and of the gene that encodes the ligand vascular endothelial growth factor A (VEGFA) [14,64]. Furthermore, HER2, BRAF, epidermal growth factor (EGFR), MET, FGFR2 and RAS mutations have been discovered in the CIN subtype [14,65] (Figure 2).

The most frequent genetic alteration of this subtype, along with their respective targeted drugs, is detailed in Table 2.

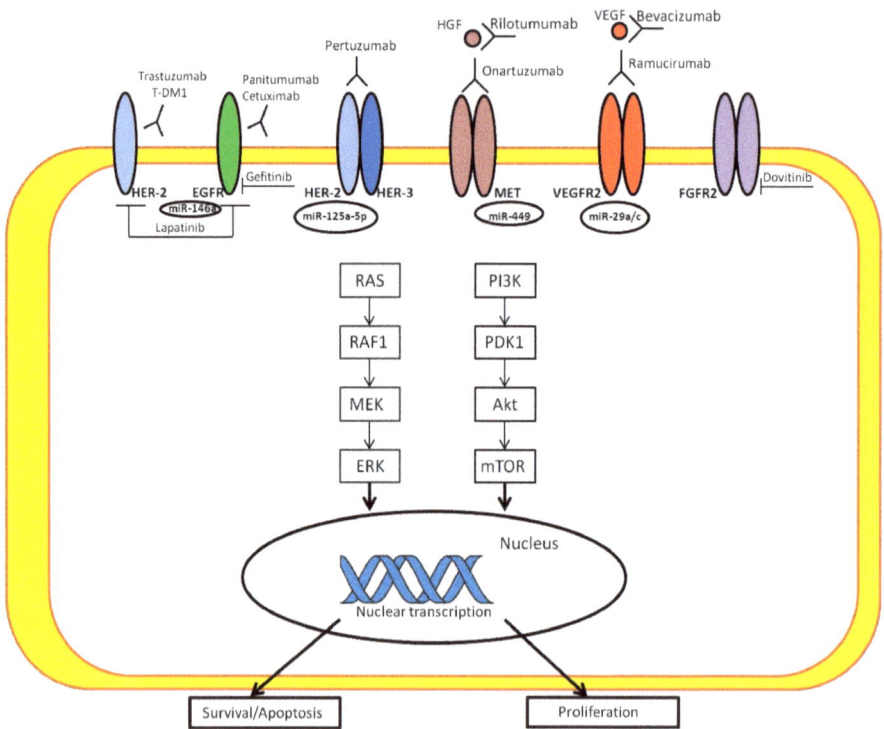

Figure 2. The most relevant targetable pathways in GC.

Table 2. Gene alteration and their respective targeted drugs.

Gene	Activity/Positivity	Molecular Alteration	Therapeutic Agents	Ref.
HER2	Member of the EGF RTK family Intestinal type (34%), diffuse type (6%) 24% in CIN, 12% in EBV and 7% in MSI subtypes	Amplification Overexpression	Trastuzumab + traditional chemotherapy (ToGA trial) Other anti-HER2 agents (lapatinib, pertuzumab and trastuzumab-emtansine) have not shown significant benefit; resistance is under investigation	[66–81]
EGFR	Member of the EGF RTK family; forms heterodimers with HER2 10% in the CIN molecular subtype	Amplification Overexpression	Panitumumab and cetuximab showed disappointing results in two large phase III trials; erlotinib and gefitinib were not effective	[82–85]
MET	RTK family; interacts with HGF 8% in the CIN molecular subtype	Amplification Overexpression	Rilotumumab was associated with significantly longer PFS and OS when added to chemotherapy in treatment-naive molecularly unselected patients with advanced GC; another anti-MET antibody, onartuzumab, did not show any advantage in combination with mFOLFOX	[86–90]
VEGF	Factors of angiogenesis 54–90% of GCs	Overexpression	Bevacizumab (AVAGAST trial) did not show increased OS Ramucirumab (RAINBOW trial) + paclitaxel confirmed OS advantage in a non-Asian population	[91–98]
FGFR	Fibroblast growth factor receptor family 9% CIN molecular subtype	Amplification	A phase II randomised trial is evaluating the activity of AZD4547, an inhibitor of FGFR 1–2 and 3, compared to paclitaxel in second-line treatment Other ongoing trials are testing dovitinib in FGFR2 amplified GC patients or in combination with docetaxel	[14,34]
KRAS	RAS GTPase; recruits the cytosolic protein RAF <5 GCs	Mutation codon 12–13	No target therapies are currently approved for this alteration in GC	[99]
CDH1	Tumour suppressor gene; encodes E-cadherin, a cell adhesion molecules 37% of the GS molecular subtype	Mutations, hypermethylation, downregulated expression	Treatments targeting EMT are under study	[100–102]
ARID1A	Tumour suppressor gene involved in chromatin remodelling 20% GS molecular subtype	Inactivating mutations	No target therapies are currently approved for this alteration in GC	[103,104]
RHOA	Rho GTPases are intracellular signaling molecules, regulating cytoskeleton organization, cell cycle and cell motility Diffuse type 30% GS molecular subtype	Mutations Interchromosomal translocation (between *CLDN18* and *ARHGAP26*)	A recent trial tested IMAB362, a chimeric IgG1 antibody against CLDN18.2 showing clinical activity in patients with 2+/3+ immunostaining	[105–109]

4.4. Genomic Stable (GS) GC

The GS subgroup included all tumours that did not fulfil appropriate criteria for inclusion in one of the other groups [14]. Patients included in this subgroup represent nearly 20% of all GC, usually show diffuse histology, have a diagnosis at an earlier age (median 59 years), distal localization and occurring equally in males and females (Figure 1). Several subtype-specific molecular changes have been described for GS tumours. The principal somatic genomic alterations observed in GS gastric tumours involve *CDH1*, *ARID1A* and *RHOA* and are described in Table 2. Moreover, an additional translocation (between *CLDN18* and *ARHGAP26*) involved in cell motility was later identified [14].

4.5. Patient-Derived Preclinical Models of GC

The lack of effective preclinical models of human tumours, reflecting the complexity and heterogeneity of cancer, has consistently limited the development of targeted drugs. In vitro and in vivo models are available: cancer cell lines; cell line xenograft mouse models (PDX), created transplanting human neoplastic fresh tissue into immunodeficient mice and organoids, which are three-dimensionally cultured tissues, mimicking human tissues [110–122]. Their advantages and disadvantages are summarised in Table 3.

Stem cell-derived gastric organoids have proven to be effective models of gastric cancer pathogenesis: *H. pylori*-activated c-Met by its virulence factor cytotoxin-associated gene A and induced a two-fold increase in epithelial cell proliferation [123]. Furthermore, epithelial dysplasia was found in gastric organoids, and adenocarcinoma quickly developed in mice having mutations in KRAS or P53 [124]. Murine epithelial-mesenchymal organoids were used also to successfully replicate hereditary GC, with short hairpin RNA knockdown of TGFBR2 [125]. The fundamental role of RHOA function in mediating anoikis in diffuse-type GC was demonstrated also in mouse organoids [126].

Table 3. Patient-derived preclinical models of GC: advantages and disadvantages.

	Cons	Pros
Cell line xenografts	- monodimensional - no tumour-microenvironment interaction - loss of architecture - genetic modifications	- rapid analysis of drug response - immortal cell lines allow unlimited source of material - low cost, low complexity
PDX models	- limited source of material - high failure rate of engraftment - long time for establishment - expensive - tissue must be rapidly processed	- reliable representation of tumour heterogeneity - includes microenvironment - can predict response to drugs
Organoids	- no tumour-microenvironment interaction	- high level of architectural and physiological similarity to native tissue - intermediate cost, easy to handle - large-scale drug screening

4.6. Role of microRNAs in Signaling Pathways of GC

MicroRNAs (miRNAs) are short, approximately 22 nucleotides in length that play key roles in the regulation of gene expression [127]. Accumulating evidence indicates that miRNAs play an important role in regulating cancer-related genes. They contribute to GC as oncogenes or tumour suppressors by inhibiting either directly or indirectly the expression of target genes, some of which are involved in signaling pathways [128]. Phosphatase and tensin homologue (PTEN) functions as a tumour suppressor by counteracting PI3K signaling [129]. miRNA-221/222 has been found to be a modulator of PTEN: by antisense or overexpression strategies, it directly affects PTEN expression [130]. PTEN is also a target gene of miRNA-21 that increases the proliferation and invasion of GC cells. A similar effect is displayed by miRNA-214 [131].

miRNA-375 is one of the most downregulated miRNAs in GC, by directly targeting PDK1, a kinase that phosphorylates Akt. Ectopic expression of miRNA-375 reduces cell viability by inducing the caspase-dependent apoptotic pathway [132]. Instead, miRNA-143 regulates the function of GC cells in the PI3K/Akt pathway because its gene target is Akt itself [133]. Down-expression of miR-181c stimulates KRAS expression and may have an important role in GC [134]. It was found that miRNA-29s could influence the Ras/Raf/MEK/ERK pathway, which acts on cell cycle progression by induction of cell cycle regulatory proteins such as CDKs and cyclins. miRNA-29c inhibits protein expression/phosphorylation of Cdc42 [135,136]. Feng et al. demonstrated that CDK6 is regulated by miRNA-107 [137]. Its expression is significantly decreased in GC, and its re-expression significantly decreases proliferation. In GC, miRNA-206 modulates downstream target

Int. J. Mol. Sci. **2018**, *19*, 1683

cyclin D2, involved in proliferation [138]. miRNA-106b and miRNA-93 could be upregulated in GC and be downstream targets of the oncogenic transcription factor E2F1, which make the tumour-suppressive function of transforming growth factor-β less effective [139]. E2F1 is a gene target of miRNA-331-3p and miRNA-106a, modulating the G1/s transition [140,141]. miRNA-331-3p is a tumour suppressor, whereas miRNA-106a promotes tumour growth. A group of researchers demonstrated that the p21 family of CDK inhibitors was suppressed by miRNA-106b-93-25 and miRNA-222-221 clusters. In particular, miRNA-25 targets p57 through the 3'-untranslated region; miRNA-106b and miRNA-93 control p21, whereas p27 and p57 are downregulated by miRNA-222 and miRNA-221 [142]. miRNA-148a has as direct target, p27, so by suppressing p27 expression, it may promote gastric cell proliferation [143]. miRNA-196a, when highly expressed, is associated with clinic-pathological parameters, such as tumour size, poor pT stage, pN stage and patients' overall survival times. In vitro and in vivo, a downregulation of miRNA-196a suppresses gastric cancer proliferation by targeting p27^{kip} [144]. Previous research has shown that miRNA-375, by targeting the JAK2 oncogene, may act as a tumour suppressor and regulate GC cell proliferation [139]. Moreover, miRNA-135 by targeting JAK2 may repress p-STAT3 activation, reduce cyclin D1 Bcl-xL expression and inhibit cell proliferation [47].

4.7. Clinical Implications of Tissue miRNAs in GC

Tissue-based GC-related miRNA biomarkers are listed in Table 4, focusing particularly on their application as diagnostic and prognostic indicators [145–159]. Dysregulated expression of miRNA can play an oncogenic or tumour-suppressor role. In fact, they can regulate different signal pathways, targeting genes involved in cell migration, angiogenesis and cell proliferation. Table 5 summarises specific miRNA targeting pathways described above [160–167].

Table 4. Diagnostic and prognostic role of tissue-based GC-related miRNAs.

miRNAs	Role	Expression in Tissue	Note	Ref.
miR-21	Diagnostic	Upregulated	Overexpressed miR-21 binds to PDCD4 and can inhibit protein expression; directly related to tumour size, depth of invasion, lymph node metastasis and vascular invasion	[145,146]
miR-21 miR-223 miR-218	Diagnostic	Upregulated Downregulated	-	[147]
miR-31	Diagnostic	Downregulated	-	[148]
miR-32 miR-182 miR-143	Diagnostic	Upregulated	-	[149]
miR-106a	Diagnostic	Upregulated	Level of miR-106a is closely related to tumour size, differentiation degree, lymph node and distant metastasis	[141]
miR-20 miR-150b miR-451	Prognostic	Upregulated Upregulated Downregulated		[150,151]
miR-29	Prognostic	Downregulated	This miRNA is associated with poor prognosis	[152]
miR-106b	Prognostic	Upregulated	This miRNA is associated with poor prognosis	[153]
miR-125a-5p	Prognostic	Downregulated	Multivariate analysis shows that its downregulation is an independent prognostic factor for survival	[154]
miR-206	Prognostic	Downregulated	mRNA-206 is an independent prognostic factor in GC patients	[155]

15

Table 4. *Cont.*

miRNAs	Role	Expression in Tissue	Note	Ref.
miR-17-5p miR-21 miR-106a miR-106b miR-7a	Prognostic	Upregulated	-	[142,156]
miR-10b miR-21 miR-223 miR-338 let-7a miR-30a-5p miR-126	Prognostic	-	These seven miRNAs are significantly related to recurrence-free periods and overall survival of patients; an overexpression of miR-223 in primary GC is associated with less survival without metastasis	[157,158]
miR-125b miR-199a miR-100	Prognostic	Upregulated	These miRNAs are associated with progression of GC	[159]
Let-7g miR-433 miR-214	Prognostic	Upregulated Upregulated Downregulated	Levels of these miRNAs are associated with tumour infiltration depth, lymph node metastasis and tumour stage.	[159]

Table 5. Expression and deregulation of miRNAs in gastric cancer.

miRNAs	Relative Expression	Target Gene	Cell Function	Ref.
miR-146a	Upregulated	EGFR	Invasion Migration	[160]
miR-449	Upregulated	MET SIRT1 CDK6	Cell proliferation Apoptosis Cell cycle	[161]
miR-29a/c	Downregulated	VEGF	Vascular cell Metastasis Growth	[162]
miR-181c	Upregulated	KRAS NOTCH4	Cell proliferation	[134]
miR-221 miR-222	Upregulated	CDKN1A CDKN1B CDKN1C	Cell Cycle	[142]
miR-200c	Upregulated	CDH RHO	Metastasis Chemoresistance	[163]
miR-150	Upregulated	EGR2	Apoptosis Cell proliferation	[150]
miR-382	Upregulated	PTEN	Angiogenesis	[164]
miR-124	Upregulated	ROCK1	Cell proliferation Invasion	[165]
miR-125a-5p	Upregulated	ERBB2 E2F3	Cell proliferation Metastasis Invasion Migration	[154,166]
miR-145	Downregulated	ETS1	Migration Invasion Angiogenesis	[167]

5. Conclusions

The recent molecular research on GC has generated large amounts of data that are currently not integrated into clinical practice.

However, they may be of help in the design of future clinical trials aiming to personalise treatment in several ways: (i) by identifying the driving pathways of tumour growth; (ii) by discovering potential drugs targeting such pathways; (iii) by finding predictable mechanisms of resistance and strategies to overcome them.

It must be emphasised that each targetable molecular alteration/pathway is not specific to a distinct subtype of GC; therefore, molecular subgroups alone are not sufficient to assign a patient to a clinical trial. On the contrary, molecular characterization of patients is useful to select a small population to be screened for protocol-eligible molecular aberrations. The implementation of GC research and the molecular classification of patients in clinical trials may be important to select the most appropriate therapies in GC. The hope is that combining histological and molecular classification will be supportive of GC therapeutics and prognosis, but also in the near future for new non-invasive diagnostic approaches such as to identify specific GC biomarker subtypes from circulating nucleic acid or tumour cells.

Conflicts of Interest: The author declares no conflicts of interest.

References

1. Siegel, R.L.; Miller, K.D.; Jemal, A. Cancer statistics, 2016. *CA Cancer J. Clin.* **2016**, *66*, 7–30. [CrossRef] [PubMed]
2. Borrmann, R. Geschwulste des margens. In *Handbuch spez pathol anat und histo*; Henke, F., Lubarsch, O., Eds.; Springer: Berlin, Germany, 1926; pp. 864–871.
3. Siewert, J.R.; Stein, H.J. Classification of adenocarcinoma of the oesophagogastric junction. *Br. J. Surg.* **1998**, *85*, 1457–1459. [CrossRef] [PubMed]
4. Lauren, P. The two histological main types of gastric carcinoma: Diffuse and so called intestinal-type carcinoma: An attempt at a histo-clinical classification. *Acta Pathol. Microbiol. Scand.* **1965**, *64*, 31–49. [CrossRef] [PubMed]
5. Lauwers, G.Y.; Carneiro, F.; Graham, D.Y. Gastric carcinoma. In *WHO Classification of Tumours of the Digestive System*, 4th ed.; Bosman, F.T., Carneiro, F., Hruban, R.H., Theise, N.D., Eds.; World Health Organization: Lyon, France, 2010; Volume 3, pp. 48–58, ISBN-13 9789283224327.
6. Kajitani, T. The general rules for the gastric cancer study in surgery and pathology I: Clinical classification. *Jpn. J. Surg.* **1981**, *1*, 127–139.
7. Tan, I.B.; Ivanova, T.; Lim, K.H.; Ong, C.W.; Deng, N.; Lee, J.; Tan, S.H.; Wu, J.; Lee, M.H.; Ooi, C.H.; et al. Intrinsic subtypes of gastric cancer, based on gene expression pattern, predict survival and respond differently to chemotherapy. *Gastroenterology* **2011**, *141*, 476–485. [CrossRef] [PubMed]
8. Choi, Y.Y.; Cheong, J.H. Beyond precision surgery: Molecularly motivated precision care for gastric cancer. *Eur. J. Surg. Oncol.* **2017**, *43*, 856–864. [CrossRef] [PubMed]
9. Lee, Y.S.; Cho, Y.S.; Lee, G.K.; Lee, S.; Kim, K.W.; Jho, S.; Kim, H.M.; Hong, S.H.; Hwang, J.H.; Kim, S.Y.; et al. Genomic profile analysis of diffuse-type gastric cancers. *Genome Biol.* **2014**, *15*, R55. [CrossRef] [PubMed]
10. Tanabe, S.; Aoyagi, K.; Yokozaki, H.; Sasaki, H. Gene expression signatures for identifying diffuse-type gastric cancer associated with epithelial-mesenchymal transition. *Int. J. Oncol.* **2014**, *44*, 1955–1970. [CrossRef] [PubMed]
11. Kim, B.; Bang, S.; Lee, S.; Kim, S.; Jung, Y.; Lee, C.; Choi, K.; Lee, S.G.; Lee, K.; Lee, Y.; et al. Expression Profiling and Subtype-Specific Expression of stomach cancer. *Cancer Res.* **2003**, *63*, 8248–8255. [PubMed]
12. Min, L.; Zhao, Y.; Zhu, S.; Qiu, X.; Cheng, R.; Xing, J.; Shao, L.; Guo, S.; Zhang, S. Integrated Analysis Identifies Molecular Signatures and Specific Prognostic Factors for Different Gastric Cancer Subtypes. *Transl. Oncol.* **2017**, *10*, 99–107. [CrossRef] [PubMed]

13. Lei, Z.; Tan, I.B.; Das, K.; Deng, N.; Zouridis, H.; Pattison, S.; Chua, C.; Feng, Z.; Guan, Y.K.; Ooi, C.H.; et al. Identification of molecular subtypes of gastric cancer with different responses to PI3-kinase inhibitors and 5-fluorouracil. *Gastroenterology* **2013**, *145*, 554–565. [CrossRef] [PubMed]

14. Cancer Genome Atlas Research Network. Comprehensive molecular characterization of gastric adenocarcinoma. *Nature* **2014**, *513*, 202–209. [CrossRef]

15. Benita, Y.; Cao, Z.; Giallourakis, C.; Li, C.; Gardet, A.; Xavier, R.J. Gene enrichment profiles reveal T-cell development, differentiation, and lineage-specific transcription factors including ZBTB25 as a novel NF-AT repressor. *Blood* **2010**, *115*, 5376–5384. [CrossRef] [PubMed]

16. Ooi, C.H.; Ivanova, T.; Wu, J.; Lee, M.; Tan, I.B.; Tao, J.; Ward, L.; Koo, J.H.; Gopalakrishnan, V.; Zhu, Y.; et al. Oncogenic pathway combinations predict clinical prognosis in gastric cancer. *PLoS Genet.* **2009**, *5*, e1000676. [CrossRef] [PubMed]

17. Cristescu, R.; Lee, J.; Nebozhyn, M.; Kim, K.M.; Ting, J.C.; Wong, S.S.; Liu, J.; Yue, Y.G.; Wang, J.; Yu, K.; et al. Molecular analysis of gastric cancer identifies subtypes associated with distinct clinical outcomes. *Nat. Med.* **2015**, *21*, 449–456. [CrossRef] [PubMed]

18. Wang, Z.; Chen, G.; Wang, Q.; Lu, W.; Xu, M. Identification and validation of a prognostic 9-genes expression signature for gastric cancer. *Oncotarget* **2017**, *10*, 73826–73836. [CrossRef] [PubMed]

19. Shinozaki-Ushiku, A.; Kunita, A.; Fukayama, M. Update on Epstein–Barr virus and gastric cancer [review]. *Int. J. Oncol.* **2015**, *46*, 1421–1434. [CrossRef] [PubMed]

20. Abe, H.; Kaneda, A.; Fukayama, M. Epstein–Barr virus associated gastric carcinoma: Use of host cell machineries and somatic gene mutations. *Pathobiology* **2015**, *82*, 212–223. [CrossRef] [PubMed]

21. Fukayama, M.; Hino, R.; Uozaki, H. Epstein–Barr virus and gastric carcinoma: Virus–host interactions leading to carcinoma. *Cancer Sci.* **2008**, *99*, 1726–1733. [CrossRef] [PubMed]

22. Song, H.J.; Srivastava, A.; Lee, J.; Kim, Y.S.; Kim, K.M.; Ki Kang, W.; Kim, M.; Kim, S.; Park, C.K.; Kim, S. Host inflammatory response predicts survival of patients with Epstein–Barr virus-associated gastric carcinoma. *Gastroenterology* **2010**, *139*, 84–92.e2. [CrossRef] [PubMed]

23. Iwai, Y.; Ishida, M.; Tanaka, Y.; Okazaki, T.; Honjo, T.; Minato, N. Involvement of PD-L1 on tumor cells in the escape from host immune system and tumor immunotherapy by PD-L1 blockade. *Proc. Natl. Acad. Sci. USA* **2002**, *99*, 12293–12297. [CrossRef] [PubMed]

24. Blank, C.; Gajewski, T.F.; Mackensen, A. Interaction of PD-L1 on tumor cells with PD-1 on tumor-specific T cells as a mechanism of immune evasion:implications for tumor immunotherapy. *Cancer Immunol. Immunother.* **2005**, *54*, 307–314. [CrossRef] [PubMed]

25. Francisco, L.M.; Sage, P.T.; Sharpe, A.H. The PD-1 pathway in tolerance and autoimmunity. *Immunol. Rev.* **2010**, *236*, 219–242. [CrossRef] [PubMed]

26. Zhang, L.; Qiu, M.; Jin, Y.; Li, B.; Wang, X.; Yan, S.; Xu, R.; Yang, D. Programmed cell death ligand 1 (PD-L1) expression on gastric cancer and its relationship with clinicopathologic factors. *Int. J. Clin. Exp. Pathol.* **2015**, *8*, 11084–11091. [PubMed]

27. Qing, Y.; Li, Q.; Ren, T.; Xia, W.; Peng, Y.; Liu, G.L.; Luo, X.Y.; Dai, X.Y.; Zhou, S.F.; Wang, D. Upregulation of PD-L1 and APE1 is associated with tumorigenesis and poor prognosis of gastric cancer. *Drug Des. Devel. Ther.* **2015**, *9*, 901–909. [CrossRef] [PubMed]

28. Kim, J.W.; Nam, K.H.; Ahn, S.H.; Park, D.J.; Kim, H.H.; Kim, S.H.; Chang, H.; Lee, J.O.; Kim, Y.J.; Lee, H.S.; et al. Prognostic implications of immunosuppressive protein expression in tumors as well as immune cell infiltration within the tumor microenvironment in gastric cancer. *Gastric Cancer* **2016**, *19*, 42–52. [CrossRef] [PubMed]

29. Thompson, E.D.; Zahurak, M.; Murphy, A.; Cornish, T.; Cuka, N.; Abdelfatah, E.; Yang, S.; Duncan, M.; Ahuja, N.; Taube, J.M.; et al. Patterns of PD-L1 expression and CD8 T cell infiltration in gastric adenocarcinomas and associated immune stroma. *Gut* **2017**, *66*, 794–801. [CrossRef] [PubMed]

30. Liu, Y.X.; Wang, X.S.; Wang, Y.F.; Hu, X.C.; Yan, J.Q.; Zhang, Y.L.; Wang, W.; Yang, R.J.; Feng, Y.Y.; Gao, S.G.; et al. Prognostic significance of PD-L1 expression in patients with gastric cancer in East Asia: A meta-analysis. *OncolTargets Ther.* **2016**, *9*, 2649–2654. [CrossRef]

31. Abe, H.; Kunita, A.; Yamashita, H.; Seto, Y.; Fukayama, M. Overexpression and gene amplification of PD-L1 in cancer cells and PD-L1+ immune cells in Epstein-Barr virus-associated gastric cancer: The prognostic implications. *Mod. Pathol.* **2017**, *30*, 427–439. [CrossRef]

32. Shankaran, V.; Muro, K.; Bang, Y.; Geva, R.; Catenacci, D.; Gupta, S.; Eder, J.P.; Berger, R.; Loboda, A.; Albright, A.; et al. Correlation of gene expression signatures and clinical outcomes in patients with advanced gastric cancer treated with pembrolizumab (MK-3475). *J. Clin. Oncol.* **2015**, *33*, 3026. [CrossRef]

33. Bang, Y.; Im, S.; Lee, K.; Cho, J.; Song, E.; Lee, K.; Kim, Y.H.; Park, J.O.; Chun, H.G.; Zang, D.Y.; et al. Randomized, double-blind phase II trial with prospective classification by ATM protein level to evaluate the efficacy and tolerability of olaparib plus paclitaxel in patients with recurrent or metastatic gastric cancer. *J. Clin. Oncol.* **2015**, *33*, 3858–3865. [CrossRef] [PubMed]

34. Fontana, E.; Smyth, E.C. Novel targets in the treatment of advanced gastric cancer: A perspective review. *Ther. Adv. Med. Oncol.* **2016**, *8*, 113–125. [CrossRef] [PubMed]

35. Liu, J.F.; Zhou, Z.X.; Chen, J.H.; Yi, G.; Chen, H.G.; Ba, M.C.; Lin, S.Q.; Qi, Y.C. Up-regulation of PIK3CA promotes metastasis in gastric carcinoma. *World J. Gastroenterol.* **2010**, *16*, 4986–4991. [CrossRef] [PubMed]

36. Tapia, O.; Riquelme, I.; Leal, P.; Sandoval, A.; Aedo, S.; Weber, H.; Letelier, P.; Bellolio, E.; Villaseca, M.; Garcia, P.; et al. The PI3K/AKT/mTOR pathway is activated in gastric cancer with potential prognostic and predictive significance. *Virchows Arch.* **2014**, *465*, 25–33. [CrossRef] [PubMed]

37. Ye, B.; Jiang, L.; Xu, H.; Zhou, D.; Li, Z. Expression of PI3K/AKT pathway in gastric cancer and its blockade suppresses tumor growth and metastasis. *Int. J. Immunopathol. Pharmacol.* **2012**, *25*, 627–636. [CrossRef] [PubMed]

38. Cinti, C.; Vindigni, C.; Zamparelli, A.; Sala, D.; Epistolato, M.; Marrelli, D.; Cevenini, G.; Tosi, P. Activated Akt as an indicator of prognosis in gastric cancer. *Virchows Arch.* **2008**, *453*, 449–455. [CrossRef] [PubMed]

39. Sangawa, A.; Shintani, M.; Yamao, N.; Kamoshida, S. Phosphorylation status of Akt and caspase-9 in gastric and colorectal carcinomas. *Int. J. Clin. Exp. Pathol.* **2014**, *7*, 3312–3317. [PubMed]

40. Welker, M.E.; Kulik, G. Recent syntheses of PI3K/Akt/mTOR signaling pathway inhibitors. *Bioorg. Med. Chem.* **2013**, *2*, 4063–4091. [CrossRef] [PubMed]

41. Janku, F.; Tsimberidou, A.M.; Garrido-Laguna, I.; Wang, X.; Luthra, R.; Hong, D.S.; Naing, A.; Falchook, G.S.; Moroney, J.W. PIK3CA mutations in patients with advanced cancers treated with PI3K/AKT/mTOR axis inhibitors. *Mol. Cancer. Ther.* **2011**, *10*, 558–565. [CrossRef] [PubMed]

42. Davies, B.R.; Greenwood, H.; Dudley, P.; Crafter, C.; Yu, D.H.; Zhang, J.; Li, J.; Gao, B.; Ji, Q.; Maynard, J.; et al. Preclinical pharmacology of AZD5363, an inhibitor of AKT: Pharmacodynamics, antitumor activity, and correlation of monotherapy activity with genetic background. *Mol. Cancer Ther.* **2012**, *11*, 873–887. [CrossRef] [PubMed]

43. Li, V.; Wong, C.; Chan, T.; Chan, A.S.; Zhao, W.; Chu, K.M.; So, S.; Chen, X.; Yuen, S.T.; Leung, S.Y. Mutations of PIK3CA in gastric adenocarcinoma. *BMC Cancer* **2005**, *5*, 29. [CrossRef] [PubMed]

44. Yu, H.G.; Ai, Y.W.; Yu, L.L.; Zhou, X.D.; Liu, J.; Li, J.H.; Xu, X.M.; Liu, S.; Chen, J.; Liu, F.; et al. Phosphoinositide 3-kinase/Akt pathway plays an important role in chemoresistance of gastric cancer cells against etoposide and doxorubicin induced cell death. *Int. J. Cancer* **2008**, *122*, 433–443. [CrossRef] [PubMed]

45. Oki, E.; Kakeji, Y.; Tokunaga, E.; Nishida, K.; Koga, T.; Egashira, A.; Morita, M.; Maehara, Y. Impact of PTEN/AKT/ PI3K signal pathway on the chemotherapy for gastric cancer. *J. Clin. Oncol.* **2006**, *24*, 4034. [CrossRef]

46. Im, S.; Lee, K.; Nam, E. Potential prognostic significance of p185HER2 overexpression with loss of PTEN expression in gastric carcinomas. *Tumori* **2005**, *91*, 513–521. [PubMed]

47. Wu, H.; Huang, M.; Cao, P.; Wang, T.; Shu, Y.; Liu, P. MiR-135a targets JAK2 and inhibits gastric cancer cell proliferation. *Cancer Biol. Ther.* **2012**, *13*, 281–288. [CrossRef] [PubMed]

48. Brooks, A.J.; Dai, W.; O'Mara, M.L.; Abankwa, D.; Chhabra, Y.; Pelekanos, R.A.; Gardon, O.; Tunny, K.A.; Blucher, K.M.; Morton, C.J.; et al. Mechanism of activation of protein kinase JAK2 by the growth hormone receptor. *Science* **2014**, *344*, 1249783. [CrossRef] [PubMed]

49. Levine, R.L.; Wadleigh, M.; Cools, J.; Ebert, B.L.; Wernig, G.; Huntly, B.J.; Boggon, T.J.; Wlodarska, I.; Clark, J.J.; Moore, S.; et al. Activating mutation in the tyrosine kinase JAK2 in polycythemia vera, essential thrombocythemia, and myeloid metaplasia with myelofibrosis. *Cancer Cell* **2005**, *7*, 387–397. [CrossRef] [PubMed]

50. Buchert, M.; Burns, C.; Ernst, M. Targeting JAK kinase in solid tumors: Emerging opportunities and challenges. *Oncogene* **2016**, *35*, 939–951. [CrossRef] [PubMed]

51. Hurwitz, H.; Uppal, N.; Wagner, S.; Bendell, J.; Beck, J.; Wade, S.; Nemunaitis, J.J.; Stella, P.J.; Pipas, J.M.; Wainberg, Z.A.; et al. A randomized doubleblind phase 2 study of ruxolitinib (RUX) or placebo (PBO) with capecitabine (CAPE) as second-line therapy in patients (pts) with metastatic pancreatic cancer (mPC). *J. Clin. Oncol.* **2015**, *32*, 4000. [CrossRef]

52. Pedrazzani, C.; Corso, G.; Velho, S.; Leite, M.; Pascale, V.; Bettarini, F.; Marrelli, D.; Seruca, R.; Roviello, F. Evidence of tumor micro satellite instability in gastric cancer with familial aggregation. *Fam. Cancer* **2009**, *8*, 215–220. [CrossRef] [PubMed]

53. Velho, S.; Fernandes, M.S.; Leite, M.; Figueiredo, C.; Seruca, R. Causes and consequences of microsatellite instability in gastric carcinogenesis. *World J. Gastroenterol.* **2014**, *20*, 16433–16442. [CrossRef] [PubMed]

54. Chung, D.C.; Rustgi, A.K. DNA mismatch repair and cancer. *Gastroenterology* **1995**, *109*, 1685–1699. [CrossRef]

55. Smyth, E.C.; Wotherspoon, A.; Peckitt, C.; Nankivell, M.G.; Eltahir, Z.; Wilson, S.H.; de Castro, D.G.; Okines, A.F.C.; Langley, R.E.; Cunningham, D. Correlation between mismatch repair deficiency (MMRd), microsatellite instability (MSI) and survival in MAGIC. *J. Clin. Oncol.* **2016**, *15*, 4064. [CrossRef]

56. Pinto, M.; Wu, Y.; Mensink, R.G.; Cirnes, L.; Seruca, R.; Hofstra, R.M. Somatic mutations in mismatch repair genes in sporadic gastric carcinomas are not a cause but a consequence of the mutator phenotype. *Cancer Genet. Cytogenet.* **2008**, *180*, 110–114. [CrossRef] [PubMed]

57. Zhu, L.; Li, Z.; Wang, Y.; Zhang, C.; Liu, Y.; Qu, X. Microsatellite instability and survival in gastric cancer: A systematic review and meta-analysis. *Mol. Clin. Oncol.* **2015**, *3*, 699–705. [CrossRef] [PubMed]

58. Le, D.; Uram, J.; Wang, H.; Bartlett, B.; Kemberling, H.; Eyring, A.; Skora, A.D.; Luber, B.S.; Azad, N.S.; Laheru, D.; et al. PD-1 blockade in tumors with mismatch-repair deficiency. *N. Engl. J. Med.* **2015**, *372*, 2509–2520. [CrossRef] [PubMed]

59. Camargo, M.C.; Kim, W.H.; Chiaravalli, A.M.; Kim, K.M.; Corvalan, A.H.; Matsuo, K.; Yu, J.; Sung, J.J.; Herrera-Goepfert, R.; Meneses-Gonzalez, F.; et al. Improved survival of gastric cancer with tumour Epstein-Barr virus positivity: An international pooled analysis. *Gut* **2014**, *63*, 236–243. [CrossRef] [PubMed]

60. Choi, Y.Y.; Bae, J.M.; An, J.Y.; Kwon, I.G.; Cho, I.; Shin, H.B.; Eiji, T.; Aburahmah, M.; Kim, H.I.; Cheong, J.H.; et al. Is microsatellite instability a prognostic marker in gastric cancer? A systematic review with meta-analysis. *J. Surg. Oncol.* **2014**, *110*, 129–135. [CrossRef] [PubMed]

61. Giam, M.; Rancati, G. Aneuploidy and chromosomal instability in cancer: A jackpot to chaos. *Cell Div.* **2015**, *10*, 3. [CrossRef] [PubMed]

62. Chia, N.Y.; Tan, P. Molecular classification of gastric cancer. *Ann. Oncol.* **2016**, *27*, 763–769. [CrossRef] [PubMed]

63. Aprile, G.; Giampieri, R.; Bonotto, M.; Bittoni, A.; Ongaro, E.; Cardellino, G.G.; Graziano, F.; Giuliani, F.; Fasola, G.; Cascinu, S.; et al. The challenge of targeted therapies for gastric cancer patients: The beginning of a long journey. *Expert Opin. Investig. Drugs* **2014**, *23*, 925–942. [CrossRef] [PubMed]

64. Chen, T.; Xu, X.Y.; Zhou, P.H. Emerging molecular classifications and therapeutic implications for gastric cancer. *Chin. J. Cancer* **2016**, *35*, 49. [CrossRef] [PubMed]

65. Tan, P.; Yeoh, K.G. Genetics and Molecular Pathogenesis of Gastric Adenocarcinoma. *Gastroenterology* **2015**, *149*, 1153–1162.e3. [CrossRef] [PubMed]

66. Gravalos, C.; Jimeno, A. HER2 in gastric cancer: A new prognostic factor and a novel therapeutic target. *Ann. Oncol.* **2008**, *19*, 1523–1529. [CrossRef] [PubMed]

67. Bang, Y.J.; Van Cutsem, E.; Feyereislova, A.; Chung, H.C.; Shen, L.; Sawaki, A.; Lordick, F.; Ohtsu, A.; Omuro, Y.; Satoh, T.; et al. Trastuzumab in combination with chemotherapy versus chemotherapy alone for treatment of HER2-positive advanced gastric or gastro-oesophageal junction cancer (ToGA): A phase 3, open-label, randomised controlled trial. *Lancet* **2010**, *376*, 687–697. [CrossRef]

68. Hecht, J.R.; Bang, Y.J.; Qin, S.K.; Chung, H.C.; Xu, J.M.; Park, J.O.; Jeziorski, K.; Shparyk, Y.; Hoff, P.M.; Sombrero, A.; et al. Lapatinib in Combination with Capecitabine Plus Oxaliplatin in Human Epidermal Growth Factor Receptor 2-Positive Advanced or Metastatic Gastric, Esophageal, or Gastroesophageal Adenocarcinoma: TRIO-013/LOGiC—A Randomized Phase III Trial. *J. Clin. Oncol.* **2016**, *34*, 443–451. [CrossRef] [PubMed]

69. Baselga, J.; Cortés, J.; Kim, S.B.; Im, S.A.; Hegg, R.; Im, Y.H.; Roman, L.; Pdrini, J.L.; Pienkowski, T.; Kontt, A.; et al. Pertuzumab plus trastuzumab plus docetaxel for metastatic breast cancer. *N. Engl. J. Med.* **2012**, *366*, 109–119. [CrossRef] [PubMed]

70. Hecht, J.R.; Bang, Y.J.; Qin, S.K.; Chung, H.C.; Xu, J.M.; Park, J.O.; Jeziorski, K.; Shparyk, Y.; Hoff, P.M.; Sombrero, A.; et al. Lapatinib in combination with capecitabine plus oxaliplatin (CapeOx) in HER2 positive advanced or metastatic gastric (A/MGC), esophageal (EAC), or astroesophageal (GEJ) adenocarcinoma: The logic trial. *J. Clin. Oncol.* **2013**, *31*, LBA4001. [CrossRef]

71. Satoh, T.; Xu, R.H.; Chung, H.C.; Sun, G.P.; Doi, T.; Xu, J.M.; Tsuji, A.; Omuro, Y.; Li, J.; Wang, J.W.; et al. Lapatinib plus paclitaxel versus paclitaxel alone in the second-line treatment of HER2-amplified advanced gastric cancer in Asian populations: TyTAN-a randomized, phase III study. *J. Clin. Oncol.* **2014**, *32*, 2039–2049. [CrossRef] [PubMed]

72. Deva, S.; Baird, R.; Cresti, N.; Garcia-Corbacho, J.; Hogarth, L.; Frenkel, E.; Kawaguchi, K.; Arimura, A.; Donaldson, K.; Posner, J.; et al. Phase I expansion of S-222611, a reversible inhibitor of EGFR and HER2, in advanced solid tumors, including patients with brain metastases. *J. Clin. Oncol.* **2015**, *33*, 2511. [CrossRef]

73. Lee, J.Y.; Hong, M.; Kim, S.T.; Park, S.H.; Kang, W.K.; Kim, K.M.; Lee, J. The impact of concomitant genomic alterations on treatment outcome for trastuzumab therapy in HER2-positive gastric cancer. *Sci. Rep.* **2015**, *5*, 9289. [CrossRef] [PubMed]

74. Zuo, Q.; Liu, J.; Zhang, J.; Wu, M.; Guo, L.; Liao, W. Development of trastuzumab-resistant human gastric carcinoma cell lines and mechanisms of drug resistance. *Sci. Rep.* **2015**, *5*, 11634. [CrossRef] [PubMed]

75. Piro, G.; Carbone, C.; Cataldo, I.; Di Nicolantonio, F.; Giacopuzzi, S.; Aprile, G.; Simionato, F.; Boschi, F.; Zanotto, M.; Mina, M.M.; et al. An FGFR3 Autocrine Loop Sustains Acquired Resistance to Trastuzumab in Gastric Cancer Patients. *Clin. Cancer Res.* **2016**, *22*, 6164–6175. [CrossRef] [PubMed]

76. Arienti, C.; Zanoni, M.; Pignatta, S.; Del Rio, A.; Carloni, S.; Tebaldi, M.; Tedaldi, G.; Tesei, A. Preclinical evidence of multiple mechanisms underlying trastuzumab resistance in gastric cancer. *Oncotarget* **2016**, *7*, 18424–18439. [CrossRef] [PubMed]

77. White, C.D.; Brown, M.D.; Sacks, D.B. IQGAPs in cancer: A family of scaffold proteins underlying tumorigenesis. *FEBS Lett.* **2009**, *583*, 1817–1824. [CrossRef] [PubMed]

78. Walch, A.; Seidl, S.; Hermannstädter, C.; Rauser, S.; Deplazes, J.; Langer, R.; von Weyhern, C.H.; Sarbia, M.; Busch, R.; Feith, M.; et al. Combined analysis of Rac1, IQGAP1, Tiam1 and E-cadherin expression in gastric cancer. *Mod. Pathol.* **2008**, *21*, 544–552. [CrossRef] [PubMed]

79. Khoury, H.; Naujokas, M.A.; Zuo, D.; Sangwan, V.; Frigault, M.M.; Petkiewicz, S.; Dankort, D.L.; Muller, W.J.; Park, M. HGF converts ErbB2/Neu epithelial morphogenesis to cell invasion. *Mol. Biol. Cell* **2005**, *16*, 550–561. [CrossRef] [PubMed]

80. Chen, C.T.; Kim, H.; Liska, D.; Gao, S.; Christensen, J.G.; Weiser, M.R. MET activation mediates resistance to lapatinib inhibition of HER2- amplified gastric cancer cells. *Mol. Cancer Ther.* **2012**, *11*, 660–669. [CrossRef] [PubMed]

81. De Silva, N.; Schulz, L.; Paterson, A.; Qain, W.; Secrier, M.; Godfrey, E.; Cheow, H.; O'Donovan, M.; Lao-Sirieix, P.; Jobanputra, M.; et al. Molecular effects of Lapatinib in the treatment of HER2 overexpressing oesophago-gastric adenocarcinoma. *Br. J. Cancer* **2015**, *113*, 1305–1312. [CrossRef] [PubMed]

82. Lordick, F.; Kang, Y.; Chung, H.; Salman, P.; Oh, S.; Bodoky, G.; Kurteva, G.; Volovat, C.; Moiseyenko, V.M.; Gorbunova, V.; et al. Capecitabine and cisplatin with or without cetuximab for patients with previously untreated advanced gastric cancer (EXPAND): A randomised, open-label phase 3 Trial. *Lancet Oncol.* **2013**, *14*, 490–499. [CrossRef]

83. Waddell, T.; Chau, I.; Cunningham, D.; Gonzalez, D.; Okines, A.F.; Okines, C.; Wotherspoon, A.; Saffert, C.; Middleton, G.; Wadsley, J.; et al. Epirubicin, oxaliplatin, and capecitabine with or without panitumumab for patients with previously untreated advanced oesophagogastric cancer (REAL3): A randomised, open-label phase 3 trial. *Lancet Oncol.* **2013**, *14*, 481–489. [CrossRef]

84. Dragovich, T.; Mccoy, S.; Fenoglio-Preiser, C.; Wang, J.; Benedetti, J.; Baker, A.F.; Hackett, C.B.; Urba, S.G.; Zaner, K.S.; Blanke, C.D.; et al. Phase II trial of erlotinib in gastroesophageal junction and gastric adenocarcinomas: SWOG 0127. *J. Clin. Oncol.* **2006**, *24*, 4922–4927. [CrossRef] [PubMed]

85. Dutton, S.J.; Ferry, D.R.; Blazeby, J.M.; Abbas, H.; Dahle-Smith, A.; Mansoor, W.; Thompson, J.; Harrison, M.; Chatteriee, A.; Falk, S.; et al. Gefitinib for oesophageal cancer progressing after chemotherapy (COG): A phase 3, multicentre, double-blind, placebocontrolled randomised trial. *Lancet Oncol.* **2014**, *15*, 894–904. [CrossRef]

86. Ha, S.Y.; Lee, J.; Kang, S.Y.; Do, I.G.; Ahn, S.; Park, J.O; Kang, W.K.; Choi, M.G.; Sohn, T.S.; Bae, J.M.; et al. MET overexpression assessed by new interpretation method predicts gene amplification and poor survival in advanced gastric carcinomas. *Mod. Pathol.* **2013**, *26*, 1632–1641. [CrossRef] [PubMed]

87. Scagliotti, G.V.; Novello, S.; Von Pawel, J. The emerging role of MET/HGF inhibitors in oncology. *Cancer Treat. Rev.* **2013**, *39*, 793–801. [CrossRef] [PubMed]

88. Cunningham, D.; Tebbutt, N.; Davidenko, I.; Murad, A.; Al-Batran, S.; Ilson, D.; Tjulandin, S.; Gotovkin, E.; Karaszewska, B.; Bondarenko, I.; et al. Phase III, randomized, double-blind, multicenter, placebo (P)-controlled trial of rilotumumab (R) plus epirubicin, cisplatin and capecitabine (ECX) as first-line therapy in patients (pts) with advanced MET-positive (pos) gastric or gastroesophageal junction (G/GEJ) cancer: RILOMET-1 study. *J. Clin. Oncol.* **2015**, *33*, 4000. [CrossRef]

89. Shah, M.; Bang, Y.; Lordick, F.; Tabernero, J.; Chen, M.; Hack, S.; Phan, S.; Shames, D.S.; Cunningham, D. Metgastric: A phase III study of onartuzumab plus mFOLFOX6 in patients with metastatic HER2-negative (HER2-) and METpositive (MET+) adenocarcinoma of the stomach or gastroesophageal junction (GEC). *J. Clin. Oncol.* **2015**, *33*, 4012. [CrossRef]

90. Iveson, T.; Donehower, R.; Davidenko, I.; Tjulandin, S.; Deptala, A.; Harrison, M.; Nirni, S.; Lakshmaiah, K.; Thomas, A.; Jiang, Y.; et al. Rilotumumab in combination with epirubicin, cisplatin, and capecitabine as first-line treatment for gastric or oesophagogastric junction adenocarcinoma: An open-label, dose de-escalation phase 1b study and a double-blind, randomised phase 2 study. *Lancet Oncol.* **2014**, *15*, 1007–1018. [CrossRef]

91. Chen, J.; Zhou, S.J.; Zhang, Y.; Zhang, G.Q.; Zha, T.Z.; Feng, Y.Z.; Zhang, K. Clinicopathological and prognostic significance of galectin-1 and vascular endothelial growth factor expression in gastric cancer. *World J. Gastroenterol.* **2013**, *19*, 2073–2079. [CrossRef] [PubMed]

92. Lee, S.J.; Kim, J.G.; Sohn, S.K.; Chae, Y.S.; Moon, J.H.; Kim, S.N.; Bae, H.I.; Chung, H.Y.; Yu, W. No association of vascular endothelial growth factor-A (VEGF-A) and VEGF-C expression with survival in patients with gastric cancer. *Cancer Res. Treat.* **2009**, *41*, 218–223. [CrossRef] [PubMed]

93. Deguchi, K.; Ichikawa, D.; Soga, K.; Watanabe, K.; Kosuga, T.; Takeshita, H.; Konishi, H.; Morimura, R.; Tsujiura, M.; Komatsu, S.; et al. Clinical significance of vascular endothelial growth factors C and D and chemokine receptor CCR7 in gastric cancer. *Anticancer Res.* **2010**, *30*, 2361–2366. [PubMed]

94. Gou, H.F.; Chen, X.C.; Zhu, J.; Jiang, M.; Yang, Y.; Cao, D.; Hou, M. Expressions of COX-2 and VEGF-C in gastric cancer: Correlations with lymphangiogenesis and prognostic implications. *J. Exp. Clin. Canc. Res.* **2011**, *30*, 14. [CrossRef] [PubMed]

95. Ohtsu, A.; Shah, M.A.; Van Cutsem, E.; Rha, S.Y.; Sawaki, A.; Park, S.R.; Lim, H.Y.; Yamada, Y.; Wu, J.; Langer, B.; et al. Bevacizumab in combination with chemotherapy as first-line therapy in advanced gastric cancer: A randomized, double-blind, placebo-controlled phase III study. *J. Clin. Oncol.* **2011**, *29*, 3968–3976. [CrossRef] [PubMed]

96. Van Cutsem, E.; de Haas, S.; Kang, Y.K.; Ohtsu, A.; Tebbutt, N.C.; Ming, X.J.; Peng Yong, W.; Langer, B.; Delmar, P.; Scherer, S.J.; et al. Bevacizumab in combination with chemotherapy as first-line therapy in advanced gastric cancer: A biomarker evaluation from the AVAGAST randomized phase III trial. *J. Clin. Oncol.* **2012**, *30*, 2119–2127. [CrossRef] [PubMed]

97. Fuchs, C.S.; Tomasek, J.; Yong, C.J.; Dumitru, F.; Passalacqua, R.; Goswami, C.; Safran, H.; dos Santos, L.V.; Aprile, G.; Ferry, D.R.; et al. Ramucirumab monotherapy for previously treated advanced gastric or gastro-oesophageal junction adenocarcinoma (REGARD): An international, randomised, multicentre, placebocontrolled, phase 3 trial. *Lancet* **2014**, *383*, 31–39. [CrossRef]

98. Li, J.; Qin, S.; Xu, J.; Guo, W.; Xiong, J.; Bai, Y.; Sun, G.; Yang, Y.; Wang, L.; Xu, N.; et al. Apatinib for chemotherapy-refractory advanced metastatic gastric cancer: Results from a randomized, placebocontrolled, parallel-arm, phase II trial. *J. Clin. Oncol.* **2013**, *31*, 3219–3225. [CrossRef] [PubMed]

99. Choi, Y.Y.; Noh, S.H.; Cheong, J.H. Molecular Dimensions of Gastric Cancer: Translational and Clinical Perspectives. *J. Pathol. Transl. Med.* **2016**, *50*, 1–9. [CrossRef] [PubMed]

100. Corso, G.; Marrelli, D.; Pascale, V.; Vindigni, C.; Roviello, F. Frequency of CDH1 germline mutations in gastric carcinoma coming from high- and low-risk areas: Metanalysis and systematic review of the literature. *BMC Cancer* **2012**, *12*, 8. [CrossRef] [PubMed]

101. Liu, Y.C.; Shen, C.Y.; Wu, H.S.; Hsieh, T.Y.; Chan, D.C.; Chen, C.J.; Yu, J.C.; Yu, C.P.; Harn, H.J.; Chen, P.J.; et al. Mechanisms inactivating the gene for E-cadherin in sporadic gastric carcinomas. *World J. Gastroenterol.* **2006**, *12*, 2168–2173. [CrossRef] [PubMed]

102. Li, X.; Wu, W.K.; Xing, R.; Wong, S.H.; Liu, Y.; Fang, X.; Zhang, Y.; Wang, M.; Wang, J.; Li, L.; et al. Distinct Subtypes of Gastric Cancer Defined by Molecular Characterization Include Novel Mutational Signatures with Prognostic Capability. *Cancer Res.* **2016**, *76*, 1724–1732. [CrossRef] [PubMed]

103. Weissman, B.; Knudsen, K.E. Hijacking the chromatin remodeling machinery: Impact of SWI/SNF perturbations in cancer. *Cancer Res.* **2009**, *69*, 8223–8230. [CrossRef] [PubMed]

104. Wang, D.D.; Chen, Y.B.; Pan, K.; Wang, W.; Chen, S.P.; Chen, J.G.; Zhao, J.J.; Lv, L.; Pan, Q.Z.; Li, Y.Q.; et al. Decreased expression of the ARID1A gene is associated with poor prognosis in primary gastric cancer. *PLoS ONE* **2012**, *7*, e40364. [CrossRef] [PubMed]

105. Shang, X.; Marchioni, F.; Evelyn, C.R.; Sipes, N.; Zhou, X.; Seibel, W.; Wortman, M.; Zheng, Y. Small-molecule inhibitors targeting G-protein-coupled Rho guanine nucleotide exchange factors. *Proc. Natl. Acad. Sci. USA* **2013**, *110*, 3155–3160. [CrossRef] [PubMed]

106. Shang, X.; Marchioni, F.; Sipes, N.; Evelyn, C.R.; Jerabek-Willemsen, M.; Duhr, S.; Seibel, W.; Wortman, M.; Zheng, Y. Rational design of small molecule inhibitors targeting RhoA subfamily Rho GTPases. *Chem. Biol.* **2012**, *19*, 699–710. [CrossRef] [PubMed]

107. Türeci, O.; Koslowski, M.; Helftenbein, G.; Castle, J.; Rohde, C.; Dhaene, K.; Seitz, G.; Sahin, U. Claudin-18 gene structure, regulation, and expression is evolutionary conserved in mammals. *Gene* **2011**, *481*, 83–92. [CrossRef] [PubMed]

108. Yao, F.; Kausalya, J.P.; Sia, Y.Y.; Teo, A.S.; Lee, W.H.; Ong, A.G.; Zhang, Z.; Tan, J.H.; Li, G.; Bertrand, D.; et al. Recurrent Fusion Genes in Gastric Cancer: CLDN18-ARHGAP26 Induces Loss of Epithelial Integrity. *Cell Rep.* **2015**, *12*, 272–285. [CrossRef] [PubMed]

109. Al Batran, S.E.; Schuler, M.H.; Zvirbule, Z.; Manikhas, G.; Lordick, F.; Rusyn, A.; Vynnyk, Y.; Vynnychenko, I.; Fadeeva, N.; Nechaeva, M.; et al. FAST: An international, multicenter, randomized, phase II trial of epirubicin, oxaliplatin, and capecitabine (EOX) with or without IMAB362, a first-in-class anti-CLDN18.2 antibody, as firstline therapy in patients with advanced CLDN18.2 gastric and gastroesophageal junction (GEJ) adenocarcinoma. *J. Clin. Oncol.* **2016**, *34*, LBA4001. [CrossRef]

110. Hidalgo, M.; Amant, F.; Biankin, AV.; Budinskà, E.; Byrne, A.T.; Caldas, C.; Clarke, R.B.; de Jong, S.; Jonkers, J.; Mælandsmo, G.M.; et al. Patient-derived xenograft models: An emerging platform for translational cancer research. *Cancer Discov.* **2014**, *4*, 998–1013. [CrossRef] [PubMed]

111. Hausser, H.J.; Brenner, R.E. Phenotypic instability of Saos-2 cells in long-term culture. *Biochem. Biophys. Res. Commun.* **2005**, *333*, 216–222. [CrossRef] [PubMed]

112. Gillet, J.P.; Calcagno, A.M.; Varma, S.; Marino, M.; Green, L.J.; Vora, M.I.; Patel, C.; Orina, J.N.; Eliseeva, T.A.; Singal, V.; et al. Redefining the relevance of established cancer cell lines to the study of mechanisms of clinical anti-cancer drug resistance. *Proc. Natl. Acad. Sci. USA* **2011**, *108*, 18708–18713. [CrossRef] [PubMed]

113. Furukawa, T.; Kubota, T.; Watanabe, M.; Kitaijma, M.; Hoffman, R.M. Orthotopic transplantation of histologically intact clinical specimens of stomach cancer to nude mice: Correlation of metastatic sites in mouse and individual patient donors. *Int. J. Cancer* **1993**, *53*, 608–612. [CrossRef] [PubMed]

114. Furukawa, T.; Fu, X.; Kubota, T.; Watanabe, M.; Kitajima, M.; Hoffman, R.M. Nude mouse metastatic models of human stomach cancer constructed using orthotopic implantation of histologically intact tissue. *Cancer Res.* **1993**, *53*, 1204–1208. [PubMed]

115. Zhang, L.; Yang, J.; Cai, J.; Song, X.; Deng, J.; Huang, H.; Chen, D.; Yang, M.; Wery, J.P.; Li, S.; et al. A subset of gastric cancers with EGFR amplification and overexpression respond to cetuximab therapy. *Sci. Rep.* **2013**, *3*, 2992. [CrossRef] [PubMed]

116. Zhu, Y.; Tian, T.; Li, Z.; Tang, Z.; Wang, L.; Wu, J.; Li, Y.; Dong, B.; Li, Y.; Dong, B.; et al. Establishment and characterization of patient-derived tumor xenograft using gastroscopic biopsies in gastric cancer. *Sci. Rep.* **2015**, *5*, 8542. [CrossRef] [PubMed]

117. Lau, W.M.; Teng, E.; Chong, H.S.; Lopez, K.A.; Tay, A.Y.; Salto-Tellez, M.; Shabbir, A.; So, J.B.; Shan, S.L. CD44v8-10 is a cancer-specific marker for gastric cancer stem cells. *Cancer Res.* **2014**, *74*, 2630–2641. [CrossRef] [PubMed]

118. Gao, H.; Korn, J.M.; Ferretti, S.; Monahan, J.E.; Wang, Y.; Singh, M.; Zhang, C.; Schnell, C.; Yang, G.; Zhang, Y.; et al. High-throughput screening using patient-derived tumor xenografts to predict clinical trial drug response. *Nat. Med.* **2015**, *21*, 1318–1325. [CrossRef] [PubMed]

119. Park, H.; Cho, S.Y.; Kim, H.; Na, D.; Han, J.Y.; Chae, J.; Park, C.; Park, O.K.; Min, S.; Kang, J.; et al. Genomic alterations in BCL2L1 and DLC1 contribute to drug sensitivity in gastric cancer. *Proc. Natl. Acad. Sci. USA* **2015**, *112*, 12492–12497. [CrossRef] [PubMed]

120. Dedhia, P.H.; Bertaux-Skeirik, N.; Zavros, Y.; Spence, J.R. Organoid models of human gastrointestinal development and disease. *Gastroenterology* **2016**, *150*, 1098–1112. [CrossRef] [PubMed]

121. Hill, D.R.; Spence, J.R. Gastrointestinal organoids: Understanding the molecular basis of the host-microbe interface. *Cell Mol. Gastroenterol Hepatol.* **2017**, *3*, 138–149. [CrossRef] [PubMed]

122. van de Wetering, M.; Francies, H.E.; Francis, J.M.; Bounova, G.; Iorio, F.; Pronk, A.; van Houdt, W.; van Gorp, J.; Taylor-Weiner, A.; Kester, L.; et al. Prospective derivation of a living organoid biobank of colorectal cancer patients. *Cell* **2015**, *161*, 933–945. [CrossRef] [PubMed]

123. McCracken, K.W.; Catá, E.M.; Crawford, C.M.; Sinagoga, K.L.; Schumacher, M.; Rocjich, B.E.; Tsai, Y.H.; Mayhew, C.N.; Spence, J.R.; Zavros, Y.; et al. Modelling human development and disease in pluripotent stemcell-derived gastric organoids. *Nature* **2014**, *516*, 400–404. [CrossRef] [PubMed]

124. Li, X.; Nadauld, L.; Ootani, A.; Corney, D.C.; Pai, R.K.; Gevaert, O.; Cantrell, M.A.; Rack, P.G.; Neal, J.T.; Chan, C.W.; et al. Oncogenic transformation of diverse gastrointestinal tissues in primary organoid culture. *Nat. Med.* **2014**, *20*, 769–777. [CrossRef] [PubMed]

125. Nadauld, L.D.; Garcia, S.; Natsoulis, G.; Bell, J.M.; Miotke, L.; Hopmans, E.S.; Xu, H.; Pai, R.K.; Palm, C.; Regan, J.F.; et al. Metastatic tumor evolution and organoid modeling implicate TGFBR2 as a cancer driver in diffuse gastric cancer. *Genome Biol.* **2014**, *15*, 428. [CrossRef] [PubMed]

126. Wang, K.; Yuen, S.T.; Xu, J.; Lee, S.P.; Yan, H.H.; Shi, S.T.; Siu, H.C.; Deng, S.; Chu, K.M.; Law, S.; et al. Whole-genome sequencing and comprehensive molecular profiling identify new driver mutations in gastric cancer. *Nat. Genet.* **2014**, *46*, 573–582. [CrossRef] [PubMed]

127. Lee, Y.; Ahn, C.; Han, J.; Choi, H.; Kim, J.; Yim, J.; Lee, J.; Provost, P.; Radmark, O.; Kim, S. The nuclear RNase III Drosha initiates microRNA processing. *Nature* **2003**, *425*, 415–419. [CrossRef] [PubMed]

128. Ruan, K.; Fang, X.; Ouyang, G. MicroRNAs: Novel regulators in the hallmarks of human cancer. *Cancer Lett.* **2009**, *285*, 116–126. [CrossRef] [PubMed]

129. Kim, R.H.; Mak, T.W. Tumours and tremors: How PTEN regulation underlies both. *Br. J. Cancer* **2006**, *94*, 620–624. [CrossRef] [PubMed]

130. Zhang, C.-Z.; Han, L.; Zhang, A.-L.; Fu, Y.-C.; Yue, X.; Wang, G.-X.; Jia, Z.-F.; Pu, P.-Y.; Zhang, Q.-Y.; Kang, C.-S. MicroRNA221 and microRNA-222 regulate gastric carcinoma cell proliferation and radioresistance by targeting PTEN. *BMC Cancer* **2010**, *10*, 367. [CrossRef]

131. Zhang, B.G.; Li, J.F.; Yu, B.Q.; Zhu, Z.G.; Liu, B.Y.; Yan, M. microRNA-21 promotes tumor proliferation and invasion in gastric cancer by targeting PTEN. *Oncol. Rep.* **2012**, *27*, 1019–1026. [CrossRef] [PubMed]

132. Tsukamoto, Y.; Nakada, C.; Noguchi, T.; Tanigawa, M.; Nguyen, L.T.; Uchida, T.; Hijina, T.; Matsuura, K.; Fujioka, T.; Seto, M.; et al. MicroRNA-375 is downregulated in gastric carcinomas and regulates cell survival by targeting PDK1 and 14-3-3zeta. *Cancer Res.* **2010**, *70*, 2339–2349. [CrossRef] [PubMed]

133. Takagi, T.; Iio, A.; Nakagawa, Y.; Naoe, T.; Tanigawa, N.; Akao, Y. Decreased expression of microRNA-143 and -145 in human gastric cancers. *Oncology* **2009**, *77*, 12–21. [CrossRef] [PubMed]

134. Hashimoto, Y.; Akiyama, Y.; Otsubo, T.; Shimada, S.; Yuasa, Y. Involvement of epigenetically silenced microRNA-181c in gastric carcinogenesis. *Carcinogenesis* **2010**, *31*, 777–784. [CrossRef] [PubMed]

135. Lang, N.; Liu, M.; Tang, Q.L.; Chen, X.; Liu, Z.; Bi, F. Effects of microRNA-29 family members on proliferation and invasion of gastric cancer cell lines. *Chin. J. Cancer* **2010**, *29*, 603–610. [CrossRef] [PubMed]

136. Lee, J.T., Jr.; McCubrey, J.A. The Raf/MEK/ERK signal transduction cascade as a target for chemotherapeutic intervention in leukemia. *Leukemia* **2002**, *16*, 486–507. [CrossRef] [PubMed]

137. Feng, L.; Xie, Y.; Zhang, H.; Wu, Y. miR-107 targets cyclin-dependent kinase 6 expression, induces cell cycle G1 arrest and inhibits invasion in gastric cancer cells. *Med. Oncol.* **2012**, *29*, 856–863. [CrossRef] [PubMed]

138. Zhang, L.; Liu, X.; Jin, H.; Guo, X.; Xia, L.; Chen, Z.; Bai, M.; Liu, J.; Shang, X.; Wu, K.; et al. MiR-206 inhibits gastric cancer proliferation in part by repressing CyclinD2. *Cancer Lett.* **2013**, *332*, 94–101. [CrossRef] [PubMed]

139. Ding, L.; Xu, Y.; Zhang, W.; Deng, Y.; Si, M.; Du, Y.; Yao, H.; Liu, X.; Ke, Y.; Si, J.; et al. MiR-375 frequently downregulated in gastric cancer inhibits cell proliferation by targeting JAK2. *Cell Res.* **2010**, *20*, 784–793. [CrossRef] [PubMed]

140. Guo, X.; Guo, L.; Ji, J.; Zhang, J.; Chen, X.; Cai, Q.; Li, J.; Gu, Q.; Liu, B.; Zhu, Z.; et al. miRNA-331-3p directly targets E2F1 and induces growth arrest in human gastric cancer. *Biochem. Biophys. Res. Commun.* **2010**, *398*, 1–6. [CrossRef] [PubMed]

141. Xiao, B.; Guo, J.; Miao, Y.; Jiang, Z.; Huan, R.; Zhang, Y.; Li, D.; Zhong, J. Detection of miR-106a in gastric carcinoma and its clinical significance. *Clin. Chim. Acta* **2009**, *400*, 97–102. [CrossRef] [PubMed]

142. Kim, Y.K.; Yu, J.; Han, T.S.; Park, S.Y.; Namkoong, B.; Kim, D.H.; Hur, K.; Yoo, M.W.; Lee, H.J.; Yang, H.K.; et al. Functional links between clustered microRNAs: Suppression of cell-cycle inhibitors by microRNA clusters in gastric cancer. *Nucleic Acids Res.* **2009**, *37*, 1672–1681. [CrossRef] [PubMed]

143. Guo, S.L.; Peng, Z.; Yang, X.; Fan, K.J.; Ye, H.; Li, Z.H.; Wang, Y.; Xu, X.L.; Li, J.; Wang, Y.L.; et al. miR-148a promoted cell proliferation by targeting p27 in gastric cancer cells. *Int. J. Biol. Sci.* **2011**, *7*, 567–574. [CrossRef] [PubMed]

144. Sun, M.; Liu, X.H.; Li, J.H.; Yang, J.S.; Zhang, E.B.; Yin, D.D.; Liu, Z.L.; Zhou, J.; Ding, Y.; Li, S.Q.; et al. MiR-196a is upregulated in gastric cancer and promotes cell proliferation by downregulating p27(kip1). *Mol. Cancer Ther.* **2012**, *11*, 842–852. [CrossRef] [PubMed]

145. Chan, S.H.; Wu, C.W.; Li, A.F.; Chi, C.W.; Lin, W.C. miR-21 microRNA expression in human gastric carcinomas and its clinical association. *Anticancer Res.* **2008**, *28*, 907–911. [PubMed]

146. Motoyama, K.; Inoue, H.; Mimori, K.; Tanaka, F.; Kojima, K.; Uetake, H.; Sugihara, K.; Mori, M. Clinicopathological and prognostic significance of PDCD4 and microRNA-21 in human gastric cancer. *Int. J. Oncol.* **2010**, *36*, 1089–1095. [CrossRef] [PubMed]

147. Li, B.; Zhao, Y.; Guo, G.; Li, W.; Zhu, E.D.; Luo, X.; Mao, X.H.; Zou, Q.M.; Yu, P.W.; Zuo, Q.F.; et al. Plasma microRNAs, miR-223, miR-21 and miR-218, as novel potential biomarkers for gastric cancer detection. *PLoS ONE* **2012**, *7*, e41629. [CrossRef] [PubMed]

148. Zhang, Y.; Guo, J.; Li, D.; Xiao, B.; Miao, Y.; Jiang, Z.; Zhuo, H. Down-regulation of miR-31 expression in gastric cancer tissues and its clinical significance. *Med. Oncol.* **2010**, *27*, 685–689. [CrossRef] [PubMed]

149. Li, X.; Luo, F.; Li, Q.; Xu, M.; Feng, D.; Zhang, G.; Wu, W. Identification of new aberrantly expressed miRNAs in intestinal-type gastric cancer and its clinical significance. *Oncol. Rep.* **2011**, *26*, 1431–1439. [CrossRef] [PubMed]

150. Katada, T.; Ishiguro, H.; Kuwabara, Y.; Kimura, M.; Mitui, A.; Mori, Y.; Ogawa, R.; Harata, K.; Fujii, Y. microRNA expression profile in undifferentiated gastric cancer. *Int. J. Oncol.* **2009**, *34*, 537–542. [CrossRef] [PubMed]

151. Bandres, E.; Bitarte, N.; Arias, F.; Agorreta, J.; Fortes, P.; Agirre, X.; Zarate, R.; Diaz-Gonzalez, J.A.; Ramirez, N.; Sola, J.J.; et al. microRNA-451 regulates macrophage migration inhibitory factor production and proliferation of gastrointestinal cancer cells. *Clin. Cancer Res.* **2009**, *15*, 2281–2290. [CrossRef] [PubMed]

152. Gong, J.; Li, J.; Wang, Y.; Liu, C.; Jia, H.; Jiang, C.; Wang, Y.; Luo, M.; Zhao, H.; Dong, L.; et al. Characterization of microRNA-29 family expression and investigation of their mechanistic roles in gastric cancer. *Carcinogenesis* **2014**, *35*, 497–506. [CrossRef] [PubMed]

153. Yang, T.S.; Yang, X.H.; Chen, X.; Wang, X.D.; Hua, J.; Zhou, D.L.; Zhou, B.; Song, Z.S. MicroRNA-106b in cancer-associated fibroblasts from gastric cancer promotes cell migration and invasion by targeting PTEN. *FEBS Lett.* **2014**, *588*, 2162–2169. [CrossRef] [PubMed]

154. Nishida, N.; Mimori, K.; Fabbri, M.; Yokobori, T.; Sudo, T.; Tanaka, F.; Shibata, K.; Ishii, H.; Doki, Y.; Mori, M. MicroRNA-125a-5p is an independent prognostic factor in gastric cancer and inhibits the proliferation of human gastric cancer cells in combination with trastuzumab. *Clin. Cancer Res.* **2011**, *17*, 2725–2733. [CrossRef] [PubMed]

155. Yang, Q.; Zhang, C.; Huang, B.; Li, H.; Zhang, R.; Huang, Y.; Wang, J. Downregulation of microRNA-206 is a potent prognostic marker for patients with gastric cancer. *Eur. J. Gastroenterol Hepatol.* **2013**, *25*, 953–957. [CrossRef] [PubMed]

156. Volinia, S.; Calin, G.A.; Liu, C.G.; Ambs, S.; Cimmino, A.; Petrocca, F.; Visone, R.; Iorio, M.; Roldo, C.; Ferracin, M.; et al. A microRNA expression signature of human solid tumors defines cancer gene targets. *Proc. Natl. Acad. Sci. USA* **2006**, *103*, 2257–2261. [CrossRef] [PubMed]

157. Li, X.; Zhang, Y.; Zhang, Y.; Ding, J.; Wu, K.; Fan, D. Survival prediction of gastric cancer by a seven-microRNA signature. *Gut* **2010**, *59*, 579–585. [CrossRef] [PubMed]

158. Li, X.; Zhang, Y.; Zhang, H.; Liu, X.; Gong, T.; Li, M.; Sun, L.; Ji, G.; Shi, Y.; Han, Z.; et al. miRNA-223 promotes gastric cancer invasion and metastasis by targeting tumor suppressor EPB41L3. *Mol. Cancer Res.* **2011**, *9*, 824–833. [CrossRef] [PubMed]

159. Ueda, T.; Volinia, S.; Okumura, H.; Shimizu, M.; Taccioli, C.; Rossi, S.; Alder, H.; Liu, C.G.; Oue, N.; Yasui, W.; et al. Relation between microRNA expression and progression and prognosis of gastric cancer: A microRNA expression analysis. *Lancet Oncol.* **2010**, *11*, 136–146. [CrossRef]

160. Kogo, R.; Mimori, K.; Tanaka, F.; Komune, S.; Mori, M. Clinical significance of miR-146a in gastric cancer cases. *Clin. Cancer Res.* **2011**, *17*, 4277–4284. [CrossRef] [PubMed]

161. Bou Kheir, T.; Futoma-Kazmierczak, E.; Jacobsen, A.; Krogh, A.; Bardram, L.; Hother, C.; Gronbaek, K.; Federspiel, B.; Lund, A.H.; Friis-Hansen, L. miR-449 inhibits cell proliferation and is down-regulated in gastric cancer. *Mol. Cancer* **2011**, *10*, 29. [CrossRef] [PubMed]

162. Tsai, M.M.; Wang, C.S.; Tsai, C.Y.; Huang, H.W.; Chi, H.C.; Lin, Y.H.; Lu, P.H. Potential diagnostic, prognostic and therapeutic targets of microRNAs in human gastric cancer. *Int. J. Mol. Sci.* **2016**, *17*. [CrossRef] [PubMed]

163. Chang, L.; Guo, F.; Wang, Y.; Lv, Y.; Huo, B.; Wang, L.; Liu, W. MicroRna-200c regulates the sensitivity of chemotherapy of gastric cancer SGC7901/DDP cells by directly targeting RhoE. *Pathol. Oncol. Res.* **2014**, *20*, 93–98. [CrossRef] [PubMed]

164. Yoon, J.H.; Swiderski, P.M.; Kaplan, B.E.; Takao, M.; Yasui, A.; Shen, B.; Pfeifer, G.P. Processing of UV damage in vistro by FEN-1 proteins aas part of an alternative DNA excision repair pathway. *Biochemistry* **1999**, *38*, 4809–4817. [CrossRef] [PubMed]

165. Hu, C.B.; Li, Q.L.; Hu, J.F.; Zhang, Q.; Xie, J.P.; Deng, L. miR-124 inhibits growth and invasion of gastric cancer by targeting ROCK1. *Asian Pac. J. Cncer Prev.* **2014**, *15*, 6543–6546. [CrossRef]

166. Xu, Y.; Huang, Z.; Liu, Y. Reduced miR-125a-5p expression is associated with gastric carcinogenesis through the targeting of E2F3. *Mol. Med. Rep.* **2014**, *10*, 2601–2608. [CrossRef] [PubMed]

167. Zheng, L.; Pu, J.; Qi, T.; Qi, M.; Li, D.; Xiang, X.; Huang, K.; Tong, Q. miRNA-145 targets v-ets erythroblastosis virus E26 oncogene homolog 1 to suppress the invasion, metastasis, and angiogenesi of gastric cancer cell. *Mol. Cancer Res.* **2013**, *11*, 182–193. [CrossRef] [PubMed]

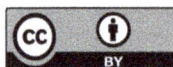

International Journal of
Molecular Sciences

MDPI

Review

What's New in Gastric Cancer: The Therapeutic Implications of Molecular Classifications and Future Perspectives

Giuseppe Tirino [1,*], Luca Pompella [1], Angelica Petrillo [1], Maria Maddalena Laterza [1],
Annalisa Pappalardo [1], Marianna Caterino [1], Michele Orditura [1], Fortunato Ciardiello [1],
Gennaro Galizia [2] and Ferdinando De Vita [1,*]

[1] Division of Medical Oncology, Department of Precision Medicine, School of Medicine, University of
    Campania "Luigi Vanvitelli", Via Pansini n.5, 80131 Naples, Italy; luca.pompella@icloud.com (L.P.);
    angelic.petrillo@gmail.com (A.P.); marilena_laterza@yahoo.it (M.M.L.);
    annalisa.pappalardo88@gmail.com (A.P.); caterinomarianna@gmail.com (M.C.);
    michele.orditura@unicampania.it (M.O.); fortunato.ciardiello@unicampania.it (F.C.)
[2] Division of GI Tract Surgical Oncology, Department of Cardio-Thoracic and Respiratory Sciences,
    School of Medicine, University of Campania "Luigi Vanvitelli", Via Pansini n.5, 80131 Naples, Italy;
    gennaro.galizia@unicampania.it
*   Correspondence: giuseppe.tirino@unicampania.it (G.T.); ferdinando.devita@unicampania.it (F.D.V.);
    Tel.: +39-081-566-6729 (G.T.); +39-081-566-6713 (F.D.V.)

Received: 18 August 2018; Accepted: 5 September 2018; Published: 7 September 2018

Abstract: Despite some remarkable innovations and the advent of novel molecular classifications the prognosis of patients with advanced gastric cancer (GC) remains overall poor and current clinical application of new advances is disappointing. During the last years only Trastuzumab and Ramucirumab have been approved and currently used as standard of care targeted therapies, but the systemic management of advanced disease did not radically change in contrast with the high number of molecular drivers identified. The Cancer Genome Atlas (TCGA) and Asian Cancer Research Group (ACRG) classifications paved the way, also for GC, to that more contemporary therapeutic approach called "precision medicine" even if tumor heterogeneity and a complex genetic landscape still represent a strong barrier. The identification of specific cancer subgroups is also making possible a better selection of patients that are most likely to respond to immunotherapy. This review aims to critically overview the available molecular classifications summarizing the main druggable molecular drivers and their possible therapeutic implications also taking advantage of new technologies and acquisitions.

Keywords: gastric cancer; molecular classifications; targeted therapy; immunotherapy

1. Introduction

During the last years, "precision medicine" has deeply changed the therapeutic landscape of several malignancies. The customization of healthcare led to a global and significant improvement in cancer management and has faded the "one size fit-all" era. However, in contrast to the steady increase in survival observed for most cancer types, advances have been slow and difficult for gastric cancer (GC).

In fact, despite some remarkable innovations there is still an urgent need for a deeper understanding of the genetic and molecular background of this cancer and for novel treatment approaches.

Several therapeutic strategies have been already investigated and new molecular classifications have been proposed, nevertheless the prognosis of patients with advanced disease remains overall poor with a median overall survival (OS) of about 11 months and disappointing five-year survival rate of approximately 25–30% [1,2], even if a correct "continuum of care" is making longer survivals less anecdotical.

Only trastuzumab (anti-HER2 monoclonal antibody) and ramucirumab (anti-VEGFR monoclonal antibody) have proven to be successful weapons among all of the several molecular drivers identified, but currently still lacking of any clinical utility; for these reasons, the standard systemic chemotherapy still represents a "forced" mainstay of the treatment of advanced disease.

All of these efforts led to a fundamental acquisition: gastric cancer should be considered to be a collection of different molecular entities, rather than a single homogeneous disease.

As a matter of fact, in contrast with the overall declining trends for the four major malignancies, gastric cancer has still one of the highest estimated mortality rate, representing the third leading cause of cancer-related death (8.8%) with alarming statistics that make it one of the most lethal disease in the world (723,000 estimated deaths out of almost one-million new cases per year worldwide) [3].

Even if its incidence significantly fell over the last decades it still represents the fifth most common cancer (6.8% of all) with 10,800 new diagnoses still expected in 2018 only in the United States (US) [4].

These numbers require the biggest effort and attention on this cancer in order to investigate its heterogeneity and to maximize treatment outcomes.

The biggest challenge for the next future will be to understand which cancer subgroup deserves a specific targeted agent, also reconsidering drugs that have failed at an early research stage through the definition of more precise molecular drivers by using new technologies, such as patient-derived xenograft (PDX) and tumor organoids or an integrated genomic analysis, and consequently to minimize the amount of patients who receive a same treatment without any molecular selection.

This review aims to critically overview the available molecular classifications and the latest findings for GC and to outline the possible future scenarios and implications of these acquisitions.

2. Where It All Began: The "Old Dear" Histology

Gastric cancer of epithelial origin (GC) is today recognized as an extremely heterogeneous disease both in the clinical presentation modes as well as histological appearances and molecular basis. A first attempt to define GC heterogeneity was to look at it by microscope as performed by Lauren P. [5], who identified two main types of GC on histological bases: the first one called "intestinal", as it displayed features characteristic of intestinal mucosa (and it was thought to arise from intestinal metaplasia of the stomach), and the other one called "diffuse" because the cancer cells, often poorly cohesive, diffusely infiltrated the gastric wall. The World Health Organization (WHO) classification of tumors of digestive system [6], on the other hand, classifies GCs, according to their histological appearance, in "tubular adenocarcinomas" (that contain dilatated and branching tubules, with cytological atipia varying from low to high-grade), "papillary adenocarcinomas" (typically well-differentiated exophytic carcinomas with elongated finger-like processes), "mucinous adenocarcinomas" (>50% of the tumor contains extracellular mucinous pool), and "signet-ring cell adenocarcinomas" (more than 50% of the tumor consists of isolated or small groups of malignant cells, highly infiltrative, containing intracytoplasmatic mucin), the latter one resembling those that are classified as "diffuse type" in the "Lauren classification".

3. Two Steps Towards Precision Medicine: Molecular Classifications

This histological heterogeneity is only the tip of the iceberg if we think about the GC underlying molecular complexity, and, as a matter of fact, many molecular classifications have succeeded over the years (immunohistochemistry based, genomic based, proteomic based, etc.): in this section, we have tried to report the most significant, also in relation to novel therapeutic possibilities.

The first molecular attempt to classify comprehensively GC at molecular level was made by Patrick Tan's group in Singapore [7]: they analyzed 60 GC samples (from 60 patients) by expression microarrays and comparative genomic hybridization and identified three molecular GC subgroups: "tumorigenic", "reactive", and "gastric-like".

Each subtype was associated to a different biological function; for example, "reactive" group highly expresses endothelial growth factors and appears more sensitive to anti-angiogenic strategies. However, no associations were found between each subtype and Lauren's histology or tumor grading, but, when survival analysis was performed, "gastric-like" tumor emerged as the most favorable subtype in a statistically significant way.

In 2011, the same Singapore group proposed another classification of GCs in G-INT (genomic intestinal) and G-DIF (genomic diffuse) [8]. Differently from others, the authors did not start their research characterizing primary human tissue, but they used a panel of 37 GC cell lines: in that way, they identified a "gene expression signature" of 171 genes that are able to distinguish these two intrinsic GC subtypes, the first one called "G-INT" because more related to Lauren's intestinal subtype and the other one "G-DIF" more related to diffuse subtype. Moreover, this classification was also validated on a clinical cohort of 270 GC patients, with important prognostic informations: G-DIF tumors showed a statistically significant worse overall survival when compared to G-INT tumors, while Lauren's histologies were not prognostic. Furthermore, predictive informations came out from in vitro experiments on 28 cell lines, with possibly relevant implications for patient's care: G-INT cell lines were more sensitive to 5-fluorouralcil and oxaliplatin, while G-DIF resulted in being more sensitive to cisplatin. On that basis, authors designed a prospective "genomic-guided" chemotherapy trial (NCT01100801) [9], in which GC patients were allocated to "oxaliplatin arm" or "cisplatin arm" based on their intrinsic subtype; indeed, trial data were recently published [10], with some disappointing results since, although G-INT GC patients allocated to Oxaliplatin arm showed a deeper level of response, overall survival was better in G-INT patients that were allocated to cisplatin arm, leaving the authors a little bit confused, as well as the readers.

In the same years, Manish Shah proposed a new GC classification that is based on epidemiological and topographic tools [11], recognizing three subtypes: diffuse, proximal non-diffuse, and distal non-diffuse GC. Proximal non-diffuse GC arises in the cardia and it is preceded by precursor glandular dysplasia in the setting of chronic inflammation, but, differently from distal non-diffuse GC where inflammation is more related to H. Pylori infection, in proximal tumors, phlogosis is caused by gastric acid reflux [12]. To note, many tyrosine kinase receptors, like HER-2 (Human epitelial growth factor receptor 2) [13,14], EGFR (Epidermal growth factor receptor) [15], and c-MET (Mesenchymal epithelial transition factor receptor) [16] are more frequently expressed or amplified in proximal tumors when compared with distal tumors. Moreover, glycolysis and gluconeogenesis pathways are also upregulated in this subtype [10]. Distal non-diffuse gastric cancers arise instead between the gastric body and pylorus, often preceded by chronic inflammation with aspects of intestinal metaplasia, both consequences of chronic H. Pylori infection. These tumors frequently display an intestinal histological appearance (according to Lauren) and upregulate vascular endothelial growth factor and many other angiogenic pathways [17]. Finally, diffuse GC is characterized by diffuse pattern of infiltration: the complete loss of adherence properties by the cancer cells generate the so called "signet ring cells" histology, which is often due to CDH1 (Cadherin 1) tumor suppressor loss at genetic level. Other molecular aberrations in diffuse GC include FGF-R2 (Fibroblast growth factor receptor 2) tyrosine kinase receptor overexpression [18], PI3K (Phosphoinositide 3-kinase) signaling activity [19] and HER3 receptor overexpression [20]. Finally, expression of some Matrix Metallo-Proteases (MMP) is more frequent in diffuse versus intestinal cancers and it could contribute to tumor aggressiveness [21].

In 2013, Patrick Tan's group again published a new attempt to molecularly classify GCs [22]: this time the authors performed a "consensus hierarchical clustering" of 248 GC samples and identified three major subtypes ("mesenchymal", "proliferative", and "metabolic"). The "mesenchymal" subgroup was so called because of the high activity of EMT (epithelial-to-mesenchymal transition) pathway: indeed, this subtype has very high levels of CDH2 (*N*-cadherin) transcripts and low levels of CDH1 (E-cadherin), typical of mesenchymal cells. However, many other pathways characterize this GC subtype:

(1)   Cancer Stem Cells (CSCs) pathway: very high levels of CD44 (a marker of CSC) are described, with a more frequent poor differentiated histology (a surrogated marker of CSC).

(2)   p53 pathway.

(3)   Transforming Growth factor Beta (TGF-B) pathway.

(4)   Vascular endothelial growth factor (VEGF) pathway.

(5)   mTOR pathway (similarly to Shah's "diffuse subtype").

(6)   Sonic Hedgehog (SHH) pathway: a very well defined pathway active in stem cells.

To note, mesenchymal subtype is more associated to Lauren's diffuse dubtype than the other two (60% of tumors in this category are diffuse type), as well as the G-DIF (92%).

The "proliferative" subtype shows the high expression of a large set of genes correlated to cell cycle (*E2F*, *MYC*, *RAS*, etc.). These tumors are frequently correlated to Lauren's intestinal type (74%) and G-INT subgroup (71%) with very high levels of p53 mutations and copy number amplifications (in CCNE1 locus, MYC locus, KRAS locus, to name a few). Lastly, the "metabolic" subtype highly expresses metabolic-related genes and digestive-related genes, the latter ones being typical also of normal gastric mucosa. Therefore the authors hypothesized that this subtype is closer to the normal gastric mucosa than the other two, even in terms of gene expression profile. An intermediate step between the normal mucosa and this cancer subgroup could be the SPEM (spasmolytic-polypeptide-expressing metaplasia), whose genes are highly expressed by the metabolic subtype.

Although these subtypes are molecularly very distinct, no differences in terms of survival were identified. However, metabolic subtype seems to be more sensitive to 5-fluorouracil than the other two, perhaps in relation to low levels of thymidylate synthetase, while the mesenchymal subtype (probably due to "oncogenic addiction" to PI3K-AKT-mTOR pathway, as we discuss above) seems to be sensitive to several drugs that block PI3K or mTOR, opening the way for a more precise therapy for GC.

In 2014 Leung et al. [23] demonstrated the multidimensional genomic landscape and the molecular complexity of gastric adenocarcinomas performing an integrative genomic analysis on a dataset of 100 diffuse and intestinal GC samples (tumor and normal tissue paired). Using four different platforms (whole-genome sequencing, DNA copy number, gene expression, and methylation profiling), they identified the main aberrant pathways and subtype-specific genetic and epigenetic perturbations. In addition to the known mutated driver genes (TP53 frequent in both subtypes, ARID1A in Epstain Barr Virus-related (EBV) or microsatellite instability-related cancers and CDH1 in diffuse-type), authors have been able to describe new highly recurrent significant mutations (i.e., MUC6, CTNNA2, GLI3, RNF4) and particularly the high prevalence of *RHOA* (Ras homolog gene family, member A) mutations in diffuse-type tumors (14.3% vs. 0% in the intestinal-type, *p* < 0.001). These mutations determines defective RHOA pathway leading to aberrations in the adhesion functionality and escape from programmed cell death that occours when anchorage-dependent normal cells detach from the extracellular matrix, also demonstrating the possible tumor suppressive role of RHOA in this subtype. The study was one of the first to prove the deep molecular differences and to highlight the specific genetic perturbations covered below different histological features.

Few months later, the Cancer Genome Atlas (TCGA) investigators published the most important and comprehensive study that we have to date on molecular GC classification [24].

The authors characterized 295 GC tumor samples using six different molecular platforms (copy number alterations, whole exoms sequencing, mRNA sequencing, miRNA sequencing, DNA methylation analysis, and phosphoproteomic analysis) and identified four molecular subtypes: EBV-related, MSI-H (Microsatellite instability-high), Genomically Stable (GS), and Chromosomal Instability (CIN). The first one (9% of cases) is called "EBV-related", because it is characterized by Epstein Barr virus infection in the cancer cells: these tumors are mainly located in the gastric fundus or body and show extensive DNA promoter hypermethylation (a marker of "gene silencing"). Moreover, they have the highest frequency of PIK3CA (encoding for the catalytic alfa subunit of PI3K kinase) mutations (80%), as well as amplifications of *JAK2* (Janus kinase 2) or *PD-L1/L2* genes, making this subtype "ideally" the most sensitive to PI3K or PD1/PDL1 inhibition (as we will see later). The second group (22% of cases) was called "MSI" because it was characterized by genomic instability, due to a deficient DNA mismatch repair system, and lacked targetable amplifications. This subtype shows hypermethylation of MLH1 promoter region (leading to MLH1 silencing)—the cause of MSI status—and a very high mutation rate with hotspot mutations involving several genes like *HER2* (5%), *EGF-R* (5%), *HER3* (14%), *JAK2* (11%), *FGFR2* (2%), *MET* (3%), and *PIK3CA* (42%). To note, the BRAF^V600E mutation commonly seen in MSI-H colorectal cancer was universally absent. Finally, gastric MSI tumors have a very high rate of PD-L1 expression that, when associated with the high number of mutation-associated neoantigens, could make them very sensitive to checkpoint inhibitors.

The third group is called "Genomically Stable" (GC) and it accounts for 20% of TCGA dataset: it lacked somatic copy number aberrations and was more related to Lauren's diffuse histology than the other ones. A pathway frequently destroyed in this subtype is that related to "cell adhesion", with the most relevant genes mutated CDH1 (26%), RHOA (15%), and chromosomal translocation involving CLDN18 and ARHGAP (15%). The last group is characterized by chromosomal instability (50% of cases), and it thus called "CIN". Gene amplifications are very frequent, with involvement of different tyrosine kinase receptors or related pathways: HER2 (24%), EGF-R (10%), HER3 (8%), JAK2 (5%), FGFR2 (8%), MET (8%), PIK3CA (10%), and KRAS/NRAS (18%).

After all, if we move to clinical significance of this classification, not reported in the original paper, Sohn et al. [25], while using gene expression data from one of the TCGA cohort (*n* = 262), developed a robust subtype-based prediction model with the EBV subtype resulting as the one associated with the best prognosis and the "GS" subtype with the worst. Moreover, MSI and CIN subtypes had an intermediate prognosis, with a poorer overall survival than those with EBV+ but better than those with GS subtype. The authors also found important predictive informations, as the CIN subgroup experienced the biggest benefit from adjuvant chemotherapy, while the GS subtype the smallest.

One year later, the Asian Cancer research group (ACRG), analyzing 300 gastric tumor samples by two molecular platforms, provided a new GC classification, and identified four subtype [26]: "MSI", "MSS/EMT", "MSS/p53+" (p53 active), and "MSS/p53−" (p53 inactive). One of the strengths of ACRG classification is to precisely correlate each molecular subtype with clinical information, like prognosis, recurrence frequency (after surgery), and pattern of recurrence (i.e., peritoneal versus hepatic).

The MSI subtype (23% of cases), as in the TCGA cohort, was found to be hypermutated due to the frequent loss of MLH1. These tumors occur mainly in gastric antrum (75%), they are preferentially of intestinal subtype (>60%) and >50% of subjects are diagnosed at an early stage (I/II). Genes frequently affected by mutations are KRAS (23%), ALK (16%), ARID1A (44%), and those related to PI3K pathway (42%). To note, this group is associated with the best overall prognosis and the lowest frequency of recurrence (22%) of the four subtypes. The MSS/EMT (epithelial to mesenchymal transition) group (15% of cases) occurs at significantly younger age and shows mainly diffuse histology. It is characterized by a very low mutation rate when compared with other MSS groups (*p* < 0.001), but with the frequent loss of CDH1 expression, especially in a large set of signet ring cells adenocarcinomas. More importantly, the majority of subjects (>80%) in this subtype are diagnosed at stage III/IV: therefore the MSS/EMT has the worst prognosis, with the highest chance of recurrence (63%), mainly at the peritoneal site.

MSS/p53+ tumors (26% of cases) show frequent EBV positivity (with some overlap with the "EBV-related" subtype of TCGA) and a preserved activity of p53 tumor suppressor gene. Frequent mutations hit APC, ARID1A, KRAS, PIK3CA, and SMAD4. This subtype is also associated with the best overall prognosis after MSI subtype.

MSS/p53− tumors (36% of cases) present overlap with the CIN group from TCGA, showing the highest prevalence of p53 mutations and recurrent focal amplifications of tyrosine kinase receptors, like ERBB2 or cell-cycle modulators, like CCNE1 or CCND1.

4. Comparison of TCGA and ACRG Data

The TCGA and ACRG classifications are partially overlapping and complementary models: they both identified an MSI group of tumors characterized by high mutation frequency and best prognosis. While CIN and GS subtypes are present across all the ACRG groups, it is noteworthy that TCGA EBV+, GS, and CIN subtypes are enriched in ACRG MSS/p53+, MSS/EMT, and MSS/p53− respectively.

However, while CDH1 and RHOA mutations are highly prevalent in the TCGA GS subtype, in ACRG MSS/EMT, these mutations are extremely rare, making these two subtypes absolutely not equivalent or synonyms.

Possible reasons for this partial overlap between these classifications include differences related to the patient population (Korea in ACRG versus USA and Western Europe in TCGA), tumor sampling (mainly diffuse in ACRG), and technological platforms (six different molecular platform in TCGA (exome sequencing, copy number analysis, mRNA-miRNA-methylation analysis), versus only mRNA expression and targeted gene sequencing in ACRG).

Although their limitations these two classifications represent today the most important groundwork for the development of targeted therapies inspired to a concept of "biologically-guided tumor treatment", as well as patients stratification for clinical trials and improved prognostication.

5. Clinical Implications of Molecular Classifications

How can we use this enormous amount of information for a clinical application? Unfortunately, neither the TCGA nor AACR classifications can be currently used for patients' stratification and selection, as for many of the identified mutated genes the functional relevance of mutation is not known and, more importantly, they are not yet druggable.

In this section, we individually consider the most relevant molecular targets that are identified in gastric cancer and we discuss their potential therapeutic implications (Table 1).

Table 1. Major target-oriented phase II/III trials in gastric and esophagogastric adenocarcinomas.

Trial	Phase	Setting	Target	Arms	N Patients	Primary Endpoint	Result
ToGA	III	1st line	HER2+	CF/CX ± Trastuzumab	594	OS	Positive
JACOB	III	1st line	HER2+	CF/CX+ Trastuzumab ± Pertuzumab	780	OS	Negative
GATSBY	II/III	2nd line	HER2+	Taxanes ± TDM-1	345	OS	Negative
LOGIC	III	1st line	HER2+	CapeOX ± Lapatinib	545	OS	Negative
TyTAN	III	2nd line	HER2+	Paclitaxel ± Lapatinib	261	OS	Negative
EXPAND	III	1st line	EGFR (unselected)	CX ± Cetuximab	894	PFS	Negative
REAL-3	III	1st line	EGFR (unselected)	EOC ± Panitumumab	553	OS	Negative
METGastric	III	1st line	MET+	Folfox ± Onartuzumab	562	OS	Negative
RILOMET-1	III	1st line	MET+	ECX ± Rilotumumab	609	OS	Negative
SHINE	II	2nd line	FGFGR2+	Paclitaxel ± AZD4546	71	PFS	Negative
FAST	IIb	1st line	CLDN18.2+	EOX ± Claudiximab	161	PFS	Positive
AVAGAST	III	1st line	VEGF	CX ± Bevacizumab	774	OS	Negative
AVATAR	III	1st line	VEGF	CX ± Bevacizumab	202	OS	Negative
REGARD	III	2nd line	VEGFR2	Ramucirumab vs. Placebo	355	OS	Positive
RAINBOW	III	2nd line	VEGFR2	Paclitaxel ± Ramucirumab	665	OS	Positive

5.1. HER2

HER2 (Human Epidermal Growth Factor Receptor II) or ERBB2 (Avian erythroblastosis oncogene B), encoded at chromosome 17q21, is a well-defined tyrosine kinase receptor often acting as proto-oncogene in many human cancers. Oncogenic mechanisms that hit HER2 are represented by gene amplification (determining protein over-expression) or less commonly activating mutations.

HER2 lacks of a known exogenous ligand and it is transactivated by the interaction with other HER family members (EGFR or HER3 overall) or other tyrosine kinase receptors. Its activation leads to a complex cascade of transduction events within the cytoplasm, that converge on two fundamental signaling pathways: the RAS-MAP (mitogen activated protein) kinase pathway and the PI3K-AKT pathway, both determining cell survival, proliferation and migration.

In GC HER2 overexpression is mainly due to gene amplification: it occurs more frequently in proximal tumors (more than 30% of cases), than in distal cancers (less than 20%), mainly arising from the gastric body. Furthermore, Lauren intestinal subtype shows a higher expression of HER2 (up to 34%) than diffuse subtype (6%), while, concerning to TCGA classification, CIN tumors more often express HER2 as consequence of gene amplification (as mentioned above).

Different strategies to target HER2 were developed over the years: monoclonal antibodies (like trastuzumab) that bind to the extracellular domain of the receptor, determining receptor down-regulation or antibody-dependent-cytotoxicity (ADCC), and TKIs (tyrosine kinase inhibitors), that inhibit signaling cascade through the blockade of receptor kinase activity.

The pivotal phase III ToGA (Trastuzumab for Gastric cancer) trial [27] showed that, in HER2 positive GCs, the addition of trastuzumab to standard platinum-based first line treatment was effective, with a median overall survival (mOS) of about 13.8 months in the experimental arm versus 11.1 in the standard one (HR: 0.74; $p = 0.0046$). This OS still represents the highest ever reached in a phase III trial recruiting GC patients. The greatest benefit was observed in high HER2 expressing patients (IHC3+ or IHC2+/FISH+), with a mOS of 16 months versus 11.8 in low HER2 expressing patients (IHC0-1+/FISH+). Therefore, this trial led to the approval of trastuzumab in HER2 positive GC, in the first line setting for patients with IHC3+ or IHC2+/FISH+.

Based on the extraordinary results of the Cleopatra Trial in HER2 positive breast cancer [28], it has been speculated that also in GC the addition of pertuzumab (another monoclonal antibody targeting a different HER2 domain than trastuzumab) to trastuzumab itself and platinum-based chemotherapy could improve the ToGA survival rates, leading to JACOB Trial design. Unfortunately, this study was almost negative [29] because the mOS was 17.5 months in experimental arm versus 14.2 in the standard (HR: 0.84; $p = 0.0565$), a difference that did not find statistical significance.

Trastuzumab-emtansine (TDM-1) is an antibody-drug conjugate that is widely used in second line setting for metastatic HER2 positive breast cancer [30]. This drug was also studied in second line therapy of HER2 positive GC (previously treated with trastuzumab) within the GATSBY phase III trial [31]: unfortunately, TDM-1 therapy was not superior to standard taxanes (mOS 7.9 months versus 8.6 respectively, HR: 1.15, $p = 0.86$), although with lower incidence of adverse events.

Another strategy to target HER2 consists of the inhibition of kinase activity with small molecules TKIs, like Lapatinib (a multi-kinase inhibitor with a strong activity against EGFR and HER2). This molecule was tested in two randomized phase III trials enrolling GC patients with advanced disease: the LOGIC and TYTAN trials.

The LOGIC trial [32] tested lapatinib in combination with capecitabine plus oxaliplatin versus chemotherapy alone in the first line setting of HER2 positive GC patient. The trial results were negative, because mOS (the study primary endpoint) was 12.2 months in experimental arm versus 10.5 in the standard (HR: 0.91, $p = 0.349$), a statistically not significant difference, although secondary endpoints like ORR or PFS were in favor of Lapatinib arm.

Furthermore, lapatinib has been tested in second line setting within the TYTAN phase III trial [33], in wich 261 previously treated Asian GC patients were enrolled to receive lapatinib plus paclitaxel or paclitaxel alone (to note only 15 patients [6%] had previously received trastuzumab in first line). Once again, the results were negative, with insignificant differences between the two arms for OS and PFS.

Due to the disappointing results of these trials (JACOB, GATSBY, TYTAN, LOGIC), many researchers began to study mechanisms of targeted therapy resistance in GC, when considering that also patients who achieved a significant response to first line trastuzumab-based treatment can develop resistance within a few months [34].

In effect, one main bias of the second-line trials, especially the GATSBY trial, seems to be the absence of tumor rebiopsy (for example at metastatic site) at screening, taking for granted that the tumor was still HER2 positive on the basis of the basal diagnostic biopsy.

An Italian study [35] clearly showed that the acquired resistance mechanism to trastuzumab-based first line treatment could be the loss of HER2 receptor, especially for patients with dubious immunohistochemistry (IHC2+/FISH+), speculating that HER2 negative clones are positively selected by the first line anti-HER2 therapy and could subsequently expand. In that way, the negative results of the GATSBY study could be related to the fact that, in a significant proportion of cases, they have treated with TDM-1 patients who were *de facto* HER2 negative at the beginning of the second line.

Another possible mechanism of acquired resistance to trastuzumab is likely due to co-existing molecular alterations within the HER2 positive tumor clones, as clearly showed by Pietrantonio et al. [36]: mutations of EGFR/MET/KRAS/PIK3CA/PTEN or the amplifications of EGFR/MET/KRAS can co-occur in HER2 positive cells and could explain the lack of trastuzumab efficacy and/or the appearance of resistance.

In any case, to date, no standard anti-HER2 treatment is available in trastuzumab refractory HER2+ patients, and standard chemotherapy with taxanes (mainly the combination of Paclitaxel plus ramucirumab) or irinotecan is recommended.

5.2. EGFR

Epidermal Growth Factor Receptor (EGFR) or ERBB1 is a transmembrane tyrosine kinase receptor, expressed approximately in 30% of GC [37], especially those with chromosomal instability ("CIN" subtype of TCGA). This molecule represents the second most important receptor (after HER2) in GC pathogenesis: its overexpression is associated with poorly differentiated histology, vascular invasion, and potentially shorter survival [38].

Several studies evaluated the safety and efficacy of different anti-EGFR drugs, on the basis of preclinical works [39]: anti-EGFR therapies include—as we just discussed for HER2—monoclonal antibodies (like cetuximab or panitumumab) and TKIs (gefitinib, erlotinib).

Initial phase II trials combining these agents with cytotoxic chemotherapy in unselected patient population identified high response rates for the first line setting (from 41 to 65%) [40,41]. Unfortunately, all of the phase III trials investigating the role of anti-EGFR therapy in GC were negative.

The EXPAND study [42] randomized GC patients in first line setting between cetuximab plus capecitabine-cisplatin versus chemotherapy alone, showing no advantage for cetuximab arm (mPFS 4.4 months versus 5.6 months, *p* = 0.32). The patient recruitment was unselected for EGFR positivity, although in a post-hoc analysis the highest survival benefit was observed in a small subset of patients with high EGFR expression (representing probably EGFR amplified tumors).

The REAL-3 trial [43] demonstrates that adding panitumumab to epirubicin-oxaliplatin-capecitabine was even detrimental, as the mOS for the experimental arm was 8.8 months versus 11.3 months for the standard one (HR: 1.37, *p* = 0.013).

The deep failure of anti-EGFR drugs in gastric cancer can be explained mainly with the lack of a proper patient selection. In fact, a recent work by Catenacci et al. [44] showed that EGF-R amplified tumors (5% in Chicago casuistry), some of which were treated with anti-EGFR drugs, seems very prone to respond to cetuximab or ABT-806 (an investigational anti-EGFR drug), with an ORR of 58%, a DCR of 100%, and a mPFS of about 10 months. Thanks to next generation sequencing (NGS) and circulating tumor DNA (ctDNA) studies, the authors also showed the mechanisms of resistance to anti-EGFR drugs, such as the presence of EGF-R negative tumor clones, KRAS mutation/amplifications, PTEN deletion, and NRAS/HER2/MYC amplifications.

This study definitively demonstrates that EGF-R amplification is able to predict response to anti-EGFR therapies, despite the negative results in prior unselected phase III trials (EXPAND and REAL-III), but also that mechanisms of resistance exist and could be detected by novel technologies, like NGS and ctDNA.

5.3. C-MET

MET (Mesenchymal-Epithelial Transition) oncogene, also called Hepatocyte Growth Factor Receptor (HGF), is a receptor tyrosine kinase that appears to be deregulated in many human cancers [45], such as breast, colorectal, lung, pancreatic, hepatic and—not least—gastric cancer.

Its activation requires binding to HGF (the soluble ligand of MET), the so-called "canonical activation", but can also occur without HGF, through a cross-talk with other receptors (the "non canonical" pathway) [46]. MET signaling in GC is related to worse prognosis [47], because HGF/MET activity is involved in cancer growth, invasion, angiogenesis, and epithelial-to-mesenchymal transition.

The main known mechanism of MET overexpression in GC is gene amplification, which occurs in about 6% of the TCGA dataset (especially in CIN tumors). However, even tumors without gene amplification can express (or overexpress) MET, although it is not clear whether these tumors really depend on MET for survival and malignant properties.

Two monoclonal antibodies, Rilotumumab (an anti-HGF antibody) and Onartuzumab (an anti-MET antibody) were tested in clinical trials in GC: early reports [48,49] suggested that MET expression could serve as a predictive biomarker for anti-MET directed therapies, but in both phase III clinical trials evaluating Onartuzumab and Rilotumumab, the results were negative.

The METGastric phase III trial [50] evaluated the addition of onartuzumab to a chemotherapy backbone (mFOLFOX6), and enrolled 562 GC patients with HER2 negative/MET positive tumors (defined as score 1+, 2+, and 3+ by immunohistochemistry). The enrollment was stopped early due to sponsor decision, for a lack of efficacy in a phase II trial also assessing contemporary the role of onartuzumab in MET positive GC [51]. Unluckily, the addition of onartuzumab to mFOLFOX6 did not result in an improvement of OS (11 months in the experimental arm versus 11.3 in standard, HR: 0.82, $p = 0.24$) and PFS (6.7 versus 6.8 months, respectively, HR: 0.90, $p = 0.43$).

Negative results were obtained also with rilotumumab within the RILOMET-1 phase III trial [52], which used a different chemotherapy backbone (Epirubicin plus Cisplatin and Capecitabine). In that case, not only results were clearly negative with a detrimental effect (mOS was 8.8 in experimental arm versus 10.7 in the placebo group, HR: 1.34, $p = 0.003$), but study treatment was also stopped early, because an independent data monitoring found a higher number of deaths in the rilotumumab group than the placebo group.

There is a great discordance between the phase II rilotumumab study [48] and the RILOMET-1 results, because the MET+ patients treated with rilotumumab within the phase II ($n = 41$) had a mOS of 10.6 months when compared with 5.7 months of patients receiving placebo. Noteworthy, despite the cutoff to define MET positivity with immunohistochemistry was the same between phase II and III (expression ≥1+ in ≥25% of tumor cells), there was a relevant difference in the number of patients screened who were considered MET positive in phase II (64%) and phase III (81%) trial, for not known reasons.

Probably the main limit of RILOMET and METGastric trials is to have included mostly patients in whom MET was not a clear "driver" of the disease, since the highest expressing tumors (MET gene amplification) are under-represented, which can explain the negative results.

5.4. FGF

FGFR2 belongs to FGFR receptor family, which includes four different receptors and almost 23 different ligands, making it an extraordinary complex system [53]. The ligand-receptor interaction leads to initiation of a signaling cascade that lead, as for the majority of RTKs, to MAPK and PI3K-AKT pathways activation.

In GC, the first evidence of FGFR2 amplification has been described in 1990 [54], analyzing KATO III cell line. Moreover in the TCGA dataset almost 9% of patients within the CIN subtype presented FGFR2 gene amplification, which convinced researchers to test the FGFR inhibitors in FGFR2 amplified GC.

One molecule tested is AZD4547, a selective FGFR1,2,3 TKI with powerful preclinical activity in FGFR2 amplified GCs [55]. This drug was evaluated in the SHINE trial [56], in which GC patients displaying FGFR2 amplification or polysomy were randomized in second line setting between AZD4547 or paclitaxel. Trial results were negative, with a median PFS of 1.8 months in experimental arm versus 3.5 in the chemotherapy one. These very disappointing results have been mainly due to great intratumor heterogeneity for FGFR2 amplification—the FGFR2 status evaluated on archival tumor tissue may not reflect the molecular status of metastatic tumor at study screening—and to poor concordance between gene amplification and receptor expression. Therefore, an alternative predictive biomarker testing for FGFR2 is urgently needed, when considering that FGFR2-amplified tumors with FGFR2 overexpression, although at very low prevalence, exist and should be appropriately treated.

5.5. CLAUDIN18.2

Claudins are a well-known family of proteins that shape the fundamental part of tight cell junctions [57]. Within the normal gastric mucosa the isoform 2 of the Claudin18 (claudin 18.2 or CLDN18.2) is highly expressed, especially in differentiated epithelial cells, while it is quite absent in the gastric stem cell zone.

Claudin18.2 is retained in malignant transformation and is expressed in a significant proportion in primary tumors and their metastasis [58]. This molecule seems to be a good target especially in TCGA "GS" tumors that in a significant proportion (15% of cases) show a chromosomal translocation involving CLDN18 and ARHGAP.

In a phase IIb study (the FAST trial) [59], the role of Claudiximab (a chimeric monoclonal antibody against CLDN18.2 also known as Zolbetuximab-IMAB362) has been evaluated in combination with chemotherapy (epirubicin, oxaliplatin, and capecitabine [EOX]) versus chemotherapy alone in the first line setting (n = 161). This trial met its primary endpoint, because claudiximab significantly improved mPFS (7.9 months versus 4.8, HR: 0.47, p = 0.0001) and mOS (13.3 months versus 8.4, HR: 0.51, p < 0.001) as compared to EOX alone. A more pronounced benefit was observed in patients with very high CLDN18.2 expression ($\geq$2+ intensity in $\geq$70% of tumor cells), making this combination a very appealing strategy for HER2 negative GC.

A notable point in the FAST study is that the outcomes in the EOX only arm were not similar to the corresponding landmark trial REAL 2 study (OS of 11.2 (REAL 2) vs. 8.7 (FAST), which could be due to patient selection.

Other trials are under development for CLDN18.2 positive gastric cancers such as the phase II trial with Zolbetuximab (NCT03505320—"ILUSTRO" trial) and a phase III trial with claudiximab is scheduled and expected.

Overall, the major limitation seems be the availability of the testing for CLDN18.2 and the finding of the ideal cut-off point for the CLDN18.2 levels, with the suggestion of studies comparing outcomes between low CLDN18.2 levels versus higher levels. The anti-claudin research is one of the best examples of how targeted therapy is clearly the future also of gastric cancer treatments.

5.6. VEGF/VEGFR

In the TCGA "CIN" subtype, vascular endothelial growth factor (VEGF), a crucial mediator of normal and pathogenic angiogenesis, is frequently amplified up to 7% of cases. Although initial studies with bevacizumab (a monoclonal antibody targeting VEGF-A) were negative, such as the AVAGAST trial [60] and the Asiatic AVATAR trial [61], in which bevacizumab was combined with platinum-based chemotherapy in first line setting, other antiangiogenic strategies continued to be investigated.

Ramucirumab, a fully human monoclonal antibody directed against VEGFR2 (Vascular endothelial growth factor receptor 2), which is the main receptor of the VEGF system implicated in oncogenic angiogenesis, has been used in the second line setting alone [62] or in combination with weekly paclitaxel [63].

Both studies were positive, with the REGARD trial showing a significant improvement in OS with ramucirumab alone versus BSC (mOS 5.2 months versus 3.8, respectively, HR: 0.776, $p = 0.047$) and the RAINBOW trial showing a significant superiority of combination arm (ramucirumab plus paclitaxel) versus paclitaxel alone (mOS 9.63 months versus 7.36 months, respectively, HR: 0.807, $p = 0.017$).

On that positive basis, ramucirumab has been tested in first line setting in combination with cisplatin-based standard chemotherapy within the RAINFALL trial [64]: although the study formally met its primary endpoint, with an improvement in mPFS from 5.4 months (placebo arm) to 5.7 months (ramucirumab arm) (HR: 0.75, $p = 0.011$), there was no survival benefit for patients treated with RAM + Capecitabin/Cisplatin versus placebo + Capecitabin/Cisplatin (mOS 11.2 months versus 10.7 months, HR: 0.96, $p = 0.68$), making the results negative *de facto* and not significant for clinical practice.

Therefore, the role of antiangiogenic agents seems to be essential in second line setting, but in the first line, like the AVAGAST and AVATAR trial, showed for bevacizumab, probably we need to better understand who are the patients that really benefit from this strategy.

5.7. PI3K Pathway

The PI3K/AKT/mTOR pathway is a fundamental promoter of cell growth, metabolism, survival, and cell migration: it is mainly activated by cell surface tyrosine kinase receptors, but in human cancer, many component of this pathway could be affected by activating mutation (PIK3CA) or inactivating genetic events (PTEN), like gene deletion.

Approximately, 80% of PIK3CA mutations occur at three recurrent hotspots: E545K and E542K in the exon 9, and H1047R in the exon 20 [65].

In gastric adenocarcinomas, PIK3CA is one of the most frequent mutated genes especially in EBV-related GC (almost 80% of cases are mutated) and "MSI" subtype (42% of cases), as shown by TCGA, making this molecule an appealing target to pharmacological inhibition.

One of the first study evaluating the block of PI3K-AKT-mTOR pathway in GC is the GRANITE-1 Trial [66], a phase III study in which 656 GC patients who progressed after previous one or two lines of systemic chemotherapy were randomized between everolimus (a mTOR inhibitor) or placebo. Results were almost negative, because the mOS (primary endpoint of the study) resulted 5.4 months with everolimus versus 4.3 with placebo (HR: 0.90, $p = 0.124$) and mPFS was 1.7 months versus 1.4, respectively (HR: 0.66, $p < 0.001$). The modest (and statistically significant) improvement in PFS suggested a potential benefit in selected patients: for example, PIK3CA/PTEN mutations could be predictive of mTOR inhibition, as suggested by Meric-Bernstam et al. [67].

Other studies with drugs that inhibit directly PI3K or AKT are in early phase clinical trials and to date no data are available.

6. Gastric Cancer in the Immunotherapy Era: A Hope for the Future

Immunotherapy deeply changed the therapeutic landscape for several malignancies (advanced melanoma, lung, urothelial, kidney cancer, etc.) determining a global outcome improvement completely unexpected until a few years ago by boosting the body's natural defenses to fight cancer [68]. Gastric cancer is still late when compared to these others cancer types, even if some relevant results have been lately scored leading to a more confident vision for the future [69].

As already reported comprehensive molecular characterization performed by the TGCA group showed a relatively high mutational load (up to 10–15 mutations per megabase) in about 34% of gastric adenocarcinomas analyzed and a subset of tumors with microsatellite instability-high (MSI-H, 22%) or with an ideally favorable immune-environment (the "EBV-related" subgroup that shows molecular hallmarks of sensitivity to immunotherapy, such as intra- or peritumoral immune cell infiltration and

PD-L-1/PD-L-2 expression), suggesting that also gastric cancer could be a promising "fertile soil" for immunotherapy, especially based on immune checkpoint inhibitors.

These checkpoints play critical roles for physiological homeostasis and for balanced immune responses and they are heavily involved in the immune escape mechanisms of GC as well.

Also, other previous preclinical evidence supports the idea that immunotherapy can be a successful anti-GC strategy, particularly regarding the T cell-based treatment protocols: cytotoxic T lymphocytes (CTL) and tumor infiltrating lymphocytes (TIL) [70,71].

Induced CTL cell culture technology (using specific peptides) led to the clinical tests based on adoptive transfer of CTLs in patients. The induced CTLs showed specific activity against tumor cells in vitro and against primary cell culture isolated from GC patients, suggesting that this strategy could be a kind of "vaccine" and adoptive immunogenic therapy as already preliminarily demonstrated in melanoma patients (up to 40% of antitumor immune responses in phase 2 trial) [72]. As a matter of fact CTLs from GC patients are able to identify specific tumor-associated antigens and to attack the autologous neoplastic cells triggering the immune responses against gastric cancer [73].

Furthermore, Kim et al. [74] also demonstrated the anti-gastric cancer activity of cytokine-induced killer cells (CIK) that are mainly T CD80+ cells isolated from human peripheral blood mononuclear cells cultured with IL-2 and anti-CD3 antibody. The CIK cells were capable of destroying human gastric cancer cells in vitro and to inhibit tumor growth in mouse model, indicating a potential role of CIK cells as adoptive immunotherapy for GC as well.

The transfer therapy with TILs requires first of all the T cell isolation from neoplastic tissue, then the in vitro expansion and finally the selection of tumor-specific T cells. The application of these protocols in GC patients is more difficult compared to melanoma because of an hardest surgical availability of adequate tumor tissue (only 30–40% of biopsies usually acceptable for the procedure) but this strategy seems particularly promising, as shown by the positive correlation between the presence of TILs and survival in ovarian, colorectal and pancreatic cancer [75–77] and it should be still encouraged and enforced. It is important to underline that in some cases TILs can even promote cancer development depending on the functional features of lymphocytic infiltrate [78]. These techniques and others (such as dendritic cell-based vaccination [79]) need to be deepened and optimized also for gastric cancer and they appear as a complex universe yet to be entirely discovered.

With regards to checkpoint inhibitors, we can find the strongest evidence that is currently available to support the approval for use of immunotherapy in GC with first promising results.

The KEYNOTE-012 trial [80] demonstrated in an early-phase the potential application of anti-PD1 therapy with pembrolizumab (humanized IgG4-k monoclonal anybody selective to bind PD1, currently approved by FDA in the US) in 39 patients that were affected by PD-L1 positive refractory advanced gastric cancer with promising overall response (22%, 95% CI 10–39). In the single arm phase 2 trial KEYNOTE-059 [81] this activity has been confirmed in an unselected population of patients with metastatic GC (cohort 1, n = 259) previously treated with two or more systemic lines of therapy. Objective response rate (ORR) was 11.6% but it reached 15.5% in patients who were PD-L1 positive (57.1% of all, cut-off of PD-L1 ≥1%) versus 6.4% in PD-L1 negative. The outcomes were significantly better when treatment were used in an early setting (third line ORR = 16.4% versus 6.4% in the fourth line), supporting the rationale to use immunotherapy as soon as possible in the natural history of the disease when the immune response is not compromised, and when population has been stratified according to MSI status (ORR = 57.1% in MSI-H; ORR = 9.0% in MSS), although only seven patients (4%) resulted with a microsatellite instability-high status. With a median OS of 5.6 months (secondary endpoint) a promising survival rate of 23.4% at 12 months has been described.

These results suggest the need for an accurate selection of patients in order to maximize the outcome of immunotherapy and to identify the subset of patients who respond favorably.

For this purpose, Kim et al. [82] designed an open label phase 2 trial with integrated genomic analysis of all baseline tumor tissue samples and genomic profiling of circulating tumor DNA (ctDNA) in order to classify the disease characteristics of responders and non-responders to immunotherapy.

61 Asian patients with metastatic or recurrent gastric cancer refractory to standard chemotherapy were enrolled and treated with Pembrolizumab, the population included six EBV-positive diseases and seven MSI-H. An ORR of 24.6% was observed but EBV-positive and MSI-H patients obtained dramatic responses to pembrolizumab (ORR, respectively, of 85.7% and 100%), furthermore activity was significantly higher in PDL-1 positive cancer (cut-off $\geq$ 1) when compared to PDL-1 negative (ORR of 50.0% versus 0.0%, $p \leq 0.001$). In addition, other cancer subtypes such as genome stable, CIN and mesenchymal (defined by positive EMT signature) demonstrated poor responses to pembrolizumab, and particularly, the EMT subtype has been demonstrated to be a negative predictor of response to immunotherapy determining a poor survival.

Investigators additionally demonstrated a strong correlation between ctDNA mutational load and tumor mutational burden (TMB) and that decreasing ctDNA levels during the treatment are a powerful predictor of prolonged PFS and good response, opening the way to the use of ctDNA to identify patients that are likely to respond to pembrolizumab.

It is important also to outline that Pembrolizumab did not improve survival as second line treatment for PDL-1 positive advanced GCs according to findings from phase 3 KEYNOTE-061 trial recently published [83], even if the approved FDA indication for patients who have received at least two previous lines of treatment remains unchanged at current time. These negative findings added interpretative complexity to the knowledge about immunotherapy in GC.

Another anti-PD-1 drug that was successfully tested in the treatment of GC has been Nivolumab (fully human IgG4 monoclonal antibody). In the large randomized Asian phase 3 trial ATTRACTION-2 [84] Nivolumab showed a significant survival benefit in heavily pretreated patients ($\geq$2 previous lines of treatment) with advanced gastric or gastro-esophageal junction cancer reaching an overall survival of 5.26 months as compared to 4.14 months in the placebo group (HR: 0.63–95% CI 0.51–0.78; $p < 0.0001$) and with an ORR of 11.2% (0% in the placebo arm). Interestingly remarkable survival rates were described at 12 months (26.2%) and at 18 months (16.2%) in the immunotherapy group, when considering the advanced setting of treatment. We could infer that there is a definite subset of patients that strongly benefits from the treatment and has durable responses.

A potential limit of this trial could be considered the lacking of molecular analysis and patients selection (the cohort was unselected according to PDL-1 status and tumor tissue samples was not mandatory at the screening). For the 26 patients for whom PDL-1 positivity assessment was available (cut-off $\geq$1%) OS did not change when compared to the overall unselected population (5.22 months in the Nivolumab group) and the activity of immunotherapy in PDL-1 negative patients was fully superimposable with an OS of 6.05 months in the Nivolumab arm. At the moment no further data are available about other biomarkers (i.e., MSI status) but it is absolutely noteworthy that this is the first positive randomized phase 3 study of an immune checkpoint inhibitor in patients with advanced gastric cancer.

Anyhow ATTRACTION-2 is a fully Asian trial and a possible debate could arise about whether its data could be transferred or not to the western population. GC patients from Asia and from western countries are known to have different clinical outcomes [85,86], these differences have been conventionally attributed to different clinical management and disease stage. Instead, recent evidences suggest that gene expression differences exist among Asian and non-Asian gastric adenocarcinomas and different molecular signatures influence clinical outcome, especially concerning tumor immunity [87].

However, we should consider that Pembrolizumab has been successfully used also in the western population (KEYNOTE-059) and even Nivolumab has been tested in a non-Asian population. As a matter of fact in the gastric cohort of phase 1/2 trial CheckMate-032 [88] a favorable and promising activity of Nivolumab +/− Ipilimumab (a fully human monoclonal IgG1-k against CTL antigen 4) has been described in a fully Western population (160 heavily pretreated patients). Even in the Nivolumab single agent arm (quite similar to Attraction-2 experimental arm), ORR was 12% in the unselected population and 19% in PDL-1 positive patients, although outcomes have been worse than in the combination arms, and a survival rate of 39% has been observed at one year.

Tan et al. [89] published a large retrospective investigation of more than 1600 gastric cancers from six Asian and three non-Asian cohorts demonstrating that tumor immunity signatures differ significantly between Asian and non-Asian cancers. These different tumor immunity signatures, especially related to T cell function, might explain the geographical differences in clinical outcome always observed and might condition different responses to immunotherapy.

In particular Non-Asian gastric cancer seemed to be associated with enrichment of tumor infiltrating T-cells as well as T-cell gene expression signatures, including CTLA-4 signaling, while Asian gastric cancers had a significantly higher numbers of cells positive for neutrophil markers.

Asian and Caucasian GCs had distinct immune-related components, intratumoral immune, and inflammation cells populations.

Investigators also analyzed whether these differences might be due to different EBV and MRR status, both conditions notoriously related to high load of infiltrating lymphocytes [90], but no significantly differences have been demonstrated between the two cohorts.

Due to the retrospective nature of this study, results need to be further validated but we should consider that western population seems to have an "immune-environment" more favorable to immunotherapy and a stronger immune-signature, even if, as already reported, the biggest immune-oncology phase 3 trial currently available (ATTRACTION-2) has been conducted only on a entirely Asian population.

Results of ongoing immune-oncology trials [91,92] on western populations are hopefully awaited, but the design of future gastric cancer trials should consider an accurate patient selection and tumor immunity differences in patients from different geographic regions.

7. Conclusions

Clinical application of new advances and recent molecular classifications is still disappointing. Tumor heterogeneity and the still imperfect understanding of the complex tumor biology represent a brake to the definitive overcoming of the "one size fit-all" era also for gastric cancer.

With the exception of first accelerated anti-PD-1 drugs approval, at current time, as mentioned above, only two target therapies have been approved and are currently used as a standard of care: Trastuzumab and Ramucirumab.

When compared to the big amount of molecular drivers identified and tested for GC, these advances represent still a small step to that more contemporary and comprehensive clinical approach, called "precision medicine", to which genomic heterogeneity is a stubborn barrier.

New treatments are urgently needed in order to give patients more benefits from new drugs and new technologies available. What molecular classifications can already teach us is that in the next future it will not be possible to give patients a same treatment in an unselective manner and that a more rigorous selection of patients will be mandatory.

For example evidence clearly identified two subgroups of GC, as characterized by MSI-H and EBV-positive status, which may benefit from immunotherapy and for whom front-line anti-PD1 drugs could be pursued, in addition to other hallmarks (PD1 status, TMB) that will drive therapeutic approaches and future research.

On the other side it is also possible to identify another subset of GCs (GS, MMT/EMT) poorly responsive to immunotherapy and in which for example the development of inhibitors of cMET pathway, Rho-kinase, PI3K/mTOR pathway should be encouraged as demonstrated by the anti-claudin line of research, which seems particularly promising in the selected population.

Another challenge is represented by the development of predictive biomarkers of response also using the ctDNA technology, a procedure that will need to be validated and studied in deep but that could help identifying patients with a high risk for progressive disease early and their possible resistance mechanisms.

Int. J. Mol. Sci. **2018**, *19*, 2659

The analysis of ctDNA might also help detecting genomic alterations not detected in primary tumors at baseline, considered the evidence of a possible significant discrepancy within a same primary tumor and between primary tumors and metastatic sites genomic alterations, a discrepancy potentially determining the targeted therapies failure [93].

As already tested in other cancer types [94], also the use of patient-derived xenograft (PDX) models could help in the search of these predictors. Analyzing non-responder PDXs, for example, we could identify those mechanisms that determine resistance to the tested therapy facilitating the ideation of dedicated prospective trials. As a matter of fact gastric PDX platforms are already available and first studies have been conducted [55,95].

A complementary interesting possibility could be represented by the use of "tumor organoids" [96] utilized as an alternative model for the research in order to verify ex vivo the sensitivity of tumor cells to targeted therapies. Furthermore PDXs and organoids can help in understanding why in different tumor contexts effective targeted agents are poorly active in different cancer types (i.e., anti-HER2 therapy in colorectal and gastric cancer).

GC is a collection of different molecular entities and its landscape is enormously complex, but recent efforts and knowledge laid the foundations for the development of more modern and solid therapeutic approaches and clinical trials, also taking advantage of new preclinical models to revalue promising drugs that failed in the past years.

Molecular classifications, especially TGCA and ACRG, opened the doors wide on the complete comprehension of the complex genetic landscape of gastric cancer and on the way to the full application of precision medicine also for this malignancy, even if at current time they still appear as separated and isolated systems, while a standardization and a "common strategy" approach would be desirable.

The biggest challenge for the next future will be to understand which cancer subgroup deserves a specific targeted agent and to design clinical trials tailored on these subgroups, in order to transfer the molecular classifications acquisitions into the clinical practice and to minimize the numbers of patients who receive a systemic treatment without any molecular selection.

Author Contributions: F.D.V. designed the general outline and the aims of the paper providing expert opinion on the topics and supervising the writing of the paper; G.T. and L.P. wrote the main paragraphs and contributed to the general outline, the original draft preparation and the literature review; A.P. (Angelica Petrillo), M.M.L., A.P. (Annalisa Pappalardo) and M.C. did the literature review and contributed to the writing of specific paragraphs and to the first revision; M.O., F.C. and G.G. provided specific expert opinion and critically contributed to the final review and the supervision.

Funding: This paper received no external funding or grants.

Conflicts of Interest: The authors declare no conflicts of interest.

References

1. Smyth, E.C.; Verheij, M.; Allum, W.; Cunningham, D.; Cervantes, A.; Arnold, A. Gastric cancer: ESMO Clinical Practice Guidelines for diagnosis, treatment and follow-up. *Ann. Oncol.* **2016**, *27*, v38–v49. [CrossRef] [PubMed]
2. Waddell, T.; Verheij, M.; Allum, W.; Cunningham, D.; Cervantes, A.; Arnold, D. Gastric cancer: ESMO-ESSO-ESTRO clinical practice guidelines for diagnosis, treatment and follow-up. *Eur. J. Surg. Oncol.* **2014**, *40*, 584–591. [CrossRef] [PubMed]
3. Ferlay, J.; Soerjomataram, I.; Dikshit, R.; Eser, S.; Mathers, C.; Rebelo, M.; Parkin, D.M.; Forman, D.; Bray, F. Cancer incidence and mortality worldwide: Sources, methods and major patterns in GLOBOCAN2012. *Int. J. Cancer* **2015**, *136*, E359–E386. [CrossRef] [PubMed]
4. Siegel, R.L.; Miller, K.D.; Jemal, A. Cancer statistics. *CA Cancer J. Clin.* **2018**, *68*, 7–30. [CrossRef] [PubMed]
5. Lauren, P. The two histological main types of gastric carcinoma: Diffuse and so-called intestinal-type carcinoma. An attempt at a histo-clinical classification. *Acta Pathol. Microbiol. Scand.* **1965**, *64*, 31–49. [CrossRef] [PubMed]

6. Bosman, F.T.; Carneiro, F.; Hruban, R.H.; Theise, N.D. *WHO Classification of Tumours of the Digestive System*, 4th ed.; WHO Classification of Tumours; Agency for Research on Cancer: Lyon, France, 2010; Volume 3, ISBN1 13-9789283224327. ISBN2 10-9283224329.
7. Tay, S.T.; Leong, S.H.; Yu, K.; Aggarwal, A.; Tan, S.Y.; Lee, C.H.; Wong, K.; Visvanathan, J.; Lim, D.; Wong, W.K.; et al. A Combined Comparative Genomic Hybridization and Expression Microarray Analysis of Gastric Cancer Reveals Novel Molecular Subtypes. *Cancer Res.* **2003**, *63*, 3309–3316. [PubMed]
8. Tan, I.B.; Ivanova, T.; Lim, K.H.; Ong, C.W.; Deng, N.; Lee, J.; Tan, S.H.; Wu, J.; Lee, M.H.; Ooi, C.H.; et al. Intrinsic subtypes of gastric cancer, based on gene expression pattern, predict survival and respond differently to chemotherapy. *Gastroenterology* **2011**, *141*, 476–485. [CrossRef] [PubMed]
9. Yong, W.-P.; Rha, S.Y.; Tan, I.B.; Choo, S.-P.; Syn, N.; Koh, V.; Tan, S.H.; So, J.; Shabbir, A.; Tan, C.S.; et al. Microarray-based tumor molecular profiling to direct choice of cisplatin plus S-1 or oxaliplatin plus S-1 for advanced gastric cancer: A multicentre, prospective, proof-of-concept phase 2 trial. *J. Clin. Oncol.* **2017**, *35*, 48. [CrossRef]
10. Yong, W.P.; Rha, S.Y.; Tan, I.B.; Choo, S.P.; Syn, N.L.; Koh, V.; Tan, S.H.; Asuncion, B.R.; Sundar, R.; So, J.B.Y.; et al. Real-time Tumor Gene Expression Profiling to Direct Gastric Cancer Chemotherapy: Proof-of-Concept '3G' Trial. *Clin. Cancer Res.* **2018**. [CrossRef] [PubMed]
11. Shah, M.A.; Khanin, R.; Tang, L.; Janjigian, Y.Y.; Klimstra, D.S.; Gerdes, H.; Kelsen, D.P. Molecular classification of gastric cancer: A new paradigm. *Clin. Cancer Res.* **2011**, *17*, 2693–2701. [CrossRef] [PubMed]
12. Crew, K.D.; Neugut, A.I. Epidemiology of Gastric cancer. *World J. Gastroenterol.* **2006**, *12*, 354–362. [CrossRef] [PubMed]
13. Tanner, M.; Hollmén, M.; Junttila, T.T.; Kapanen, A.I.; Tommola, S.; Soini, Y.; Helin, H.; Salo, J.; Joensuu, H.; Sihvo, E.; et al. Amplification of HER-2 in gastric carcinoma: Association with Topoisomerase II alpha gene amplification, intestinal type, poor prognosis and sensitivity to trastuzumab. *Ann. Oncol.* **2005**, *16*, 273–278. [CrossRef] [PubMed]
14. Gravalos, C.; Márquez, A.; García-Carbonero, R.; Rivera, F.; Colomer, R.; Sastre, J. Correlation between Her2/NEU Overexpression/Amplification and Clinicopathological Parameters in Advanced Gastric Cancer Patients: A Prospective Study 2007. Presented at: Gastrointestinal Cancers Symposium 130. Abstract 89. Available online: http://www.asco.org/ASCOv2/Meetings/Abstracts?&vmview=abst_detail_view&confID=45&abstractID=10315 (accessed on 20 June 2006).
15. Chen, Y.; Guo, S.Y.; Guo, W. The association between EGFR expression and clinical pathology characteristics in gastric cancer. *Open Life Sci.* **2016**, *11*, 318–321. [CrossRef]
16. Janjigian, Y.Y.; Tang, L.H.; Coit, D.G.; Kelsen, D.P.; Francone, T.D.; Weiser, M.R.; Jhanwar, S.C.; Shah, M.A. MET expression and amplification in patients with localized gastric cancer. *Cancer Epidemiol. Biomark. Prev.* **2011**, *20*, 1021–1027. [CrossRef] [PubMed]
17. Takahashi, Y.; Cleary, K.R.; Mai, M.; Kitadai, Y.; Bucana, C.D.; Ellis, L.M. Significance of vessel count and vascular endothelial growth factor and its receptor (KDR) in intestinal-type gastric cancer. *Clin. Cancer Res.* **1996**, *2*, 1679–1684. [PubMed]
18. Yashiro, M.; Matsuoka, T. Fibroblast growth factor receptor signaling as therapeutic targets in gastric cancer. *World J. Gastroenterol.* **2016**, *22*, 2415–2423. [CrossRef] [PubMed]
19. Feng, W.; Brown, R.E.; Trung, C.D.; Li, W.; Wang, L.; Khoury, T.; Alrawi, S.; Yao, J.; Xia, K.; Tan, D. Morphoproteomic profile of mTOR, Ras/Raf kinase/ERK, and NF-kappaB pathways in human gastric adenocarcinoma. *Ann. Clin. Lab. Sci.* **2008**, *38*, 195–209. [PubMed]
20. Zhang, X.L.; Yang, Y.S.; Xu, D.P.; Qu, J.H.; Guo, M.Z.; Gong, Y.; Huang, J. Comparative study on overexpression of, HER2/NEU and HER3 in gastric cancer. *World J. Surg.* **2009**, *33*, 2112–2118. [CrossRef] [PubMed]
21. Kitoh, T.; Yanai, H.; Saitoh, Y.; Nakamura, Y.; Matsubara, Y.; Kitoh, H.; Yoshida, T.; Okita, K. Increased expression of matrix metalloproteinase-7 in invasive early gastric cancer. *J. Gastroenterol.* **2004**, *39*, 434–440. [CrossRef] [PubMed]
22. Lei, Z.; Tan, I.B.; Das, K.; Deng, N.; Zouridis, H.; Pattison, S.; Chua, C.; Feng, Z.; Guan, Y.K.; Ooi, C.H.; et al. Identification of molecular subtypes of gastric cancer with different responses to PI3-kinase inhibitors and 5-fluorouracil. *Gastroenterology* **2013**, *145*, 554–565. [CrossRef] [PubMed]

23. Wang, K.; Yuen, S.T.; Xu, J.; Lee, S.P.; Yan, H.H.; Shi, S.T.; Siu, H.C.; Deng, S.; Chu, K.M.; Leung, S.Y.; et al. Whole-genome sequencing and comprehensive molecular profiling identify new driver mutations in gastric cancer. *Nat. Genet.* **2014**, *46*, 573–582. [CrossRef] [PubMed]

24. Bass, A.J.; Thorsson, V.; Shmulevich, I.; Reynolds, S.M.; Miller, M.; Bernard, B.; Cancer Genome Atlas Research Network. Comprehensive molecular characterization of gastric adenocarcinoma. *Nature* **2014**, *513*, 202–209. [CrossRef] [PubMed]

25. Sohn, B.H.; Hwang, J.E.; Jang, H.J.; Lee, H.S.; Oh, S.C.; Shim, J.J.; Lee, K.W.; Kim, E.H.; Yim, S.Y.; Lee, S.H.; et al. Clinical Significance of Four Molecular Subtypes of Gastric Cancer Identified by the Cancer Genome Atlas Project. *Clin. Cancer Res.* **2017**, *26*. [CrossRef] [PubMed]

26. Cristescu, R.; Lee, J.; Nebozhyn, M.; Kim, K.M.; Ting, J.C.; Wong, S.S.; Liu, J.; Yue, Y.G.; Wang, J.; Yu, K.; et al. Molecular analysis of gastric cancer identifies subtypes associated with distinct clinical outcomes. *Nat. Med.* **2015**, *21*, 449–456. [CrossRef] [PubMed]

27. Bang, Y.J.; Van Cutsem, E.; Feyereislova, A.; Chung, H.C.; Shen, L.; Sawaki, A.; Lordick, F.; Ohtsu, A.; Omuro, Y.; Satoh, T.; et al. ToGA Trial Investigators. Trastuzumab in combination with chemotherapy versus chemotherapy alone for treatment of HER2-positive advanced gastric or gastro-oesophageal junction cancer (ToGA): A phase 3, open-label, randomised controlled trial. *Lancet* **2010**, *376*, 687–697. [CrossRef]

28. Swain, S.M.; Baselga, J.; Kim, S.B.; Ro, J.; Semiglazov, V.; Campone, M.; Ciruelos, E.; Ferrero, J.M.; Schneeweiss, A.; Heeson, S.; et al. Pertuzumab, trastuzumab, and docetaxel in HER2-positive metastatic breast cancer. *N. Engl. J. Med.* **2015**, *372*, 724–734. [CrossRef] [PubMed]

29. Tabernero, J.; Hoff, P.M.; Shen, L.; Ohtsu, A.; Shah, M.A.; Cheng, K.; Song, C.; Wu, H.; Eng-Wong, J.; Kang, Y.-K. Pertuzumab (P) + Trastuzumab (H) + Chemotherapy (CT) for, H.E.R2-Positive Metastatic Gastric or Gastro-Oesophageal Junction Cancer (mGC/GEJC): Final Analysis of a Phase III Study (JACOB). *Ann. Oncol.* **2017**, *28*, v209–v268. [CrossRef]

30. Diéras, V.; Miles, D.; Verma, S.; Pegram, M.; Welslau, M.; Baselga, J.; Krop, I.E.; Blackwell, K.; Hoersch, S.; Xu, J.; et al. Trastuzumab emtansine versus capecitabine plus lapatinib in patients with previously treated HER2-positive advanced breast cancer (EMILIA): A descriptive analysis of final overall survival results from a randomised, open-label, phase 3 trial. *Lancet Oncol.* **2017**, *18*, 732–742. [CrossRef]

31. Thuss-Patience, P.C.; Shah, M.A.; Ohtsu, A.; Van Cutsem, E.; Ajani, J.A.; Castro, H.; Mansoor, W.; Chung, H.C.; Bodoky, G.; Shitara, K.; et al. Trastuzumab emtansine versus taxane use for previously treated HER2-positive locally advanced or metastatic gastric or gastro-oesophageal junction adenocarcinoma (GATSBY): An international randomised, open-label, adaptive, phase 2/3 study. *Lancet Oncol.* **2017**, *18*, 640–653. [CrossRef]

32. Randolph Hecht, J.; Bang, Y.J.; Qin, S.K.; Chung, H.C.; Xu, J.M.; Park, J.O.; Jeziorski, K.; Shparyk, Y.; Hoff, P.M.; Sobrero, A.F.; et al. Lapatinib in Combination With Capecitabine Plus Oxaliplatin in Human Epidermal Growth Factor Receptor 2–Positive Advanced or Metastatic Gastric, Esophageal, or Gastroesophageal Adenocarcinoma: TRIO-013/LOGiC—A Randomized Phase III Trial. *J. Clin. Oncol.* **2016**, *5*, 443–451. [CrossRef] [PubMed]

33. Satoh, T.; Xu, R.H.; Chung, H.; Sun, G.P.; Doi, T.; Xu, J.M.; Tsuji, A.; Omuro, Y.; Li, J.; Wang, J.W.; et al. Lapatinib plus paclitaxel versus paclitaxel alone in the second-line treatment of, H.E.R2-amplified advanced gastric cancer in Asian populations: TyTAN—A randomized, phase III study. *J. Clin. Oncol.* **2014**, *32*, 2039–2049. [CrossRef] [PubMed]

34. Shimoyama, S. Unraveling trastuzumab and lapatinib inefficiency in gastric cancer: Future steps (Review). *Mol. Clin. Oncol.* **2014**, *2*, 175–181. [CrossRef] [PubMed]

35. Pietrantonio, F.; Caporale, M.; Morano, F.; Scartozzi, M.; Gloghini, A.; De Vita, F.; Giommoni, E.; Fornaro, L.; Aprile, G.; Melisi, D.; et al. HER2 loss in HER2-positive gastric or gastroesophageal cancer after trastuzumab therapy: Implication for further clinical research. *Int. J. Cancer.* **2016**, *139*, 2859–2864. [CrossRef] [PubMed]

36. Pietrantonio, F.; Fucà, G.; Morano, F.; Gloghini, A.; Corso, S.; Aprile, G.; Perrone, F.; De Vita, F.; Tamborini, E.; Tomasello, G.; et al. Biomarkers of Primary Resistance to Trastuzumab in HER2-Positive Metastatic Gastric Cancer Patients: The AMNESIA Case-Control Study. *Clin. Cancer Res.* **2018**, *24*, 1082–1089. [CrossRef] [PubMed]

37. Kim, M.A.; Lee, H.S.; Lee, H.E.; Jeon, Y.K.; Yang, H.K.; Kim, W.H. EGFR in gastric carcinomas: Prognostic significance of protein overexpression and high gene copy number. *Histopathology* **2008**, *52*, 738–746. [CrossRef] [PubMed]

38. Wang, K.L.; Wu, T.T.; Choi, I.S.; Wang, H.; Resetkova, E.; Correa, A.M.; Hofstetter, W.L.; Swisher, S.G.; Ajani, J.A.; Rashid, A.; et al. Expression of epidermal growth factor receptor in esophageal and esophagogastric junction adenocarcinomas: Association with poor outcome. *Cancer* **2007**, *109*, 658–667. [CrossRef] [PubMed]

39. Zhang, L.; Yang, J.; Cai, J.; Song, X.; Deng, J.; Huang, X.; Chen, D.; Yang, M.; Wery, J.P.; Li, S.; et al. A subset of gastric cancers with EGFR amplification and overexpression respond to cetuximab therapy. *Sci. Rep.* **2013**, *3*, 2992. [CrossRef] [PubMed]

40. Wainberg, Z.A.; Lin, L.S.; DiCarlo, B.; Dao, K.M.; Patel, R.; Park, D.J.; Wang, H.J.; Elashoff, R.; Ryba, N.; Hecht, J.R.; et al. Phase II trial of modified FOLFOX6 and erlotinib in patients with metastatic or advanced adenocarcinoma of the oesophagus and gastro-oesophageal junction. *Br. J. Cancer* **2011**, *105*, 760–765. [CrossRef] [PubMed]

41. Lordick, F.; Luber, B.; Lorenzen, S.; Hegewisch-Becker, S.; Folprecht, G.; Wöll, E.; Decker, T.; Endlicher, E.; Röthling, N.; Schuster, T.; et al. Cetuximab plus oxaliplatin/leucovorin/5-fluorouracil in first-line metastatic gastric cancer: A phase II study of the Arbeitsgemeinschaft Internistische Onkologie (AIO). *Br. J. Cancer* **2010**, *102*, 500–505. [CrossRef] [PubMed]

42. Lordick, F.; Kang, Y.K.; Chung, H.C.; Salman, P.; Oh, S.C.; Bodoky, G.; Kurteva, G.; Volovat, C.; Moiseyenko, V.M.; Gorbunova, V.; et al. Capecitabine and cisplatin with or without cetuximab for patients with previously untreated advanced gastric cancer (EXPAND): A randomised, open-label phase 3 trial. *Lancet Oncol.* **2013**, *14*, 490–499. [CrossRef]

43. Waddell, T.; Chau, I.; Cunningham, D.; Gonzalez, D.; Okines, A.F.; Okines, C.; Wotherspoon, A.; Saffery, C.; Middleton, G.; Wadsley, J.; et al. Epirubicin, oxaliplatin, and capecitabine with or without panitumumab for patients with previously untreated advanced oesophagogastric cancer (REAL3): A randomised, open-label phase 3 trial. *Lancet Oncol.* **2013**, *14*, 481–489. [CrossRef]

44. Maron, S.B.; Alpert, L.; Kwak, H.A.; Lomnicki, S.; Chase, L.; Xu, D.; O'Day, E.; Nagy, RJ.; Lanman, R.B.; Cecchi, F.; et al. Targeted Therapies for Targeted Populations: Anti-EGFR Treatment for EGFR-Amplified Gastroesophageal Adenocarcinoma. *Cancer Discov.* **2018**, *8*, 696–713. [CrossRef] [PubMed]

45. Peters, S.; Adjei, A.A. MET: A promising anticancer therapeutic target. *Nat. Rev. Clin. Oncol.* **2012**, *9*, 314–326. [CrossRef] [PubMed]

46. Jo, M.; Stolz, D.B.; Esplen, J.E.; Dorko, K.; Michalopoulos, G.K.; Strom, S.C. Cross-talk between epidermal growth factor receptor and c-Met signal pathways in transformed cells. *J. Biol Chem.* **2000**, *275*, 8806–8811. [CrossRef] [PubMed]

47. Peng, Z.; Zhu, Y.; Wang, Q.; Gao, J.; Li, Y.; Li, Y.; Ge, S.; Shen, L. Prognostic significance of MET amplification and expression in gastric cancer: A systematic review with meta-analysis. *PLoS ONE* **2014**, *9*, e84502. [CrossRef] [PubMed]

48. Iveson, T.; Donehower, R.C.; Davidenko, I.; Tjulandin, S.; Deptala, A.; Harrison, M.; Nirni, S.; Lakshmaiah, K.; Thomas, A.; Jiang, Y.; et al. Rilotumumab in combination with epirubicin, cisplatin, and capecitabine as first-line treatment for gastric or oesophagogastric junction adenocarcinoma: An open-label, dose de-escalation phase 1b study and a doubleblind, randomised phase 2 study. *Lancet Oncol.* **2014**, *15*, 1007–1018. [CrossRef]

49. Catenacci, D.V.; Henderson, L.; Xiao, S.Y.; Patel, P.; Yauch, R.L.; Hegde, P.; Zha, J.; Pandita, A.; Peterson, A.; Salgia, R.; et al. Durable complete response of metastatic gastric cancer with anti-Met therapy followed by resistance at recurrence. *Cancer Discov.* **2011**, *1*, 573–579. [CrossRef] [PubMed]

50. Shah, M.A.; Bang, Y.J.; Lordick, F.; Alsina, M.; Chen, M.; Hack, S.P.; Bruey, J.M.; Smith, D.; McCaffery, I.; Shames, D.S.; et al. Effect of Fluorouracil, Leucovorin, and Oxaliplatin with or without Onartuzumab in, H.E.R2-Negative, MET-Positive Gastroesophageal Adenocarcinoma: The METGastric Randomized Clinical Trial. *JAMA Oncol.* **2017**, *3*, 620–627. [CrossRef] [PubMed]

51. Shah, M.A.; Cho, J.Y.; Huat, I.T.B.; Tebbutt, N.C.; Yen, C.J.; Kang, A.; Shames, D.S.; Bu, L.; Kang, Y.-K. Randomized phase II study of FOLFOX+/−MET inhibitor, onartuzumab (O.), in advanced gastroesophageal adenocarcinoma(GEC). *J. Clin Oncol.* **2015**. [CrossRef]

52. Catenacci, D.V.T.; Tebbutt, N.C.; Davidenko, I.; Murad, A.M.; Al-Batran, S.E.; Ilson, D.H.; Tjulandin, S.; Gotovkin, E.; Karaszewska, B.; Bondarenko, I.; et al. Rilotumumab plus epirubicin, cisplatin, and capecitabine as first-line therapy in advanced MET-positive gastric or gastro-oesophageal junction cancer (RILOMET-1): A randomised, double-blind, placebo-controlled, phase 3 trial. *Lancet Oncol.* **2017**, *18*, 1467–1482. [CrossRef]

53. Hierro, C.; Alsina, M.; Sánchez, M.; Serra, V.; Rodon, J.; Tabernero, J. Targeting the fibroblast growth factor receptor 2 in gastric cancer: Promise or pitfall? *Ann. Oncol.* **2017**, *28*, 1207–1216. [CrossRef] [PubMed]

54. Nakatani, H.; Sakamoto, H.; Yoshida, T.; Yokota, J.; Tahara, E.; Sugimura, T.; Terada, M. Isolation of an amplified, DNA sequence in stomach cancer. *Jpn. J. Cancer Res.* **1990**, *81*, 707–710. [CrossRef] [PubMed]

55. Xie, L.; Su, X.; Zhang, L.; Yin, X.; Tang, L.; Zhang, X.; Xu, Y.; Gao, Z.; Liu, K.; Zhou, M.; et al. FGFR2 gene amplification in gastric cancer predicts sensitivity to the selective FGFR inhibitor AZD4547. *Clin. Cancer Res.* **2013**, *19*, 2572–2583. [CrossRef] [PubMed]

56. Van Cutsem, E.; Bang, Y.J.; Mansoor, W.; Petty, R.D.; Chao, Y.; Cunningham, D.; Ferry, D.R.; Smith, N.R.; Frewer, P.; Ratnayake, J.; et al. A randomized, open-label study of the efficacy and safety of AZD4547 monotherapy versus paclitaxel for the treatment of advanced gastric adenocarcinoma with FGFR2 polysomy or gene amplification. *Ann. Oncol.* **2017**, *28*, 1316–1324. [CrossRef] [PubMed]

57. Furuse, M.; Fujita, K.; Hiiragi, T.; Fujimoto, K.; Tsukita, S. Claudin-1 and -2: Novel integral membrane proteins localizing at tight junctions with no sequence similarity to occludin. *J. Cell Biol.* **1998**, *141*, 1539–1550. [CrossRef] [PubMed]

58. Singh, P.; Toom, S.; Huang, Y. Anti-claudin 18.2 antibody as new targeted therapy for advanced gastric cancer. *J. Hematol. Oncol.* **2017**, *10*, 105. [CrossRef] [PubMed]

59. Al-batran, S.; Schuler, M.; Zvirbule, Z.; Manikhas, G.; Lordick, F.; Rusyn, A.; Vynnyk, Y.; Vynnychenko, I.; Fadeeva, N.; Nechaeva, M.; et al. FAST: An international, multicenter, randomized, phase II trial of epirubicin, oxaliplatin, and capecitabine (EOX) with or without IMAB362, a first-in-class anti-CLDN18.2 antibody, as first-line therapy in patients with advanced cldn18.2+ gastric and gastroesophageal junction (GEJ) adenocarcinoma. *J. Clin. Oncol.* **2016**, *34*, LBA4001. [CrossRef]

60. Ohtsu, A.; Shah, M.A.; Van Cutsem, E.; Rha, S.Y.; Sawaki, A.; Park, S.R.; Lim, H.Y.; Yamada, Y.; Wu, J.; Langer, B.; et al. Bevacizumab in combination with chemotherapy as first-line therapy in advanced gastric cancer: A randomized, double-blind, placebo-controlled phase III study. *J. Clin. Oncol.* **2011**, *29*, 3968–3976. [CrossRef] [PubMed]

61. Shen, L.; Li, J.; Xu, J.; Pan, H.; Dai, G.; Qin, S.; Wang, L.; Wang, J.; Yang, Z.; Shu, Y.; et al. Bevacizumab plus capecitabine and cisplatin in Chinese patients with inoperable locally advanced or metastatic gastric or gastroesophageal junction cancer: Randomized, double-blind, phase III study (AVATAR study). *Gastric Cancer* **2015**, *18*, 168–176. [CrossRef] [PubMed]

62. Fuchs, C.; Tomasek, J.; Yong, C.J.; Dumitru, F.; Passalacqua, R.; Goswami, C.; Safran, H.; Dos Santos, L.V.; Aprile, G.; Ferry, D.R.; et al. Ramucirumab monotherapy for previously treated advanced gastric or gastro-oesophageal junction adenocarcinoma (REGARD): An international, randomised, multicentre, placebo-controlled, phase 3 trial. *Lancet* **2014**, *383*, 31–39. [CrossRef]

63. Wilke, H.; Muro, K.; Van Cutsem, E.; Oh, S.C.; Bodoky, G.; Shimada, Y.; Hironaka, S.; Sugimoto, N.; Lipatov, O.; Kim, T.Y.; et al. RAINBOW Study Group. Ramucirumab plus paclitaxel versus placebo plus paclitaxel in patients with previously treated advanced gastric or gastro-oesophageal junction adenocarcinoma (RAINBOW): A double-blind, randomised phase 3 trial. *Lancet Oncol.* **2014**, *15*, 1224–1235. [CrossRef]

64. Fuchs, C.S.; Shitara, K.; Di Bartolomeo, M.; Lonardi, S.; Al-Batran, S.E.; Van Cutsem, E.; Ilson, D.H.; Tabernero, J.; Chau, I.; Ducreux, M.; et al. RAINFALL: A randomized, double-blind, placebo-controlled phase, I.I.I study of cisplatin (Cis) plus capecitabine (Cape) or 5FU with or without ramucirumab (RAM) as first-line therapy in patients with metastatic gastric or gastroesophageal junction (G-GEJ) adenocarcinoma. *J. Clin. Oncol.* **2018**, *36*. [CrossRef]

65. Markman, B.; Atzori, F.; Pérez-García, J.; Tabernero, J.; Baselga, J. Status of PI3K inhibition and biomarker development in cancer therapeutics. *Ann. Oncol.* **2010**, *21*, 683–691. [CrossRef] [PubMed]

66. Ohtsu, A.; Ajani, J.A.; Bai, Y.X.; Bang, Y.J.; Chung, H.C.; Pan, H.M.; Sahmoud, T.; Shen, L.; Yeh, K.H.; Chin, K.; et al. Everolimus for previously treated advanced gastric cancer: Results of the randomized, double-blind, phase III GRANITE-1 study. *J. Clin. Oncol.* **2013**, *31*, 3935–3943. [CrossRef] [PubMed]

67. Meric-Bernstam, F.; Akcakanat, A.; Chen, H.; Do, K.A.; Sangai, T.; Adkins, F.; Gonzalez-Angulo, A.M.; Rashid, A.; Crosby, K.; Dong, M.; et al. PIK3CA/PTEN mutations and AKT activation as markers of sensitivity to allosteric mTOR inhibitors. *Clin. Cancer Res.* **2012**, *18*, 1777–1789. [CrossRef] [PubMed]

68. Yang, Y. Cancer immunotherapy: Harnessing the immune system to battle cancer. *J. Clin. Investig.* **2015**, *125*, 3335–3337. [CrossRef] [PubMed]

69. Niccolai, E.; Taddei, A.; Prisco, D.; Amedei, A. Gastric cancer and the epoch of immunotherapy approaches. *World J. Gastroenterol.* **2015**, *21*, 5778–5793. [CrossRef] [PubMed]

70. Wang, M.; Yin, B.; Wang, H.Y.; Wang, R.F. Current advances in T-cell-based cancer immunotherapy. *Immunotherapy* **2014**, *6*, 1265–1278. [CrossRef] [PubMed]

71. Disis, M.L.; Bernhard, H.; Jaffee, E.M. Use of tumour-responsive T cells as cancer treatment. *Lancet* **2009**, *373*, 673–683. [CrossRef]

72. Argonex Pharmaceuticals. *Cytotoxic T Lymphocyte-Stimulation Peptides for Prevention, Treatment, and Diagnosis of Melanoma*; WO/2001/032193; Argonex Pharmaceuticals: Charlottesville, VA, USA, 2001. [CrossRef]

73. Amedei, A.; Niccolai, E.; Della Bella, C.; Cianchi, F.; Trallori, G.; Benagiano, M.; Bencini, L.; Bernini, M.; Farsi, M.; Moretti, R.; et al. Characterization of tumor antigen peptidespecific T cells isolated from the neoplastic tissue of patients with gastric adenocarcinoma. *Cancer Immunol. Immunother.* **2009**, *58*, 1819–1830. [CrossRef] [PubMed]

74. Kim, Y.J.; Lim, J.; Kang, J.S.; Kim, H.M.; Lee, H.K.; Ryu, H.S.; Kim, J.Y.; Hong, J.T.; Kim, Y.; Han, S.B. Adoptive immunotherapy of human gastric cancer with ex vivo expanded T cells. *Arch. Pharm. Res.* **2010**, *33*, 1789–1795. [CrossRef] [PubMed]

75. Galon, J.; Costes, A.; Sanchez-Cabo, F.; Kirilovsky, A.; Mlecnik, B.; Lagorce-Pagès, C.; Tosolini, M.; Camus, M.; Berger, A.; Wind, P.; et al. Type, density, and location of immune cells within human colorectal tumors predict clinical outcome. *Science* **2006**, *313*, 1960–1964. [CrossRef] [PubMed]

76. Tomsová, M.; Melichar, B.; Sedláková, I.; Steiner, I. Prognostic significance of CD3+ tumor-infiltrating lymphocytes in ovarian carcinoma. *Gynecol. Oncol.* **2008**, *108*, 415–420. [CrossRef] [PubMed]

77. Amedei, A.; Niccolai, E.; Benagiano, M.; Della Bella, C.; Cianchi, F.; Bechi, P.; Taddei, A.; Bencini, L.; Farsi, M.; Cappello, P.; et al. Ex vivo analysis of pancreatic cancerinfiltrating T lymphocytes reveals that ENO-specific Tregs accumulate in tumor tissue and inhibit Th1/Th17 effector cell functions. *Cancer Immunol. Immunother.* **2013**, *62*, 1249–1260. [CrossRef] [PubMed]

78. Amedei, A.; Munari, F.; Bella, C.D.; Niccolai, E.; Benagiano, M.; Bencini, L.; Cianchi, F.; Farsi, M.; Emmi, G.; Zanotti, G.; et al. Helicobacter pylori secreted peptidylprolyl cis, trans-isomerase drives Th17 inflammation in gastric adenocarcinoma. *Intern. Emerg. Med.* **2014**, *9*, 303–309. [CrossRef] [PubMed]

79. Gilboa, E. DC-based cancer vaccines. *J. Clin. Investig.* **2007**, *117*, 1195–1203. [CrossRef] [PubMed]

80. Muro, K.; Chung, H.C.; Shankaran, V.; Geva, R.; Catenacci, D.; Gupta, S.; Eder, J.P.; Golan, T.; Le, D.T.; Burtness, B.; et al. Pembrolizumab for patients with PD-L1-positive advanced gastric cancer (KEYNOTE-012): A. multicentre, open-label, phase 1b trial. *Lancet Oncol.* **2016**, *17*, 717–726. [CrossRef]

81. Fuchs, C.S.; Doi, T.; Woo-Jun Jang, R.; Muro, K.; Satoh, T.; Machado, M.; Sun, W.; Jalal, S.I.; Shah, M.A.; Metges, J.P.; et al. KEYNOTE-059 cohort 1: Efficacy and safety of pembrolizumab (pembro) monotherapy in patients with previously treated advanced gastric cancer. *J. Clin. Oncol.* **2017**, *35*, 4003. [CrossRef]

82. Kim, S.T.; Cristescu, R.; Bass, A.J.; Kim, K.M.; Odegaard, J.I.; Kim, K.; Liu, X.Q.; Sher, X.; Jung, H.; Lee, M.; et al. Comprehensive molecular characterization of clinical responses to PD-1 inhibition in metastatic gastric cancer. *Nat. Med.* **2018**. [CrossRef] [PubMed]

83. Shitara, K.; Özgüroğlu, M.; Bang, Y.J.; Di Bartolomeo, M.; Mandalà, M.; Ryu, M.H.; Fornaro, L.; Olesiński, T.; Caglevic, C.; Chung, H.C.; et al. KEYNOTE-061 investigators. Pembrolizumab versus paclitaxel for previously treated, advanced gastric or gastro-oesophageal junction cancer (KEYNOTE-061): A randomised, open-label, controlled, phase 3 trial. *Lancet* **2018**, *392*, 123–133. [CrossRef]

84. Kang, Y.K.; Boku, N.; Satoh, T.; Ryu, M.H.; Chao, Y.; Kato, K.; Chung, H.C.; Chen, J.S.; Muro, K.; Kang, W.K.; et al. Nivolumab in patients with advanced gastric or gastrooesophageal junction cancer refractory to, or intolerant of, at least two previous chemotherapy regimens (ONO-4538-12, ATTRACTION-2): A. randomised, double-blind, placebo-controlled, phase 3 trial. *Lancet* **2017**, *390*, 2461–2471. [CrossRef]

85. Chen, Y.; Haveman, J.W.; Apostolou, C.; Chang, D.K.; Merrett, N.D. Asian gastric cancer patients show superior survival: The experiences of a single Australian center. *Gastric Cancer* **2015**, *18*, 256–261. [CrossRef] [PubMed]

86. Jin, H.; Pinheiro, P.S.; Callahan, K.E.; Altekruse, S.F. Examining the gastric cancer survival gap between Asians and whites in the United States. *Gastric Cancer* **2017**, *20*, 573–582. [CrossRef] [PubMed]

87. Marrelli, D.; Polom, K.; Roviello, F. Ethnicity-related differences in tumor immunity: A new possible explanation for gastric cancer prognostic variability? *Transl. Gastroenterol. Hepatol.* **2016**, *1*, 11. [CrossRef] [PubMed]

88. Janjigian, Y.Y.; Bendell, J.; Calvo, E.; Kim, J.W.; Ascierto, P.A.; Sharma, P.; Ott, P.A.; Peltola, K.; Jaeger, D.; Evans, J.; et al. CheckMate-032 Study: Efficacy and Safety of Nivolumab and Nivolumab Plus Ipilimumab in Patients with Metastatic Esophagogastric Cancer. *J. Clin. Oncol.* **2018**. [CrossRef] [PubMed]

89. Lin, S.J.; Gagnon-Bartsch, J.A.; Tan, I.B.; Earle, S.; Ruff, L.; Pettinger, K.; Ylstra, B.; van Grieken, N.; Rha, S.Y.; Chung, H.C.; et al. Signatures of tumour immunity distinguish Asian and non-Asian gastric adenocarcinomas. *Gut* **2015**, *64*, 1721–1731. [CrossRef] [PubMed]

90. Chiaravalli, A.M.; Feltri, M.; Bertolini, V.; Bagnoli, E.; Furlan, D.; Cerutti, R.; Novario, R.; Capella, C.; Intratumour, T. Cells, their activation status and survival in gastric carcinomas characterised for microsatellite instability and Epstein-Barr virus infection. *Virchows Arch.* **2006**, *448*, 344–353. [CrossRef] [PubMed]

91. Tabernero, J.; Bang, Y.J.; Fuchs, C.S.; Ohtsu, A.; Kher, U.; Lam, B.; Koshiji, M.; Cutsem, E.V. KEYNOTE-062: Phase III study of pembrolizumab (MK-3475) alone or in combination with chemotherapy versus chemotherapy alone as first-line therapy for advanced gastric or gastroesophageal junction (GEJ) adenocarcinoma. *J. Clin. Oncol.* **2016**, *34*. [CrossRef]

92. Efficacy Study of Nivolumab Plus Ipilimumab or Nivolumab Plus Chemotherapy Against Chemotherapy in Stomach Cancer or Stomach/Esophagus Junction Cancer (CheckMate649). Available online: https://clinicaltrials.gov/ct2/show/NCT02872116 (accessed on 31 August 2018).

93. Pectasides, E.; Stachler, M.D.; Derks, S.; Liu, Y.; Maron, S.; Islam, M.; Alpert, L.; Kwak, H.; Kindler, H.; Polite, B.; et al. Genomic Heterogeneity as a Barrier to Precision Medicine in Gastroesophageal Adenocarcinoma. *Cancer Discov.* **2018**, *8*, 37–48. [CrossRef] [PubMed]

94. Bertotti, A.; Migliardi, G.; Galimi, F.; Sassi, F.; Torti, D.; Isella, C.; Corà, D.; Di Nicolantonio, F.; Buscarino, M.; Petti, C.; et al. A molecularly annotated platform of patient-derived xenografts ("xenopatients") identifies HER2 as an effective therapeutic target in cetuximab-resistant colorectal cancer. *Cancer Discov.* **2011**, *1*, 508–523. [CrossRef] [PubMed]

95. Gavine, P.R.; Ren, Y.; Han, L.; Lv, J.; Fan, S.; Zhang, W.; Xu, W.; Liu, Y.J.; Zhang, T.; Fu, H.; et al. Volitinib, a potent and highly selective c-Met inhibitor, effectively blocks c-Met signaling and growth in c-MET amplified gastric cancer patient-derived tumor xenograft models. *Mol. Oncol.* **2015**, *9*, 323–333. [CrossRef] [PubMed]

96. Gao, M.; Lin, M.; Rao, M.; Thompson, H.; Hirai, K.; Choi, M.; Georgakis, G.V.; Sasson, A.R.; Bucobo, J.C.; Tzimas, D.; et al. Development of Patient-Derived Gastric Cancer Organoids from Endoscopic Biopsies and Surgical Tissues. *Ann. Surg. Oncol.* **2018**. [CrossRef] [PubMed]

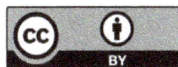

International Journal of
Molecular Sciences

MDPI

Review

The Pattern of Signatures in Gastric Cancer Prognosis

Julita Machlowska [1], Ryszard Maciejewski [1] and Robert Sitarz [1,2,*]

[1] Department of Human Anatomy, Medical University of Lublin, 20-090 Lublin, Poland;
    julita.machlowska@gmail.com (J.M.); maciejewski.r@gmail.com (R.M.)
[2] Department of Surgery, St. John's Cancer Center, 20-090 Lublin, Poland
*   Correspondence: r.sitarz@umlub.pl; Tel.: +48-81-448-60-20; Fax: +48-81-448-60-21

Received: 28 April 2018; Accepted: 30 May 2018; Published: 4 June 2018

Abstract: Gastric cancer is one of the most common malignancies worldwide and it is a fourth leading cause of cancer-related death. Carcinogenesis is a multistage disease process specified by the gradual procurement of mutations and epigenetic alterations in the expression of different genes, which finally lead to the occurrence of a malignancy. These genes have diversified roles regarding cancer development. Intracellular pathways are assigned to the expression of different genes, signal transduction, cell-cycle supervision, genomic stability, DNA repair, and cell-fate destination, like apoptosis, senescence. Extracellular pathways embrace tumour invasion, metastasis, angiogenesis. Altered expression patterns, leading the different clinical responses. This review highlights the list of molecular biomarkers that can be used for prognostic purposes and provide information on the likely outcome of the cancer disease in an untreated individual.

Keywords: gastric cancer; HER2; cell cycle regulators; microsatellite instability; apoptosis; mucins; multidrug resistance proteins; invasiveness; peritoneal spreading; neovascularization

1. Introduction

Gastric cancer (GC) is an aggressive disease that is still a global health problem with its heterogeneous nature. In the last several decades, the decrease of gastric cancer incidence has been noted, however it is still the fourth leading cause of cancer-related death worldwide [1]. Alternative prevention, as food preservation, earlier diagnosis, and therefore, prior treatments cause abatement of recorded incidents, although the prognosis is still bad. The standard therapies include surgical resection with chemotherapy, and in suitable cases, chemoradiation [2]. To treat advanced gastric cancers and metastasis, it is still a huge barrier to be overlapped; however, little progress has been reported [3]. Gastric cancer is a heterogeneous disease; therefore, new investigation and approaches need to be considered including prevention, early detection, as well as innovative and effective therapeutic efforts.

Neoadjuvant therapy as the dosing of therapeutic agents before a major treatment of cancer, became more popular in recent studies on gastric cancer combating. The first approach in this field was reported in 1989, concerning gastric cancer patients, where cisplatin (EAP) was confirmed as an effective agent in locally advanced gastric cancer, and therefore it was a chance for surgery in patients with poor prognosis [4]. Nowadays, the importance of neoadjuvant therapy is an interesting investigation for many researchers for extension of survival time in advanced GC cases. The randomized controlled trials have been implemented; nevertheless, the final outcomes are still not consistent [5,6]. The study that was conducted by Songun et al., 1999 [7] showed that more active regimens than methotrexate (FAMTX) are required for future randomized trials.

Gastric cancer immunotherapy is another powerful approach due to better understanding of immunological networks and molecular mechanisms of immunosuppression in the cancer environment. Vaccination strategies based on protein and peptide vaccines, which can be identified by cytotoxic

T and helper T lymphocytes. Currently, there are several immunotherapy-based approaches like adoptive cell therapy, where various cell types can be implemented, like lymphokine-activated killer cells [8], tumor infiltration lymphocytes (TILs) [9], and anti-CD3 monoclonal antibody-induced killer cells [10]. Dendritic cells incubated with mRNA can show the encoded antigen, which making them another vaccine type based on mRNA gene transfer [11]. Both protein and peptide targets are useful tool for stimulation of immune response, HER2/neu-derived peptide [12] and MAGE [13] which are related to MHC class I and induce cytotoxic T cells against GC cancers.

Discovering the pattern of signatures could be used as a biomarker to guide targeted therapy for gastric cancer. This heading will individualize the cancer therapy relay on integrated and global recognition of dysfunctional signalling pathways. The presented review pays attention on the currently available biomarkers for prognosis of gastric cancer. Nowadays, there are many different signatures that can provide the division of gastric carcinoma by taking in consideration age, histopathological type, *Helicobacter pylori* infection, microsatellite instability, module of HER2 expression, molecular markers of cell cycle regulators, factors that regulate apoptosis, multidrug resistance proteins, agents that influence cell membrane properties, and agents with an impact on the progression of gastric cancer and peritoneal metastasis. Radical patient selection, appropriate combinations of targeted therapies, and deployment of emerging immunotherapeutic investigations will for sure hone the treatment of this global disease.

2. Screening for *Epstein–Barr viruses*

Infection with *Epstein-Barr virus* (*EBV*) is associated with a wide spectrum of malignant diseases, like Hodgkin and non-Hodgkin lymphomas, post-transplant lymphoproliferative disorder (PTLD), and gastric cancer [14]. It must be clarified that *EBV* infects basically all humans by the time that they reach adulthood and the viral genome is detained in a low number of B lymphocytes. To assess *EBV* as a marker for cancer development, it is strongly advised to quantify the number of infected cells and to indicate their types. Upon primary infection, it transiently runs a short lytic program and after predominantly establishes latent infection [15]. Serological tests are commonly used to confirm the primary infection and report remote infection [16]. One of the most popular serological assays is heterophile antibody test. Cancer related to *EBV* infection is correlated with high titers against Early Antigen (EA) and IgG Viral Capsid Antigen Antibody (VCA) with low *EBV* Nuclear Antigen Antibody (EBNA) titer. Unfortunately, analogous patterns are probable in autoimmune disease and this test is not decisive when the immune system is defective, for instance, acquired immunodeficiency syndrome (AIDS) or allogeneic transplant patients.

EBER in Situ Hybridization Assay is a gold standard for localization of *EBV* in biopsied tumor [17]. *EBER1* and *EBER2* are non-polyadenylated viral transcripts, which are conjointly called *Epstein–Barr* virus-encoded small RNA (*EBER*), which are expressed at a very high level in infected cells. They have been labelled as a natural marker for latent type of infection. DNA of *EBV* is evidential within malignant epithelial cells in 10% of gastric adenocarcinomas, mostly in those arising in the stump after surgical gastrectomy and in undifferentiated with abundant tumor-infiltrating lymphocytes [18]. *EBV* positive gastric cancer patients have specific genetic mutations and epigenetic patterns profile, which is assigned to the clinical phenotype of the malignancy. It was postulated that some genes, like *BcLF1, BHRF1, BARF0, BARF1, BZLF1, EBNA1, BLLF1*, and *BRLF1* are overexpressed in GC cases with positive *EBV* infection [19–21]. *EBV* occurs as episomes in nuclei of host cell and averagely 205 host cell genes are altered in patients with *EBV*-positive GCs, embracing *TGFBR1, AKT2, MAP3K4*, and *CCNA1* [21]. Epigenetic alterations are also connected to the *EBV* positive gastric carcinoma. Zhao et al., 2013 [21] showed that 216 genes were hypermethylated and were transcriptionally down-regulated, and 46 were demethylated and transcriptionally up-regulated in the study that was conducted on cultured *EBV* positive GC cells. The hypermethylation status of the *IHH, ACSS1, TRABD*, and *FAM3B* genes was also found among analysed tumor samples. Targeted therapies in advanced GC with *Epstein-Barr virus* positive patients, can be applied to the *PIK3CA/Akt* pathway, *JAK2* and *PD-1/PD-L1*, and *PD-L2* pathway [22].

3. HER2 Status in Gastric Cancer

The HER2 receptor is a member of the Epidermal Growth Factor Receptor (EGFR) family. Its activation is going through its spontaneous homo/heterodimerization with the other EGFR family receptors [23]. Many studies have been investigated on HER2 amplification and high expression in gastric cancer, applying a different method, showing the range of positive cases between 6% and 30% [24–26]. GC very often displays heterogeneity of the HER2 genotype and phenotype, which can have impact on testing inaccuracy [27]. The EMEA (European Medicines Agency) recommended the IHC immunohistochemistry method (IHC) as a first screening, adding the scoring criteria, with 3+ samples to be positive and 2+ only positive, when approved by Fluorescence in situ hybridization (FISH). When considering the increased frequency of overexpression/amplification of *HER2* among GC cases, preclinical and early phase clinical studies have been conducted to assess the therapeutic value for targeted approaches [28,29]. Tanner et al., 2005 [29] investigated the occurrence and the clinical importance of *HER-2/neu* amplification in gastric carcinoma. The frequency of *HER2/neu* amplification was, respectively, 12.2% of the gastric and 24.0% of the gastroesophageal adenocarcinomas. *HER-2/neu* amplification was higher in the intestinal histologic type of gastric cancer (21.5%) in comparison to the diffuse (2%), it was not associated with age and gender, but with the poor survival of GC patients. Trastuzumab antibody that was targeting HER-2/neu inhibited the growth of a p185 (HER-2/neu) overexpressing gastric. Accuracy of trastuzumab was tested as a single dose or in combination with other chemotherapeutic agents in human gastric cancer xenograft models with high HER2 expression [28]. Trastuzumab, while added as a single drug, inhibited the tumor expansion in HER2-overexpressing models, but not in the HER2-negative. Trastuzumab with combinations of any other agents, like docetaxel, paclitaxel, capecitabine, irinotecan, and cisplatin, displayed higher anticancer action than being administrated separately. Other molecular agents targeting HER2 have been analyzed, such as pertuzumab, lapatinib, and the antibody-drug conjugate trastuzumab-emtansine (TDM-1) [28,30,31]. Unfortunately, the final effect of them has been displayed to be poor in comparison to trastuzumab, which is the first agent of targeted therapy confirmed as a standard treatment in gastric cancer.

4. Gastric Cancers with Microsatellite Instability

Microsatellite instability (MSI) is an important indication of the DNA mismatch repair deficiency, and therefore it is perceived as a factor in the expeditive collection of genetic changes in the gastric carcinogenesis process [32]. Hang et al., 2018 [33] presented the molecular mechanisms of of microsatellite instability (MSI) and its importance in GC prognosis. Next generation sequencing data of the whole transcriptome were investigated from The Cancer Genome Atlas (TCGA), covering 64 high-level MSI (MSI-H) gastric cancer samples, 44 low-level MSI (MSI-L) and 187 stable microsatellite (MSI-S) gastric cancer samples [33]. The results showed that MSI status might have impact on the prognosis of GC patients, partially through the inflammatory bowel disease, antigen processing and presentation, measles, toxoplasmosis, and herpes simplex infection pathways. *HLA-DRA*, *HLA-DRB5*, *JAK2*, *HLA-DQA1*, *HLA-DMA*, *CASP8*, and *Fas* could be predictive factors for gastric cancer prognosis.

Although MSI cases in general are deprived of targeted alterations, mutations in *PIK3CA*, *EGFR*, *ERBB3*, and *ERBB2* were detected [22]. Additionally, MSI tumors alteration status of genes showed common mutations in major histocompatibility complex class I genes, including *B2M* and *HLA-B*. To reveal a precise association between human mutL homolog 1 (*hMLH1*) promoter methylation and gastric cancer, a meta-analysis study was investigated by Ye et al., 2018 [34]. It was postulated that *hMLH1* promoter methylation had significant correlation with not only microsatellite instability, but also with lymph node metastasis and the low expression of hMLH1 protein. Polom K et al., 2018 [35] investigated the analysis of MSI status among cases with marginal involvement after gastrectomy, and the establishment of an association between MSI, margin status, and survival rate They displayed that patients with MSI-H gastric cancer might possess long-term survival despite positive resection margin (RM+) status. This might be important step towards surgical treatments that are based on to clinical and pathological factors [35].

5. CDX2 Expression in the Intestinal Type of Gastric Epithelial Dysplasia and Its Correlation with CD10

CDX2 is a Drosophila caudal-related homeobox transcription factor, and it is a member of the caudal-related homeobox gene family. It is perceived as an important factor in mammalian early intestinal development and the regulation of intestine-characteristic gene transcription [36]. The role of CDX2 in gastric cancer has been reported as responsible for the proliferation and differentiation of intestinal type of epithelial cells by controlling transcriptional activation of intestine specific proteins, like sucrase-isomaltase, carbonic anhydrase I, or Mucin 2 (MUC2) [37]. It also acts through the inhibition of growth by the activation of WAF1 (cyclin-dependent kinase inhibitor) [38]. In the study that was conducted by Park et al., 2010 [39], CDX2 is expressed mostly among adenomatous-type gastric epithelial dysplasia in comparison to the hybrid or foveolar types. CDX2 expression level is the lowest in the advanced gastric cancers, and it is also very decreased in the early onset of gastric cancers, indicating the possibility to act as a tumor suppressor. The study also showed that an increasing expression of CDX2 is correlated with an increased expression of CD10, which is cell surface zinc-dependent metalloprotease, also called as endopeptidase (NEP) (EC 3.4.24.11), enkephalinase, or acute lymphoblastic leukemia antigen, which in this case is promoting intestinal metaplasia of gastric epithelium. The study that was performed by Huang et al., 2005 [40] reported that CD10 expression by stromal cells was meaningfully increased in the primary gastric carcinomas in comparison to normal mucosas. CD10 expression was detected more frequently in differentiated carcinomas and it seems to cause the promotion of invasion and lymph node metastasis processes of differentiated gastric carcinoma.

6. Abnormalities in Cell Cycle Regulators

Genetic alterations in several regulators of the cell cycle have a significant impact on the gastric carcinogenesis process. Cyclin D1 and retinoblastoma protein (pRb) are important factors in the progression from G1 phase to S phase, which is crucial in the cell cycle [41]. In general, cyclins are positive regulators of the cell cycle process and their overexpression is linked to uncontrolled cell growth and cancer development. The main targets of cyclin D1-Cdk complexes are the retinoblastoma family of protein Rb [42]. The study that was conducted by Arici et al., 2009 [43] intimated the higher expression of Rb and cyclin D1 among nonneoplastic mucosa comprising dysplasia, intestinal metaplasia, atrophy, and gastritis to carcinoma, which indicates that the expression of pRb and cyclin D1 can occur in early stages of gastric carcinogenesis. Cyclin D1 is expressed among genetic alterations in gastric carcinomas, including advanced gastric carcinomas and early stage, using immunohistochemistry as a good standard method for the detection of early stage gastric cancers and their differentiation from hyperplastic polyp patients [44].

Another very important cell cycle regulatory protein is p16, which is cyclin-dependent kinase inhibitor (CDKI) [45]. The *p16* gene acts as a tumor suppressor gene and negatively regulates cell growth and proliferation. The relation between the inactivation of *p16* and the evolution of gastric cancer has been reported by several study groups. Deletion of *p16* gene exon 2 is related to the carcinogenesis process and progression of gastric carcinoma, which was reported by Hayashi et al., 1997 [46]. Wu et al., 1998 [47] showed that deletion of *p16* gene was oftentimes present in intestinal type of gastric cancer in comparison to the diffuse type. Hypermethylation of the *p16* locus, which causes functional inactivation, plays a relevant role in the pathogenesis of sporadic gastric cancer [48].

Cyclin-dependent kinase inhibitor 1B, called p27^{Kip1}, is referred to play a role as a cell cycle inhibitor protein with the main function to slow down or even stop the cell division cycle [49].

Nitti et al., 2002 [50] showed that low p27^{Kip1} protein expression in gastric adenocarcinoma relates to advanced tumours, it is significantly higher in weakly differentiated cases and is perceived as a negative prognostic agent for patient's survival. Zheng et al., 2005 [51] first reported that p27^{Kip1} expression, cell cycle arrest, and apoptosis are strongly correlated in the SGC7901 cell line. Overexpression of p27^{KIP1} was associated with the induction of apoptosis and the extension of cell cycle in G1 phase of SGC7901 cells.

p21^{Cip1}, also known as cyclin-dependent kinase (CDK) inhibitor 1, which can inhibit all cyclin/CDK complexes and it is a main target of p53 operations [52]. p21 protein expression progressive decreases from normal gastric mucosa, chronic superficial gastritis, and precancerous gastric lesions to gastric cancer was reported by Luo et al., 2014 [53]. They also suggested that the loss of p21 expression was very closely correlated with stadium of tumour differentiation, area of invasion, vascular invasion, Lauren classification, and metastasis to lymph node. It seems that p21 occurs in a role of tumour suppressor in the development and expansion of gastric cancer.

7. Factors that Regulate Apoptosis Process

Many studies have been investigated on *p53* genetic alterations in gastric carcinomas. It became clear that *p53* mutational changes show up in early stages of cancer development and their frequency is much higher with the cancer development process [54]. *P53* mutations are detected in 0–77% of gastric cancer cases [55] and they are significantly more frequent in proximal lesions than in distal. They mostly occur in exons 4–11, and they have several hot spots at codons 175, 245, 248, 273, 282, and 213. G:C > A:T transitions at CpG sites and are therefore are very popular types of alterations in GC patients [56]. P53 immunoreactivity is observed in 17–90.7% of invasive gastric cancer cases. Nuclear staining of p53 is not similar between diffuse and intestinal gastric carcinomas, with distinctly higher appearance in intestinal types [57]. Molecular analysis of gastric cancer that was performed by Cristescu et al., 2015 [58] showed the different gastric cancer subtypes are assigned to the different clinical outcomes and the TP53 is also a part of division of molecular gastric cancer. The group revealed that the tumor protein 53 active and TP53-inactive subtypes incorporate patients with intermediate prognosis and recurrence rates, however TP53-active group displays more promising prognosis.

The cell surface receptor programmed death-1 (PD1) and its ligand (PDL1) have been described in gastric tumours as markers assigned to poor prognosis of the patient [59]. Screening of clinical importance of PD1 and its ligands' expression, as well as T cell infiltration might be a future perspective for using this as biomarkers in GC immunotherapy [60]. Correlation with clinical features showed that PDL1 membranous expression was in around 38% of tumour cells among the analysed cases, as well as 75% of infiltrating immune cells. The expression of PDL1 was visibly higher in a group of patients without metastasis, with PCNA and C-met expression, as well as *EBV* positive group. The study that was conducted by Böger et al., 2016 [61] displayed that PD-L1 expression was importantly dominated among men with GC, *Her2/neu* positive, *Epstein Barr* virus positive, microsatellite instable, *PIK3CA*-mutated, GCs of the proximal stomach, unclassified, and papillary. The significantly better patient's outcome was correlated with the high PD-L1/PD-1 expression was associated with a significantly better patient outcome. The connection of PD-L1/PD-1 expression with various clinico-pathological characteristics might supply as a surrogate marker of PD-L1-positive gastric carcinomas, as well as can allow for improving the immune checkpoint treatment possibilities [61].

The *p73* gene encodes for a protein with high similarity to this displayed by *p53*. Kang et al., 2000 [62] described the expression of p73 in gastric carcinoma tissues. Importantly, low levels of p73 expression were detected in noncancerous gastric tissues and analysed cell lines, whereas p73 was detected in 94.9% of carcinoma tissues. The study demonstrated that p73 is not an aim of genetic modifications in gastric carcinogenesis. Wild-type p73 is very often overexpressed in gastric cancer tissues by the activation of a silent allele or transcriptional induction of an active allele.

Murine double minute gene 2 (*mdm2*) is a newly described oncogene that is placed at chromosome 12q13-14 [63]. Studies on the expression of mdm2 revealed that it is increasing in gastric cancer [64].

Moreover, expression level of the MDM2 protein is significantly higher in intestinal metaplasia in comparison to chronic gastritis [65]. Subtypes of intestinal metaplasia show different patterns of expression of the mdm2 and p53 protein [66]. Their expression is increased in atypical intestinal metaplasia (AIM) and gastric carcinomas in comparison to simple intestinal metaplasia (SIM). AIM may display the precancerous nature of gastric carcinoma more largely than SIM or the conventional IM subtypes. Moreover, AIM may be concerned as a preneoplastic lesion and be a significant indicator in the clinical follow-up of GC patients.

B-cell lymphoma 2 (Bcl-2) expression and increased risk of gastric carcinoma recurrence was studied by Wu et al., 2014 [67]. There is still a lack of predictive indicators for GC recurrence, therefore, the determination of such factors, like it was performed for bcl-2 expression, might be applicable after curative resection in patients with gastric cancer. In fact, the researchers displayed that peritoneal recurrence occurred as the mostly observed type after curative gastrectomy. Moreover Wu et al., 2014 [67] showed that lymph node metastases, depth of invasion, as well as negative expression of bcl-2 were correlated with a higher probability of recurrence action.

8. Multidrug Resistance Related Proteins

DNA repair protein complementing XP-A cells is a protein that in humans is encoded by the *XPA* gene [68]. *XPA* A23G and *XPC* exon 8 Val499Ala polymorphisms were explored to be effective markers for the recognition of individuals at risk of developing gastric cardiac adenocarcinoma (GCA) [69]. D'Errico et al., 2006 [70] have displayed that mutation in the *XPC* gene are responsible for accumulation of oxidative damage in human cells. 'A' allele of *XPA*-23G > A has been correlated with increased levels of places tender to formamidopyrimidine DNA glycosylase that shows oxidative DNA damage in the lymphocytes of carriers [71]. Polymorphisms in both genes can impact on destroying the capability to look for bulky adducts and oxidative DNA damage. This might promote the accumulation of DNA lesions, and therefore increased gastric cancer risk.

Expression of multidrug resistance-associated protein 2 (MRP2) was detected in several carcinomas, which was reported by Sandusky et al., 2002 [72]. High expression of MRP2 is important in the in initial absence of reaction to chemotherapy treatment of tumor, and therefore, it might be a significant biomarker for chemotherapy response. Immunohistochemistry was conducted on zinc formalin-fixed tissue. Immunostaining was detected in neoplastic cells on the cell membrane with M2-lll-6 antibody against MRP2 and cell membrane and cytoplasm with EAG5 against MRP2. Among examined cancers MPR2 was localized in eight of 13 gastric carcinomas and the expression was increased in well differentiated tumours. MRP2 is associated with irinotecan and anthracyclines transport, therefore the clinical applications of pharmacogenetics might allow for accurately defining the appropriate drug and dose for individual treatment [73].

The multidrug resistance 1 gene (*MDR1*) is very important candidate gene in developing gastric cancer susceptibility [74]. A total 365 gastric cancer patients and 367 controls were genotyped using the designed restriction site-polymerase chain reaction method to look for single genetic polymorphisms (SNPs) of the *MDR1* gene. The outcome showed the allele and genotype frequencies of c.159G > T and c.1564A > T to be statistically different among both analysed groups in the Chinese Han population. Detected variants could play a role as molecular markers in early gastric cancer diagnosis. Zhu et al., 2013 [75] reported that MDR1 has a significant impact on drug resistance answer, and the knockdown of MDR1 might reverse this phenotype among gastric cancer cells. To present the exact role of MDR1, the group performed knockdown of MDR1 expression using shRNA in gastric cancer cells that are resistant to drugs. The results were reviewed to assess Adriamycin (ADR) accumulation and drug sensitivity. Using two shRNAs it was possible to inhibit the expression of mRNA and protein of MDR1 in SGC7901-MDR1 cells. In final observation the group concluded *MDR1* knockdown to cause decreasing of ADR collection in cells and increment of susceptibility to ADR treatment.

The expression of Glutathione S-transferases Pi (GST-P), also known as GST-π, is readily higher in tumours chemically induced. In response to the tumor creation, GST-π is expressed as a resistance mechanism by which cells can survive [76]. The expression of GST-π in patients with gastric carcinoma was increased in comparison to normal mucosa (51.3% versus 23.2%), which was reported by Yu et al., 2014 [77]. The correlation of GST-π expression was observed with sex (male versus female, 59.7% versus 35.7%, $p < 0.05$) and differentiation (well, moderately, and poorly, 40.5%, 41.9%, and 64.7%, respectively, $p < 0.05$). Moreover, high expression of GST-π was connected to the tumor invasion, recurrence, as well as poor prognosis.

9. Mucins with Impact on Cell Membrane Properties

Mucins are a family of extracellular large molecular weight, heavily glycosylated proteins (glycoconjugates). Both membrane bound mucins and secreted mucin possess many shared features [78]. Their important properties have related to capability to form gels, with main functions regarding lubrication, cell signalling, and the creation of chemical barriers. Mucins are frequently engaged in an inhibitory role [79]. Overexpression of mucin proteins, MUC1, MUC2, MUC5AC, and MUC6 have been reported in to be present in the gastric carcinogenesis process [80]. The correlation between the expression of several mucins and clinicopathologic profiles and patient's survival are presented in Table 1.

Table 1. Mucins and their impact on patient's survival with gastric cancer.

MUC Type	Function	Expression Patterns in Gastric Cancer	Authors
MUC1	Protective role by binding to pathogens, functions in a cell signalling capacity, presented in the nucleus regulation the activity of transcription factor complexes, which take part in tumor-induced changes of host immunity system	MUC1 positive cases highly overexpressed in intestinal-type carcinomas, increased rate of vascular invasion and lymph node metastasis, lower 5-year survival rate	Wang et al., 2016 [81]
MUC2	The major intestinal mucin, expressed by goblet cells of the small intestine and colon, important role in organizing the intestinal mucus layers at the epithelial surface; forming trimers that crosslink with TFF3 and Fcγbp, allow to highly viscous extracellular layer	Strongly correlated with the intestinal histological type, the correlation between MUC2 and HER2 expression is possible to demonstrate the connection between the intestinal differentiation of cancer cells and HER2 expression	Park et al., 2015 [82]
MUC5AC	Glycoprotein of gastric and respiratory tract epithelium guards the mucosa from infection and chemical damage, thanks to binding to inhaled microorganisms and particles, which are later removed by the mucociliary system	Decreased Muc5AC expression was importantly correlated with poor overall survival, additionally, decreased Muc5AC expression was also meaningfully reported to the tumour invasion depth and lymph node metastasis	Zhang et al., 2015 [83]
MUC6	Might deliver a mechanism for modulation of the composition of the protective mucus layer connected to acid secretion or the presence of bacteria and noxious agents in the lumen, involvement in the cytoprotection of epithelial surfaces	MUC6 is a marker of gastric foveolar cells and antral/cardiac mucous glandular cells, reflect to gastric phenotypes	Kim et al., 2013 [84]

10. Factors that Influence High Progression of Gastric Cancer and Peritoneal Metastasis

In metastatic gastric cancer, expansion into the peritoneal cavity is present in more than 55–60% of patients [85]. Peritoneal dissemination is an important clinical indication, resulting in poor prognosis [86]. Recently, Cristescu et al., 2015 [58] investigated a gene expression dataset of 300 primary gastric tumors to sectionalize four molecular subtypes of GC, which were connected with different patterns of molecular alteration, prognosis of GC patients, progression, and cancer prognosis, which encompass MSS/TP53$^+$ subtype, MSS/TP53$^-$ subtype, MSI subtype, and MSS/EMT subtype. The MSS/EMT subtype includes diffuse tumors type of GC with very poor prognosis, with the disposition to come up in young age and the highest recurrence frequency (63%) of the four classified subtypes is present [58]. An insightful view of the molecular occurrence of each step of peritoneal dissemination is shown in Figure 1, indicating markers of prognosis that are described in the next four sections. Described molecules may contribute to the multiple steps; we tried to highlight their impact on each process while taking into consideration their putative primary involvement to peritoneal dissemination.

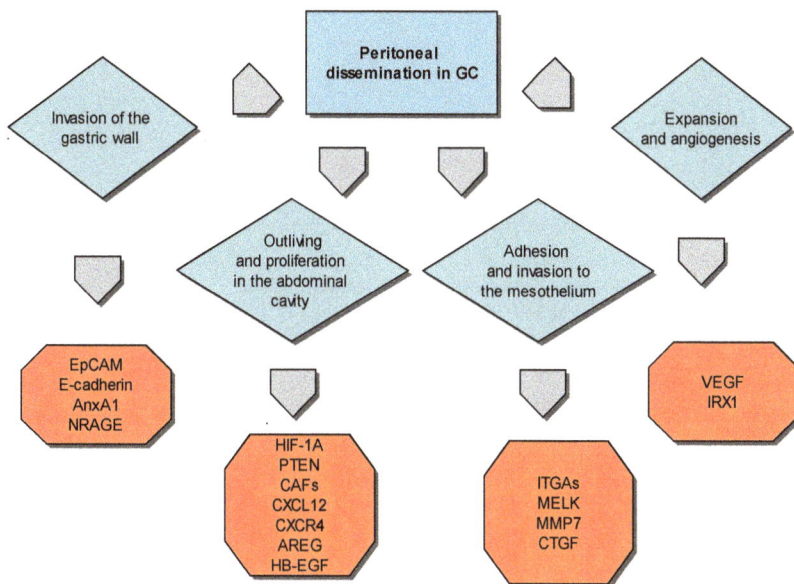

Figure 1. Peritoneal dissemination steps and molecular markers.

10.1. Gastric Cancer Cells Invasiveness

Epithelial cellular adhesion molecule (EpCAM) is a factor that is involved in physical homophilic interaction between intestinal epithelial cells (IECs) and intraepithelial lymphocytes (IELs) at the mucosal epithelium, and it is involved in first line of defence against mucosal infection [87]. The EpCAM expression has been investigated in GC patients with peritoneal metastasis (PM) [88]. They reported that the expression of EpCAM was visibly higher in the PM lesions when compared to the primary lesions. Therefore, the intraperitoneally dosed EpCAM antibody may possibly play a role to contribute to the anti-cancer outcome in PM lesions of GC. In conclusion, the authors gave the suggestion that only GC cells with an increased level of EpCAM have a potential to metastasize to the peritoneum.

E-cadherin (epithelial-cadherin), which was encoded by the *CDH1* gene, is a transmembrane glycoprotein that takes part mainly in cell-cell adhesion maintenance. Its role is regarded to the signalling pathways, which controls cell proliferation, migration, survival, and invasion [89]. Dysregulation of E-cadherin allows for gastric carcinoma development by disturbing gastric epithelial cells [90]. E-cadherin is a tumor suppressor that has been described to be downregulated in gastric cancer [22]. They highlighted the abnormal E-cadherin expression and some connections with tumor stage, grade, depth of invasion, and therefore it might be useful as a predictor for tumor invasiveness in gastric cancer patients. Moreover, genetic alterations in the *CDH1* gene and epigenetic factors, such as DNA hypermethylation, are significant factors to decrease E-cadherin in GC development [91]. The authors observed high correlation of promoter hypermethylation of *CDH1* with gastric cancer, which shows that epigenetics and *CDH1* are important to GC ethology. The group also mentioned that genetic variant C-160A in *CDH1* was associated with cardia, intestinal and diffuse GC. The association between *H. pylori* infection and promoter methylation of *CDH1* gene were studied by Perri et al., 2007 [92] and *CDH1* methylation was categorized as an early event in *H. pylori* gastritis. The environmental effect of *H. pylori* infection on methylation status was assigned to the *H. pylori* eradication therapy in reversal methylation profile among patients with chronic gastritis [93]. In 1998, the linkage between germline mutation in *CDH1* gene and the genetic cause of hereditary diffuse GC (HDGC) was revealed [94]. Germline *CDH1* mutations are connected to the increased lifetime risk of occurring diffuse gastric (DGC). Intestinal-type GC cases do not belong to the HDGC type, and among these families there is no evidence to analyze the *CDH1* mutation [95].

Annexin A1 (AnxA1) is well described glucocorticoid-regulated anti-inflammatory protein. The exogenous and endogenous form of annexin A1 counter-regulate the actions of inborn immune cells, specifically extravasation and the formation of proinflammatory mediators, which control the appropriate level of activation to be reached but not overstepped [96]. The role of AnxA1 in GC survival was described by Cheng et al., 2012 [97]. High expression of AnxA1 was correlated with peritoneal metastasis and serosal invasion. Additionally, AnxA1 expression was certainly associated with invasiveness of human gastric cancer cells both in vitro and in vivo studies. The regulation of cell invasion by AnxA1 was also observed in this study, by the formyl peptide receptor (FPR)/extracellular signal-regulated kinase/integrin beta-1-binding protein pathway, in which all three FPRs (FPR1-FPR3) were committed in this regulation process.

Neurotrophin receptor-interacting melanoma antigen-encoding gene homolog (NRAGE) induces cell apoptosis and suppresses cell metastasis [98]. To understand the role and the clinical importance of NRAGE in GC, Kanda et al., 2016 [99] reported the expression levels of *NRAGE* and its putative interacting genes. Their studies showed the correlation between a higher level of *NRAGE* mRNA expression in GC patients in comparison to normal tissues. Both NRAGE mRNA and protein levels were strictly correlated. Increased NRAGE expression in GCs was connected to the disease-free survival and described as an autonomous marker for GC prognosis. Additionally, expression of *NRAGE* mRNA was observed to be correlated with that of apoptosis antagonizing transcription factor (*AATF*), as well as *NRAGE* knockdown importantly reduced the proliferation, migration, and invasion actions of GC cells.

10.2. Expansion of Peritoneal Dissemination

Peritoneal dissemination very often shows in late-stage GC and it is perceived as a crucial problem that shortens the survival time of patients with gastric carcinoma [100]. Peritoneal milky spots (PMSs) are omentum-associated lymphoid tissues that have been described as the area of origin of immature PMS macrophages [101]. The hypoxic microenvironment is engaged in supervising the tumor stem cell phenotype and is connected to the patient's prognosis through hypoxia-inducible factor-1α (HIF-1α), which is a major transcriptional factor that corresponds to hypoxic stimuli. While the peritoneal dissemination is expanding, the gastric cancer stem/progenitor cells (GCSPCs) are eligible to come into PMSs, in which the hypoxia is maintained. Miao et al., 2014 [102] displayed the correlation of the higher expression of HIF-1α and gastric cancer peritoneal dissemination (GCPD) among GC cases. The GCSPC population expanded in primary gastric cancer cells when hypoxia was present in vitro, also hypoxic GCSPCs displayed intensified self-renewal action, but decreased differentiation ability, which was interceded by HIF-1α. The authors concluded the results to PMSs role, which is assigned to serve a hypoxic niche and favour GCSPCs peritoneal dissemination through HIF-1α.

The tumor suppressor gene phosphatase and tensin homolog (PTEN) is one of the major factors in decreasing tumor growth, expansion, and metastasis [103]. Zhang et al., 2014 [104] revealed a unique action by which PTEN can prohibit the growth and invasion of gastric carcinoma. This mechanism is regarding the downregulation of focal adhesion kinase (FAK) expression and highlights that exploiting *PTEN/PI3K/NF-κB/FAK* axis is an auspicious direction to treat gastric cancer metastasis. The results of this investigation showed that the high expression of PTEN or knockdown in GC cells in consequence provoked the downregulation or the upregulation of FAK, and lowered or raised cell invasion, appropriately. Additionally, FAK increased expression might redeem the inhibition of cell invasion by PTEN. PTEN can inhibit PI3K/NF-κB pathway and reduce the DNA binding of NF-κB on the FAK promoter. Ma et al., 2017 [105] have been reported that low expression of PTEN was detected in a large part of GC tissues, which displayed important associations with differentiation grade in GC patients. PTEN knockdown encouraged the expansion and invasion of cells and could lead to an expected increase in p-AKT, p-GSK-3β, β-catenin, E-cadherin, MMP-7, MMP-2, and MMP-9 in GC cells.

Cancer-associated fibroblasts (CAFs) are apparently responsible for the invasion process and metastatic actions in some cancers, among them gastric cancer is titled, through the activation of CXCL12/CXCR4 signalling [106]. The group investigated increased CXCL12 expression levels, which correlated with grater tumor size, higher tumor depth, lymphatic invasion, and poor prognosis in GC. Stimulation CXCL12/CXCR4 by CAFs interceded integrin β1 clustering at the cell surface increases invasiveness of GC cells. Yasumoto et al., 2006 [107] visibly showed the CXCR4/CXC12 axis actions in the development of peritoneal carcinomatosis from gastric carcinoma. They conducted the calculation of *CXCR4* mRNA expression levels among NUGC4 cells, and it was increased, also the cells displayed sprightly migratory actions, answering to its ligand CXCL12. The CXCL12 intensified proliferation and fast escalations in the phosphorylation of protein kinase B/Akt and extracellular signal-regulated kinase of NUGC4 cells. Analysis showed that 67% primary tumours of the stomach with peritoneal metastasis were positive for CXCR4 expression, in comparison to 25% with another distant metastasis were positive. Explicitly, 85% of CXCR4-expressing primary tumours raised peritoneal metastases. CXCR4 positivity of primary gastric carcinomas meaningfully was associated with the evolution of peritoneal carcinomatosis.

Yasumoto et al., 2011 [108] were interested in whether epidermal growth factor receptor (EGFR) ligands play any role in the expansion of peritoneal spread from gastric cancer. According to their observations, an increased concentration of the EGFR ligands amphiregulin, heparin-binding EGF-like growth factor (HB-EGF) and CXCL12, occurred in malignant ascites. High expression levels of EGFR and CXCR4 mRNA and protein were observed among primary tumours and human gastric cancer cell lines, with an upraised possibility to evoke peritoneal carcinomatosis. Amphiregulin AREG and HB-EGF were provoking factors of intensified proliferation, migration, and functional CXCR4 expression in gastric cancer NUGC4 cells, with the overexpression of CXCR4. These observations drew attention to the EGFR ligands amphiregulin and HB-EGF as important factors, interacting with the CXCL12/CXCR4 axis, in the development of peritoneal spread from gastric cancer.

10.3. Adhesion of Gastric Carcinoma Cells to the Peritoneum

The connection between peritoneal lining and GC cells is a major move in peritoneal dissemination. Takatsuki H et al., 2004 [109] showed that, the peritoneal implantation of NUGC-4 human gastric carcinoma cells in athymic mice, dosing of the cells with anti-alpha2 or anti-alpha3 integrin antibody decreased the number of disseminated nodules. Moreover, suppression by the anti-alpha3 integrin antibody was more powerful than that by the anti-α2 integrin antibody. The cDNAs to human α2 and α3 integrins (ITGAs) were applied into K562 leukemic cells. Those cells displayed a positive occurrence of the integrin beta1 subunit and negative of the α2 or α3 subunit. The α3 integrin-transfected cells were adhered to the monolayer of peritoneal mesothelial cells intensely in comparison to others. Reverse transcription-PCR was applied to detect the expression of laminin-5 and laminin-10/11, which were both high-affinity ligands for alpha3beta1 integrin. mRNA for these isoforms was observed in mesothelial cells from the diaphragm and parietal peritoneum. To conclude, α3β1 integrin is important factor in activation the first steps in attachment of cancer cells to the peritoneum, and therefore allowing for the creation of peritoneal metastasis.

Maternal embryonic leucine zipper kinase (MELK) is a serine/threonine-protein kinase that is engaged in multiple processes, including cell cycle regulation, self-renewal of stem cells, apoptosis and splicing regulation. It has a significant impact on cell proliferation and carcinogenesis [110]. Du et al.,

2014 [111] described the expression of mRNA and protein level of MELK in gastric cancer. Reduction the proliferation, migration, and invasion actions of GC cells were observed after the knockdown of MELK activity, as well as lower number of cells in the G1/G0 phase and higher those in the G2/M and S phases. Further knocking down of the MELK expression was assigned to the decreased quantity of actin stress fibers and inhibited RhoA operations. At the end, the scientists reported that the knockdown of MELK reduced the phosphorylation of the FAK and paxillin, and prevented gastrin-stimulated FAK/paxillin phosphorylation. To summarize the MELK importance, it is an essential factor for causing cell migration and invasion via the FAK/Paxillin pathway, and therefore, it is crucial in GC development.

Matrix metalloproteinase-7 (MMP-7) is an enzyme that plays a role in matrix degrading and impacts on the occurring of invasion and metastasis in gastric cancer patients [112]. Yonemura et al., 2000 [113] investigated experiments to check the machinery creation of peritoneal dissemination among GC cases. The MMP-7 protein level and mRNA expression were studied in primary gastric cancers and peritoneal dissemination. The obtained results revealed the overexpression of *MMP-7* mRNA in 53% of cases regarding primary gastric tumours, whereas in the normal gastric mucosa, fibroblasts, and mesothelial cells, there was negative expression of this marker. Immunohistochemistry analysis displayed the MMP-7 immunoreactivity on the cell membrane and the cytoplasm of GC cancerous cells. The higher MMP-7 protein level was observed among 53% of primary cancers and MMP-7 tissue status had a statistically relevant correlation with lymph node metastasis, weak differentiation, and peritoneal dissemination. Examined GC cases with MMP-7 expression had a worse survival rate and an increased risk of death of peritoneal recurrence. The 100% of investigated peritoneal disseminations expressed *MMP-7* mRNA and 93% revealed immunoreactivity to anti-human MMP-7 monoclonal antibody. The results suggested the substantial role of MMP-7 in the creation of peritoneal dissemination in gastric cancer.

Connective tissue growth factor (CTGF) has been reported to be involved in peritoneal metastasis and gastric cancer progression [114]. High expression of CTGF, as well as treatment with the recombinant protein considerably reduced cell adhesion [115]. CTGF enduring transfectants displayed a lower number and size of tumor nodules in the mesentery, during in vivo peritoneal metastasis. Overexpression of CTGF among GC patients was significantly correlated with the earlier TNM staging and an increased survival rate after the surgery. Coimmunoprecipitation analysis showed that CTGF binds to integrin $\alpha 3$. These results demonstrated that the mediation of GC peritoneal metastasis is occurring through integrin $\alpha 3\beta 1$ attaching to laminin, and CTGF efficiently stops the cooperation by binding to integrin $\alpha 3\beta 1$.

10.4. Peritoneal Spreading and Neovascularization

High expression of *IRX1* gene, which codes iroquois-class homeodomain protein IRX1, was strongly connected with the growth arrest in GC cases. Additionally, the overexpression of *IRX1* gene suppresses peritoneal expansion and spread the tumor metastasis [116]. Human umbilical vein endothelial cells (HUVECs) and chick embryo and SGC-7901 gastric cancer cells were operated for angiogenesis and vasculogenic mimicry (VM) tests. For detecting the function of the downstream target gene of *IRX1*, the bradykinin receptor B2 (*BDKRB2*), small interfering RNA was applied. Results showed the suppression of peritoneal spreading with the reduction of angiogenesis as well as VM creation. The supernatant from SGC-7901/*IRX1* cells, revealed a strong inhibiting effect on angiogenesis both in vitro and in chick embryo.Reduction of tube formation, cell proliferation, and migration, as well as invasion in vitro, were reported by gene-specific RNA interference for *BDKRB2*, or its effector *PAK1*, which codes serine/threonine-protein kinase PAK1. It is now proved that enforcing *IRX1* expression, importantly suppresses peritoneal expansion and pulmonary metastasis via anti-angiogenesis and anti-VM mechanisms.

The important role of angiogenesis in cancer and the cloning of vascular endothelial growth factor (VEGF) in 1989 focused the research studies on this issue and allowed for the important clinical translation of VEGF—directed therapies to the clinic [117]. VEGFR2 receptor expression is limited to vasculature and it is a very significant factor in angiogenesis. Its activation in consequences allow for actuation a complex cascade of downstream signalling pathways that are caused by VEGF receptors, which further results in neovascularization, vasodilation, higher vascular permeability, and migration of bone marrow endothelial cells [118]. VEGF blockade inhibits these pathways and effects tumor survival, migration, and invasion. Advanced gastric cancer is still a huge challenge to find an effective treatment. Monoclonal antibody Ramucirumab can block VEGFR2 activation by binding to it. Randomized phase III trial, called REGARD, was using ramucirumab treatment in comparison to the placebo for patients with advanced, pre-treated gastric cancer, which achieves its initial endpoint of increased total survival [119]. Another RAINBOW trial of paclitaxel with ramucirumab versus paclitaxel with placebo for advanced pre-treated gastric cancer approved the increased survival benefit of ramucirumab, as an antiangiogenic cure among GC patients. Therefore, ramucirumab is the first FDA approved treatment for advanced gastric cancer after previously applied chemotherapy. Recently Roviello et al., 2017 [120] performed a meta-analysis to check the efficacy and the safety of the novel VEGFR-2 inhibitors among cases with metastatic gastric and gastroesophageal junction cancer. A meta-analysis that is based on the literature of randomized controlled trials (RCTs) was investigated. A significant impact of overall survival, which was increased, was detected. This study confirmed the anti-VEGFR-2 inhibitors, like apatinib and ramucirumab positive action [120].

Cyclooxygenase-2 (COX-2) expression is connected to the angiogenesis and *Helicobacter pylori* infection among gastric cancer patients [121]. Immunohistochemical stain against cyclooxygenase 1 and 2 has been investigated among samples that were resected from patients with GC. Among the 72 analysed patients, cases with cyclooxygenase 2-positive staining were tightly correlated with vascular invasion and *H. pylori* infection, as well as poorer prognosis. On the other hand, multivariate analysis displayed that vascular invasion, serosal invasion, and lymph node metastasis were autonomous prognostic factors for patients with gastric cancer, but cyclooxygenase 2 expression was not.

Knowing the apoptotic and proliferative levels among gastric cancer patients may be helpful to find better treatment options and prevention of developing GC. The importance of Ki-67, caspase-3, and p53 expression levels were demonstrated by Xiao et al., 2013 [122], and were correlated with clinical data among patients with GC. The Ki-67 and p53 expression was correlated with tumor-node-metastasis staging. Detection of increased caspase-3 and p53 expression were assigned to the intestinal-type of GC. Correlation between three tested agents: Ki-67, caspase-3, and p53 was statistically significant. Positive correlation among caspase-3 expression and adverse prognosis of GC patients was displayed by the Kaplan-Meier analysis. Additionally, the Cox's proportional hazards model was used to show that several clinical data, such as: age, gender, depth of invasion, lymphatic invasion, lymph node metastasis, TNM staging, Lauren's classification, and caspase-3 expression were autonomous prognostic agents for gastric cancer patients. In conclusion, expression of Ki-67, caspase-3, and p53 can be perceived as factors that influence the differentiation and progression of GC.

11. Conclusions

Gastric cancer is a highly heterogeneous disease. Advantageous studies of the molecular biomarkers of gastric cancer have been deeply investigated, in outcome provided a wide spectrum of signatures in this area. This review summarized the recognition patterns of gastric cancer, including cell cycle regulators, factors that regulates apoptosis, microsatellite instability, multidrug resistance proteins, factors that influence cell membrane properties, module of HER2 expression, and agents with impact on the progression of gastric cancer and peritoneal metastasis. Novel investigation must be done to display specific signatures for the early diagnosis of gastric cancer and for the prediction of chemo/radiotherapy. Nowadays, is it possible to apply high throughput technologies, such as whole genome and exome sequencing, to find various biomarkers with prognostic and diagnosis potential. It is a promising tool to obtain auspicious outcomes to further clinical applications.

Conflicts of Interest: The authors declare no conflict of interest.

References

1. Zhang, X.; Zhang, P. Gastric cancer: Somatic genetics as a guide to therapy. *J. Med. Genet.* **2017**, *54*, 305–312. [CrossRef] [PubMed]
2. Franz, J.L.; Cruz, A.B., Jr. The treatment of gastric cancer with combined surgical resection and chemotherapy. *J. Surg. Oncol.* **1977**, *9*, 131–137. [CrossRef] [PubMed]
3. Coburn, N.; Cosby, R.; Klein, L.; Knight, G.; Malthaner, R.; Mamazza, J.; Mercer, C.D.; Ringash, J. Staging and surgical approaches in gastric cancer: A systematic review. *Cancer Treat. Rev.* **2018**, *63*, 104–115. [CrossRef] [PubMed]
4. Wilke, H.; Preusser, P.; Fink, U.; Gunzer, U.; Meyer, H.J.; Meyer, J.; Siewert, J.R.; Achterrath, W.; Lenaz, L.; Knipp, H. Preoperative chemotherapy in locally advanced and nonresectable gastric cancer: A phase II study with etoposide, doxorubicin, and cisplatin. *J. Clin. Oncol.* **1989**, *7*, 1318–1326. [CrossRef] [PubMed]
5. Kelsen, D.; Karpeh, M.; Schwartz, G.; Gerdes, H.; Lightdale, C.; Botet, J.; Lauers, G.; Klimstra, D.; Huang, Y.; Saltz, L.; et al. Neoadjuvant therapy of high-risk gastric cancer: A phase II trial of preoperative FAMTX and postoperative intraperitoneal fluorouracil-cisplatin plus intravenous fluorouracil. *J. Clin. Oncol.* **1996**, *14*, 1818–1828. [CrossRef] [PubMed]
6. Newman, E.; Marcus, S.G.; Potmesil, M.; Sewak, S.; Yee, H.; Sorich, J.; Hayek, M.; Muggia, F.; Hochster, H. Neoadjuvant chemotherapy with CPT-11 and cisplatin downstages locally advanced gastric cancer. *J. Gastrointest. Surg.* **2002**, *6*, 212–223. [CrossRef]
7. Songun, I.; Keizer, H.J.; Hermans, J.; Klementschitsch, P.; de Vries, J.E.; Wils, J.A.; van der Bijl, J.; van Krieken, J.H.; van de Velde, C.J. Chemotherapy for operable gastric cancer: Results of the Dutch randomised FAMTX trial. The Dutch Gastric Cancer Group (DGCG). *Eur. J. Cancer* **1999**, *35*, 558–562. [CrossRef]
8. Rosenberg, S. Lymphokine-activated killer cells: A new approach to immunotherapy of cancer. *J. Natl. Cancer Inst.* **1985**, *75*, 595–603. [PubMed]
9. Rosenberg, S.A.; Spiess, P.; Lafreniere, R. A new approach to the adoptive immunotherapy of cancer with tumor-infiltrating lymphocytes. *Science* **1986**, *233*, 1318–1321. [CrossRef] [PubMed]
10. Yun, Y.S.; Hargrove, M.E.; Ting, C.C. In vivo antitumor activity of anti-CD3-induced activated killer cells. *Cancer Res.* **1989**, *49*, 4770–4774. [PubMed]
11. Kyte, J.A.; Gaudernack, G. Immuno-gene therapy of cancer with tumour-mRNA transfected dendritic cells. *Cancer Immunol. Immunother.* **2006**, *55*, 1432–1442. [CrossRef] [PubMed]
12. Kono, K.; Rongcun, Y.; Charo, J.; Ichihara, F.; Celis, E.; Sette, A.; Appella, E.; Sekikawa, T.; Matsumoto, Y.; Kiessling, R. Identification of HER2/neu-derived peptide epitopes recognized by gastric cancer-specific cytotoxic T lymphocytes. *Int. J. Cancer* **1998**, *78*, 202–208. [CrossRef]
13. Traversari, C.; van der Bruggen, P.; Luescher, I.F.; Lurquin, C.; Chomez, P.; Van Pel, A.; de Plaen, E.; Amar-Costesec, A.; Boon, T. A nonapeptide encoded by human gene MAGE-1 is recognized on HLA-A1 by cytolytic T lymphocytes directed against tumor antigen MZ2-E. *J. Exp. Med.* **1992**, *176*, 1453–1457. [CrossRef] [PubMed]
14. Gulley, M.L.; Tang, W. Laboratory assays for Epstein–Barr virus-related disease. *J. Mol. Diagn.* **2008**, *10*, 279–292. [CrossRef] [PubMed]
15. Tsurumi, T.; Fujita, M.; Kudoh, A. Latent and lytic *Epstein-Barr virus* replication strategies. *Rev. Med. Virol.* **2005**, *15*, 3–15. [CrossRef] [PubMed]
16. Klutts, J.S.; Ford, B.A.; Perez, N.R.; Gronowski, A.M. Evidence-Based Approach for Interpretation of *Epstein-Barr virus* Serological Patterns. *J. Clin. Microbiol.* **2009**, *47*, 3204–3210. [CrossRef] [PubMed]
17. Weiss, L.M.; Chen, Y.Y. EBER in situ hybridization for *Epstein-Barr virus*. *Methods Mol. Biol.* **2013**, *999*, 223–230. [PubMed]
18. Zur Hausen, A.; van Rees, B.P.; van Beek, J.; Craanen, M.E.; Bloemena, E.; Offerhaus, G.J.; Meijer, C.J.; van den Brule, A.J. *Epstein-Barr virus* in gastric carcinomas and gastric stump carcinomas: A late event in gastric carcinogenesis. *J. Clin. Pathol.* **2004**, *57*, 487–491. [CrossRef] [PubMed]

19. Kim, J.; Lee, H.S.; Bae, S.I.; Lee, Y.M.; Kim, W.H. Silencing and CpG island methylation of GSTP1 is rare in ordinary gastric carcinomas but common in *Epstein-Barr virus*-associated gastric carcinomas. *Anticancer Res.* **2005**, *25*, 4013–4019. [PubMed]

20. Sudo, M.; Chong, J.M.; Sakuma, K.; Ushiku, T.; Uozaki, H.; Nagai, H.; Funata, N.; Matsumoto, Y.; Fukayama, M. Promoter hypermethylation of E-cadherin and its abnormal expression in *Epstein-Barr virus*-associated gastric carcinoma. *Int. J. Cancer* **2004**, *109*, 194–199. [CrossRef] [PubMed]

21. Zhao, J.; Liang, Q.; Cheung, K.F.; Kang, W.; Lung, R.W.; Tong, J.H.; To, K.F.; Sung, J.J.; Yu, J. Genome-wide identification of *Epstein-Barr virus*-driven promoter methylation profiles of human genes in gastric cancer cells. *Cancer* **2013**, *119*, 304–312. [CrossRef] [PubMed]

22. Bass, A.J.; Thorsson, V.; Shmulevich, I.; Reynolds, S.M.; Miller, M.; Bernard, B.; Hinoue, T.; Laird, P.W.; Curtis, C.; Shen, H.; et al. Comprehensive molecular characterization of gastric adenocarcinoma. *Nature* **2014**, *513*, 202–209. [CrossRef] [PubMed]

23. Akiyama, T.; Sudo, C.; Ogawara, H.; Toyoshima, K.; Yamamoto, T. The product of the human c-erbB-2 gene: A 185-kilodalton glycoprotein with tyrosine kinase activity. *Science* **1986**, *232*, 1644–1646. [CrossRef] [PubMed]

24. Kim, M.A.; Jung, E.J.; Lee, H.S.; Lee, H.E.; Jeon, Y.K.; Yang, H.K.; Kim, W.H. Evaluation of *HER-2* gene status in gastric carcinoma using immunohistochemistry, fluorescence in situ hybridization, and real-time quantitative polymerase chain reaction. *Hum. Pathol.* **2007**, *38*, 1386–1393. [CrossRef] [PubMed]

25. Takehana, T.; Kunitomo, K.; Kono, K.; Kitahara, F.; Iizuka, H.; Matsumoto, Y.; Fujino, M.A.; Ooi, A. Status of c-erbB-2 in gastric adenocarcinoma: A comparative study of immunohistochemistry, fluorescence in situ hybridization and enzyme-linked immuno-sorbent assay. *Int. J. Cancer* **2002**, *98*, 833–837. [CrossRef] [PubMed]

26. Tsapralis, D.; Panayiotides, I.; Peros, G.; Liakakos, T.; Karamitopoulou, E. Human epidermal growth factor receptor-2 gene amplification in gastric cancer using tissue microarray technology. *World J. Gastroenterol.* **2012**, *18*, 150–155. [CrossRef] [PubMed]

27. Hofmann, M.; Stoss, O.; Shi, D.; Büttner, R.; van de Vijver, M.; Kim, W.; Ochiai, A.; Rüschoff, J.; Henkel, T. Assessment of a HER2 scoring system for gastric cancer: Results from a validation study. *Histopathology* **2008**, *52*, 797–805. [CrossRef] [PubMed]

28. Fujimoto-Ouchi, K.; Sekiguchi, F.; Yasuno, H.; Moriya, Y.; Mori, K.; Tanaka, Y. Antitumor activity of trastuzumab in combination with chemotherapy in human gastric cancer xenograft models. *Cancer Chemother. Pharmacol.* **2007**, *59*, 795–805. [CrossRef] [PubMed]

29. Tanner, M.; Hollmén, M.; Junttila, T.T.; Kapanen, A.I.; Tommola, S.; Soini, Y.; Helin, H.; Salo, J.; Joensuu, H.; Sihvo, E. Amplification of HER-2 in gastric carcinoma: Association with Topoisomerase IIα gene amplification, intestinal type, poor prognosis and sensitivity to trastuzumab. *Ann. Oncol.* **2005**, *16*, 273–278. [CrossRef] [PubMed]

30. Kasprzyk, P.G.; Song, S.U.; Di Fiore, P.P.; King, C.R. Therapy of an animal model of human gastric cancer using a combination of anti-erbB-2 monoclonal antibodies. *Cancer Res.* **1992**, *52*, 2771–2776. [PubMed]

31. Nicholas, G.; Cripps, C.; Au, H.J.; et al. Early results of a trial of trastuzumab, cisplatin and docetaxel (TCD) for the treatment of metastatic gastric cancer overexpressing HER2. *Ann. Oncol.* **2006**, *17*, 316.

32. Yuza, K.; Nagahashi, M.; Watanabe, S.; Takabe, K.; Wakai, T. Hypermutation and microsatellite instability in gastrointestinal cancers. *Oncotarget* **2017**, *8*, 112103–112115. [CrossRef] [PubMed]

33. Hang, X.; Li, D.; Wang, J.; Wang, G. Prognostic significance of microsatellite instability-associated pathways and genes in gastric cancer. *Int. J. Mol. Med.* **2018**, *42*, 149–160. [CrossRef] [PubMed]

34. Ye, P.; Shi, Y.; Li, A. Association between hMLH1 Promoter Methylation and Risk of Gastric Cancer: A Meta-Analysis. *Front. Physiol.* **2018**, *9*, 368. [CrossRef] [PubMed]

35. Polom, K.; Marrelli, D.; Smyth, E.C.; Voglino, C.; Roviello, G.; Pascale, V.; Varas, J.; Vindigni, C.; Roviello, F. The Role of Microsatellite Instability in Positive Margin Gastric Cancer Patients. *Surg. Innov.* **2018**, *25*, 99–104. [CrossRef] [PubMed]

36. Beck, F.; Chawengsaksophak, K.; Waring, P.; Playford, R.J.; Furness, J.B. Reprogramming of intestinal differentiation and intercalary regeneration in Cdx2 mutant mice. *Proc. Natl. Acad. Sci. USA* **1999**, *96*, 7318–7323. [CrossRef] [PubMed]

37. Freund, J.N.; Domon-Dell, C.; Kedinger, M.; Duluc, I. The *Cdx-1* and *Cdx-2* homeobox genes in the intestine. *Biochem. Cell Biol.* **1998**, *76*, 957–969. [CrossRef] [PubMed]

38. Bai, Y.Q.; Miyake, S.; Iwai, T.; Yuasa, Y. CDX2, a homeobox transcription factor, upregulates transcription of the p21/WAF1/CIP1 gene. *Oncogene* **2003**, *22*, 7942–7949. [CrossRef] [PubMed]

39. Park, D.Y.; Srivastava, A.; Kim, G.H.; Mino-Kenudson, M.; Deshpande, V.; Zukerberg, L.R.; Song, G.A.; Lauwers, G.Y. CDX2 expression in the intestinal-type gastric epithelial neoplasia: Frequency and significance. *Mod. Pathol.* **2010**, *23*, 54–61. [CrossRef] [PubMed]

40. Huang, W.B.; Zhou, X.J.; Chen, J.Y.; Zhang, L.H.; Meng, K.; Ma, H.H.; Lu, Z.F. CD10-positive stromal cells in gastric carcinoma: Correlation with invasion and metastasis. *Jpn. J. Clin. Oncol.* **2005**, *35*, 245–250. [CrossRef] [PubMed]

41. You, J.; Bird, R.C. Selective induction of cell cycle regulatory genes *cdk1* (*p34cdc2*), cyclins A/B, and the tumor suppressor gene *Rb* in transformed cells by okadaic acid. *J. Cell. Physiol.* **1995**, *164*, 424–433. [CrossRef] [PubMed]

42. Rafferty, M.A.; Fenton, J.E.; Jones, A.S. An overview of the role and inter-relationship of epidermal growth factor receptor, cyclin D and retinoblastoma protein on the carcinogenesis of squamous cell carcinoma of the larynx. *Clin. Otolaryngol. Allied Sci.* **2001**, *26*, 317–320. [CrossRef] [PubMed]

43. Arici, D.S.; Tuncer, E.; Ozer, H.; Simek, G.; Koyuncu, A. Expression of retinoblastoma and cyclin D1 in gastric carcinoma. *Neoplasma* **2009**, *56*, 63–67. [CrossRef] [PubMed]

44. Gao, P.; Zhou, G.Y.; Liu, Y.; Li, J.S.; Zhen, J.H.; Yuan, Y.P. Alteration of cyclin D1 in gastric carcinoma and its clinicopathologic significance. *World J. Gastroenterol.* **2004**, *10*, 2936–2939. [CrossRef] [PubMed]

45. Serrano, M.; Hannon, G.J.; Beach, D. A new regulatory motif in cell-cycle control causing specific inhibition of cyclin D/CDK4. *Nature* **1993**, *366*, 704–707. [CrossRef] [PubMed]

46. Hayashi, K.; Metzger, R.; Salonga, D.; Danenberg, K.; Leichman, L.P.; Fink, U.; Sendler, A.; Kelsen, D.; Schwartz, G.K.; Groshen, S.; et al. High frequency of simultaneous loss of p16 and p16beta gene expression in squamous cell carcinoma of the esophagus but not in adenocarcinoma of the esophagus or stomach. *Oncogene* **1997**, *15*, 1481–1488. [CrossRef] [PubMed]

47. Wu, M.S.; Shun, C.T.; Sheu, J.C.; Wang, H.P.; Wang, J.T.; Lee, W.J.; Chen, C.J.; Wang, T.H.; Lin, J.T. Overexpression of mutant p53 and c-erbB-2 proteins and mutations of the *p15* and *p16* genes in human gastric carcinoma: With respect to histological subtypes and stages. *J. Gastroenterol. Hepatol.* **1998**, *13*, 305–310. [CrossRef] [PubMed]

48. Ficorella, C.; Cannita, K.; Ricevuto, E.; Toniato, E.; Fusco, C.; Sinopoli, N.T.; De Galitiis, F.; Di Rocco, Z.C.; Porzio, G.; Frati, L.; et al. P16 hypermethylation contributes to the characterization of gene inactivation profiles in primary gastric cancer. *Oncol. Rep.* **2003**, *10*, 169–173. [CrossRef] [PubMed]

49. Cuesta, R.; Martinez-Sanchez, A.; Gebauer, F. miR-181a regulates cap-dependent translation of p27(kip1) mRNA in myeloid cells. *Mol. Cell. Biol.* **2009**, *29*, 2841–2851. [CrossRef] [PubMed]

50. Nitti, D.; Belluco, C.; Mammano, E.; Marchet, A.; Ambrosi, A.; Mencarelli, R.; Segato, P.; Lise, M. Low level of p27(Kip1) protein expression in gastric adenocarcinoma is associated with disease progression and poor outcome. *J. Surg. Oncol.* **2002**, *81*, 167–175. [CrossRef] [PubMed]

51. Zheng, J.Y.; Wang, W.Z.; Li, K.Z.; Guan, W.X.; Yan, W. Effect of p27(KIP1) on cell cycle and apoptosis in gastric cancer cells. *World J. Gastroenterol.* **2005**, *11*, 7072–7077. [CrossRef] [PubMed]

52. Tsai, L.H.; Harlow, E.; Meyerson, M. Isolation of the human *cdk2* gene that encodes the cyclin A- and adenovirus E1A-associated p33 kinase. *Nature* **1991**, *353*, 174–177. [CrossRef] [PubMed]

53. Luo, D.H.; Zhou, Q.; Hu, S.K.; Xia, Y.Q.; Xu, C.C.; Lin, T.S.; Pan, Y.T.; Wu, J.S.; Jin, R. Differential expression of Notch1 intracellular domain and p21 proteins, and their clinical significance in gastric cancer. *Oncol. Lett.* **2014**, *7*, 471–478. [CrossRef] [PubMed]

54. Gonçalves, A.R.; Carneiro, A.J.; Martins, I.; de Faria, P.A.; Ferreira, M.A.; de Mello, E.L.; Fogaça, H.S.; Elia, C.C.; de Souza, H.S. Prognostic significance of p53 protein expression in early gastric cancer. *Pathol. Oncol. Res.* **2011**, *17*, 349–355. [CrossRef] [PubMed]

55. Gomyo, Y.; Osaki, M.; Kaibara, N.; Ito, H. Numerical aberration and point mutation of *p53* gene in human gastric intestinal metaplasia and well-differentiated adenocarcinoma: Analysis by fluorescence in situ hybridization (FISH) and PCR-SSCP. *Int. J. Cancer* **1996**, *66*, 594–599. [CrossRef]

56. Hongyo, T.; Buzard, G.S.; Palli, D.; Weghorst, C.M.; Amorosi, A.; Galli, M.; Caporaso, N.E.; Fraumeni, J.F., Jr.; Rice, J.M. Mutations of the *K-ras* and *p53* genes in gastric adenocarcinomas from a high-incidence region around Florence, Italy. *Cancer Res.* **1995**, *55*, 2665–2672. [PubMed]

57. Kushima, R.; Müller, W.; Stolte, M.; Borchard, F. Differential p53 protein expression in stomach adenomas of gastric and intestinal phenotypes: Possible sequences of p53 alteration in stomach carcinogenesis. *Virchows Arch.* **1996**, *428*, 223–227. [CrossRef] [PubMed]

58. Cristescu, R.; Lee, J.; Nebozhyn, M.; Kim, K.M.; Ting, J.C.; Wong, S.S.; Liu, J.; Yue, Y.G.; Wang, J.; Yu, K.; et al. Molecular analysis of gastric cancer identifies subtypes associated with distinct clinical outcomes. *Nat. Med.* **2015**, *21*, 449–456. [CrossRef] [PubMed]

59. Tamura, T.; Ohira, M.; Tanaka, H.; Muguruma, K.; Toyokawa, T.; Kubo, N.; Sakurai, K.; Amano, R.; Kimura, K.; Shibutani, M.; et al. Programmed Death-1 Ligand-1 (PDL1) Expression Is Associated with the Prognosis of Patients with Stage II/III Gastric Cancer. *Anticancer Res.* **2015**, *35*, 5369–5376. [PubMed]

60. Xing, X.; Guo, J.; Wen, X.; Ding, G.; Li, B.; Dong, B.; Feng, Q.; Li, S.; Zhang, J.; Cheng, X.; et al. Analysis of PD1, PDL1, PDL2 expression and T cells infiltration in 1014 gastric cancer patients. *Oncoimmunology* **2017**, *7*, e1356144. [CrossRef] [PubMed]

61. Böger, C.; Behrens, H.M.; Mathiak, M.; Krüger, S.; Kalthoff, H.; Röcken, C. PD-L1 is an independent prognostic predictor in gastric cancer of Western patients. *Oncotarget* **2016**, *7*, 24269–24283. [CrossRef] [PubMed]

62. Kang, M.J.; Park, B.J.; Byun, D.S.; Park, J.I.; Kim, H.J.; Park, J.H.; Chi, S.G. Loss of imprinting and elevated expression of wild-type p73 in human gastric adenocarcinoma. *Clin. Cancer Res.* **2000**, 1767–1771.

63. Oliner, J.D.; Kinzler, K.W.; Meltzer, P.S.; George, D.L.; Vogelstein, B. Amplification of a gene encoding a p53-associated protein in human sarcomas. *Nature* **1992**, *358*, 80–83. [CrossRef] [PubMed]

64. Günther, T.; Schneider-Stock, R.; Häckel, C.; Kasper, H.U.; Pross, M.; Hackelsberger, A.; Lippert, H.; Roessner, A. *Mdm2* gene amplification in gastric cancer correlation with expression of Mdm2 protein and p53 alterations. *Mod. Pathol.* **2000**, *13*, 621–626. [CrossRef] [PubMed]

65. Nakajima, N.; Ito, Y.; Yokoyama, K.; Uno, A.; Kinukawa, N.; Nemoto, N.; Moriyama, M. The expression of murine double minute 2 (MDM2) on helicobacter pylori-infected intestinal metaplasia and gastric cancer. *J. Clin. Biochem. Nutr.* **2009**, *44*, 196–202. [CrossRef] [PubMed]

66. Wang, L.; Zhang, X.Y.; Xu, L.; Liu, W.J.; Zhang, J.; Zhang, J.P. Expression and significance of p53 and mdm2 in atypical intestinal metaplasia and gastric carcinoma. *Oncol. Lett.* **2011**, *2*, 707–712. [CrossRef] [PubMed]

67. Wu, J.; Liu, X.; Cai, H.; Wang, Y. Prediction of tumor recurrence after curative resection in gastric carcinoma based on bcl-2 expression. *World J. Surg. Oncol.* **2014**, *12*, 40. [CrossRef] [PubMed]

68. Sugitani, N.; Sivley, R.M.; Perry, K.E.; Capra, J.A.; Chazin, W.J. XPA: A key scaffold for human nucleotide excision repair. *DNA Repair* **2016**, *44*, 123–135. [CrossRef] [PubMed]

69. Dong, Z.; Guo, W.; Zhou, R.; Wan, L.; Li, Y.; Wang, N.; Kuang, G.; Wang, S. Polymorphisms of the DNA repair gene XPA and XPC and its correlation with gastric cardiac adenocarcinoma in a high incidence population in North China. *J. Clin. Gastroenterol.* **2008**, *42*, 910–915. [CrossRef] [PubMed]

70. D'Errico, M.; Parlanti, E.; Teson, M.; de Jesus, B.M.; Degan, P.; Calcagnile, A.; Jaruga, P.; Bjørås, M.; Crescenzi, M.; Pedrini, A.M.; et al. New functions of XPC in the protection of human skin cells from oxidative damage. *EMBO J.* **2006**, *25*, 4305–4315. [CrossRef] [PubMed]

71. Dusinská, M.; Dzupinková, Z.; Wsólová, L.; Harrington, V.; Collins, A.R. Possible involvement of XPA in repair of oxidative DNA damage deduced from analysis of damage, repair and genotype in a human population study. *Mutagenesis* **2006**, *21*, 205–211. [CrossRef] [PubMed]

72. Sandusky, G.E.; Mintze, K.S.; Pratt, S.E.; Dantzig, A.H. Expression of multidrug resistance-associated protein 2 (MRP2) in normal human tissues and carcinomas using tissue microarrays. *Histopathology* **2002**, *41*, 65–74. [CrossRef] [PubMed]

73. Toffoli, G.; Cecchin, E. Pharmacogenetics of stomach cancer. *Suppl. Tumori* **2003**, *2*, S19–S22. [PubMed]

74. Qiao, W.; Wang, T.; Zhang, L.; Tang, Q.; Wang, D.; Sun, H. Association between single genetic polymorphisms of MDR1 gene and gastric cancer susceptibility in Chinese. *Med. Oncol.* **2013**, *30*, 643. [CrossRef] [PubMed]

75. Zhu, C.Y.; Lv, Y.P.; Yan, D.F.; Gao, F.L. Knockdown of MDR1 increases the sensitivity to adriamycin in drug resistant gastric cancer cells. *Asian Pac. J. Cancer Prev.* **2013**, *14*, 6757–6760. [CrossRef] [PubMed]

76. Hayes, P.C.; Bouchier, I.A.; Beckett, G.J. Glutathione S-transferase in humans in health and disease. *Gut* **1991**, *32*, 813–818. [CrossRef] [PubMed]

77. Yu, P.; Du, Y.; Cheng, X.; Yu, Q.; Huang, L.; Dong, R. Expression of multidrug resistance-associated proteins and their relation to postoperative individualized chemotherapy in gastric cancer. *World J. Surg. Oncol.* **2014**, *12*, 307. [CrossRef] [PubMed]

78. Dekker, J.; Rossen, J.W.; Büller, H.A.; Einerhand, A.W. The MUC family: An obituary. *Trends Biochem. Sci.* **2002**, *27*, 126–131. [CrossRef]

79. Marin, F.; Luquet, G.; Marie, B.; Medakovic, D. Molluscan shell proteins: Primary structure, origin, and evolution. *Curr. Top. Dev. Biol.* **2008**, *80*, 209–276. [PubMed]

80. Lee, H.S.; Lee, H.K.; Kim, H.S.; Yang, H.K.; Kim, Y.I.; Kim, W.H. MUC1, MUC2, MUC5AC, and MUC6 expressions in gastric carcinomas: Their roles as prognostic indicators. *Cancer* **2001**, *92*, 1427–1434. [CrossRef]

81. Wang, X.T.; Kong, F.B.; Mai, W.; Li, L.; Pang, L.M. MUC1 Immunohistochemical Expression as a Prognostic Factor in Gastric Cancer: Meta-Analysis. *Dis. Mark.* **2016**, *2016*, 9421571. [CrossRef] [PubMed]

82. Park, K.K.; Yang, S.I.; Seo, K.W.; Yoon, K.Y.; Lee, S.H.; Jang, H.K.; Shin, Y.M. Correlations of Human Epithelial Growth Factor Receptor 2 Overexpression with MUC2, MUC5AC, MUC6, p53, and Clinicopathological Characteristics in Gastric Cancer Patients with Curative Resection. *Gastroenterol. Res. Pract.* **2015**, *2015*, 946359. [CrossRef] [PubMed]

83. Zhang, C.T.; He, K.C.; Pan, F.; Li, Y.; Wu, J. Prognostic value of Muc5AC in gastric cancer: A meta-analysis. *World J. Gastroenterol.* **2015**, *21*, 10453–10460. [CrossRef] [PubMed]

84. Kim, D.H.; Shin, N.; Kim, G.H.; Song, G.A.; Jeon, T.Y.; Kim, D.H.; Lauwers, G.Y.; Park, D.Y. Mucin expression in gastric cancer: Reappraisal of its clinicopathologic and prognostic significance. *Arch. Pathol. Lab. Med.* **2013**, *137*, 1047–1053. [CrossRef] [PubMed]

85. Siegel, R.; Naishadham, D.; Jemal, A. Cancer statistics, 2012. *CA Cancer J. Clin.* **2012**, *62*, 10–29. [CrossRef] [PubMed]

86. Shen, L.; Shan, Y.S.; Hu, H.M.; Price, T.J.; Sirohi, B.; Yeh, K.H.; Yang, Y.H.; Sano, T.; Yang, H.K.; Zhang, X.; et al. Management of gastric cancer in Asia: Resource-stratified guidelines. *Lancet Oncol.* **2013**, *14*, e535–e547. [CrossRef]

87. Trzpis, M.; McLaughlin, P.M.; de Leij, L.M.; Harmsen, M.C. Epithelial cell adhesion molecule: More than a carcinoma marker and adhesion molecule. *Am. J. Pathol.* **2007**, *171*, 386–395. [CrossRef] [PubMed]

88. Imano, M.; Itoh, T.; Satou, T.; Yasuda, A.; Nishiki, K.; Kato, H.; Shiraishi, O.; Peng, Y.F.; Shinkai, M.; Tsubaki, M.; et al. High expression of epithelial cellular adhesion molecule in peritoneal metastasis of gastric cancer. *Target. Oncol.* **2013**, *8*, 231–235. [CrossRef] [PubMed]

89. Van Roy, F.; Berx, G. The cell-cell adhesion molecule E-cadherin. *Cell. Mol. Life Sci.* **2008**, *65*, 3756–3788. [CrossRef] [PubMed]

90. Till, J.E.; Yoon, S.S.; Ryeom, S. E-cadherin and K-ras: Implications of a newly developed model of gastric cancer. *Oncoscience* **2017**, *4*, 162–163. [PubMed]

91. Lee, H.S.; Choi, S.I.; Lee, H.K.; Kim, H.S.; Yang, H.K.; Kang, G.H.; Kim, Y.I.; Lee, B.L.; Kim, W.H. Distinct clinical features and outcomes of gastric cancers with microsatellite instability. *Mod. Pathol.* **2002**, *15*, 632–640. [CrossRef] [PubMed]

92. Perri, F.; Cotugno, R.; Piepoli, A.; Merla, A.; Quitadamo, M.; Gentile, A.; Pilotto, A.; Annese, V.; Andriulli, A. Aberrant DNA methylation in non-neoplastic gastric mucosa of H. Pylori infected patients and effect of eradication. *Am. J. Gastroenterol.* **2007**, *102*, 1361–1371. [CrossRef] [PubMed]

93. Chan, A.O.; Peng, J.Z.; Lam, S.K.; Lai, K.C.; Yuen, M.F.; Cheung, H.K.; Kwong, Y.L.; Rashid, A.; Chan, C.K.; Wong, B.C. Eradication of Helicobacter pylori infection reverses E-cadherin promoter hypermethylation. *Gut* **2006**, *55*, 463–468. [CrossRef] [PubMed]

94. Guilford, P.; Hopkins, J.; Harraway, J.; McLeod, M.; McLeod, N.; Harawira, P.; Taite, H.; Scoular, R.; Miller, A.; Reeve, A.E. E-cadherin germline mutations in familial gastric cancer. *Nature* **1998**, *392*, 402–405. [CrossRef] [PubMed]

95. Van der Post, R.S.; Vogelaar, I.P.; Carneiro, F.; Guilford, P.; Huntsman, D.; Hoogerbrugge, N.; Caldas, C.; Schreiber, K.E.; Hardwick, R.H.; Ausems, M.G.; et al. Hereditary diffuse gastric cancer: Updated clinical guidelines with an emphasis on germline *CDH1* mutation carriers. *J. Med. Genet.* **2015**, *52*, 361–374. [CrossRef] [PubMed]

96. Perretti, M.; D'Acquisto, F. Annexin A1 and glucocorticoids as effectors of the resolution of inflammation. *Nat. Rev. Immunol.* **2009**, *9*, 62–70. [CrossRef] [PubMed]

97. Cheng, T.Y.; Wu, M.S.; Lin, J.T.; Lin, M.T.; Shun, C.T.; Huang, H.Y.; Hua, K.T.; Kuo, M.L. Annexin A1 is associated with gastric cancer survival and promotes gastric cancer cell invasiveness through the formyl peptide receptor/extracellular signal-regulated kinase/integrin beta-1-binding protein 1 pathway. *Cancer* **2012**, *118*, 5757–5767. [PubMed]

98. Zhang, G.; Zhou, H.; Xue, X. Complex roles of NRAGE on tumor. *Tumour Biol.* **2016**, *37*, 11535–11540. [CrossRef] [PubMed]

99. Kanda, M.; Shimizu, D.; Fujii, T.; Tanaka, H.; Tanaka, Y.; Ezaka, K.; Shibata, M.; Takami, H.; Hashimoto, R.; Sueoka, S.; et al. Neurotrophin Receptor-Interacting Melanoma Antigen-Encoding Gene Homolog is Associated with Malignant Phenotype of Gastric Cancer. *Ann. Surg. Oncol.* **2016**, *23* (Suppl. S4), 532–539. [CrossRef] [PubMed]

100. Yan, T.D.; Black, D.; Sugarbaker, P.H.; Zhu, J.; Yonemura, Y.; Petrou, G.; Morris, D.L. A systematic review and meta-analysis of the randomized controlled trials on adjuvant intraperitoneal chemotherapy for resectable gastric cancer. *Ann. Surg. Oncol.* **2007**, *14*, 2702–2713. [CrossRef] [PubMed]

101. Mebius, R.E. Lymphoid organs for peritoneal cavity immune response: Milky spots. *Immunity* **2009**, *30*, 670–672. [CrossRef] [PubMed]

102. Miao, Z.F.; Wang, Z.N.; Zhao, T.T.; Xu, Y.Y.; Gao, J.; Miao, F.; Xu, H.M. Peritoneal milky spots serve as a hypoxic niche and favor gastric cancer stem/progenitor cell peritoneal dissemination through hypoxia-inducible factor 1α. *Stem Cells* **2014**, *32*, 3062–3074. [CrossRef] [PubMed]

103. Chu, E.C.; Tarnawski, A.S. PTEN regulatory functions in tumor suppression and cell biology. *Med. Sci. Monit.* **2004**, *10*, RA235–RA241. [PubMed]

104. Zhang, L.L.; Liu, J.; Lei, S.; Zhang, J.; Zhou, W.; Yu, H.G. PTEN inhibits the invasion and metastasis of gastric cancer via downregulation of FAK expression. *Cell Signal.* **2014**, *26*, 1011–1020. [CrossRef] [PubMed]

105. Ma, J.; Guo, X.; Zhang, J.; Wu, D.; Hu, X.; Li, J.; Lan, Q.; Liu, Y.; Dong, W. PTEN Gene Induces Cell Invasion and Migration via Regulating AKT/GSK-3β/β-Catenin Signaling Pathway in Human Gastric Cancer. *Dig. Dis. Sci.* **2017**, *62*, 3415–3425. [CrossRef] [PubMed]

106. Izumi, D.; Ishimoto, T.; Miyake, K.; Sugihara, H.; Eto, K.; Sawayama, H.; Yasuda, T.; Kiyozumi, Y.; Kaida, T.; Kurashige, J.; et al. CXCL12/CXCR4 activation by cancer-associated fibroblasts promotes integrin β1 clustering and invasiveness in gastric cancer. *Int. J. Cancer* **2016**, *138*, 1207–1219. [CrossRef] [PubMed]

107. Yasumoto, K.; Koizumi, K.; Kawashima, A.; Saitoh, Y.; Arita, Y.; Shinohara, K.; Minami, T.; Nakayama, T.; Sakurai, H.; Takahashi, Y.; et al. Role of the CXCL12/CXCR4 axis in peritoneal carcinomatosis of gastric cancer. *Cancer Res.* **2006**, *66*, 2181–2187. [CrossRef] [PubMed]

108. Yasumoto, K.; Yamada, T.; Kawashima, A.; Wang, W.; Li, Q.; Donev, I.S.; Tacheuchi, S.; Mouri, H.; Yamashita, K.; Ohtsubo, K.; et al. The EGFR ligands amphiregulin and heparin-binding egf-like growth factor promote peritoneal carcinomatosis in CXCR4-expressing gastric cancer. *Clin. Cancer Res.* **2011**, *17*, 3619–3630. [CrossRef] [PubMed]

109. Takatsuki, H.; Komatsu, S.; Sano, R.; Takada, Y.; Tsuji, T. Adhesion of gastric carcinoma cells to peritoneum mediated by alpha3beta1 integrin (VLA-3). *Cancer Res.* **2004**, *64*, 6065–6070. [CrossRef] [PubMed]

110. Nakano, I.; Paucar, A.A.; Bajpai, R.; Dougherty, J.D.; Zewail, A.; Kelly, T.K.; Kim, K.J.; Ou, J.; Groszer, M.; Imura, T.; et al. Maternal embryonic leucine zipper kinase (MELK) regulates multipotent neural progenitor proliferation. *J. Cell Biol.* **2005**, *170*, 413–427. [CrossRef] [PubMed]

111. Du, T.; Qu, Y.; Li, J.; Li, H.; Su, L.; Zhou, Q.; Yan, M.; Li, C.; Zhu, Z.; Liu, B. Maternal embryonic leucine zipper kinase enhances gastric cancer progression via the FAK/Paxillin pathway. *Mol. Cancer* **2014**, *13*, 100. [CrossRef] [PubMed]

112. Kitoh, T.; Yanai, H.; Saitoh, Y.; Nakamura, Y.; Matsubara, Y.; Kitoh, H.; Yoshida, T.; Okita, K. Increased expression of matrix metalloproteinase-7 in invasive early gastric cancer. *J. Gastroenterol.* **2004**, *39*, 434–440. [CrossRef] [PubMed]

113. Yonemura, Y.; Endou, Y.; Fujita, H.; Fushida, S.; Bandou, E.; Taniguchi, K.; Miwa, K.; Sugiyama, K.; Sasaki, T. Role of MMP-7 in the formation of peritoneal dissemination in gastric cancer. *Gastric Cancer* **2000**, *3*, 63–70. [CrossRef] [PubMed]

114. Jiang, C.G.; Lv, L.; Liu, F.R.; Wang, Z.N.; Liu, F.N.; Li, Y.S.; Wang, C.Y.; Zhang, H.Y.; Sun, Z.; Xu, H.M. Downregulation of connective tissue growth factor inhibits the growth and invasion of gastric cancer cells and attenuates peritoneal dissemination. *Mol. Cancer* **2011**, *10*, 122. [CrossRef] [PubMed]

115. Chen, C.N.; Chang, C.C.; Lai, H.S.; Jeng, Y.M.; Chen, C.I.; Chang, K.J.; Lee, P.H.; Lee, H. Connective tissue growth factor inhibits gastric cancer peritoneal metastasis by blocking integrin α3β1-dependent adhesion. *Gastric Cancer* **2015**, *18*, 504–515. [CrossRef] [PubMed]

116. Jiang, J.; Liu, W.; Guo, X.; Zhang, R.; Zhi, Q.; Ji, J.; Zhang, J.; Chen, X.; Li, J.; Zhang, J.; et al. IRX1 influences peritoneal spreading and metastasis via inhibiting BDKRB2-dependent neovascularization on gastric cancer. *Oncogene* **2011**, *30*, 4498–4508. [CrossRef] [PubMed]

117. Leung, D.W.; Cachianes, G.; Kuang, W.J.; Goeddel, D.V.; Ferrara, N. Vascular endothelial growth factor is a secreted angiogenic mitogen. *Science* **1989**, *246*, 1306–1309. [CrossRef] [PubMed]

118. Kowanetz, M.; Ferrara, N. Vascular endothelial growth factor signaling pathways: Therapeutic perspective. *Clin. Cancer Res.* **2006**, *12*, 5018–5022. [CrossRef] [PubMed]

119. Javle, M.; Smyth, E.C.; Chau, I. Ramucirumab: Successfully targeting angiogenesis in gastric cancer. *Clin. Cancer Res.* **2014**, *20*, 5875–5881. [CrossRef] [PubMed]

120. Roviello, G.; Polom, K.; Roviello, F.; Marrelli, D.; Multari, A.G.; Paganini, G.; Pacifico, C.; Generali, D. Targeting VEGFR-2 in Metastatic Gastric Cancer: Results from a Literature-Based Meta-Analysis. *Cancer Investig.* **2017**, *35*, 187–194. [CrossRef] [PubMed]

121. Yamac, D.; Ayyildiz, T.; Coşkun, U.; Akyürek, N.; Dursun, A.; Seckin, S.; Koybasioglu, F. Cyclooxygenase-2 expression and its association with angiogenesis, Helicobacter pylori, and clinicopathologic characteristics of gastric carcinoma. *Pathol. Res. Pract.* **2008**, *204*, 527–536. [CrossRef] [PubMed]

122. Xiao, L.J.; Zhao, S.; Zhao, E.H.; Zheng, X.; Gou, W.F.; Takano, Y.; Zheng, H.C. Clinicopathological and prognostic significance of Ki-67, caspase-3 and p53 expression in gastric carcinomas. *Oncol. Lett.* **2013**, *6*, 1277–1284. [CrossRef] [PubMed]

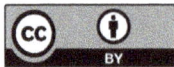

International Journal of
Molecular Sciences

MDPI

Article

Characterizing Metastatic *HER2*-Positive Gastric Cancer at the *CDH1* Haplotype

Laura Caggiari [1,†], Gianmaria Miolo [2], Angela Buonadonna [2], Debora Basile [2,3],
Davide A. Santeufemia [4], Antonio Cossu [5], Giuseppe Palmieri [6], Mariangela De Zorzi [1],
Mara Fornasarig [7], Lara Alessandrini [8], Vincenzo Canzonieri [8], Giovanni Lo Re [9],
Fabio Puglisi [2,3], Agostino Steffan [1], Renato Cannizzaro [7] and Valli De Re [1,†,*]

[1] Immunopathology and Cancer Biomarkers, IRCCS CRO National Cancer Institute, 33081 Aviano, Italy;
   lcaggiari@cro.it (L.C.); mdezorzi@cro.it (M.D.Z.); asteffan@cro.it (A.S.)
[2] Medical Oncology, IRCCS, CRO National Cancer Institute, 33081 Aviano, Italy; gmiolo@cro.it (G.M.);
   abuonadonna@cro.it (A.B.); deborabasile1090@gmail.com (D.B.); fabio.puglisi@cro.it (F.P.)
[3] Department of Medicine, School of Medical Oncology, University of Udine, 0432 Udine, Italy
[4] SSD Oncology, Ospedale Civile Alghero, 07041 Alghero, Italy; davidesanteufemia@gmail.com
[5] Operative Unit of Pathology Department of Surgical, Microsurgical and Medical Sciences,
   University of Sassari, 07100 Sassari, Italy; cossu@uniss.it
[6] Institute of Biomolecular Chemistry, Cancer Genetics Unit, C.N.R., 07100 Sassari, Italy; g.palmieri@icb.cnr.it
[7] Gastroenterology, IRCCS CRO National Cancer Institute, 33081 Aviano, Italy; mfornasarig@cro.it (M.F.);
   rcannizzaro@cro.it (R.C.)
[8] Pathology, IRCCS CRO National Cancer Institute, 33081 Aviano, Italy; lara.alessandrini@cro.it (L.A.);
   vcanzonieri@cro.it (V.C.)
[9] Medical Oncology Department, Santa Maria degli Angeli Hospital, 33170 Pordenone, Italy;
   Giovanni.lore@aopn.fvg.it
*   Correspondence: vdere@cro.it; Tel.: +39-0434-659672
†   These authors contributed equally to this work.

Received: 28 November 2017; Accepted: 21 December 2017; Published: 23 December 2017

Abstract: The *CDH1* gene, coding for the E-cadherin protein, is linked to gastric cancer (GC) susceptibility and tumor invasion. The human epidermal growth factor receptor 2 (*HER2*) is amplified and overexpressed in a portion of GC. *HER2* is an established therapeutic target in metastatic GC (mGC). Trastuzumab, in combination with various chemotherapeutic agents, is a standard treatment for these tumors leading to outcome improvement. Unfortunately, the survival benefit is limited to a fraction of patients. The aim of this study was to improve knowledge of the *HER2* and the E-cadherin alterations in the context of GC to characterize subtypes of patients that could better benefit from targeted therapy. An association between the P7-*CDH1* haplotype, including two polymorphisms (rs16260A-rs1801552T) and a subset of *HER2*-positive mGC with better prognosis was observed. Results indicated the potential evaluation of *CDH1* haplotypes in mGC to stratify patients that will benefit from trastuzumab-based treatments. Moreover, data may have implications to understanding the *HER2* and the E-cadherin interactions in vivo and in response to treatments.

Keywords: E-cadherin; *CDH1*; *HER2*; metastatic gastric cancer; rs16260; rs1801552

1. Introduction

Gastric cancer (GC) is a serious health problem worldwide. This year 28,000 new cases, with approximately 10,960 related deaths, are expected in the United States [1]. Even though surgery is the primary treatment option for early stage GC, diagnosis is often late in Western countries. This is probably due to the lack of proper screening programs and a lack of symptoms for a long time. About 35% of patients present with "de novo" metastatic GC (mGC) and approximately 70% that underwent surgery for the primary tumor will have disease recurrence or develop distant metastases, with a median survival of about one year, despite palliative chemotherapy [2–4].

In selected small tumors (i.e., stage Tis or T1) endoscopic resection may be performed, mainly in experienced centers. However, complete tumor resection with adequate margins and lymph node dissection remains the only potentially curative therapy for patients with non-metastatic GC. Furthermore, perioperative chemotherapy can improve survival outcomes for patients with operable disease [5].

In metastatic or recurrent disease, chemotherapy is the standard treatment, although it is not curative. However, despite the introduction in clinical practice of new drugs and chemotherapeutic schedules, only little progress has been made in recent years. The most important advance came from the international (24 countries) phase 3 randomized "ToGA" study (NCT01041404) [6]. In this trial, the addition of the trastuzumab, a monoclonal antibody, to the chemotherapy with cisplatin and capecitabine was compared to the same chemotherapy combination alone, in a population of *HER2*-positive metastatic gastric or gastro-esophageal junction cancers. The *HER2* is a transmembrane protein with tyrosine kinase activity implicated by its interaction with epidermal growth factor (EGF) family in cell growth and differentiation (Figure 1). In the ToGA study the median overall survival (OS) was found to be higher in patients who received trastuzumab plus chemotherapy compared with those who received the only chemotherapy (13.8 vs. 11.1 months). Immunohistochemical (IHC) scoring evaluates both the *HER2* membranous staining (absent, weak or detected in only one part of the membrane, moderate/weak complete or basolateral membranous staining and strong) and the percentage of the tumor cells staining (<10% or ≥ 10% of cells). A greater survival benefit was detected in patients whose tumors were IHC-positive (score 3+) or IHC-equivocal (score 2+), but in situ hybridization-positive (16 vs. 11.8 months; hazard ratio (HR) = 0.65). In addition, it was seen that the addition of the trastuzumab to chemotherapy did not compromise patient quality of life. Unfortunately, in a substantial proportion of mGC patient who progress after initial response to chemotherapy the death occurs in a few months [4]. Furthermore, the prognostic significance of the *HER2* expression in GC remains to be elucidated.

Breakthroughs in the GC biology are currently changing the landscape of GC. More specifically, the understanding of molecular mechanisms underlying the different pathological features has led to new GC classifications [7,8]. Originally GC was categorized according to anatomical presentation [9,10], and to histological classes (WHO classification and Lauren classification) [11,12]. More recently, the characterization of GC includes the *HER2* status and the HER-positive disease is reported in about 18% (range 4.4% to 53.4%) of patients [13].

In 2014, the Cancer Genome Atlas (TGCA) project [14] subdivided GC according to different molecular biology tests in four subgroups: EBV-positive (about 8% of all GC), Microsatellite Instable (MSI, about 22%), Chromosomal Instable (CIN, about 50%), and Genomically Stable (GS, about 20%) cancers. Additionally, in 2015 the Asian Cancer Research Group (ACRG) [15] proposed an alternative molecular classification due to the different biological characteristics of Asian patients. This classification divided GC in four subgroups represented by: Microsatellite Stable/epithelial-to-mesenchymal transition (MSS/EMT), Microsatellite Stable TP53-positive (MSS/TP53+, somehow overlapping with EBV type of TCGA classification), Microsatellite Stable TP53-negative (MSS/TP53−, similar to CIN by TCGA), and Microsatellite Instable (MSI).

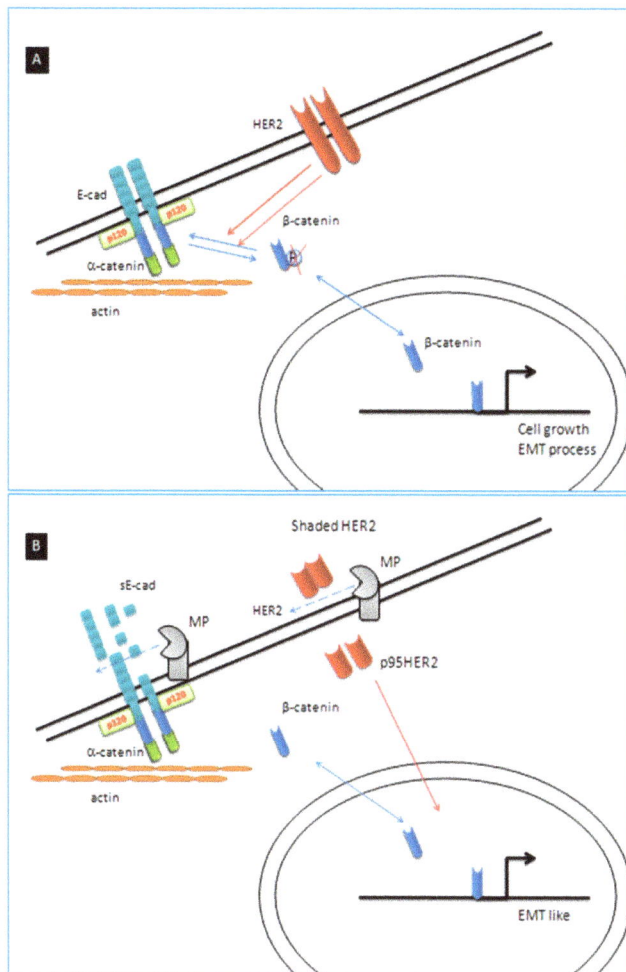

Figure 1. Schematic diagram of E-cadherin-*HER2* interaction. The E-cadherin present three different domains: the conserved cytoplasmic domain, a transmembrane domain, and an extracellular domain. The E-cadherin cytoplasmic tail presents two regions: the catenin-binding domain and the juxtamembrane domain. β-catenin binds to the E-cadherin domain and this complex via α-catenin connects and regulates E-cad interaction with the actin cytoskeleton. p120-catenin binds the *CDH1* juxtamembrane domain and stabilizes E-cad expression at the cell surface. (**A**) Activation of the *HER2* by inducing the phosphorylation of β-catenin directs the dissociation of β-catenin from the E-cad complex, thus leading to a decrease of E-cad-mediated cell adhesion, facilitate epithelial-mesenchymal transition (EMT), and the translocation of β-catenin to the nucleus where it acts as a transcriptional regulator of genes involved in cell growth and the EMT process; (**B**) *HER2* activation increases metalloproteinase (MP) activity, which leads to an increased production of soluble E-cadherin (sE-cad) through the cleavage of E-cad. Metalloproteinase also cleaves *HER2* into a cytoplasmic tail domain, p95*HER2*, and a shaded soluble *HER2* fragment. The p95*HER2* fragment maintains the phosphokinase activity, thus favoring the dissociation of the β-catenin/E-cad complex leading to GC progression and metastasis. The production of the sE-cad causes a reduction in cell adhesion and, by its diffusion into the microenvironment, acts as a paracrine/autocrine signaling molecule that regulates numerous signaling pathways implicated in tumor progression, including a key role in the *HER2* interaction/activation and phosphorylation of β-catenin.

In the present study, our attention is focused on tumors with *CDH1* mutation, which could be included in the GS subtype of TCGA classification, mostly represented by GC of diffused histotype widely distributed to all the anatomical sites of the stomach and tending to a metastatic process linked to EMT [14]. *CDH1* encodes the E-cadherin (E-cad), a transmembrane glycoprotein especially abundant in epithelial tissues that mediate calcium-dependent adhesion between epithelial cells. Several *CDH1* mutations with a reduced activity/expression of the E-cad [16], as well as the *HER2* overexpression [17], have been associated with shorter GC patient survival. More recent evidence points to β-catenin as a common link between the *HER2* overexpression and the E-cad repression in influencing EMT, the metastatic process, and outcome [18].

A deep understanding of molecular characterization of patients with mGC focusing on both the *HER2*-positive and the *CDH1* polymorphisms could provide the scientific background to develop modern clinical trial protocols in order to maximize the benefit of novel biological agents in a proper patient population [7]. The present study was designed to characterize *CDH1* in mGC subtypes according to the *HER2*-expression and to evaluate the association between the *CDH1* and the prognosis.

2. Results

2.1. Patient Characteristics

Fifty-nine consecutive patients with mGC were enrolled in this study; patients meeting the criteria for hereditary diffuse GC have been excluded. In total, 44 patients were males and 15 were females, and the mean age at diagnosis was 60 years (range, 40–76 years). Twelve cases (20.3%; (N = 10 males, median age 56.5 years) were classified at diagnosis as *HER2*-positive by an IHC score of 2+/neu amplification or by an IHC score of 3. All mGC patients received the same chemotherapeutic regimen with the addition of trastuzumab in mGC *HER2*-positive tumors (mGC-*HER2*).

At a median follow-up time of two years, a trend for a better OS was showed in the mGC-*HER2* positive group of patients although due to the limited number of cases the difference did not reach a statistical significance (468 days, standard deviation (SD) 389 vs. 584 days, SD 336; p = 0.20) (Figure 2). These data are in accord with previous studies reported in the literature, which used targeted treatment [6,19].

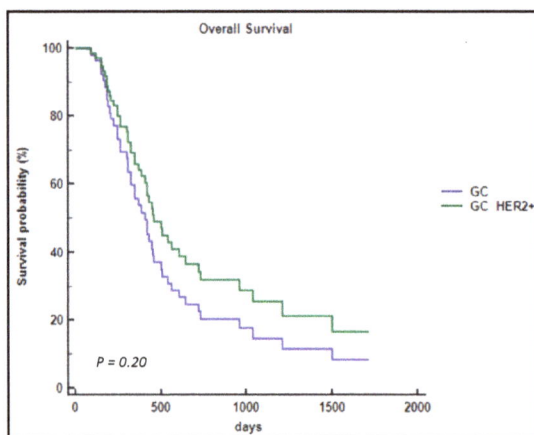

Figure 2. Cox regression for overall survival (OS) analysis for the mGC patient subgroup based on the *HER2*-expression.

2.2. CDH1 Mutations

A summary of *CDH1* mutations found in the promoter/5′UTR region and in all 16 exons and their surrounding sequences, are reported in Table 1, stratified on the basis of the *HER2* status. Mutations resulted in: (i) missense variant in three cases (mGC-*HER2* P296, mGC P310, P623); (ii) a frameshift variant in one case resulting in a truncating protein (mGC-*HER2* P586) [20]; (iii) synonymous mutations in seven cases, including a new mutation (GeneBank accession number: KT820428.1) (mGC-*HER2* P586, mGC P310, P295, P311, P476, P368, P490); and (iv) eight in the non-coding region (i.e., promoter/5′UTR/surrounding regions) (mGC-*HER2* P586, mGC P377, P304, P294, P376, P479, P368, P490). Six among these mutations resulted in a polymorphic site (≥5% allele frequency) (Table 1) (rs5030625 c.-472delA, rs16260 c.-285C>A, rs3743674 c.48+6C>T, rs2276330 c.1937-13T>C, rs1801552 c.2076T>C and rs33964119 c.2253C>T). Allele and genotype frequencies of the six polymorphic variants are reported in Table 2 stratified based on the mGC-*HER2* expression. A significant association was found between the rs16260 c.-285 A-allele and *HER2*-positive mGC (p = 0.0009).

2.3. Association between CDH1 P7-Haplotype and mGC-HER2

We investigated the association between mGC stratified by *HER2* expression and the *CDH1* haplotype resulting from the six polymorphic sites dispersed over the entire *CDH1* gene. A total of 11 different *CDH1* haplotypes were identified and their frequencies reported in Table 3. Haplotype P7 was exclusively present in six mGC-*HER2* patients, one of them showing a P7 haplotype in homozygous cases (Table 4). Linkage disequilibrium (LD) analysis in mGC patients showed a tight association between rs16260 and rs1801552 (D′ = 1.0000, R^2 = 0.1731, χ^2 = 16.2759, p = 0.0001), which was not present in mGC-*HER2* (D′ = 0.3555, R^2 = 0.0721, χ^2 = 1.7311, p = 0.1883). The contemporary presence of the rs16260-A allele and rs1801552-T-allele, both included in the P7 haplotype, was strictly associated with mGC-*HER2* disease (Table 3).

2.4. Association between the CDH1 P7 Haplotype and the Survival of mGC-HER2 Patients

The relationship between the P7 haplotype and OS was statistically analyzed by using Cox regression curves. The P5, P6, and P8–P11 haplotypes with less than two cases in mGC-*HER2* (Table 3) were combined in a unique group, and designed them as haplotype "matched". Figure 3A shows the OS of all GC cases (independent of the *HER2*-expression) stratified on haplotype-based approaches. The haplotype P7 was associated with better outcome (median OS: 1037 days) compared to the other haplotypes (median OS: 312 to 448 days). Notably, a significantly worse prognosis was observed with the "matched" haplotype (median OS: 312 days; HR 2.79, 95% CI 1.032–7.548) and the haplotype P1 (median OS: 419 days; HR 2.54, 95% CI 1.049–6.169). The haplotype P7 was present only in the mGC-*HER2* group where it distinguished patients with better survival compared to those with the "matched" haplotype and haplotype P1 (HR 4.33, 95% CI 1.033–7.548; HR 2.58, 95% CI 0.328–20.275, respectively). The "matched" haplotype and haplotype P1 were also associated with poorer prognosis in mGC group when compared to haplotype P3 (HR 1.412, 95% CI 0.717–2.779). Figure 3B indicates the OS distribution according to the restricted GC haplotype (i.e., rs16260 and rs1801552), specifically associated with the mGC-*HER2* patients as reported above. Data confirmed the better outcome was associated with the restricted AT haplotype (median OS: 1037 days, 95% CI 371–1037) which, in our series, is supported by the observation of a statistically significant difference in the OS compared to the CC haplotype (median OS: 420 days, 95% CI 312–500; HR 2.374, 95% CI 1.077–5.229).

Table 1. *CDH1* germline mutations found in mGC according to the *HER2*-expression.

CDH1 Region Gene	Reference Polymorphism	cDNA Change	Amino Acid Change	Type of Variant	Genotype	
					mGC-HER2 (n)	mGC (n)
Promoter	rs5030625	c.-472delA		Polymorphic variant	A/A (4)	A/A (10)
Promoter	rs16260	c.-285C>A		Polymorphic variant	G/A (1) A/C (6)	G/A (1) A/A (3) A/C (16)
Promoter	rs34149581	c.-276T>C				T/C (1)
5'UTR	rs34033771	c.-71C>G				C/G (1)
IV1	rs3743674	c.48+6C>T		Polymorphic variant	C/C (1)	T/C (9) C/C (1)
EXON3	rs1801023	c.345G>A	p.Thr115=	Synonymous variant		G/A (1)
IV4	rs33963999	c.531+10G>C				G/C (2)
IV5	rs189969617	c.688-14C>T				C/T (1)
EXON7	rs142822590	c.892G>A	p.Ala298Thr	Missense variant		G/A (1)
EXON11	SCV000588228.1	c.1612delG	p.Asp538Thrfs*19	Frameshift mutation	delG (1)	
EXON12	rs35187787	c.1774G>A	p.Ala592Thr	Missense variant	G/A (1)	
EXON12	rs33969373	c.1896C>T	p.HIS632=	Synonymous variant		C/T (2)
IV12	rs2276330	c.1937-13T>C		Polymorphic variant	C/T (2)	C/T (10)
EXON13	rs1801552	c.2076T>C	p.Ala692=	Polymorphic synonymous variant	C/T (5) T/T (3)	C/T (24) T/T (5)
IV13	rs35686369	c.2164+15_2164+16insA			insA (1)	insA (2)
EXON14	rs879026401	c.2232A>G	p.Pro744=	Synonymous variant		A/G (1)
EXON14	rs33964119	c.2253C>T	p.Asn751=	Synonymous variant	C/T (1)	C/T (2)
EXON15	rs587782549	c.2204G>A	p.Arg796Gln	Missense variant		G/A (1)

Abbreviations: *HER2*, human epidermal growth factor receptor 2; mGC, metastatic gastric cancer. Filled boxes correspond to the polymorphic variants.

Table 2. Allele and genotype frequencies of *CDH1* polymorphic sites in patients with mGC according to the *HER2*-expression.

Reference Polymorphism	Allele/Genotype	mGC-*HER2*	Frequency	mGC	Frequency	*p*	OR (95% CI)
			rs5030625				
Allele	G	23	0.96	84	0.89	0.33	2.738 (0.33–22.51)
	A	1	0.04	10	0.11		
	G/G	11	0.92	37	0.79		
Genotype	G/A	1	0.08	10	0.21		
	A/A	0	0.00	0	0.00		
Dominant model	GG/AA+AG	11/1	0.92/0.08	37/10	0.79/0.21	0.30	2.973 (0.34–25.86)
Recessive model	AA/AG+GG	0/12	0.00/1.00	0/47	0.00/1.00	nv	
			rs16260				
Allele	**A**	**14**	**0.58**	**22**	**0.23**	**≤0.001**	**4.582 (1.79–11.75)**
	C	**10**	**0.42**	**72**	**0.77**		
	A/A	**4**	**0.33**	**3**	**0.06**		
Genotype	**A/C**	**6**	**0.50**	**16**	**0.34**		
	C/C	**2**	**0.17**	**28**	**0.60**		
Recessive model	**CC/AA+AC**	**2/10**	**0.17/0.83**	**28/19**	**0.60/0.40**	**≤0.01**	**7.368 (1.45–37.46)**
Dominant model	**AA/AC+CC**	**4/8**	**0.33/0.67**	**3/44**	**0.06/0.94**	**0.01**	**7.333 (1.37–39.18)**
			rs3743674				
Allele	T	22	0.92	83	0.88	0.64	1.457 (0.30–7.07)
	C	2	0.08	11	0.12		
	T/T	11	0.92	37	0.79		
Genotype	T/C	0	0.00	9	0.19		
	C/C	1	0.08	1	0.02		
Recessive model	CC/CT+TT	1/11	0.08/0.92	1/46	0.02/0.98	0.29	4.182 (0.24–72.21)
Dominant model	TT/CC+CT	11/1	0.92/0.08	37/10	0.79/0.21	0.30	2.973 (0.34–25.86)
			rs2276330				
Allele	T	22	0.92	84	0.90	0.74	1.309 (0.27–6.42)
	C	2	0.08	10	0.11		
	T/T	10	0.83	37	0.79		
Genotype	T/C	2	0.17	10	0.21		
	C/C	0	0.00	0	0.00		
Dominant model	TT/CT+CC	10/2	0.83/0.17	37/10	0.79/0.21	0.72	1.351 (0.25–7.19)
Recessive model	CC/TT+CT	0/12	0.00/1.00	0/47	0.00/1.00	nv	
			rs1801552				
Allele	C	13	0.54	60	0.64	0.39	0.670 (0.27–1.66)
	T	11	0.46	34	0.36		
	C/C	4	0.33	18	0.38		
Genotype	T/C	5	0.42	24	0.51		
	T/T	3	0.25	5	0.11		
Recessive model	TT/CC+CT	3/9	0.25/0.75	5/42	0.11/0.89	0.19	2.800 (0.56–13.90)
Dominant model	CC/CT+TT	4/8	0.33/0.67	18/29	0.38/0.62	0.75	1.241 (0.33–4.72)
			rs33964119				
	C	23	0.96	92	0.98	0.58	0.500 (0.04–5.76)
Allele	T	1	0.04	2	0.02		
	C/C	11	0.92	45	0.96		
Genotype	T/C	1	0.08	2	0.04		
	T/T	0	0.00	0	0.00		
Recessive model	CC/CT+TT	11/1	0.92/0.08	45/2	0.96/0.04	0.57	2.045 (0.17–24.66)
Dominant model	TT/CC+CT	0/12	0.00/1.00	0/47	0.00/1.00	nv	

Abbreviations: *HER2*, the human epidermal growth factor receptor 2; OR, odds ratio; is the relative measure of the number of an allele or a genotype in the mGC-*HER2* group relative to the comparison of the number of allele/genotype in the mGC, by considering as the reference the most frequent allele in the mGC-*HER2*. If the OR is >1 the allele or genotype having the greatest frequency in the mGC-*HER2* is higher than that found in the mGC group. 95% CI (confidence interval) is the probability that the confidence interval contains the true odds ratio. Statistically significant *p* values are reported in bold type.

Table 3. Haplotype analysis in patients with mGC according to *HER2* expression.

Haplotype	rs5030625	rs16260	rs3743674	rs2276330	rs1801552	rs33964119	mGC (N 94)	Frequency	mGC-HER2 (N 24)	Frequency	p	OR (95% CI)
P1	G	C	T	T	C	C	19	0.20	2	0.08	0.24	0.359 (0.08–1.67)
P2	G	A	T	T	C	C	22	0.23	6	0.25	1.00	1.091 (0.39–3.09)
P3	G	C	T	T	T	C	31	0.33	4	0.17	0.14	0.406 (0.13–1.29)
P4	C	C	C	C	C	C	9	0.09	2	0.08	1.00	0.859 (0.17–4.26)
P5	A	C	C	C	C	C	7	0.07	1	0.04	0.69	0.540 (0.06–4.61)
P6	C	A	T	T	T	C	1	0.01	0	0.00	1.00	
P7	**G**	**C**	**T**	**T**	**T**	**C**	**0**	**0.00**	**7**	**0.29**	**≤0.001**	
P8	G	C	C	C	T	C	1	0.01	0	0.00	1.00	
P9	A	C	C	T	T	T	2	0.02	0	0.00	1.00	
P10	G	C	T	T	C	T	2	0.02	1	0.04	0.50	2.00 (0.17–23.03)
P11	G	A	C	C	C	C	0	0.00	1	0.04	0.20	

Abbreviations: *HER2*, human epidermal growth factor receptor 2; mGC, metastatic gastric cancer; OR, odds ratio; is the relative measure of the number of the mGC haplotype relative to the comparison of the number of the same haplotype in the mGC-*HER2*, by considering as the reference the most frequent haplotype in the mGC. If the OR is >1 the haplotype having the most frequency in the mGC is higher than that found in the mGC-*HER2* group. 95% CI (confidence interval) is the probability that the confidence interval contains the true odds ratio. Statistically significant p values are highlighted and reported in bold type.

Table 4. *CDH1* haplotype plus germline mutation found in patients with *HER2*-mGC.

Patient Identifier	Haplotype	CDH1 Germline Mutation			
		EXON11 c.1612delG	EXON12 c.1774G>A	IV13 c.2164+15_2164+16insA	EXON14 c.2253C>T
P287	P5–P11				
P291	P2–P7				
P292	P4–P7				
P296	P2–P7		■		
P297	P3–P7				
P301	P2–P3				
P303	P2–P4				
P380	P1–P2				
P391	P2–P7				
P486	P7–P7				
P582	P3–P3				
P586	P1–P10			■	■

mGC, metastatic gastric cancer. Filled boxes indicate the presence of the *CDH1* germline mutations, open boxes indicate their absence.

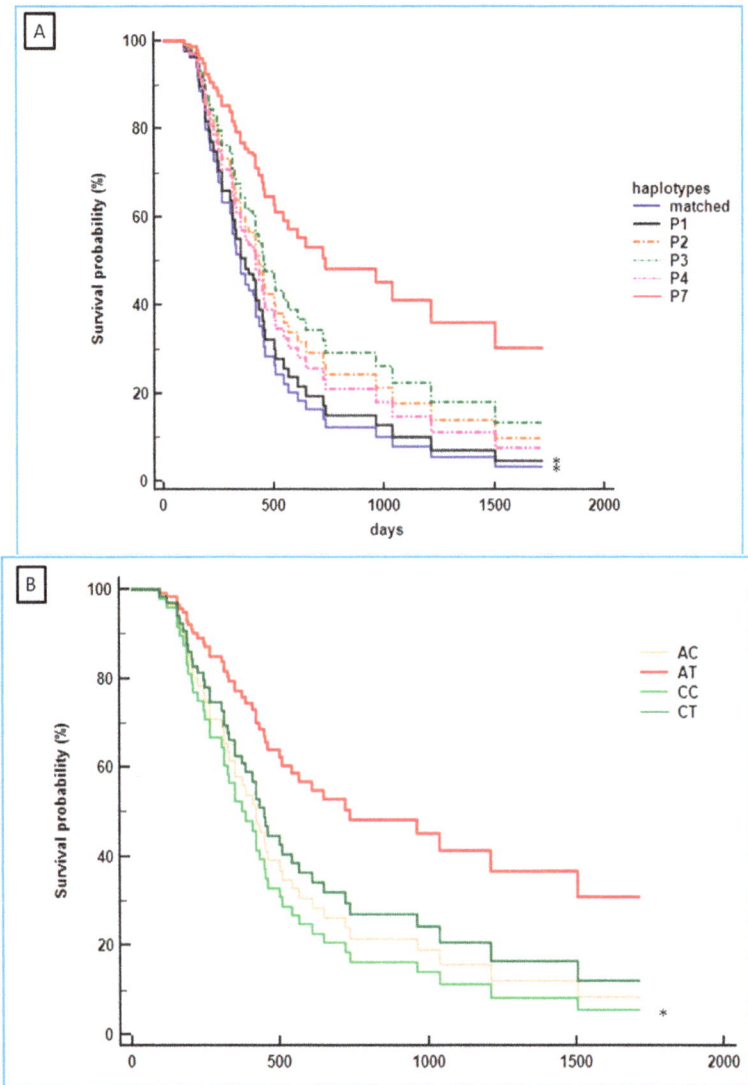

Figure 3. Cox regression for overall survival analysis according to the *CDH1* haplotypes (**A**) and the restricted *CDH1* haplotype model (**B**). (**A**) Overall survival curves of all patients with mGC (*n* = 59) based on their different *CDH1* haplotype; (**B**) Overall survival curves of all patients with mGC (*n* = 59) according to coupled rs16260 and rs1801552 polymorphisms. * indicates a significant difference compared to the P7 haplotype (panel **A**) and coupled AT polymorphism (panel **B**).

3. Discussion

Targeted *HER2* therapy for mGC works differently due to the heterogeneity of the tumor. Positivity for the *HER2* status (by IHC or by fluorescence in situ hybridization) is a prerequisite for the *HER2* targeted therapy, but it is not sufficient to predict the treatment response. In the present study, we found an association between specific *CDH1* polymorphisms with a subset of *HER2*-positive mGC that, in turn, are associated with distinct prognosis behavior (Figure 3A). The association between the haplotype P7 with the better OS is not due to the presence of additional mutations to the P7-related *CDH1* mutations since, among the *HER2* patients carrying haplotype P7, only one had an additional non-polymorphic *CDH1* mutation (i.e., pt P296 with a missense variant); of note, this patient experienced a poor prognosis (median OS: 164 days). Notably, analysis of LD in mGC showed a specific association with two polymorphisms (i.e., *CDH1* rs16260 and rs1801552) that were not found in the *HER2*-positive mGC. In fact, these polymorphisms showed minor allele frequency (MAF) variants in mGC-*HER2*: rs16260-A and rs1801552-T alleles. By using these two polymorphisms (i.e., rs16260/rs1801552) Cox regression analysis was simplified from 11 to four haplotypes and confirmed the association of haplotype P7, including the rs16260-A and the rs1801552-T alleles, with the mGC-*HER2* subtype with the best OS (Figure 3B). Functionally, the rs16260-A polymorphism located in the *CDH1* promoter region had been associated with an alteration in the *CDH1* transcriptional efficiency. In vitro testing using luciferase reporter gene revealed that the rs16260-A allele decreased *CDH1* transcriptional activity by 68% compared to the C-allele. However, the effect of rs16260-A variant on *CDH1* expression in vivo is still unknown [21] and a significant decrease of *CDH1* production in the peripheral blood cells of mutation carrier patients compared to that produced in the control-cohort was not found [22]. Additionally, the potential contribution of rs16260-A allele to GC risk remains controversial [23,24], while the potential prognostic value of this variant in breast cancer and in metastatic colon cancer did not reach statistical significance [25,26].

With regard to the second polymorphism, the rs1801552-T, a protective association between this variant in homozygous and non-syndromic cleft lip has been reported [27]. Recent studies indicated that patients with cleft lip had a higher incidence of tumors than the general population [28,29] and, moreover, family members with pathogenetic *CDH1* mutation showed a higher incidence of cleft lip/palate than the general population (6–7% versus about 0.1%) [28,30,31]. In addition, a previous study by using rs1801552 heterozygous individuals with GC compared to controls demonstrated a *CDH1* allelic expression imbalance in hereditary GC family members with an increase of the ratio of the *CDH1* RNA rs1801552 T-allele/C-allele that was not found in cancer-free individuals [32]. Results had suggested, for some unknown reason, the reduction of *CDH1* C-allele-specific expression in patients at risk for GC.

In our series we found relationship between the *CDH1* variants and patient survival in the setting of mGC, particularly in the *HER2*-positive disease. Previous studies supported a functional interaction between the *HER2* and the E-cad. Briefly, the β-catenin binds the C-terminal cytoplasmic domain of the E-cad and this complex via the α-catenin connects and regulates the E-cad interaction with the actin cytoskeleton, while association of the p120-catenin with the juxtamembrane domain of the E-cad stabilizes the E-cad expression at the cell surface (Figure 1). Activation of the *HER2* by inducing the phosphorylation of the β-catenin directs the dissociation of β-catenin from the E-cad complex, thus leading to a decrease of the E-cad-mediated cell adhesion facilitating tumor cells invasion and migration. In addition, the dissociation of the β-catenin from the E-cad complex causes the translocation of the β-catenin to the nucleus which drives the transcription of various target genes associated with cell survival, proliferation and metastasis. E-cad can also be solubilized (sE-cad) by membrane E-cad cleavage and be released into the extracellular environment [33] (Figure 1). The production of sE-cad not only undermines adherence junctions, but, by its diffusion into the micro environment, it regulates numerous signals implicated in tumor progression, including a key role in *HER2* interaction/activation and phosphorylation of the β-catenin [18]. Furthermore, *HER2* activation was known to increase metalloproteinase activity and, thus, it further leads to high increased production of the sE-cad by the cleavage of the E-cad. Through the specific cleavage of its cytoplasmic tail domain into the p95*HER2* fragment, it maintains the phosphokinase activity of the *HER2* favoring the dissociation of the β-catenin/E-cad complex that, overall, both promote GC progression and metastasis (Figure 1).

Overall, these findings support a possible functional role of the E-cad in response to the anti-*HER2* treatment in mGC-*HER2* subtype. However, the role of the *CDH1* mutations in this context requires elucidation through further studies. Interestingly, in human transfected breast epithelial cell lines over-expressing the *HER2* receptor resulted in inhibition of E-cad expression [34]. Lapatinib resistance in *HER2*-positive breast cancer cells was also associated with a EMT and the EMT-related down-regulation of E-cad [35]. Moreover, treatment with the *HER2*-specific tyrosine kinase inhibitors (AG285 and *HER2* siRNA) was found to produce a down-regulation of the E-cad in ovarian cancer cells [36]. Overall, these studies demonstrate the important connection between *HER2* and E-cad in human cancers.

The determination of the *HER2* status in patients with advanced GC is crucial in order to select patients who may benefit from the new anti-*HER2* agents; the results of this study, if confirmed in a prospective larger series, could improve the understanding of molecular interactions between *HER2* and E-cad and define their role as predictive factors for targeted therapy.

4. Materials and Methods

4.1. Study Population

For the present study, between 2011 and 2017 we enrolled 59 consecutive patients with confirmatory of metastatic GC. Forty-four were males and 15 were females, and the mean age at diagnosis was 60 years (range, 40–76 years). Patients were grouped according to confirmed *HER2*-status at diagnosis. Patients agreed to participate to the study and provided informed consent (CRO-2011-2012 Code EUDRACT: 2011-001720-37).

4.2. Genotyping Analysis

Genomic DNA was extracted from each subject's peripheral blood lymphocytes using an EZ1 DNA blood kit (QIAGEN, Hilden, Germany) according to the manufacturer's instructions.

Screening for mutations of *CDH1* exons and neighboring intronic sequences was performed using the polymerase chain reaction (PCR) with previously-described primers and the reaction conditions [37]. In short, 15 individual PCR reactions were performed on each sample for a full mutational screen of all 15 exons and splice junctions of the *CDH1* gene. Amplified PCR products were sequenced on an Applied Biosystems 3130 automated sequencer (Applied Biosystems, Foster City, CA, USA) using the Big Dye v3.1 Terminator Cycle Sequencing Kit (Life Technologies, Monza, Italy) and sequence data were aligned and analyzed using CodonCode Aligner software.

The promoter, 5'UTR and the exon 1 polymorphisms were genotyped by PCR method. A 581-bp fragment containing this region was amplified with the following primers: the forward *CDH1FPRO* 5'-TCCCAGGTCTTAGTGAGCCA-3' and the reverse *CDH1Exon1REV* 5'-TGACGACGGGAGAGGAAG-3'. The amplification was performed in a programmable thermal cycler as follows: touchdown (hold (94 °C 4 min) eight cycles (94 °C 45 s; 58 °C 50 s; 72 °C 1 min; reducing the annealing temperature by 1 °C each cycle)), three cycles (94 °C 45 s; 53 °C 50 s; 72 °C 1 min), and a final cycle of 72 °C for 10 min. After amplification the PCR product was sequenced using the primer *CDH1FPRO*.

We screened each of the above samples for the c.-472delA *CDH1* polymorphism using a new PCR method in place of current genotyping analysis by the PCR-RFLP method. DNA fragments containing the promoter region of interest were amplified with two distinct PCR reaction using the following primers: 1° reaction (forward, *CDH1G347proFor* 5'-CAGCTTGGGTGAAAGAGTGAGC-3'; reverse ECad347Rev 5'-GGCCACAGCCAATCAGCA-3'); 2° reaction (forward, *CDH1GA347proFor* 5'-CAGCTTGGGTGAAAGAGTGAGA-3'; reverse ECad347Rev 5'-GGCCACAGCCAATCAGCA-3'). The PCR conditions were set as follows: initial denaturation at 94 °C for 4 min; 10 cycles at 94 °C for 30 s, 65 °C for 1 min, 20 cycles at 94 °C for 30 s, 62 °C for 30 s and 72 °C for 1 min; and a final extension at 72 °C for 8 min, in a Veriti Thermal Cycler (Life Technologies). PCR products were analyzed on a 2.5% agarose gel stained with ethidium bromide and photographed under UV light. G/G homozygous cases were represented by DNA bands in the 1° reaction, GA/GA homozygous cases were represented by DNA bands in the 2° reaction. G/GA heterozygous cases display a combination of both bands. To validate this new PCR method the promoter region of same samples was amplified using the following primers: forward, 5'-GCCCCGACTTGTCTCTCTAC-3'; reverse, 5'-GGCCACAGCCAATCAGCA-3' and PCR products were sequenced.

4.3. Immunohistochemistry

A formalin-fixed, paraffin-embedded tumor block was cut into 4-μm-thick sections for H and E and immunostaining. Immunohistochemistry was performed by using the rabbit monoclonal antibodies against HER 2 (clone 4B5, Ventana Medical System, Tucson, AZ, USA).

4.4. Statistical Analysis

The frequencies of allele and genotype were compared between mGC-*HER2* and mGC patients by means of chi-squared test (VassarStats, http://faculty.vassar.edu/lowry/VassarStats.html).

The haplotype frequencies were analyzed with the SNPator [38] and Arlequin software [39].

Survival analysis was performed at the time of the first treatment by using Cox regression analysis.

5. Conclusions

In conclusion, the evaluation of a restricted *CDH1* haplotype in mGC could help to select the patients that gain greater benefit from the anti-*HER2* treatments. Furthermore, since a high level of the sE-cadherin may modulate sensitivity to RTK inhibitors, the evaluation of its serum concentration in different phases of treatment could have a role in monitoring the therapeutic response overtime.

Acknowledgments: The authors would like to thank Gianna Tabaro for providing an invaluable assistance during the conduct of this study. The study was supported by CRO 5x1.000_2010_MdS and the Centro di Riferimento Oncologico, CRO Intramural Grant.

Author Contributions: Laura Caggiari and Valli De Re conceived and designed the experiments and supervised the whole project, interpreted the results and wrote and prepared the manuscript; Laura Caggiari, Gianmaria Miolo, Mariangela De Zorzi, Lara Alessandrini, and Vincenzo Canzonieri, performed experiments and data preparation; Gianmaria Miolo, Debora Basile, Davide A. Santeufemia, Antonio Cossu, and Giuseppe Palmieri analyzed the data and contributed to the manuscript preparation; Gianmaria Miolo, Angela Buonadonna, Mara Fornasarig, Giovanni Lo Re, Agostino Steffan, and Renato Cannizzaro collected and characterized the samples; and Valli De Re and Fabio Puglisi interpreted the results and critically evaluated the manuscript. All authors read and approved the final manuscript for publication.

Conflicts of Interest: The authors declare no conflict of interest.

Abbreviations

GC	Gastric cancer
mGC	Metastatic gastric cancer
HER2	Human epidermal growth factor receptor 2
E-cad	E-cadherin
IHC	Immunohistochemical
EBV	Epstein-barr virus
EMT	Epithelial-to-mesenchymal transition
MP	Metalloproteinase

References

1. Siegel, R.L.; Miller, K.D.; Jemal, A. Cancer statistics, 2017. *CA Cancer J. Clin.* **2017**, *67*, 7–30. [CrossRef] [PubMed]

2. Santeufemia, D.A.; Lumachi, F.; Fadda, G.M.; Lo Re, G.; Miolo, G.; Basso, S.M.M.; Chiara, G.B.; Tumolo, S. Comment on "Repetitive transarterial chemoembolization (TACE) of liver metastases from gastric cancer: Local control and survival results": Will there be clinical implications in the future? *Eur. J. Radiol.* **2013**, *82*, 1591–1592. [CrossRef] [PubMed]

3. Romano, F.; Garancini, M.; Uggeri, F.; Degrate, L.; Nespoli, L.; Gianotti, L.; Nespoli, A.; Uggeri, F. Surgical treatment of liver metastases of gastric cancer: State of the art. *World J. Surg. Oncol.* **2012**, *10*, 157. [CrossRef] [PubMed]

4. Catalano, V.; Graziano, F.; Santini, D.; D'Emidio, S.; Baldelli, A.M.; Rossi, D.; Vincenzi, B.; Giordani, P.; Alessandroni, P.; Testa, E.; et al. Second-line chemotherapy for patients with advanced gastric cancer: Who may benefit? *Br. J. Cancer* **2008**, *99*, 1402–1407. [CrossRef] [PubMed]

5. Orditura, M.; Galizia, G.; Sforza, V.; Gambardella, V.; Fabozzi, A.; Laterza, M.M.; Andreozzi, F.; Ventriglia, J.; Savastano, B.; Mabilia, A.; et al. Treatment of gastric cancer. *World J. Gastroenterol.* **2014**, *20*, 1635–1649. [CrossRef] [PubMed]

6. Bang, Y.-J.; Van Cutsem, E.; Feyereislova, A.; Chung, H.C.; Shen, L.; Sawaki, A.; Lordick, F.; Ohtsu, A.; Omuro, Y.; Satoh, T.; et al. Trastuzumab in combination with chemotherapy versus chemotherapy alone for treatment of *HER2*-positive advanced gastric or gastro-oesophageal junction cancer (ToGA): A phase 3, open-label, randomised controlled trial. *Lancet* **2010**, *376*, 687–697. [CrossRef]

7. Garattini, S.K.; Basile, D.; Cattaneo, M.; Fanotto, V.; Ongaro, E.; Bonotto, M.; Negri, F.V.; Berenato, R.; Ermacora, P.; Cardellino, G.G.; et al. Molecular classifications of gastric cancers: Novel insights and possible future applications. *World J. Gastrointest. Oncol.* **2017**, *9*, 194–208. [CrossRef] [PubMed]

8. Bonotto, M.; Garattini, S.K.; Basile, D.; Ongaro, E.; Fanotto, V.; Cattaneo, M.; Cortiula, F.; Iacono, D.; Cardellino, G.G.; Pella, N.; et al. Immunotherapy for gastric cancers: Emerging role and future perspectives. *Expert Rev. Clin. Pharmacol.* **2017**, *10*, 609–619. [CrossRef] [PubMed]

9. Lubarsch, O.; Henke, F.; Rössle, R. Handbuch der Speziellen Pathologischen Anatomie und Histologie. *Springer* **1937**, *9* (part 3). Available online: http://www.springer.com/series/206 (accessed on 30 November 2017).

10. Siewert, J.R.; Stein, H.J. Carcinoma of the gastroesophageal junction—Classification, pathology and extent of resection. *Dis. Esophagus* **1996**, *9*, 173–182. [CrossRef]

11. WHO Classification of Tumours of the Digestive System, Fourth Edition. Available online: http://apps.who.int/bookorders/WHP/detart1.jsp?sesslan=1&codlan=1&codcol=70&codcch=4003 (accessed on 14 November 2017).

12. Lauren, P. The two histological main types of gastric carcinoma: Diffuse and so-called intestinal-type carcinoma. An attempt at a histo-clinical classification. *Acta Pathol. Microbiol. Scand.* **1965**, *64*, 31–49. [CrossRef] [PubMed]

13. Shan, L.; Ying, J.; Lu, N. *HER2* expression and relevant clinicopathological features in gastric and gastroesophageal junction adenocarcinoma in a Chinese population. *Diagn. Pathol.* **2013**, *8*, 76. [CrossRef] [PubMed]

14. The Cancer Genome Atlas Research Network. Comprehensive molecular characterization of gastric adenocarcinoma. *Nature* **2014**, *513*, 202–209. [CrossRef]

15. Ye, X.S.; Yu, C.; Aggarwal, A.; Reinhard, C. Genomic alterations and molecular subtypes of gastric cancers in Asians. *Chin. J. Cancer* **2016**, *35*, 42. [CrossRef] [PubMed]

16. Chu, C.-M.; Chen, C.-J.; Chan, D.-C.; Wu, H.-S.; Liu, Y.-C.; Shen, C.-Y.; Chang, T.-M.; Yu, J.; Harn, H.-J.; Yu, C.-P.; et al. *CDH1* polymorphisms and haplotypes in sporadic diffuse and intestinal gastric cancer: A case–control study based on direct sequencing analysis. *World J. Surg. Oncol.* **2014**, *12*, 80. [CrossRef] [PubMed]

17. Dang, H.-Z.; Yu, Y.; Jiao, S.-C. Prognosis of *HER2* over-expressing gastric cancer patients with liver metastasis. *World J. Gastroenterol.* **2012**, *18*, 2402–2407. [CrossRef] [PubMed]

18. Nami, B.; Wang, Z. *HER2* in breast cancer stemness: A negative feedback loop towards trastuzumab resistance. *Cancers* **2017**, *9*, 40. [CrossRef] [PubMed]

19. Namikawa, T.; Munekage, E.; Munekage, M.; Maeda, H.; Yatabe, T.; Kitagawa, H.; Sakamoto, K.; Obatake, M.; Kobayashi, M.; Hanazaki, K. Evaluation of a trastuzumab-containing treatment regimen for patients with unresectable advanced or recurrent gastric cancer. *Mol. Clin. Oncol.* **2016**, *5*, 74–78. [CrossRef] [PubMed]

20. Caggiari, L.; Miolo, G.; Canzonieri, V.; De Zorzi, M.; Alessandrini, L.; Corona, G.; Cannizzaro, R.; Santeufemia, D.A.; Cossu, A.; Buonadonna, A.; et al. A new mutation of the *CDH1* gene in a patient with an aggressive signet-ring cell carcinoma of the stomach. *Cancer Biol. Ther.* **2017**, 1–6. [CrossRef] [PubMed]

21. Pisignano, G.; Napoli, S.; Magistri, M.; Mapelli, S.N.; Pastori, C.; Marco, S.D.; Civenni, G.; Albino, D.; Enriquez, C.; Allegrini, S.; et al. A promoter-proximal transcript targeted by genetic polymorphism controls E-cadherin silencing in human cancers. *Nat. Commun.* **2017**, *8*, 15622. [CrossRef] [PubMed]

22. Zhan, Z.; Wu, J.; Zhang, J.-F.; Yang, Y.-P.; Tong, S.; Zhang, C.-B.; Li, J.; Yang, X.-W.; Dong, W. *CDH1* gene polymorphisms, plasma *CDH1* levels and risk of gastric cancer in a Chinese population. *Mol. Biol. Rep.* **2012**, *39*, 8107–8113. [CrossRef] [PubMed]

23. Jiang, B.; Zhu, K.; Shao, H.; Bao, C.; Ou, J.; Sun, W. Lack of association between the *CDH1* polymorphism and gastric cancer susceptibility: A meta-analysis. *Sci. Rep.* **2015**, *5*, 7891. [CrossRef] [PubMed]

24. Chen, B.; Zhou, Y.; Yang, P.; Liu, L.; Qin, X.-P.; Wu, X.-T. *CDH1* -160C>A gene polymorphism is an ethnicity-dependent risk factor for gastric cancer. *Cytokine* **2011**, *55*, 266–273. [CrossRef] [PubMed]

25. Memni, H.; Macherki, Y.; Klayech, Z.; Ben-Haj-Ayed, A.; Farhat, K.; Remadi, Y.; Gabbouj, S.; Mahfoudh, W.; Bouzid, N.; Bouaouina, N.; et al. E-cadherin genetic variants predict survival outcome in breast cancer patients. *J. Transl. Med.* **2016**, *14*, 320. [CrossRef] [PubMed]

26. Matsusaka, S.; Zhang, W.; Cao, S.; Hanna, D.L.; Sunakawa, Y.; Sebio, A.; Ueno, M.; Yang, D.; Ning, Y.; Parekh, A.; et al. TWIST1 polymorphisms predict survival in patients with metastatic colorectal cancer receiving first-line bevacizumab plus oxaliplatin-based chemotherapy. *Mol. Cancer Ther.* **2016**, *15*, 1405–1411. [CrossRef] [PubMed]

27. Song, H.; Wang, X.; Yan, J.; Mi, N.; Jiao, X.; Hao, Y.; Zhang, W.; Gao, Y. Association of single-nucleotide polymorphisms of *CDH1* with nonsyndromic cleft lip with or without cleft palate in a northern Chinese Han population. *Medicine (Baltimore)* **2017**, *96*, e5574. [CrossRef] [PubMed]

28. Kluijt, I.; Siemerink, E.J.M.; Ausems, M.G.E.M.; van Os, T.A.M.; de Jong, D.; Simões-Correia, J.; van Krieken, J.H.; Ligtenberg, M.J.; Figueiredo, J.; van Riel, E.; et al. Dutch working group on hereditary gastric cancer *CDH1*-related hereditary diffuse gastric cancer syndrome: Clinical variations and implications for counseling. *Int. J. Cancer* **2012**, *131*, 367–376. [CrossRef] [PubMed]

29. Benusiglio, P.R.; Malka, D.; Rouleau, E.; De Pauw, A.; Buecher, B.; Noguès, C.; Fourme, E.; Colas, C.; Coulet, F.; Warcoin, M.; et al. *CDH1* germline mutations and the hereditary diffuse gastric and lobular breast cancer syndrome: A multicentre study. *J. Med. Genet.* **2013**, *50*, 486–489. [CrossRef] [PubMed]

30. Frebourg, T.; Oliveira, C.; Hochain, P.; Karam, R.; Manouvrier, S.; Graziadio, C.; Vekemans, M.; Hartmann, A.; Baert-Desurmont, S.; Alexandre, C.; et al. Cleft lip/palate and *CDH1*/E-cadherin mutations in families with hereditary diffuse gastric cancer. *J. Med. Genet.* **2006**, *43*, 138–142. [CrossRef] [PubMed]

31. Mossey, P.A.; Little, J.; Munger, R.G.; Dixon, M.J.; Shaw, W.C. Cleft lip and palate. *Lancet* **2009**, *374*, 1773–1785. [CrossRef]

32. Pinheiro, H.; Bordeira-Carrico, R.; Seixas, S.; Carvalho, J.; Senz, J.; Oliveira, P.; Inacio, P.; Gusmao, L.; Rocha, J.; Huntsman, D.; et al. Allele-specific *CDH1* downregulation and hereditary diffuse gastric cancer. *Hum. Mol. Genet.* **2010**, *19*, 943–952. [CrossRef] [PubMed]

33. Repetto, O.; De Paoli, P.; De Re, V.; Canzonieri, V.; Cannizzaro, R. Levels of Soluble E-Cadherin in Breast, Gastric, and Colorectal Cancers. Available online: https://www.hindawi.com/journals/bmri/2014/408047/ (accessed on 17 November 2017).

34. D'souza, B.; Taylor-Papadimitriou, J. Overexpression of ERBB2 in human mammary epithelial cells signals inhibition of transcription of the E-cadherin gene. *Proc. Natl. Acad. Sci. USA* **1994**, *91*, 7202–7206. [CrossRef] [PubMed]

35. Liu, J.; Chen, X.; Mao, Y.; Qu, Q.; Shen, K. Association of epithelial-mesenchymal transition with lapatinib resistance through multipe pathways activation in *HER2*-positive breast cancer. *J. Clin. Oncol.* **2014**, *32*, e11579. [CrossRef]

36. Cheng, J.-C.; Qiu, X.; Chang, H.-M.; Leung, P.C.K. *HER2* mediates epidermal growth factor-induced down-regulation of E-cadherin in human ovarian cancer cells. *Biochem. Biophys. Res. Commun.* **2013**, *434*, 81–86. [CrossRef] [PubMed]

37. Garziera, M.; Canzonieri, V.; Cannizzaro, R.; Geremia, S.; Caggiari, L.; Zorzi, M.D.; Maiero, S.; Orzes, E.; Perin, T.; Zanussi, S.; et al. Identification and characterization of *CDH1* germline variants in sporadic gastric cancer patients and in individuals at risk of gastric cancer. *PLoS ONE* **2013**, *8*, e77035. [CrossRef] [PubMed]
38. Morcillo-Suarez, C.; Alegre, J.; Sangros, R.; Gazave, E.; de Cid, R.; Milne, R.; Amigo, J.; Ferrer-Admetlla, A.; Moreno-Estrada, A.; Gardner, M.; et al. SNP analysis to results (SNPator): A web-based environment oriented to statistical genomics analyses upon SNP data. *Bioinformatics* **2008**, *24*, 1643–1644. [CrossRef] [PubMed]
39. Excoffier, L.; Laval, G.; Schneider, S. Arlequin (version 3.0): An integrated software package for population genetics data analysis. *Evol. Bioinform. Online* **2007**, *1*, 47–50. [CrossRef] [PubMed]

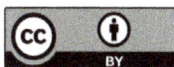

International Journal of
Molecular Sciences

MDPI

Article

Quantitative Proteomic Approach Targeted to Fibrinogen β Chain in Tissue Gastric Carcinoma

Ombretta Repetto [1], Stefania Maiero [2], Raffaella Magris [2], Gianmaria Miolo [3], Maria Rita Cozzi [4], Agostino Steffan [4], Vincenzo Canzonieri [5], Renato Cannizzaro [2] and Valli De Re [1,*]

[1] Facility of Bio-Proteomics, Immunopathology and Cancer Biomarkers, CRO Aviano National Cancer Institute, 33081 Aviano, Italy; orepetto@cro.it
[2] Gastroenterology, CRO Aviano National Cancer Institute, 33081 Aviano, Italy; smaiero@cro.it (S.M.); raffaella.magris@cro.it (R.M.); rcannizzaro@cro.it (R.C.)
[3] Medical Oncology, CRO Aviano National Cancer Institute, 33081 Aviano, Italy; gmiolo@cro.it
[4] Immunopathology and Cancer Biomarkers, CRO Aviano National Cancer Institute, 33081 Aviano, Italy; mrcozzi@cro.it (M.R.C.); asteffan@cro.it (A.S.)
[5] Pathology, CRO Aviano National Cancer Institute, 33081 Aviano, Italy; vcanzonieri@cro.it
* Correspondence: vdere@cro.it; Tel.: +39-0434-659-672

Received: 22 January 2018; Accepted: 5 March 2018; Published: 7 March 2018

Abstract: Elevated plasma fibrinogen levels and tumor progression in patients with gastric cancer (GC) have been largely reported. However, distinct fibrinogen chains and domains have different effects on coagulation, inflammation, and angiogenesis. The aim of this study was to characterize fibrinogen β chain (FGB) in GC tissues. Retrospectively we analyzed the data of matched pairs of normal (N) and malignant tissues (T) of 28 consecutive patients with GC at diagnosis by combining one- and two-dimensional electrophoresis (1DE and 2DE) with immunoblotting and mass spectrometry together with two-dimensional difference in gel electrophoresis (2D-DIGE). 1DE showed bands of the intact FGB at 50 kDa and the cleaved forms containing the fragment D at ~37–40 kDa, which corresponded to 19 spots in 2DE. In particular, spot 402 at ~50 kDa and spots 526 and 548 at ~37 kDa were of interest by showing an increased expression in tumor tissues. A higher content of spot 402 was associated with stomach antrum, while spots 526 and 548 amounts correlated with corpus and high platelet count ($>208 \times 10^9$/L). The quantification of FGB and cleaved products may help to further characterize the interconnections between GC and platelet/coagulation pathways.

Keywords: DIGE; comparative proteomics; gastric cancer; fibrinogen β chain; FGB; coagulation; platelets; biomarker

1. Introduction

Gastric cancer (GC) is the fifth most common cancer and the third leading cause of cancer death in the world [1]. Therefore, there is a great interest in deciphering the molecular pathways associated with its progression and prognosis. Environment and lifestyles are general risk factors for GC, but interaction of diet with multiple genetic and epigenetic alterations also occur during GC development [2–5]. Proteomics provided consistent information in revealing proteome alterations associated with GC, dissected some of the mechanisms underlying gastric cancerogenesis, and enabled the identification of several diagnostic, prognostic, and predictive biomarkers [6–9].

Hemostasis systemic perturbations are well known to occur in GC [10]. In particular, venous thromboembolism (VTE) has been implicated in GC progression and metastasis [11–14]. Clinically relevant VTE in GC patients shows an incidence of >5% at 1 year post diagnosis and 12–17% at 2 years, increasing to 24.4% in metastatic advanced GC [15–17].

Most recently, by using a two-dimensional difference in gel electrophoresis (2D-DIGE)-based comparative proteomic approach on human tissues we identified the fragment D of fibrinogen ß chain (FGB) as marker of preoperative response to neoadjuvant chemo-radiotherapy in rectal cancer [18]. FGB protein is linked to α and γ chains by numerous disulfide bonds to form fibrinogen, a key molecular player of both coagulation and inflammation [10,19,20]. The mean pre-treatment plasma fibrinogen level has been correlated with a hyper-coagulable status, tumor progression and prognosis of several types of malignancies (ovarian [21], biliary [22], esophageal [23], pancreatic [24]), including GC [10–14].

At present, the complex molecular interplay between fibrinogen and cancer has not been fully analyzed locally within the tumor tissue.

In the present study, we investigated differential FGB protein expression levels in biopsies of non-metastatic GC patients, to assess interconnections between GC and platelet/coagulation pathways, and to propose FGB as molecular marker for GC diagnosis. Correlations among the means of platelet (PLT) count, white blood cell count (WBC), neutrophil-to-lymphocyte ratio (NLR) and FGB cleaved products were also analyzed.

2. Results

2.1. Patients and Disease Characteristics

A total of 28 consecutive patients with GC were included in our analysis. Characteristics of both patients and the disease are reported in Tables 1 and A1. Patients' tumors were mostly characterized by corpus location (65%), diffuse histotype (65%), and T3–T4 pathological stages (68%).

Table 1. Clinicopathological characteristics of the 28 patients affected by gastric cancer included in the study (n.s., statistically not significant for $p > 0.05$).

Characteristic	uT1–T2	uT3–T4	p-Value
Gender			n.s.
Male	4	9	
Female	5	10	
Age, years			n.s.
<50	3	4	
>50	6	15	
Histological type			n.s.
Intestinal	4	4	
Diffuse	4	13	
Other	1	2	
Location			n.s.
Corpus	4	14	
Antrum	4	4	
Cardias	1	1	

uT, endoscopic ultrasound evaluation of tumor depth: uT1, invasion of lamina propria, muscolaris mucosae or submucosa; uT2, invasion of muscolaris propria; uT3, invasion of subserosa; uT4, penetration of serosa or invasion of adjacent structures.

The means of plasma routine blood count parameters at diagnosis are reported in Table 2 (detailed information in Table A2).

Table 2. Blood count parameters of gastric cancer (GC)-affected patients (WBC, white blood cells; ANC, absolute neutrophil count; ALC, absolute lymphocyte count; N/R, ANC/ALC ratio; PLT, platelet count; PT-INR, prothrombin time–international normalized ratio; FIB, fibrinogen level; APTT, activated partial thromboplastin time). Values at diagnosis refer to 22 patients.

Parameter	Mean (±SD)
WBC ($\times 10^9$/L)	6.33 ± 1.96
ANC($\times 10^9$/L)	3.93 ± 1.54
ALC ($\times 10^9$/L)	1.83 ± 0.74
N/R	2.54 ± 1.71
PLT ($\times 10^9$/L)	258 ± 114.90
PT-INR	1.00 ± 0.05
FIB g/L	2.97 ± 46
APTTs	29 ± 3

2.2. One-Dimension Immunoblotting

The quantitative proteomics workflow adopted is illustrated in Figure A1.

In T versus N tissues of patients belonging to both groups of tumor staging (Group I: T1 and T2; Group II: T3 and T4), a higher content of a band at ~50 kDa, corresponding to the weight of the entire FGB (UniProtKB entry: P02675; Figure A2), occurred (Figure 1b). Two additional bands of ~37 and ~40 kDa were detected in T tissues, with a higher content in Group II patients especially for the 37 kDa band (Figure 1b). One-dimensional electrophoresis revealed that the amount of total protein loading among samples was homogeneous (Figure 1a).

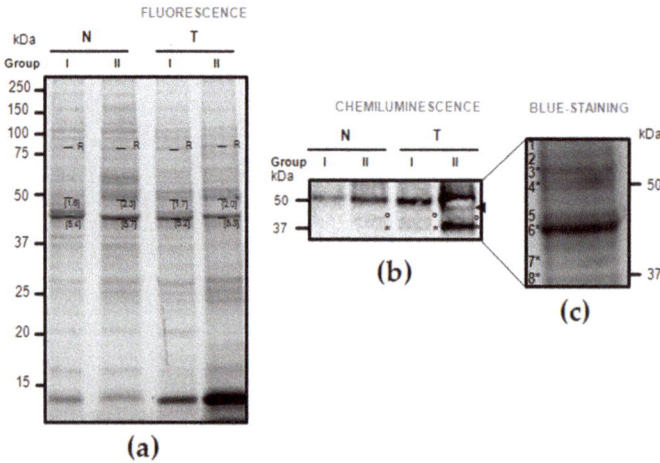

Figure 1. One-dimensional electrophoresis (1DE) and immunoblotting of fibrinogen ß chain (FGB) in normal (N) versus tumor-affected (T) gastric tissues belonging to patients divided according to their tumor stage (Group I: T1–T2; Group II: T3–T4). (**a**) Image of the 1DE stain-free gel fluorescence acquired upon excitation with the Chemidoc system before its transfer to nitrocellulose membrane. Numbers refer to the relative quantity of the band calculated with the Image Lab^{TM} software (R, reference band for which quantity is 1); (**b**) Chemiluminescence signals of proteins cross-reacting with the anti-FGB antibody. Circles and asterisks evidence a band at ~40 and 37 kDa, respectively, while the arrow shows a band at <50 kDa; (**c**) From the blue-stained 1DE gel in (**a**), an area of ~37–60 kDa was excised, and gel portions numbered 1 to 8 submitted to analysis by mass spectrometry for protein identification. Asterisks confirmed the presence of FGB product(s) in the gel portions.

2.3. Validation of Fibrinogen β Chain (FGB) by Mass Spectrometry

The presence of FGB in the 1DE portions of the ~37–60 kDa area (Figure 1c) was validated by mass spectrometry. FGB peptides were identified at ~50 kDa (Figure 1c, gel portions nr 3 and 4), ~40 kDa (Figure 1c, gel portions nr 6), and ~37 kDa (Figure 1c, gel portions nr 7 and 8) (Table A3). The FGB identified at ~50 kDa was the entire form after release of fibrinopeptide B by thrombin in 44–45, and the identified peptides covered from 45 to 491 (Table A3, Figure A2). The FGB identified at ~37 kDa corresponded to the fragment D, after plasmin cleavage of FGB in 163–164, and the identified peptides covered from 164 to 491 (Table A3). Fragment D of FGB was also identified in the band at ~40 kDa, and its slightly different molecular weight (MW) may be related to possible post-translational modifications such as glycosylation, as evidenced after interrogation with iPTMnet bioinformatic resource (Figure A2).

2.4. Cross-Reaction of FGB on Two-Dimensional Electrophoresis (2DE) Maps of Gastric Tissue

An immunoblotting performed to detect FGB on 2DE proteome map of gastric tissues is illustrated in Figure 2. The matching between the spots cross-reacting with anti-FGB antibody on the nitrocellulose membrane and the protein profiles of the 2DE gel, from which the membrane was obtained, was digitally performed. A total of 19 matched spots were individuated, and their differential patterns analyzed in a 2D-DIGE project comparing all the 25 gels (Figure 2c; Table A1).

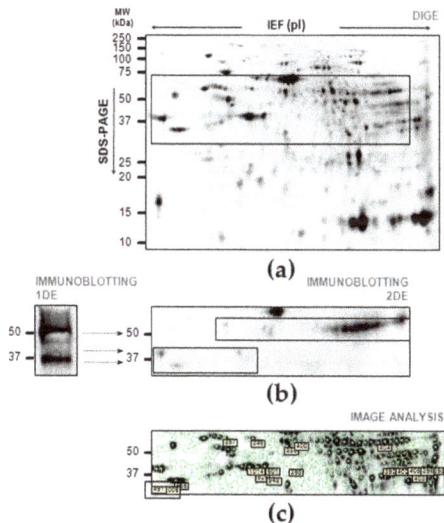

Figure 2. Two-Dimensional Electrophoresis (2DE) and immunoblotting of FGB from proteins pooled from normal and tumor-affected gastric tissues. (**a**) After labelling with cyanines, proteins were resolved by isoelectrofocusing (IEF) over the pI 3–10, followed by 8–16% gradient Sodium Dodecyl Sulfate—PolyAcrylamide Gel Electrophoresis (SDS-PAGE). The gel image was acquired and added to a Decyder project before its transfer to a nitrocellulose membrane. The frame corresponds to the gel area shown in (**b**); (**b**) Visualization of spots cross-reacting with the anti-FGB antibody ([1F9], GeneTex) in the gel area corresponding to the rectangle in (**a**). The 2DE protein map showed FGB cross-reacting spots in the same molecular weights (MWs) as those evidenced by immunoblotting on 1DE gel, here visualized on the left (for more details, see Figure 1b). The frames corresponds to the gel area containing the FGB cross-reacting spots shown in (**c**), on which our image analysis focussed; (**c**) FGB cross-reactive spots were identified, numbered, and analyzed using the Decyder software for quantitative analysis and comparison, as described in Methods section.

Among the 19 spots cross-reacting with the FGB antibody, a part of them was present in the MW region of ~50 kDa and another one in the MW region of ~37–40 kDa (Figure 2b).

In particular, a total of 10 cross-reacting spots (numbered as spots 392, 393, 396, 397, 398, 100, 402, 403, 404 and 405) were found in the MW of 50 kDa as multiple pI isoforms, coming from different phosphorylation status, as evidenced after interrogation with iPTMnet bioinformatic resource (Figure A2). The interrogation of P02675 sequence (UniProtKB) with PhosphoSite Plus evidenced a total of 43 possible different pI values depending on 43 different phoshorylated residues (results in: https://www.phosphosite.org/isoelectricCalcAction.action?id=20774&residues=43&x=41&y=3; accessed on 18 December 2017). The MW/pI position of spots/isoforms corresponding to the entire FGB form in our 2D map fitted with others' published findings as well as with the calculated MW/pI 52.314/7.15. While the position of the FGB cleaved spots/isoforms fitted with our previous findings in rectal tissues [18], as well as with the calculated MW/pI 37.649/5.85.

2.5. Differential Expression of FGB in Gastric Cancer Tissues

Among the 19 spots cross-reacting with the FGB antibody, a total of 13 spots (numbered as spot 383, 393, 396–398, 402–405, 501, 526 and 548) were present in all the gels and, thus, further analyzed.

The results of variation in their abundance between normal and tumor tissues are reported in Table 3, where significant changes at $p < 0.05$ are evidenced in bold. Six among these spots (393, 402, 404, 405, 526 and 548) were differentially expressed between N and T tissue in both Group I and Group II.

Table 3. Comparison of 13 fibrinogen β chain (FGB) spot abundance between tumor-affected (T) and not-affected (N) gastric tissues of patients grouped into "Group I" or "Group II" according to their uT stage ("Group I": T1 and T2; "Group II": T3 and T4).

Comparison Groups	Spots												
	383	397	398	400	393	396	402	403	404	405	501	526	548
• N "Group II" versus N "Group I"	1	−1.6	−1.3	−1.0	1.1	1.1	1.5	1.2	−1.0	1.1	1.1	1.0	1.4
• T "Group I" versus N "Group I"	−1.3	−1.5	−1.5	−1.1	**1.5**	**1.5**	**2.0**	1.3	**1.8**	**1.6**	1.6	**1.5**	**1.6**
• T "Group II" versus N "Group II"	−1.3	−1.2	−1.2	−1.3	**1.5**	1.2	**3.2**	1.1	**2.8**	**1.8**	1.22	**1.82**	**1.75**

Spot variation in abundance is expressed as average spot volume ratio; values >1 refer to an increase, while values <−1 refer to a decrease. Statistically significant average spot volume ratios <1.5 or >1.5 (One-way Anova; $p < 0.05$) are indicated in bold.

In particular, three spots at ~50 kDa (nr. 402, 404 and 405) and two spots at ~37 kDa (nr. 526 and 548) significantly increased in content in T versus N tissues, as well as, if not statistically significantly, in T of Group II versus T of Group I (Figure 3a,c,e). These spots were, thus, globally associated with tumor and, particularly, in tumor at advanced stages (i.e., T3–T4).

Regarding tumor anatomical sites, spot 402, similarly to spots 403, 404, 405, 393 and 396, showed a significantly higher content in T of antrum (Figure 3b), while spots 526 and 548 showed a significantly higher content in T of corpus (Figure 3d,f).

Regarding tumor histological classification, only the spot 501 showed an association with the diffuse type (Figure 3g).

There was no significant difference in FGB abundance depending on either age (except for spot 402) or sex gender (except for spot 501), in any of the spots analyzed (Table 4).

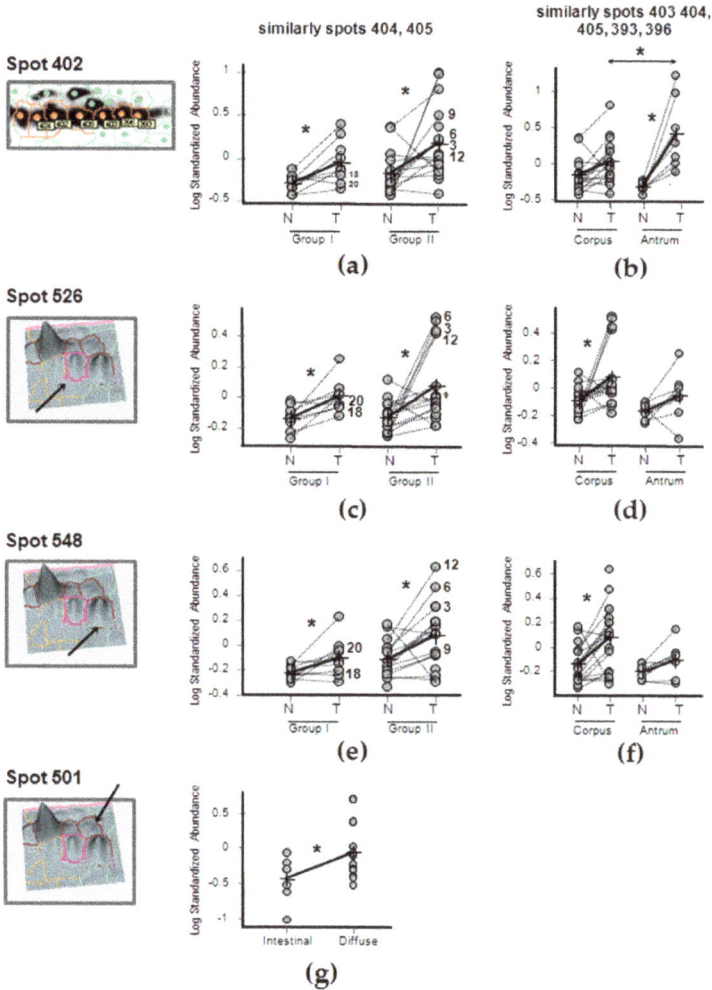

Figure 3. Graphical visualization of abundance distribution of spots 402, 526, 548 and 501 in tumor non-affected (N) and tumor-affected (T) gastric tissue biopsies, according to their tumor stage (Group I: T1–T2; Group II: T3–T4), anatomical site (corpus, antrum) or histological type (intestinal, diffuse). (a) Abundance of Spot 402, similarly to spots 404, 405, 526 (c) and 548 (d), increased in T versus N tissues both in Group I and II, and more even in T-tissue of Group II. (b) Spot 402 abundance, similarly to spots 403, 404, 405, 393 and 396 was particularly higher in T than N in the antrum location, while spots 526 and 548, showed the highest abundance associated with corpus location. (e) Spot 548, similarly to spots 402 (a) and 526 (c), increased in content in T versus N tissues both in Group I and II, its abundance being higher in T-tissues of Group II. (f) Spot 548 content was significantly higher in T versus N tissues in corpus. (g) Spot 501 content was higher in diffuse than intestinal histological type. In each graph, a single circle represents the Log standardized abundance of the spot calculated for a single gel/patient. Asterisks indicate a statistically significant difference at paired *t*-test $p < 0.05$ or between T tissues of different groups (**b**,**g**) at Student's *t*-test $p < 0.05$. Dotted lines combine N and T samples belonging to the same patient and co-migrated within the same gel, while arrows indicate a detail of the Decyder tridimensional 3D view of the graphically visualized spots.

Table 4. Intergroup comparison of FGB spots abundance in affected tumor-samples.

Groups	Spots												
	383	397	398	400	393	396	402	403	404	405	501	526	548
"Tumor staging" Group II (nr = 19) versus Group I (nr = 9)	−1.3	1.0	−1.2	−1.3	1.4	1.2	**3.2**	1.1	**2.8**	1.8	1.2	**1.8**	**1.8**
"Anatomical subsites" Antrum (nr = 8) versus. corpus (nr = 18)	−1.0	**−1.9**	**−2.0**	1.4	**1.7**	**1.7**	**3.4**	**1.9**	**2.8**	**2.3**	1.9	−1.5	−1.7
"Histological subtypes" Diffuse (nr = 18) versus intestinal (nr = 7)	−1.1	1.0	−1.3	−1.3	−1.3	−1.1	−2.1	1.0	−2	−1.7	**3.0**	1.3	−1.1
"Age" >50 years (nr = 19) versus <50 years (nr = 7)	1.1	1.4	1.2	1.1	1.1	−1.1	**3.6**	−1.0	1.8	2.0	−1.1	1.1	1.2
"Sex" Female (nr = 15) versus male (nr = 13)	1.3	2.0	1.8	1.3	−1.0	1.0	−1.0	−1.1	1.2	1.1	−2	−1.3	1.0

Spot variation in abundance is expressed as average spot volume ratio. Statistically significant spot volume ratio <1.5 or >1.5 (Student's *t*-test; $p < 0.05$) were indicated in bold. Values >1.5 refer to an increase, while values <−1.5 refer to a decrease in the average spot volume ratio.

2.6. Correlation of Blood Count Parameters and FGB Abundance

We first analyzed the differences in blood cell count and coagulation markers with each of the 13 spots of interest. Among these, an inverse correlation between the activated partial thromboplastin time (APTT-sec) and the spot 548 log abundance was found ($p = 0.05$, Figure 4). No significant difference was found between the other blood coagulation markers and FGB spot abundance.

We further analyzed the association between changes in blood cell count and FGB spot abundance. By focusing on the only tumor stage Group II, there was a significant correlation between PLT count and spot 526 and 548 log abundances ($p = 0.0006$ and $p = 0.021$, Figure 5a,b, respectively).

In a cohort of healthy blood donors (24 females and 22 males), the optimum cut-off value for PLT count was fixed at 280×10^9/L, estimating the sample mean (208×10^9/L) and two standard deviations ($\pm 70 \times 10^9$/L).

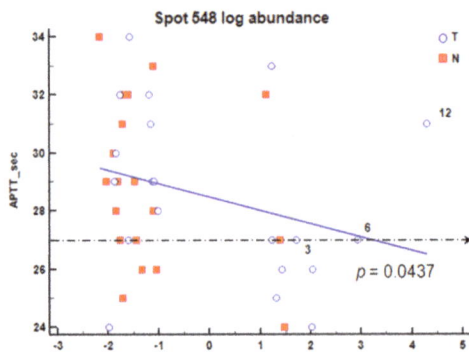

Figure 4. Graphical visualization of the correlation between the activated partial thromboplastin time (APTT) and the log abundance of spot 548 in normal (N, ■) together with malignant (T, ○) tissues of patients belonging to T stage Group II (T3–T4). The broken line indicates the low value considered to be normal. Regression line values were: intercept 28.3 (SE 0.46) and slope −0.55 (SE 0.26).

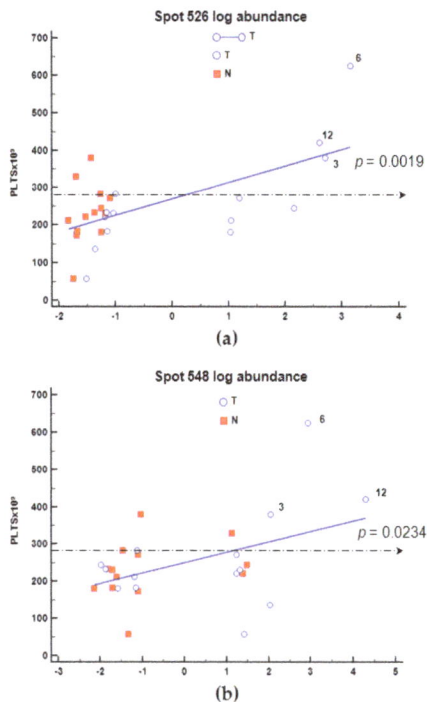

Figure 5. Graphical visualization of the correlation between platelet counts (PLT) and the log abundance of spot 526 in malignant (T, ¡) tissues (**a**), and spots 548 in normal (N, ■) together with malignant (T, ○) tissues of patients (**b**) belonging to Group II (T3–T4). The optimum PLT cut-off of 280×10^9/L(mean $\pm 70 \times 10^9$/L), calculated in the cohort of healthy individuals, is indicated with a broken line. Regression line values were: intercept 260.5 (SE 20.6) and slope 45.0 (SE 12.35) (**a**); intercept 258.4 (SE 15.45) and slope 20.9 (SE 8.85) (**b**).

In GC-affected patients, we individuated 5 patients with PLT count $>280 \times 10^9$/L (patients nr. 3, 6, 9, 12, 18 and 20; Table A2). We excluded patient nr. 11 (PLT count $= 330 \times 10^9$/L) because it was not possible to separate her low abundant T protein extracts. For both spots, the highest PLT count was found in patients nr. 3, 12 and 6, who showed the highest spot abundance (Figure 5a,b,e).

A positive trend between the other blood parameters and FGB spot abundance was found but without statistical significance.

3. Discussion

The present study evidences the differential expression of FGB and its cleaved forms in the biopsies of not-metastatic GC patients. Higher protein contents of the entire form of FGB (~50 kDa) and isoforms containing plasmin-cleavage product "fragment D" of FGB (~37–40 kDa) were found in tumoral gastric tissues compared with non tumoral adjacent tissues, at both early (Group I: T1–T2) and advanced tumor depth (Group II: T3–T4). Even not statistically significant, these increases in content were more evident in patients with advanced GC (Group II: T3–T4) compared with patients at early pathological stages (Group I: T1–T2).

Together with α and β polypeptides, FGB is part of fibrinogen, a disulfide cross-linked homodimer of 340 kDa composed by two outer D domains connected to a central E one. Fibrinogen is known as a principal factor in the maintenance of hemostasis through its conversion from a soluble, plasma protein to an insoluble fibrin gel [18]. During fibrinolysis, both soluble and cross-linked fibrin is enzymatically degraded into fragments, among which the D-dimers typically contains two D domains and one E domain of the original FGB molecule [10].

In malignancies, the presence of fibrin(ogen) is known to affect the progression of tumor cell growth and their metastasis. Globally, the assessment of fibrinogen content and fibrinolysis products in plasma is known to help in cancer diagnosis but also to evaluate both therapeutic effects and prognosis. In the particular case of GC, the preoperative plasma content of fibrinogen is clinically relevant as predictor of lymphatic and hematogenous metastasis, tumor progression, as well as tumor stage and survival [10].

Our data evidencing an up-regulation of both FGB and its cleaved fragments in GC tumors versus the adjacent non-tumoral tissues agree with the 2D results from Wang et al. [25] and the label-free quantitative proteomics findings of Dai et al. [26] in six pairs of primary and advanced poorly differentiated gastric adenocarcinoma tissues. On a larger cohort of patients, our study succeeded in confirming this increase in content and strengthening the hypothesis of an association between the accumulation of both FGB and its cleaved products and gastric malignancy directly in tumor tissues.

Our work allowed to evidence a differential accumulation of FGB in gastric tissues of GC patients depending on the anatomical site affected by cancer: the entire FGB was found to be more abundant in the antrum of the stomach, while its cleaved forms showed a higher content in the corpus. This different content of FGB in different stomach regions may reflect different roles played by FGB in tumorigenesis depending on gastric microenvironments and/or their pathogenesis [27]. For instance, *Helicobacter pylori* infection, one of the most important risk factor of GC, is associated with GC of antrum and intestinal type, and it also causes inflammation and gastritis [28], thus it could have an impact on the production of fibrinogen which is strictly related to the inflammatory response(s).

In the majority of tumor types, abundant fibrinogen, further assembled into fibrin, within the stroma has been proposed to originate from plasma exudation deposition [29]. In solid tumor tissues, the so-called microvascular "enhanced permeability" leads to extravasation and tumoritropic accumulation within the cancer of macromolecules such as plasma proteins, including all those necessary for clot formation (e.g., fibrinogen) [10]. At the same time, an extra-hepatic synthesis of fibrinogen is also known to occur, even if there is still a paucity of information regarding both its structure and function [30–32]. The extra-hepatic fibrinogen synthesis may be important for tissue repair at local sites of injury, and/or may have a pathogenetic role, but it is not known whether extra-hepatic synthesis of FGB significantly contributes to the normal plasma fibrinogen concentration. The deposition of fibrin/ogen into the extracellular matrix may form a provisional matrix on which new blood vessels extend, and serve as a scaffold to support binding of tumor growth factors influencing tumor growth, malignant transformation, and migration [33–37].

Interestingly, a study aimed at defining the role of coagulation proteins in tumor progression by immunohistochemistry highly localized fibrin II and fragment D of FGB in the stroma at tumor periphery near the host-tumor interface, and co-localized hemostatic proteins with the "vascular endothelial growth factor" (VEGF), activated by the "tissue factor" (TF) produced by tumor cells [38].

In addition, factors involved in the regulation of fibrin activation/degradation expressed on cancer cell surfaces may also play a role in tumor invasion, proliferation, and metastasis [39,40]. It may thus be tempting in the future to localize FGB and its D fragment in situ in gastric tissues of our cohort of patients, to better understand a possible role played by FGB in cancer progression.

Globally, hyperfibrinogenemia before treatment is increasingly recognized as an important risk factor influencing the survival of patients with solid tumors [41]. In the particular case of GC, hyperfibrinogenemia has been analyzed as prognostic factor of lymphatic and hematogenous metastasis, tumor progression, adjacent organ involvement and survival [42–50]. In our cohort of patients, there was a positive trend between fibrinogen level in plasma and FGB spot abundance in the tissues, but this correlation did not reach a statistical significance. Our data are thus insufficient to provide a clear information about a correlation between plasma fibrinogen level and FGB spot content in situ in the tumor microenvironment.

Nonetheless, we found a negative correlation between spot 548 and APTT, and a positive correlation between spots 526 and 548 and PLT count, with a better correlation between PLTs and spot 526 in the only malignant T tissues. These associations were particularly evident in T tissues of patients with the highest tumor depth (Group II), this suggesting that by increasing tumor depth the content of peptides included in spots 526 and 548 also increased. Normal value of APTT ranged between 27 to 40 s, and measures the time necessary to generate fibrin from initiation of the intrinsic coagulation pathway, thus short APTT is indicative of an increased risk of hypercoagulability. Several studies indicated that hypercoagulability affect tumor cell adhesion and migration across endothelial junctions [51]. Thus, in our series, patients with lower APTT and higher spot 548 values could be considered at higher risk for tumor growth and metastatic dissemination. Of interest, it has been reported that plasma D-dimer, the smallest product resulting from fibrin degradation by enzymes including plasmin, can also interfere with cellular signaling systems, cell proliferation and angiogenesis, but can also affect PLTs and extra-cellular matrix [52–55]. It has been demonstrated that activation of the coagulation cascade occurring in a cancer such as GC may arise from the direct capacity of tumor cells to express and release pro-coagulant factors, including TF, and to activate the host hemostatic system [56].

In our series, patients showing the highest content of the two degraded forms of FGB containing the fragment D have a significant correlation with PLT count $>280 \times 10^9$/L suggesting a possible role between the increase in content of cleaved FGB in T tissues and PLT count at plasma level. Platelet activation and aggregation, in addition to accelerating coagulation, provide a bolus of secreted proteins, including fibrinogen, and granule contents to the immediate area, all of which help to initiate and accelerate the inflammatory response(s) by the host. It is interesting to note that soluble fibrin monomers have been proposed to enhance PLT adhesion to circulating tumor cells and, thus, facilitate metastatic spread [36,57]. In particular, activated PLTs, similarly to tumor cells, have receptors specific for binding with fibrinogen and fibrin fibers (GPIIb/IIIa). It cannot be excluded that these interactions may also occur in our tissues.

Results of the present study added new information regarding the association of blood parameters and hypercoagulability in GC with the FGB and its cleaved products, which we found differentially expressed in situ in our samples. The FGB forms we found may thus represent new candidate molecules for GC diagnosis, which could be further exploited in terms of possible interconnections between cancer and platelet/coagulation pathways. Recent proposals of many coagulation assays for prognostic value strengthen the importance of coagulation-related investigations in cancer clinics [42,43,58,59].

4. Materials and Methods

4.1. Patients and Tissues

A total of 28 tumor (T) and corresponding adjacent healthy normal (N) gastric tissue biopsies were collected at diagnosis from 28 patients enrolled at the CRO-IRCCS, National Cancer Institute of Aviano (PN), Italy CRO National Cancer institute (Table 1), following the approval by the Institutional Review Board (IRB) of CRO-IRCCS, National Cancer Institute of Aviano (PN), Italy (IRB number CRO-2014-03, 3 March 2014) and written informed consent of all the participating patients. These paired biopsies were stored at −80 °C until analyses. Clinical and laboratory evaluations of all patients are reported in Tables 1 and 2, Tables A1 and A2.

Patients were enrolled between April 2014 and December 2016 and stratified dependently on tumor depth according to the stomach TNM clinical classification [60], evaluated by ultrasound endoscopy.

4.2. Blood Sample Analysis

Venous blood samples in citrated tubes (0.109 M) were collected at diagnosis before the initiation of the treatments. Test performed were: prothrom-bin time–international normalized ratio (PT-INR), activated partial thromboplastin time (APTT), fibrinogen by Clauss clotting method (Siemens-Dade

Behring Healthcare Diagnostics, Marburg, Germany). White blood cells (WBC) and platelet count were measured in EDTA blood samples with a ADVIA2120 Analyser (Siemens).

We considered the following blood biomarker data: white blood cells (WBC); absolute neutrophil count (ANC); absolute lymphocyte count (ALC); ANC/ALC ratio (N/R); platelet count (PLT); prothrombin time (PT-INR); fibrinogen (FIB); activated partial thromboplastin time (APTT).

For 6 patients these analyses were not performed because plasma was not available.

4.3. Sample Preparation and Grouping

Soluble proteins were extracted from the frozen biopsies as previously reported [61]. Briefly, frozen tissue samples were lysed in 200 μL cold lysis buffer (4% (w/v) CHAPS, 7 M Urea, 2 M Thiourea, 30 mM Tris, pH 8.5) with a protease inhibitor cocktail (Sigma-Aldrich, St. Louis, MO, USA), homogenated with a sample grinding kit (GE Healthcare, Uppsala, Sweden) and prepared for two-dimensional electrophoresis (2DE) with 2D Clean-Up Kit (GE Healthcare, Uppsala, Sweden). Protein concentrations were determined with the commercial Bradford reagent (Bio-Rad, Milan, Italy).

Samples were grouped into two groups: "Group I" and "Group II", including patients with primary tumors classified as either "T1 or T2", or "T3 or T4", respectively. Other comparison groupings were based on: (i) anatomical subsite (corpus or antrum); (ii) histological type (diffuse or intestinal); (iii) age (< or >50 years); and (iv) sex (male or female).

4.4. One-Dimensional Electrophoresis (1DE) and Immunoblotting Anti-Fibrinogen β Chain

The presence of FGB and its possible differential abundance were first investigated by immunoblotting analyses. Within each T group (I and II), proteins extracted from either GC or C tissues were pooled (3 patients per pool). Ten μg of proteins per pool were fractionated on 12% Criterion TGX Stain-Free gels and, after gel image acquisition upon fluorescence excitation with the Chemidoc system (Bio-Rad, Milan, Italy), electrotransferred onto nitrocellulose membranes. Membranes were incubated with the monoclonal antibody anti-FGB [1F9] (1:500; GeneTex, Irvine, CA, USA). Antibody-bound proteins were detected by enhanced chemiluminescence using the Chemidoc system after incubation with ECL HRP-conjugated secondary antibodies (1:10,000 dilution, Santa-Cruz, CA, USA) and reaction with ClarityTM Western ECL Substrate (Bio-Rad, Milan, Italy). Because of the lack of universal house-keeping genes to be used as sample loading control in GC [62], image of the stain-free gel acquired before its transfer was used as control for equal protein loading among samples.

4.5. Validation of the 1DE Bands Cross-Reacting with Fibrinogen β Chain

Pooled protein T extracts (10 μg per lane) were separated by 1DE, and images of blue-stained gel were acquired with the Chemidoc system. A total of 10 gel portions in the MW range between 75 and 37 kDa containing proteins cross-reacting with the FGB antibody (Figure 2, rectangle and numbered lanes) were excised, reduced by incubation with 10 mM dithiothreitol (1 h at 57 °C), and alkylated with 55 mM iodoacetamide (45 min at room temperature). Samples were further washed with NH_4HCO_3, dehydrated, trypsin digested and processed for LC-MS/MS analyses using a LTQ XL-Orbitrap ETD equipped with a HPLC NanoEasy-PROXEON (Thermo Fisher Scientific, Waltham, MA, USA). Database searches were done with the MASCOT search engine version 2.3 against SwissProt and NCBInr (Matrix Science, London, UK), and the presence of FGB was searched among first 15 report hits.

4.6. Two-Dimensional Difference in Gel Electrophoresis (2D-DIGE) and Immunoblotting Anti-Fibrinogen β Chain

The entire project consisted of 25 gels detailed in Table A1, each gel containing two protein extracts (25 μg per extract) from both T and N tissues of the same patient, respectively, each labeled with Cy3 or Cy5 with the internal standard (Cy2) representative of the all samples analyzed. In two gels, when protein tissue concentration was not sufficient (gels 5 and 10, Table A1), only proteins from one type of biopsy were analyzed per patient, and protein extracts from two different patients were comigrated.

Cyanine dyes were used for protein labeling (CyDye DIGE Fluor minimal dyes; GE Healthcare, Uppsala, Sweden). Proteins were separated by isoelectrofocusing (IEF) on 3–10 pH gradient dry strips (IPG, GE Healthcare, Uppsala, Sweden) and then on 8–16% Criterion TGX precast midi protein gels (Bio-Rad, Milan, Italy). After 2DE and image gel acquisition (Amersham Typhoon; GE Healthcare, Uppsala, Sweden), differential analysis (DeCyder software version 6.5, GE Healthcare, Uppsala, Sweden) was performed.

One 2DE gel containing 50 µL of two protein extracts (N and T) labeled with cyanines was scanned, its image being loaded to the Decyder project, and immediately after electrotransferred onto a nitrocellulose membrane, which was then processed for revelation of FGB as described above. The 2DE spots visualized in the nitrocellulose membrane as cross-reacting with the anti-FGB antibody were then found in the corresponding Decyder gel, and further image differential gel analyses focused on these only spots of interest. This immunoblotting analysis was performed in triplicate.

4.7. Database Searches for Fibrinogen β Chain Sequence and Post-Translational Modifications

To better interpret the experimental data about FGB isoforms, we focused FGB amino acid sequence and its possible enzymatic cleavage available in UniProtKB (http://www.uniprot.org/uniprot/P02675). Possible post-translational modifications were searched with the iPTMnet integrated resource ([63]; http://proteininformationresource.org/iPTMnet) and GeneCards® human gene database (http://www.genecards.org), using FGB as substrate. The profiles of FGB-spots were compared with those either found after searches in the bibliographic database PubMed (https://www.ncbi.nlm.nih.gov/pubmed/) or available on-line on databases of 2D gel reference maps (DOSAC-COBS-2DPAGE, OGP, REPRODUCTION-2DPAGE, SWISS-2DPAGE, UCD-2DPAGE).

4.8. Image Analysis and Statistics

First, in intragroup comparisons within Groups I and II, we compared the abundances of a selected set of spots in N versus T tissues of the same patient (Table 3). While in intergroup comparisons, N tissue proteome profiles of Group I were compared with N ones of Group II (Table 3) and, similarly, T tissue proteome profiles of Group I were compared with T ones of Group II (Table 4). Secondly, we focused on the only T gastric tissues, and we compared the expressions of our spots of interest among patients depending on: (i) anatomical subsites (corpus versus antrum), (ii) histological types (intestinal versus diffuse) and (iii) age (> versus <50 years old) (Table 4).

Gel image pairs were processed by the Decyder Differential In-gel Analysis (DIA) module to co-detect and differentially quantify the protein spots in the images; the internal standard sample was used as a reference to normalize the data, so the rest of the normalized spot maps could be compared among them. While the Biological variation analysis (BVA) module allowed to perform a gel-to-gel matching of spots across multiple gels, allowing quantitative comparison of protein expression.

The BVA workspace was imported in the Decyder EDA (Extended Data Analysis) module to perform univariate statistical analyses of FGB spot expression. Paired t-test was performed to compare spot expression in normal versus tumor samples collected from the same patient. While Group I (N and T) to Group II (N and T) comparison of spot differential expression was analyzed using independent statistical tests based on average spot volume ratio with One-way Anova corrected with false discovery rate (default setting). Intergroup comparison depending on (i) gender, (ii) age, (iii) cancer histological type and (iv) location were performed using independent statistical tests with Student's t-test, since these factors between Groups I and II were not statistically different. Based on average spot volume ratio, spots for which relative expression changed at least 1.5-fold (increase or decrease) at 95% confidence level ($p < 0.05$) were considered to be significant. Sample size was calculated considering an intergroup spot fold change of 1.5, a σ value of 50, an α value of 0.05, and a power of the test of 0.80. The sample size for each group resulted 8, and it was enlarged in the case of Group II where preliminary analyses showed a higher FGB content.

4.9. Correlation Analysis of Blood Parameters

Log standard abundance data of spots 402, 526, 548 and 501 in both T and N tissue proteomes of Group I and II patients were correlated with blood markers.

We focused on the only 5 patients of our cohort having the abundance of FGB spots in their T tissue proteome maps and PLT count $>280 \times 10^9$/L (asterisks in Table A2).

We used a PLT cut-off value of 280×10^9/L estimating the sample mean (208×10^9/L) and two standard deviations ($\pm 70 \times 10^9$/L) in a cohort of healthy subjects.

5. Conclusions

By a targeted comparative proteomics, we succeeded in revealing an *in situ* differential expression of both the entire and the cleaved FGB forms in GC tissues, depending on cancer development, location, as well as pathological stage. Some of the found FGB forms were associated with blood parameters linked to hypercoagulability. The FGB-related proteins may thus represent new candidate(s) for GC diagnosis, which may be further exploited in terms of possible interconnections between cancer and coagulation pathways.

Acknowledgments: Ombretta Repetto fellowship is funded by 5X1000_2010_MdS. The funder had no role in study design, data collection and analysis, decision to publish, or preparation of the manuscript.

Author Contributions: Ombretta Repetto and Valli De Re conceived and designed the experiments; Ombretta Repetto performed the proteomics experiments; Maria Rita Cozzi and Agostino Steffan collected and analyzed plasma parameters; Ombretta Repetto, Maria Rita Cozzi and Valli De Re analyzed the data; Raffaella Magris contributed to biopsy and clinical data collections; Vincenzo Canzonieri was involved in anatomical and cytological evaluation; Renato Cannizzaro, Stefania Maiero and Gianmaria Miolo acquired clinical data and enrolled patients; Ombretta Repetto, Valli De Re and Maria Rita Cozzi wrote the paper.

Conflicts of Interest: The authors declare no conflict of interest. The founding sponsors had no role in the design of the study; in the collection, analyses, or interpretation of data; in the writing of the manuscript, and in the decision to publish the results.

Abbreviations

1DE	one-dimensional electrophoresis
2DE	two-dimensional electrophoresis
ALC	absolute lymphocyte count
ANC	absolute neutrophil count
APTT	activated partial thromboplastin time
APTT RATIO	ratio of APPT
BVA	biological variation analysis
DIA	decyder differential in-gel analysis
DIGE	difference gel electrophoresis
FGB	fibrinogen β chain
FIB	fibrinogen level
GC	gastric cancer
IEF	isoelectrofocusing
N/R	ANC/ALC ratio
PLT	platelet count
PT	prothrombin time
WBC	white blood cells

Appendix A

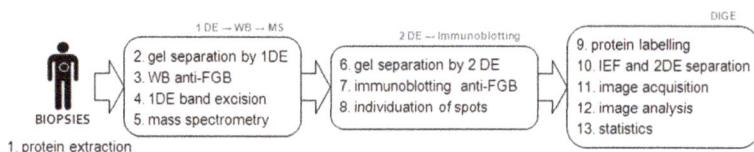

Figure A1. A schematic illustration of the proteomic workflow adopted. Proteins have been extracted from both gastric tumor-affected (T) and normal (N) biopsies of 28 patients. After extraction (1), some protein pools were separated by one-dimensional electrophoresis (1DE) (2), the presence of fibrinogen β chain (FGB) was investigated by western blotting (WB) (3), and the presence of FGB in the cross-reacting 1DE bands was validated by mass spectrometry (4,5). Some protein extracts resulted to contain high levels of FGB were separated by two-dimensional electrophoresis (2DE) (6), and the presence of FGB was successfully individuated to some spots after 2DE immunoblotting on gels (7, 8). For comparative analyses by DIGE, all the protein extracts were labelled (9), separated by isoelectric focusing (IEF) and molecular weight (2DE) (10), images were acquired (11) and targeted image analyses were performed on the only spots of interest containing FGB (12,13). Details are explained in Methods section.

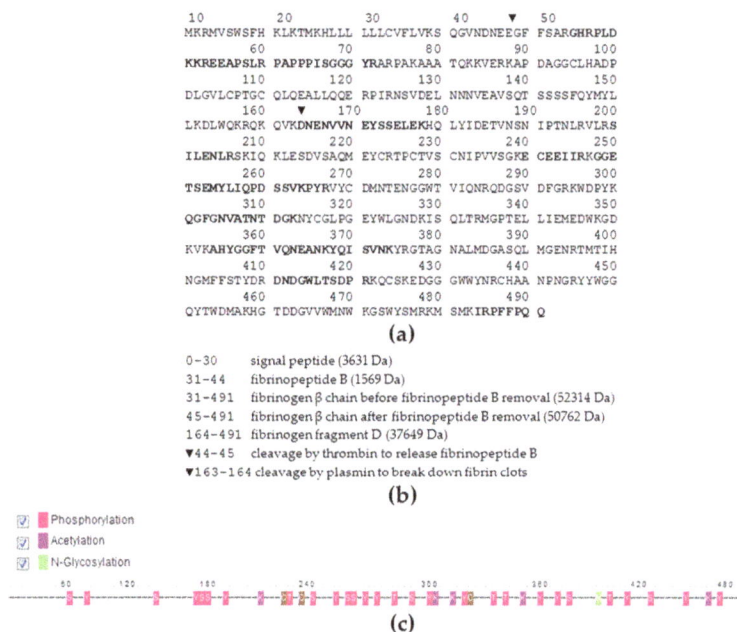

Figure A2. The complete amino acid sequence of fibrinogen β chain (FGB) immature form (http://www.uniprot.org/uniprot/P02675), where the peptides identified by mass spectrometry in gel portions of Figure 1c are evidenced in bold (a). The FGB immature form of 56 kDa is processed into a mature form of ~52 kDa after signal peptide removal. During the conversion of fibrinogen into fibrin, thrombin cleaves fibrinopeptide B from β chains and releases FGB forms of ~51 kDa, which can be further cleaved by plasmin into fibrinogen fragments D of ~37 kDa to break down fibrin clots. These processes are summarized in (b). All the possible post-translational modifications (phosphorylation, acetylation and N-glycosilation) are shown as interactive sequence in (c), after interrogation of P02675 as substrate with iPTMnet bioinformatic resource (http://proteininformationresource.org/iPTMnet).

Table A1. Clinical details of the gastric cancer (GC)-affected patients and corresponding protein pairs extracted from both normal (N) and gastric cancer-affected (T) tissues, labelled with either Cy3 or Cy5 dyes and mixed with the Cy2-labelled internal standard for two-dimensional difference in gel electrophoresis, as described in 'Material and methods' section.

Patient nr.	Age	Male/Female [a]	uT	uN [b]	Histological Classification [b]	Anatomical Subsites	Tissue [c]	Cye Dye	Gel nr.
1	54	M	3	N+	diffuse	corpus	N	cy3	1
							T	cy5	
2	50	F	3	N+	diffuse	antrum	N	cy3	2
							T	cy5	
3	44	F	3	N+	diffuse	corpus	N	cy3	3
							T	cy5	
4	39	F	3	N+	diffuse	corpus	N	cy3	4
							T	cy5	
5	68	M	3	N0	diffuse	corpus	N	cy3	5
6	52	M	3	N+	n.a.	corpus	T	cy5	
7	55	M	3	N+	diffuse	corpus	N	cy5	6
							T	cy3	
8	81	F	3	N+	intestinal	antrum	N	cy5	7
							T	cy3	
9	74	M	3	N+	diffuse	antrum	N	cy5	8
							T	cy3	
10	65	M	4	N+	diffuse	corpus	N	cy5	9
							T	cy3	
11	71	F	3	N0	diffuse	antrum	N	cy5	10
12	69	M	3	N+	intestinal	corpus	T	cy3	
13	60	F	4	n.a.	other	corpus	N	cy5	11
							T	cy3	
14	68	F	4	N0	intestinal	corpus	N	cy5	12
							T	cy3	
15	54	M	3	N+	diffuse	cardia	N	cy5	13
							T	cy3	
16	70	F	2	n.a.	intestinal	antrum	N	cy5	14
							T	cy3	
17	76	F	1	N0	intestinal	antrum	N	cy3	15
							T	cy5	
18	59	M	1	N0	other	cardia	N	cy3	16
							T	cy5	
19	66	F	1	N0	diffuse	corpus	N	cy5	17
							T	cy3	
20	48	M	2	N0	intestinal	corpus	N	cy5	18
							T	cy3	
21	36	F	1	N0	intestinal	corpus	N	cy5	19
							T	cy3	
22	59	M	1	N+	diffuse	corpus	N	cy5	19
							T	cy3	
23	69	F	3	N0	n.a.	corpus	N	cy3	20
							T	cy5	
24	58	M	3	N+	diffuse	corpus	N	cy3	21
							T	cy5	
25	45	F	3	N+	diffuse	corpus	N	cy5	22
							T	cy3	
26	68	M	1	N0	diffuse	antrum	N	cy5	23
							T	cy3	
27	50	F	1	N0	diffuse	antrum	N	cy5	24
							T	cy3	
28	55	F	3	N+	diffuse	corpus	N	cy5	25
							T	cy3	

[a] M, male, F, female; [b] n.a., not available; [c] N, normal tissue; T, GC-affected tissue.

Table A2. Blood biomarkers of gastric cancer-affected patients (WBC, white blood cells; ANC, absolute neutrophil count; ALC, absolute lymphocyte count; N/R, ANC/ALC ratio; PLT, platelet count; PT, prothrombin time; FIB, fibrinogen level; APTT activated partial thromboplastin time; APTT RATIO, the ratio of APPT). Values at diagnosis refer to 22 patients.

Patient nr. [a]	WBC × 10^9/L	PLT × 10^9/L	ANC × 10^9/L	ALC × 10^9/L	N/R	PT-INR	FIB g/L [b]	APTTs	APTT RATIO
1	4.65	221	3	1.3	2.31	0.93	2.91	27	0.83
2	1.19	57	0.7	0.4	1.75	0.93	2.76	26	0.86
3 *	5.23	379	4.5	0.7	6.43	1.13	2.76	26	0.88
4	7.9	272	4.2	2.6	1.62	1	3.54	33	1.1
5	7.61	174	4.1	2.9	1.41	0.99	2.20	28	0.93
6 *	8.95	624	5.3	2.7	1.96	0.95	n.a.	27	0.89
7	6.29	182	3.4	2	1.70	0.99	2.95	34	1.14
8	4.74	184	2.6	1.8	1.44	1	2.76	31	1.03
9 *	7.19	283	4.3	2	2.15	0.96	3.34	29	0.95
10	9.61	137	7.8	1.1	7.09	1.03	3.01	24	0.79
11	7.92	330	5.3	2	2.65	0.99	n.a.	32	1.04
12 *	7.57	421	3.9	3.1	1.26	0.95	2.96	31	1.03
13	8.12	231	6.1	1.2	5.08	1.02	3.37	25	0.83
14	5.11	245	2.7	1.9	1.42	0.92	3.57	24	0.79
15	6.74	212	5.1	1.1	4.64	1.04	3.68	32	1.06
16	4.8	234	2.4	2	1.20	1.06	3.03	29	0.95
17	4,1	215	2.4	1.3	1.85	1.03	3.45	30	1.01
18 *	7.72	283	4.1	2.8	1.46	1.03	3.37	32	1.07
19	7.63	233	5.5	1.6	3.44	0.97	2.16	27	0.89
20 *	6.71	345	3.3	2.7	1.22	1.02	2.56	29	0.97
21	5.05	235	3.2	1.6	2.00	0.95	2.56	27	0.91
22	4.51	177	2.6	1.5	1.73	1.01	2.26	28	0.95

[a] asterisk indicates patients with PLT count upper the cut-off value: 280×10^9/L; [b] n.a., not available.

Table A3. Details of fibrinogen β chain identification by mass spectrometry and database searches in protein extracts of gastric cancer tissues separated by one-dimensional electrophoresis. The MASCOT scores are reported for the only gel portions resulting to contain fibrinogen β chain.

Gel Portion nr.[a]	Database	Accession	Description	Score/Seq. Coverage %	Start–End	Peptide	Matches/Sequences
4	NCBInr	gi|119625336	Fibrinogen β chain, isoform CRA_b	239/29	42–48	R.GHRPLDK.K	11/7
					50–69	K.REEAPSLRPAPPPISGGGYR.A	
					161–175	K.DNENVVNEYSSELEK.H	
					197–203	R.SILENLR.S	
					220–226	K.ECEEIIR.K	
					228–244	K.GGETSEMYLIQPDSSVK.D	
5	SwissProt	FIBB_HUMAN	Fibrinogen β chain	376/28	45–51	R.GHRPLDK.K	19/12
					53–72	K.REEAPSLRPAPPPISGGGYR.A	
					164–178	K.DNENVVNEYSSELEK.H	
					200–206	R.SILENLR.S	
					212–224	K.LESDVSAQMEYCR.T	
					240–246	K.ECEEIIR.K	
					248–267	K.GGETSEMYLIQPDSSVKPYR.V	
					301–313	K.QGFGNVATNTDGK.N	
					354–367	K.AHYGGFTVQNEANK.Y	
					368–374	K.YQISVNK.Y	
					411–421	R.DNDGWLTSDPR.K	
					484–491	K.IRPFFPQQ.-	
7 *	SwissProt	FIBB_HUMAN	Fibrinogen β chain	269/15	164–178	K.DNENVVNEYSSELEK.H	6/5
					212–224	K.LESDVSAQMEYCR.T	
					225–239	R.TPCTVSCNIPVVSGK.E	
					301–313	K.QGFGNVATNTDGK.N	
					354–367	K.AHYGGFTVQNEANK.Y	
					484–491	K.IRPFFPQQ.-	
8 *	SwissProt	FIBB_HUMAN	Fibrinogen β chain	340/19	164–178	K.DNENVVNEYSSELEK.H	8/7
					212–224	K.LESDVSAQMEYCR.T	
					225–239	R.TPCTVSCNIPVVSGK.E	
					240–246	K.ECEEIIR.K	
					248–267	K.GGETSEMYLIQPDSSVKPYR.V	
					301–313	K.QGFGNVATNTDGK.N	
					354–367	K.AHYGGFTVQNEANK.Y	
9 *	SwissProt	FIBB_HUMAN	Fibrinogen β chain	477/21	164–178	K.DNENVVNEYSSELEK.H	13/11
					212–224	K.LESDVSAQMEYCR.T	
					225–239	R.TPCTVSCNIPVVSGK.E	
					240–246	K.ECEEIIR.K	
					248–267	K.GGETSEMYLIQPDSSVKPYR.V	
					301–313	K.QGFGNVATNTDGK.N	
					354–367	K.AHYGGFTVQNEANK.Y	
					484–491	K.IRPFFPQQ.-	

[a] gel portion nr., gel portion numbers refer to Figure 1c; *, gel portions containing the protein sequence 164–491, the fragment D of FGB, coming from plasmin cleavage in 163–164.

References

1. Ferlay, J.; Soerjomataram, I.; Dikshit, R.; Eser, S.; Mathers, C.; Rebelo, M.; Parkin, D.M.; Forman, D.; Bray, F. Cancer incidence and mortality worldwide: Sources, methods and major patterns in GLOBOCAN 2012. *Int. J. Cancer* **2015**, *136*, E359–E386. [CrossRef] [PubMed]
2. Fakhri, B.; Lim, K.H. Molecular landscape and sub-classification of gastrointestinal cancers: A review of literature. *J. Gastrointest. Oncol.* **2017**, *8*, 379–386. [CrossRef] [PubMed]
3. Gigek, C.O.; Calcagno, D.Q.; Rasmussen, L.T.; Santos, L.C.; Leal, M.F.; Wisnieski, F.; Burbano, R.R.; Lourenço, L.G.; Lopes-Filho, G.J.; Smith, M.A.C. Genetic variants in gastric cancer: Risks and clinical implications. *Exp. Mol. Pathol.* **2017**, *103*, 101–111. [CrossRef] [PubMed]
4. Nishikawa, J.; Iizasa, H.; Yoshiyama, H.; Nakamura, M.; Saito, M.; Sasaki, S.; Shimokuri, K.; Yanagihara, M.; Sakai, K.; Suehiro, Y.; et al. The role of epigenetic regulation in Epstein-Barr virus-Associated gastric cancer. *Int. J. Mol. Sci.* **2017**, *18*, E1606. [CrossRef] [PubMed]
5. Patel, T.N.; Roy, S.; Ravi, R. Gastric cancer and related epigenetic alterations. *Ecancermedicalscience* **2017**, *11*, 714. [CrossRef] [PubMed]
6. Kang, C.; Lee, Y.; Lee, J.E. Recent advances in mass spectrometry-based proteomics of gastric cancer. *World J. Gastroenterol.* **2016**, *22*, 8283–8293. [CrossRef] [PubMed]
7. Leal, M.F.; Wisnieski, F.; de Oliveira Gigek, C.; do Santos, L.C.; Calcagno, D.Q.; Burbano, R.R.; Smith, M.C. What gastric cancer proteomic studies show about gastric carcinogenesis? *Tumour Biol.* **2016**, *37*, 9991–10010. [CrossRef] [PubMed]
8. Mohri, Y.; Toiyama, Y.; Kusunoki, M. Progress and prospects for the discovery of biomarkers for gastric cancer: A focus on proteomics. *Expert Rev. Proteom.* **2016**, *13*, 1131–1139. [CrossRef] [PubMed]
9. Sheikh, I.A.; Mirza, Z.; Ali, A.; Aliev, G.; Ashraf, G.M. A proteomics based approach for the identification of gastric cancer related markers. *Curr. Pharm. Des.* **2016**, *22*, 804–811. [CrossRef] [PubMed]
10. Repetto, O.; De Re, V. Coagulation and fibrinolysis in gastric cancer. *Ann. N. Y. Acad. Sci.* **2017**, *1404*, 27–48. [CrossRef] [PubMed]
11. Lee, K.W.; Bang, S.M.; Kim, S.; Lee, H.J.; Shin, D.Y.; Koh, Y.; Lee, Y.G.; Cha, Y.; Kim, Y.J.; Kim, J.H.; et al. The incidence, risk factors and prognostic implications of venous thromboembolism in patients with gastric cancer. *J. Thromb. Haemost.* **2010**, *8*, 540–547. [CrossRef] [PubMed]
12. Kovacova, E.; Kinova, S.; Duris, I.; Remkova, A. Local changes in hemostasis in patients with gastric cancer. *Bratisl. Lek. Listy* **2009**, *110*, 280–284. [PubMed]
13. Kovacova, E.; Kinova, S.; Duris, I.; Remkova, D.A. General changes in hemostasis in gastric cancer. *Bratisl. Lek. Listy* **2009**, *110*, 215–221. [PubMed]
14. Di Micco, P.; Romano, M.; Niglio, A.; Nozzolillo, P.; Federico, A.; Petronella, P.; Nunziata, L.; Di Micco, B.; Torella, R. Alteration of haemostasis in non-metastatic gastric cancer. *Dig. Liver Dis.* **2001**, *33*, 546–550. [CrossRef]
15. Larsen, A.C.; Frøkjær, J.B.; Fisker, R.V.; Iyer, V.; Mortensen, P.B.; Yilmaz, M.K.; Møller, B.; Kristensen, S.R.; Thorlacius-Ussing, O. Treatment-related frequency of venous thrombosis in lower esophageal, gastro-esophageal and gastric cancer—A clinical prospective study of outcome and prognostic factors. *Thromb. Res.* **2015**, *135*, 802–808. [CrossRef] [PubMed]
16. Lee, S.E.; Lee, J.H.; Ryu, K.W.; Nam, B.H.; Cho, S.J.; Lee, J.Y.; Kim, C.G.; Choi, I.J.; Kook, M.C.; Park, S.R.; et al. Preoperative plasma fibrinogen level is a useful predictor of adjacent organ involvement in patients with advanced gastric cancer. *J. Gastric Cancer* **2012**, *12*, 81–87. [CrossRef] [PubMed]
17. Khorana, A.A.; Streiff, M.B.; Farge, D.; Mandala, M.; Debourdeau, P.; Cajfinger, F.; Marty, M.; Falanga, A.; Lyman, G.H. Venous thromboembolism prophylaxis and treatment in cancer: A consensus statement of major guidelines panels and call to action. *J. Clin. Oncol.* **2009**, *27*, 4919–4926. [CrossRef] [PubMed]
18. Repetto, O.; De Re, V.; De Paoli, A.; Belluco, C.; Alessandrini, L.; Canzonieri, V.; Cannizzaro, R. Identification of protein clusters predictive of tumor response in rectal cancer patients receiving neoadjuvant chemo-radiotherapy. *Oncotarget* **2017**, *8*, 28328–28341. [CrossRef] [PubMed]
19. Weisel, J.W.; Litvinov, R.I. Fibrin Formation, Structure and Properties. *Subcell. Biochem.* **2017**, *82*, 405–456. [CrossRef] [PubMed]
20. Mosesson, M.W. Fibrinogen and fibrin structure and functions. *J. Thromb. Haemost.* **2005**, *3*, 1894–1904. [CrossRef] [PubMed]

21. Feng, Z.; Wen, R.; Bi, R.; Duan, Y.; Yang, W.; Wu, X. Thrombocytosis and hyperfibrinogenemia are predictive factors of clinical outcomes in high-grade serous ovarian cancer patients. *BMC Cancer* **2016**, *16*, 43. [CrossRef] [PubMed]

22. Li, H.; Zhao, T.; Ji, X.; Liang, S.; Wang, Z.; Yang, Y.; Yin, J.; Wang, R. Hyperfibrinogenemia predicts poor prognosis in patients with advanced biliary tract cancer. *Tumour Biol.* **2016**, *37*, 3535–3542. [CrossRef] [PubMed]

23. Zhang, S.S.; Lei, Y.Y.; Cai, X.L.; Yang, H.; Xia, X.; Luo, K.J.; Su, C.H.; Zou, J.Y.; Zeng, B.; Hu, Y.; et al. Preoperative serum fibrinogen is an independent prognostic factor in operable esophageal cancer. *Oncotarget* **2016**, *7*, 25461–25469. [CrossRef] [PubMed]

24. Wang, H.; Gao, J.; Bai, M.; Liu, R.; Li, H.; Deng, T.; Zhou, L.; Han, R.; Ge, S.; Huang, D.; et al. The pretreatment platelet and plasma fibrinogen level correlate with tumor progression and metastasis in patients with pancreatic cancer. *Platelets* **2014**, *25*, 382–387. [CrossRef] [PubMed]

25. Wang, K.J.; Wang, R.T.; Zhang, J.Z. Identification of tumor markers using two-dimensional electrophoresis in gastric carcinoma. *World J. Gastroenterol.* **2004**, *10*, 2179–2183. [CrossRef] [PubMed]

26. Dai, P.; Wang, Q.; Wang, W.; Jing, R.; Wang, W.; Wang, F.; Azadzoi, K.M.; Yang, J.H.; Yan, Z. Unraveling Molecular differences of gastric cancer by label-free quantitative proteomics analysis. *Int. J. Mol. Sci.* **2016**, *17*, E69. [CrossRef] [PubMed]

27. Smith, M.; Morton, D. *The Digestive System*, 2nd ed.; Churchill Livingstone: London, UK, 2010; eBook ISBN 9780702048418; Paperback ISBN 9780702033674.

28. Zhang, X.Y.; Zhang, P.Y.; Aboul-Soud, M.A. From inflammation to gastric cancer: Role of *Helicobacter pylori*. *Oncol. Lett.* **2017**, *13*, 543–548. [CrossRef] [PubMed]

29. Dvorak, H.F.; Harvey, V.S.; Estrella, P.; Brown, L.F.; McDonagh, J.; Dvorak, A.M. Fibrin containing gels induce angiogenesis. Implications for tumor stroma generation and wound healing. *Lab. Investig.* **1987**, *57*, 673–686. [PubMed]

30. Lawrence, S.O.; Simpson-Haidaris, P.J. Regulated de novo biosynthesis of fibrinogen in extrahepatic epithelial cells in response to inflammation. *Thromb. Haemost.* **2004**, *92*, 234–243. [CrossRef] [PubMed]

31. Haidaris, P.J. Induction of fibrinogen biosynthesis and secretion from cultured pulmonary epithelial cells. *Blood* **1997**, *89*, 873–882. [PubMed]

32. Molmenti, E.P.; Ziambaras, T.; Perlmutter, D.H. Evidence for an acute phase response in human intestinal epithelial cells. *J. Biol. Chem.* **1993**, *268*, 14116–14124. [PubMed]

33. Stewart, D.A.; Cooper, C.R.; Sikes, R.A. Changes in extracellular matrix (ECM) and ECM-associated proteins in the metastatic progression of prostate cancer. *Reprod. Biol. Endocrinol.* **2004**, *2*, 2. [CrossRef] [PubMed]

34. Simpson-Haidaris, P.J.; Rybarczyk, B. Tumors and fibrinogen. The role of fibrinogen as an extracellular matrix protein. *Ann. N. Y. Acad. Sci.* **2001**, *936*, 406–425. [CrossRef] [PubMed]

35. Palumbo, J.S.; Kombrinck, K.W.; Drew, A.F.; Grimes, T.S.; Kiser, J.H.; Degen, J.L.; Bugge, T.H. Fibrinogen is an important determinant of the metastatic potential of circulating tumor cells. *Blood* **2000**, *96*, 3302–3309. [PubMed]

36. Biggerstaff, J.P.; Seth, N.; Amirkhosravi, A.; Amaya, M.; Fogarty, S.; Meyer, T.V.; Siddiqui, F.; Francis, J.L. Soluble fibrin augments platelet/tumor cell adherence in vitro and in vivo, and enhances experimental metastasis. *Clin. Exp. Metastasis* **1999**, *17*, 723–730. [CrossRef] [PubMed]

37. Sahni, A.; Odrljin, T.; Francis, C.W. Binding of basic fibroblast growth factor to fibrinogen and fibrin. *J. Biol. Chem.* **1998**, *273*, 7554–7559. [CrossRef] [PubMed]

38. Wojtukiewicz, M.Z.; Sierko, E.; Zacharski, L.R.; Zimnoch, L.; Kudryk, B.; Kisiel, W. Tissue factor-dependent coagulation activation and impaired fibrinolysis in situ in gastric cancer. *Semin. Thromb. Hemost.* **2003**, *29*, 291–300. [CrossRef] [PubMed]

39. Lou, X.; Sun, J.; Gong, S.; Yu, X.; Gong, R.; Den, H. Interaction between circulating cancer cells and platelets: Clinical implication. *Chin. J. Cancer Res.* **2015**, *27*, 450–460. [CrossRef] [PubMed]

40. Jurasz, P.; Alonso-Escolano, D.; Radomski, M.W. Platelet-cancer interactions: Mechanisms and pharmacology of tumour cell-induced platelet aggregation. *Br. J. Pharmacol.* **2004**, *143*, 819–826. [CrossRef] [PubMed]

41. Perisanidis, C.; Psyrri, A.; Cohen, E.E.; Engelmann, J.; Heinze, G.; Perisanidis, B.; Stift, A.; Filipits, M.; Kornek, G.; Nkenke, E. Prognostic role of pretreatment plasma fibrinogen in patients with solid tumors: A systematic review and meta-analysis. *Cancer Treat. Rev.* **2015**, *41*, 960–970. [CrossRef] [PubMed]

42. Arigami, T.; Uenosono, Y.; Ishigami, S.; Okubo, K.; Kijima, T.; Yanagita, S.; Okumura, H.; Uchikado, Y.; Kijima, Y.; Nakajo, A.; et al. A novel scoring system based on fibrinogen and the neutrophil-lymphocyte ratio as a predictor of chemotherapy response and prognosis in patients with advanced gastric cancer. *Oncology* **2016**, *90*, 186–192. [CrossRef] [PubMed]

43. Arigami, T.; Uenosono, Y.; Matsushita, D.; Yanagita, S.; Uchikado, Y.; Kita, Y.; Mori, S.; Kijima, Y.; Okumura, H.; Maemura, K.; et al. Combined fibrinogen concentration and neutrophil-lymphocyte ratio as a prognostic marker of gastric cancer. *Oncol. Lett.* **2016**, *11*, 1537–1544. [CrossRef] [PubMed]

44. Palaj, J.; Kečkéš, Š.; Marek, V.; Dyttert, D.; Waczulíková, I.; Durdík, Š. Fibrinogen levels are associated with lymph node involvement and overall survival in gastric cancer patients. *Anticancer Res.* **2018**, *38*, 1097–1104. [CrossRef] [PubMed]

45. Suzuki, T.; Shimada, H.; Nanami, T.; Oshima, Y.; Yajima, S.; Ito, M.; Washizawa, N.; Kaneko, H. Hyperfibrinogenemia is associated with inflammatory mediators and poor prognosis in patients with gastric cancer. *Surg. Today* **2016**, *46*, 1394–1401. [CrossRef] [PubMed]

46. Wu, C.; Luo, Z.; Tang, D.; Liu, L.; Yao, D.; Zhu, L.; Wang, Z. Identification of carboxyl terminal peptide of fibrinogen as a potential serum biomarker for gastric cancer. *Tumour Biol.* **2016**, *37*, 6963–6970. [CrossRef] [PubMed]

47. Yamashita, H.; Kitayama, J.; Kanno, N.; Yatomi, Y.; Nagawa, H. Hyperfibrinogenemia is associated with lymphatic as well as hematogenous metastasis and worse clinical outcome in T2 gastric cancer. *BMC Cancer* **2006**, *6*, 147. [CrossRef] [PubMed]

48. Yu, W.; Wang, Y.; Shen, B. An elevated preoperative plasma fibrinogen level is associated with poor overall survival in Chinese gastric cancer patients. *Cancer Epidemiol.* **2016**, *42*, 39–45. [CrossRef] [PubMed]

49. Yu, X.; Hu, F.; Yao, Q.; Li, C.; Zhang, H.; Xue, Y. Serum fibrinogen levels are positively correlated with advanced tumor stage and poor survival in patients with gastric cancer undergoing gastrectomy: A large cohort retrospective study. *BMC Cancer* **2016**, *16*, 480. [CrossRef] [PubMed]

50. Yamashita, H.; Kitayam, J.; Nagawa, H. Hyperfibrinogenemia is a useful predictor for lymphatic metastasis in human gastric cancer. *Jpn. J. Clin. Oncol.* **2005**, *35*, 595–600. [CrossRef] [PubMed]

51. Caine, G.J.; Stonelake, P.S.; Lip, G.Y.; Kehoe, S.T. The hypercoagulable state of malignancy: Pathogenesis and current debate. *Neoplasia* **2002**, *4*, 465–473. [CrossRef] [PubMed]

52. Altiay, G.; Ciftci, A.; Demir, M.; Kocak, Z.; Sut, N.; Tabakoglu, E.; Hatipoglu, O.N.; Caglar, T. High plasma D-dimer level is associated with decreased survival in patients with lung cancer. *Clin. Oncol.* **2007**, *19*, 494–498. [CrossRef] [PubMed]

53. Buller, H.R.; van Doormaal, F.F.; van Sluis, G.L.; Kamphuisen, P.W. Cancer and thrombosis: From molecular mechanisms to clinical presentations. *J. Thromb. Haemost.* **2007**, *5*, 246–254. [CrossRef] [PubMed]

54. Buccheri, G.; Torchio, P.; Ferrigno, D. Plasma levels of D-dimer in lung carcinoma: Clinical and prognostic significance. *Cancer* **2003**, *97*, 3044–3052. [CrossRef] [PubMed]

55. Dupuy, E.; Hainaud, P.; Villemain, A.; Bodevin-Phèdre, E.; Brouland, J.P.; Briand, P.; Tobelem, G.J. Tumoral angiogenesis and tissue factor expression during hepatocellular carcinoma progression in a transgenic mouse model. *J. Hepatol.* **2003**, *38*, 793–802. [CrossRef]

56. Coussens, L.M.; Werb, Z. Inflammation and cancer. *Nature* **2002**, *420*, 860–867. [CrossRef] [PubMed]

57. Menter, D.G.; Kopetz, S.; Hawk, E.; Sood, A.K.; Loree, J.M.; Gresele, P.; Honn, K.V. Platelet "first responders" in wound response, cancer, and metastasis. *Cancer Metastasis Rev.* **2017**, *36*, 199–213. [CrossRef] [PubMed]

58. Kanda, M.; Tanaka, C.; Kobayashi, D.; Mizuno, A.; Tanaka, Y.; Takami, H.; Iwata, N.; Hayashi, M.; Niwa, Y.; Yamada, S.; et al. Proposal of the Coagulation Score as a Predictor for Short-Term and Long-Term Outcomes of Patients with Resectable Gastric Cancer. *Ann. Surg. Oncol.* **2017**, *24*, 502–509. [CrossRef] [PubMed]

59. Tas, F.; Ciftci, R.; Kilic, L.; Serilmez, M.; Karabulut, S.; Duranyildiz, D. Clinical and prognostic significance of coagulation assays in gastric cancer. *J. Gastrointest. Cancer* **2013**, *44*, 285–292. [CrossRef] [PubMed]

60. Brierley, D.; Gospodarowicz, M.K.; Wittekind, C. *Classification of Malignant Tumours*, 8th ed.; Wiley Blackwell: Hoboken, NJ, USA, 2016; pp. 63–66. ISBN 978-1-119-26357-9.

61. Repetto, O.; Zanussi, S.; Casarotto, M.; Canzonieri, V.; De Paoli, P.; Cannizzaro, R.; De Re, V. Differential proteomics of *Helicobacter pylori* associated with autoimmune atrophic gastritis. *Mol. Med.* **2014**, *20*, 57–71. [CrossRef] [PubMed]

62. Zhao, L.M.; Zheng, Z.X.; Zhao, X.; Shi, J.; Bi, J.J.; Pei, W.; Feng, Q. Optimization of reference genes for normalization of the quantitative polymerase chain reaction in tissue samples of gastric cancer. *Asian Pac. J. Cancer Prev.* **2014**, *15*, 5815–5818. [CrossRef] [PubMed]

63. Huang, H.; Arighi, C.N.; Ross, K.E.; Ren, J.; Li, G.; Chen, S.C.; Wang, Q.; Cowart, J.; Vijay-Shanker, K.; Wu, C.H. iPTMnet: An integrated resource for protein post-translational modification network discovery. *Nucleic Acids Res.* **2017**, *56*, D542–D550. [CrossRef] [PubMed]

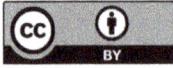

International Journal of
Molecular Sciences

MDPI

Article

The Transcriptomic Landscape of Gastric Cancer: Insights into Epstein-Barr Virus Infected and Microsatellite Unstable Tumors

Irene Gullo [1,2,3,4], Joana Carvalho [3,4], Diana Martins [3,4], Diana Lemos [3,4], Ana Rita Monteiro [3,4], Marta Ferreira [3,4], Kakoli Das [5], Patrick Tan [5,6,7], Carla Oliveira [3,4], Fátima Carneiro [1,2,3,4] and Patrícia Oliveira [3,4,*]

1   Department of Pathology, Centro Hospitalar de São João, Porto 4200-319, Portugal; irene.gullo12@gmail.com (I.G.); fcarneiro@ipatimup.pt (F.C.)
2   Department of Pathology, Faculty of Medicine of the University of Porto (FMUP), Porto 4200-319, Portugal
3   Institute of Molecular Pathology and Immunology, University of Porto (Ipatimup), Porto 4200-135, Portugal; jcarvalho@ipatimup.pt (J.C.); dianam@ipatimup.pt (D.M.); dlemos@ipatimup.pt (D.L.); anaritapatriciomonteiro@gmail.com (A.R.M.); martaf@ipatimup.pt (M.F.); carlaol@ipatimup.pt (C.O.)
4   Instituto de Investigação e Inovação em Saúde (i3S), University of Porto, Porto 4200-135, Portugal
5   Cancer and Stem Cell Biology Program, Duke-NUS Medical School, Singapore 169857, Singapore; kakoli.das@duke-nus.edu.sg (K.D.); gmstanp@duke-nus.edu.sg (P.T.)
6   Genome Institute of Singapore, Biopolis, Singapore 138672, Singapore
7   Cancer Science Institute of Singapore, National University of Singapore, Singapore 117599, Singapore
*   Correspondence: poliveira@ipatimup.pt; Tel.: +351-220-408-800

Received: 30 May 2018; Accepted: 13 July 2018; Published: 17 July 2018

Abstract: Background: Epstein-Barr Virus (EBV) positive and microsatellite unstable (MSI-high) gastric cancer (GC) are molecular subgroups with distinctive molecular profiles. We explored the transcriptomic differences between EBV+ and MSI-high GCs, and the expression of current GC immunotherapy targets such as PD-1, PD-L1, CTLA4 and Dies1/VISTA. Methods: Using Nanostring Technology and comparative bioinformatics, we analyzed the expression of 499 genes in 46 GCs, classified either as EBV positive (EBER in situ hybridization) or MSI-high (PCR/fragment analysis). PD-L1 protein expression was assessed by immunohistochemistry. Results: From the 46 GCs, 27 tested MSI-high/EBV−, 15 tested MSS/EBV+ and four tested MSS/EBV−. The Nanostring CodeSet could segregate GCs according to MSI and, to a lesser extent, EBV status. Functional annotation of differentially expressed genes associated MSI-high/EBV− GCs with mitotic activity and MSS/EBV+ GCs with immune response. PD-L1 protein expression, evaluated in stromal immune cells, was lower in MSI-high/EBV− GCs. High mRNA expression of *PD-1*, *CTLA4* and *Dies1/VISTA* and distinctive *PD-1/PD-L1* co-expression patterns ($PD-1^{high}/PD-L1^{low}$, $PD-1^{high}/PDL1^{high}$) were associated with MSS/EBV+ molecular subtype and gastric cancer with lymphoid stroma (GCLS) morphological features. Conclusions: EBV+ and MSI-high GCs present distinct transcriptomic profiles. GCLS/EBV+ cases frequently present co-expression of multiple immunotherapy targets, a finding with putative therapeutic implications.

Keywords: gastric cancer; transcriptomic profiling; Epstein-Barr Virus; EBV; microsatellite instability; MSI

---

1. Introduction

Gastric Cancer (GC) is a heterogeneous disease at the morphological and molecular levels [1]. Numerous somatic gene mutations, copy-number variations, translocations/inversions, as well as epigenetic and transcriptional changes have been described so far in this disease [2]. However, very few prognostic and predictive biomarkers of therapy response have been introduced into clinical practice [3], and the "one-size-fits-all" is currently the main approach to treat GC patients. Understanding GC molecular heterogeneity and deciphering its players is urgently needed to define more homogenous and targetable biological subtypes.

Recently, several groups [4–6] were able to uncover distinct molecular subtypes with potential clinical significance and therapeutic implications, through the integrative analysis of large-scale genomic and proteomic data. The landmark study of GC that attempted to determine a molecular-based stratification was carried out by The Cancer Genome Atlas (TCGA) research network [4]. By investigating exome sequences, copy-number alterations, DNA methylation, gene expression and proteomic data, TCGA classified GC into four subtypes: (1) Epstein-Barr Virus positive (EBV+) GCs, (2) GCs with microsatellite instability (MSI-high), (3) genomically stable GCs and (4) GCs with chromosomal instability.

The current study focuses on the EBV+ and MSI-high molecular subtypes. The TCGA study has shown that EBV+ GCs display distinctive molecular characteristics: high genomic-wide hypermethylation with *CDKN2A* silencing, amplification of *JAK2*, *CD274*, *PDCD1LG2*, and *ERBB2*, mutations of *PIK3CA*, *ARID1A* and *BCOR*, and very rarely *TP53* mutations. Most EBV+ GCs were in the proximal stomach (fundus/body), affecting mainly male patients and had a better prognosis than other subtypes [4,6]. MSI-high GCs are characterized by: a hypermethylation phenotype associated with *MLH1* silencing, and accordingly a hypermutated status often targeting *TP53*, *KRAS*, *ARID1A*, *PIK3CA*, *ERBB3*, *PTEN* and *HLA-B* [4]. Patients with MSI-high tumors are generally diagnosed at older age, are mainly females and display better prognosis than patients with the genomically stable subtype, but worse than EBV+ GC patients [4–7].

Based on gene expression analysis, the TCGA study revealed four clusters of differentially expressed (DE)-genes, which have to some extent correspondence with specific molecular subtypes [4], thus demonstrating the robustness of the proposed classification. An mRNA cluster enriched in genes involved in mitotic pathways was associated with the MSI-high subtype, while for EBV+ GCs an enrichment in genes associated with immune signaling was observed [4]. In-depth studies based on TCGA transcriptomic data confirmed that genes related to T-cell cytotoxic function, pro-inflammatory cytokines signaling and interferon gamma (IFNγ) response were highly expressed in EBV+ GCs and, to a lesser extent, in MSI-high GCs [2,6,8,9]. Moreover, PD-1/PD-L1 mRNA and protein expression are frequently present in both EBV+ and MSI-high molecular subtypes [8,9]. Accordingly, EBV+ and MSI-high GCs are frequently characterized by prominent immune infiltrate and may display the morphological features of GC with lymphoid stroma (GCLS) [9–13], a rare histological phenotype characterized by prominent lymphoid infiltration [14].

These molecular data offer a rationale to investigate the value of EBV and MSI molecular status in predicting the efficacy of immunotherapy in GC. Currently, the only predictive biomarkers used to select GC patients for targeted immunotherapy, i.e., Pembrolizumab (anti-PD-1 antibody) [15–17] are MSI-high status and/or the expression of PD-L1 by immunohistochemistry (IHC) in cancer epithelial cells and/or in immune cells of the tumor microenvironment. However, several clinical trials have shown that GC patients benefit from PD-1/PD-L1 immune checkpoint inhibitors regardless of PD-L1 expression [18–20]. Therefore, the investigation of morphological and new molecular profiles in this context might help optimizing treatment selection. A recent clinical trial with Pembrolizumab across different cancer types, including GC, demonstrated that tumors with an expression signature enriched in genes related to cytotoxic effector signaling, pro-inflammatory cytokines/chemokines and IFNγ response, showed a T-cell inflamed phenotype associated with better response to targeted immunotherapies [21]. These and other recent evidences suggest that measuring multiple immunological determinants may be relevant to predict who will respond to targeted immunotherapies [22]. Therefore, in this context, the presence of EBV positivity and MSI-high status in GC may serve to select patients for immune checkpoint inhibitor therapy [8,9,13].

Although a growing number of publications have focused on the study of EBV+ and MSI-high molecular subtypes separately or as a group, an in-depth analysis of the contribution of EBV infection and MSI status to the transcriptomic landscape of GC is still lacking. In this study, we performed an unbiased analysis, aimed at uncovering differences within the gene expression profiles of EBV+ and MSI-high molecular subtypes, and at analyzing the expression profile of current targets for immunotherapy in GC.

2. Results

We studied 46 GCs characterized for two molecular features: (1) EBV infection and, (2) MSI-high status (Figure 1). Fifteen out of 46 GC (32.6%) displayed EBV positivity (EBV+) and the remaining 31/46 (67.4%) were negative (EBV−). Concerning MSI status, 27/46 (58.7%) were MSI-high while 19/46 (41.3%) were microsatellite stable (MSS). All EBV+ GC cases were MSS, while most (27/31) EBV− cases were MSI-high (Figure 1).

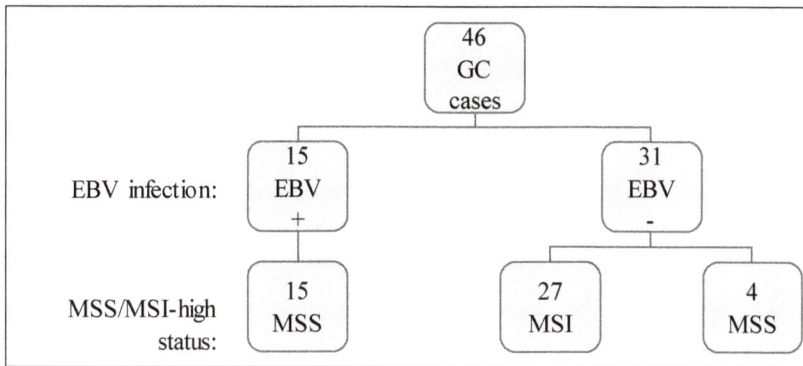

Figure 1. Cohort characterization for EBV infection and MSI status.

2.1. EBV+ and MSI-High GCs Displayed Distinct Transcriptomic Signatures

We analyzed the transcriptomic landscape of the 46 GC cases, aimed at unveiling differences between EBV+ and MSI-high GC subtypes. For this, we have used a previously published Nanostring nCounter CodeSet [23], which comprised 499 genes associated with oncogenic signaling pathways, GC molecular subtype signatures and immune response. After adequate data analysis and normalization, the expression of the 499 genes was plotted in a heatmap and non-hierarchical clustering and principal component analysis (PCA) were performed (Figure 2).

Concerning MSI-high status, we observed that 26/27 MSI-high cases were clustered in clusters 2A and 2B, and 17/19 MSS cases were clustered together in cluster 2C (Figure 2a). Using a PCA, we observed a clear separation between MSI-high and MSS cases (circles vs. squares, Figure 2b). Concerning EBV infection, we observed that most EBV+ cases (13/15) were clustered together in cluster 2C, with the remaining two EBV+ cases found within/close to cluster 2B (Figure 2a). With the PCA, almost all EBV+ cases were separated from EBV− cases (black vs. gray, Figure 2b).

As we correlated the information from the heatmap and dendrogram and the PCA, we could observe the clear separation of two MSS/EBV+ cases in the PCA, which likely reflects overall higher expression in these two cases (black squares with asterisk, Figure 2). Furthermore, we observed the MSI-high/EBV− case in MSS-rich cluster 2C, however clustered among MSI-high cases in the PCA, highlighting the differences in the clustering strategies (gray circle with asterisk, Figure 2). These results suggested that the transcriptomic landscape assessed can clearly distinguish GC cases with an MSS phenotype from those with MSI-high phenotype, and, to a lesser degree, EBV+ from EBV− cases.

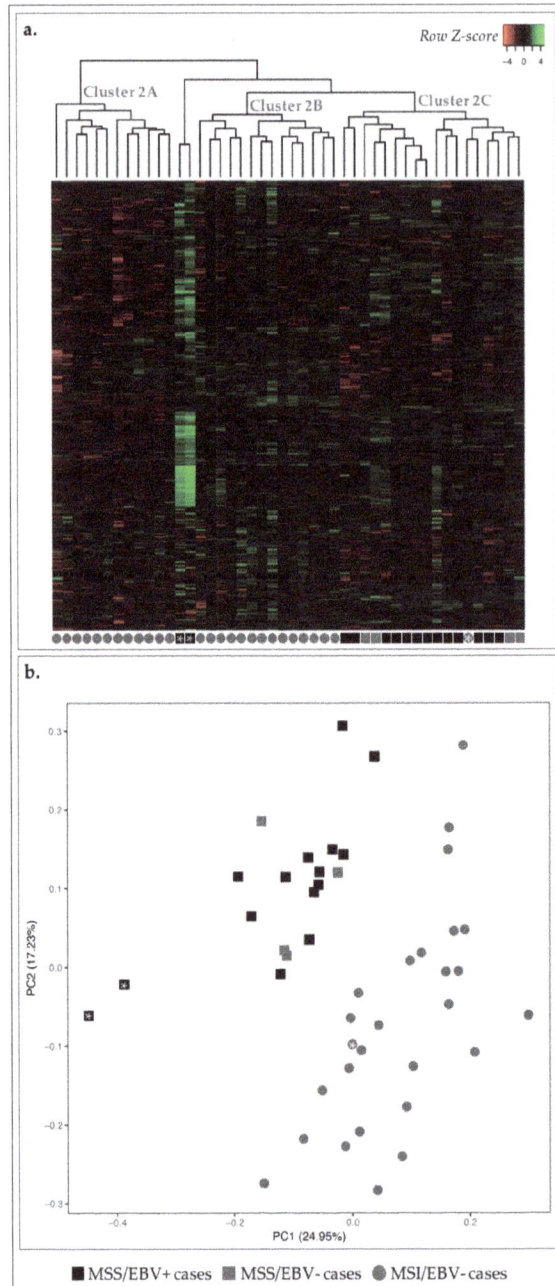

Figure 2. Transcription profile of 46 GC cases for 499 genes in the Nanostring CodeSet. Asterisks are used for cross-reference between the two figures and as links to the main text. (**a**) Heatmap for the expression of all genes in all GC cases (log 2 and Z-score scaled). Indicated are three main clusters: 2A–C. (**b**) PCA for principal components 1 and 2 for the 46 GC samples. Black squares correspond to MSS/EBV+ cases (*n* = 15), gray squares to MSS/EBV− cases (*n* = 4), gray circles to MSI-high/EBV− cases (*n* = 27).

To further reinforce these findings, we used the partitioning method *k-means* and several values of *k* to understand how strongly the gene expression profile followed the classification MSI-high or EBV+. The best results were observed for a value of *k* = 3, as the clusters calculated were the most homogeneous in terms of molecular subtypes, particularly for the MSS/MSI-high status. In fact, all MSI-high cases fell into cluster I and were perfectly separated from MSS cases that fell into clusters II and III (Table 1). For EBV− cases, the clustering was more heterogeneous, spreading across two different clusters (I and III). Of notice, if we disregard the two samples in cluster II, which correspond to those previously shown to display an abnormally high global expression profile (black squares with asterisk, Figure 2), homogeneity in cluster III becomes evident.

Table 1. Clustering results using a *k*-means approach. Represented is the number of MSI-high/MSS and EBV+/EBV− cases obtained in each cluster for each *k* value.

Value of *k*	Cluster ID	MSI Status		EBV Infection	
		MSI-High (*n* = 27)	MSS (*n* = 19)	EBV+ (*n* = 15)	EBV− (*n* = 31)
2	I	25	1	1	26
	II	2	18	14	6
3	I	27	0	0	27
	II	0	2	2	0
	III	0	17	13	4
4	I	13	0	0	13
	II	14	0	0	14
	III	0	17	13	4
	IV	0	2	2	0
5	I	0	12	9	3
	II	12	0	0	12
	III	0	2	2	0
	IV	12	0	0	12
	V	3	5	4	4

Our observations show that the gene expression profile assessed with the Nanostring CodeSet was sufficient to illustrate the molecular separation of MSS and MSI-high molecular subtypes. This analysis also provides the *rationale* to derive a smaller specific gene expression signature that strongly discriminates MSS and MSI-high phenotypes and, to a lesser extent, EBV infection status. To better understand this, we next studied each molecular subtype independently, aiming at uncovering the biological meaning of the gene expression profiles associated with each phenotype.

2.2. MSI-High GC Cases Displayed a Mitotic Signature, While MSS GC Cases Showed an Immune Response Signature

We first compared the transcriptomic landscape of MSS and MSI-high cases and detected 193 genes DE-genes (False Discovery Rate (FDR) $\leq$ 0.05 and 1.5 $\leq$ fold-change $\leq$ 0.6). By performing a non-hierarchical clustering using specifically these DE-genes, we observed that all MSS cases (*n* = 19/19) and the majority of MSI-high cases (*n* = 25/27), were clustered together (cluster 3A and cluster 3B, respectively) (Figure 3a), while two MSI-high outlier cases clustered together with the MSS cases (cluster 3A, circles with cross, Figure 3a). However, these two cases were clustered closer to the remaining MSI-high cases than MSS with PCA, with over 50% of data variability considered (Figure 3b). In fact, PCA exhibited a clear separation of cases according to MSS/MSI-high status.

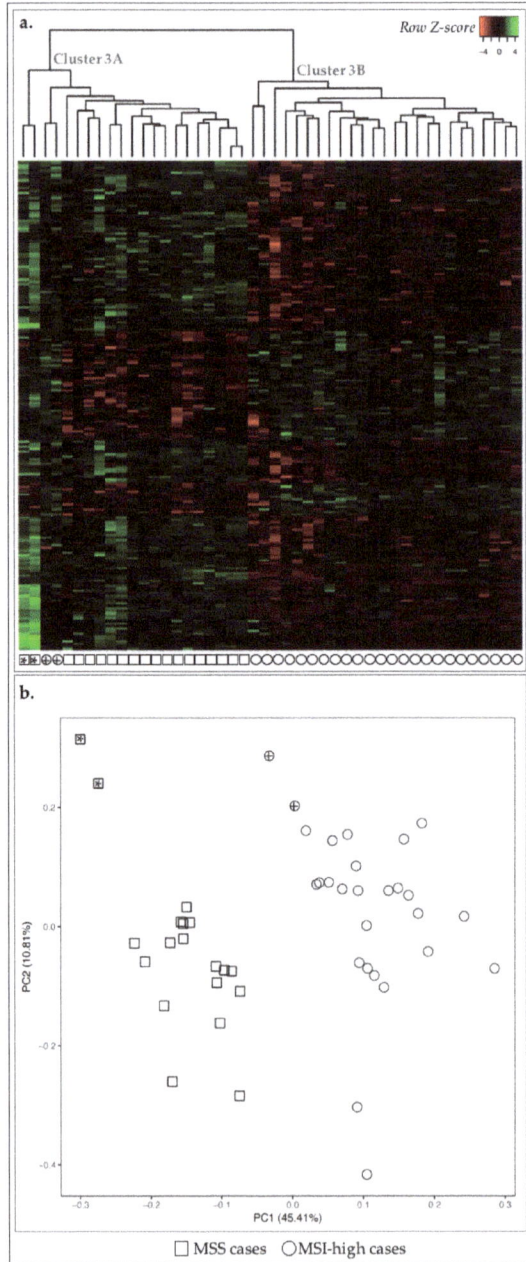

Figure 3. Expression profile of the 46 GC cases for 193 DE-genes between MSS and MSI-high cases. Asterisks and crosses are used for cross-reference between the two figures and as links to the main text. (**a**) Heatmap for the expression of the 193 DE-genes (log 2 and Z-score scaled). Indicated are two main clusters: 3A and 3B. (**b**) PCA for principal components 1 and 2 for the 46 GC samples. Squares correspond to MSS cases (*n* = 19) and circles to MSI-high (*n* = 27). Circles with cross or squares with asterisk for correspondence between panels (**a**) and (**b**) and described in the main text.

We next searched for biological annotations among the 193 DE-genes between MSS and MSI-high cases [24,25]. We observed enrichment in the more generalist terms such as signal peptide and disulfide bond, as well as in regulation of cell proliferation and chemotaxis (Table 2).

Table 2. FDR-ranked top 10 biological terms significantly enriched in the set of 193 DE-genes when comparing the expression profile for 499 genes between MSS and MSI-high cases.

Biological Term	Count	FDR
Signal Peptide	73	1.24×10^{-11}
Disulfide bond	64	1.05×10^{-09}
Secreted	44	2.67×10^{-7}
GO:0042127~regulation of cell proliferation	31	1.77×10^{-6}
GO:0006935~chemotaxis	15	3.16×10^{-6}
GO:0042330~taxis	15	3.16×10^{-6}
IPR001811:Small chemokine, interleukin-8-like	9	8.69×10^{-6}
GO:0007626~locomotory behavior	18	1.08×10^{-5}
GO:0045321~leukocyte activation	17	1.26×10^{-5}
GO:0008009~chemokine activity	9	2.10×10^{-5}

Count: number of DE-genes associated with a given biological term; FDR: False Discovery Rate.

From the 193 DE-genes, 55 were upregulated in MSI-high cases and annotated to terms associated with cell division. The remaining 138 DE-genes, downregulated in MSI-high cases, were related to chemotaxis and immune response. The 55 upregulated DE-genes in MSI-high cases were significantly associated with three annotation clusters: cluster 1 associated with cell cycle and cell division; cluster 2 with cytoskeleton and; cluster 3 associating more specific terms such as 'mitotic spindle organization' (Table 3). For the 138 downregulated DE-genes, eight clusters were significantly enriched associated with the terms: signal peptide and disulfide bond; chemotaxis; leukocyte and lymphocyte activation; chemokine activity; response to stimuli; regulation of cell death; cell migration and motility, and; polysaccharide binding (Table 3). Taken together, these results showed that MSI-high cases likely present increased cell division and decreased immune response and cell migration.

Table 3. Functional annotation clustering results for DE-genes separated according to the expression profile in MSS vs. MSI-high cases. Three clusters of associated biological terms were detected for upregulated DE-genes, while only one was detected for downregulated DE-genes. Notice that some terms among clusters are not significantly enriched (FDR > 0.05).

Cluster ID	Term	Count	FDR
	Upregulated DE-genes in MSI-high vs. MSS cases ($n = 55$)		
	GO:0022402~cell cycle process	17	1.46×10^{-8}
	GO:0000279~M phase	14	3.24×10^{-8}
	GO:0000280~nuclear division	12	1.17×10^{-7}
	GO:0007067~mitosis	12	1.17×10^{-7}
	GO:0000278~mitotic cell cycle	14	1.40×10^{-7}
Cluster 1:	GO:0000087~M phase of mitotic cell cycle	12	1.43×10^{-7}
ES = 9.5	GO:0048285~organelle fission	12	1.81×10^{-7}
	GO:0022403~cell cycle phase	14	5.62×10^{-7}
	mitosis	10	1.09×10^{-6}
	GO:0007049~cell cycle	17	1.62×10^{-6}
	cell division	11	1.48×10^{-6}
	cell cycle	12	2.50×10^{-5}
	GO:0051301~cell division	11	4.02×10^{-5}
Cluster 2:	GO:0005819~spindle	9	2.00×10^{-5}
ES = 4.3	GO:0015630~microtubule cytoskeleton	10	5.42×10^{-2}
	GO:0044430~cytoskeletal part	10	3.05
	GO:0005856~cytoskeleton	12	3.72

Table 3. *Cont.*

Cluster ID	Term	Count	FDR
Cluster 3: ES = 3.7	GO:0007052~mitotic spindle organization	4	2.13×10^{-2}
	GO:0007051~spindle organization	4	6.18×10^{-1}
	GO:0000226~microtubule cytoskeleton organization	5	1.92
	Downregulated DE-genes in MSI-high vs. MSS cases ($n = 138$)		
Cluster 1: ES = 16.0	disulfide bond	57	1.67×10^{-13}
	signal peptide	61	1.67×10^{-13}
	signal	61	1.44×10^{-13}
	disulfide bond	57	5.66×10^{-13}
Cluster 2: ES = 9.7	GO:0007626~locomotory behavior	17	2.98×10^{-7}
	GO:0042330~taxis	14	3.03×10^{-7}
	GO:0006935~chemotaxis	14	3.03×10^{-7}
Cluster 3: ES = 8.2	GO:0046649~lymphocyte activation	14	4.51×10^{-6}
	GO:0045321~leukocyte activation	15	5.12×10^{-6}
	GO:0001775~cell activation	15	4.50×10^{-5}
Cluster 4: ES = 5.4	IPR001811: Small chemokine, interleukin-8-like	8	1.75×10^{-5}
	GO:0008009~chemokine activity	8	5.02×10^{-5}
	GO:0042379~chemokine receptor binding	8	7.91×10^{-5}
	SM00199:SCY	8	1.88×10^{-4}
	cytokine	9	2.47×10^{-2}
	109.Chemokine_families	8	6.13×10^{-2}
	GO:0005125~cytokine activity	9	1.18×10^{-1}
	hsa04062:Chemokine signaling pathway	10	4.13×10^{-1}
	hsa04060:Cytokine-cytokine receptor interaction	11	1.19
Cluster 5: ES = 5.1	GO:0009719~response to endogenous stimulus	15	2.99×10^{-3}
	GO:0009725~response to hormone stimulus	14	5.54×10^{-3}
	GO:0010033~response to organic substance	17	1.38×10^{-1}
Cluster 6: ES = 4.9	GO:0043067~regulation of programmed cell death	20	1.27×10^{-2}
	GO:0010941~regulation of cell death	20	1.34×10^{-2}
	GO:0042981~regulation of apoptosis	19	4.16×10^{-2}
Cluster 7: ES = 4.9	GO:0016477~cell migration	12	1.10×10^{-2}
	GO:0006928~cell motion	15	1.88×10^{-2}
	GO:0048870~cell motility	12	2.99×10^{-2}
	GO:0051674~localization of cell	12	2.99×10^{-2}
Cluster 8: ES = 4.3	GO:0030247~polysaccharide binding	9	2.18×10^{-2}
	GO:0001871~pattern binding	9	2.18×10^{-2}
	GO:0005539~glycosaminoglycan binding	8	9.63×10^{-2}
	GO:0030246~carbohydrate binding	11	3.40×10^{-1}

ES: enrichment score per cluster calculated by DAVID. FDR: False Discovery Rate.

2.3. EBV+ GC Cases Were Associated with Immune Response Signature

Next, we compared the transcriptomic landscape of EBV+ and EBV− GC cases. We detected 142 DE-genes and non-hierarchical clustering revealed two major clusters: cluster 4A with 22/31 cases EBV− and; cluster 4B constituted by all 15 EBV+ cases plus the remaining 9 EBV− cases (Figure 4a). This separation between EBV+ and EBV− cases was partially recapitulated by PCA: 4/9 EBV− cases clustered together with EBV+ cases in the non-hierarchical clustering, were similarly grouped with PCA (gray diamonds with asterisk, Figure 4). This showed an overall less homogenous clustering according to EBV status, demonstrating that the MSI-high status was a stronger marker in GC.

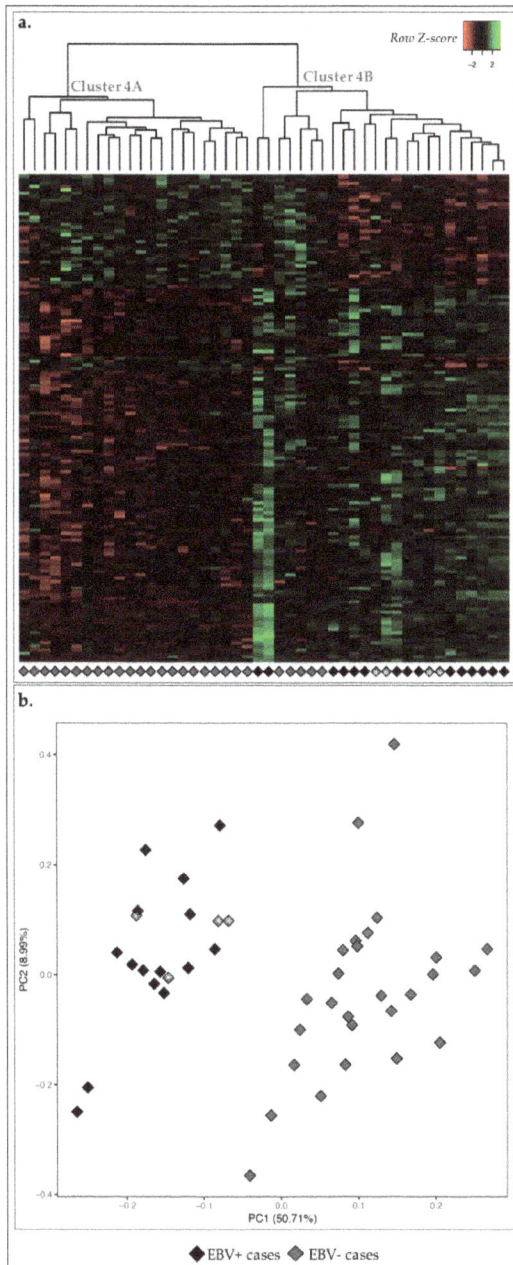

Figure 4. Expression profile of the 46 GC cases for 142 DE-genes between EBV positive and negative cases. (**a**) Heatmap for the expression of the 142 DE-genes (log 2 and Z-score scaled). Indicated are two main clusters: A and B. (**b**) PCA for principal components 1 and 2 for the 46 GC samples. Black diamonds correspond to EBV+ cases (*n* = 15) and white diamonds to EBV− cases (*n* = 31). Diamonds with asterisk for correspondence between panels (**a**) and (**b**) and described in the main text.

We then performed biological annotation of the 142 DE-genes and observed a significant enrichment in terms such as chemotaxis and immune response (Table 4).

Table 4. FDR-ranked top 10 biological terms significantly enriched in the set of 142 DE-genes when comparing the expression profile for 499 genes between EBV+ and EBV− GC cases.

Biological Term	Count	FDR
signal peptide	54	1.38×10^{-8}
IPR001811:Small chemokine, interleukin-8-like	10	1.40×10^{-8}
GO:0042330~taxis	15	3.13×10^{-8}
GO:0006935~chemotaxis	15	3.13×10^{-8}
disulfide bond	49	5.16×10^{-8}
GO:0008009~chemokine activity	10	6.98×10^{-8}
GO:0042379~chemokine receptor binding	10	1.28×10^{-7}
SM00199:SCY	10	1.99×10^{-7}
GO:0007626~locomotory behavior	17	4.65×10^{-7}
GO:0006955~immune response	25	5.25×10^{-7}

Count: number of DE-genes associated with a given biological term; FDR: False Discovery Rate.

From the 142 DE-genes, 105 were upregulated EBV+ cases vs. EBV− cases and belonged to six enriched clusters: signal peptide and disulfide bond; chemotaxis and motility; leukocyte and T-cell activation; chemokines and chemokine activity; immune system development; and T-cell differentiation (Table 5). The 37 genes downregulated in this comparison were enriched in two clusters: cell division, mitosis, and cell cycle (Table 5).

Table 5. Functional annotation clustering results for the 141 DE-genes upregulated in EBV+ cases. Six clusters of associated biological terms were detected for upregulated DE-genes and two clusters for downregulated DE-genes. Notice that some terms among clusters are not significantly enriched (FDR > 0.05).

Cluster ID	Term	Count	FDR
	Upregulated DE-genes in EBV+ vs. EBV− cases ($n = 105$)		
Cluster 1: ES = 12.2	disulfide bond	44	1.36×10^{-10}
	disulfide bond	44	3.56×10^{-10}
	signal	45	2.94×10^{-9}
	signal peptide	45	4.07×10^{-9}
Cluster 2: ES = 10.3	GO:0042330~taxis	14	5.99×10^{-9}
	GO:0006935~chemotaxis	14	5.99×10^{-9}
	GO:0007626~locomotory behavior	16	3.41×10^{-8}
	GO:0007610~behavior	16	5.57×10^{-5}
Cluster 3: ES = 10	GO:0045321~leukocyte activation	15	8.26×10^{-8}
	GO:0046649~lymphocyte activation	14	9.54×10^{-8}
	GO:0042110~T-cell activation	12	1.43×10^{-7}
	GO:0001775~cell activation	15	7.88×10^{-7}
Cluster 4: ES = 7.4	IPR001811:Small chemokine, interleukin-8-like	9	3.94×10^{-8}
	GO:0008009~chemokine activity	9	1.52×10^{-7}
	GO:0042379~chemokine receptor binding	9	2.60×10^{-7}
	SM00199:SCY	9	4.73×10^{-7}
	cytokine	10	2.20×10^{-4}
	GO:0005125~cytokine activity	10	1.39×10^{-3}
	hsa04062:Chemokine signaling pathway	11	1.09×10^{-2}
	109.Chemokine_families	9	1.22×10^{-2}
	hsa04060:Cytokine-cytokine receptor interaction	12	3.67×10^{-2}
Cluster 5: ES = 5.2	GO:0002520~immune system development	11	4.50×10^{-3}
	GO:0030097~hemopoiesis	10	9.75×10^{-3}
	GO:0002521~leukocyte differentiation	8	1.28×10^{-2}
	GO:0048534~hemopoietic or lymphoid organ development	10	2.13×10^{-2}

Table 5. *Cont.*

Cluster ID	Term	Count	FDR
Cluster 6: ES = 5.2	GO:0030217~T-cell differentiation	7	2.48×10^{-3}
	GO:0002521~leukocyte differentiation	8	1.28×10^{-2}
	GO:0030098~lymphocyte differentiation	7	3.64×10^{-2}
Downregulated DE-genes in EBV+ vs. EBV− cases ($n = 137$)			
Cluster 1: ES = 5.2	GO:0000279~M phase	8	5.32×10^{-3}
	cell division	7	4.85×10^{-3}
	GO:0007067~mitosis	7	7.12×10^{-3}
	GO:0000280~nuclear division	7	7.12×10^{-3}
	GO:0000087~M phase of mitotic cell cycle	7	7.90×10^{-3}
	GO:0048285~organelle fission	7	8.97×10^{-3}
	cell cycle	8	9.93×10^{-3}
	mitosis	6	1.38×10^{-2}
	GO:0051301~cell division	7	3.79×10^{-2}
Cluster 2: ES = 5	GO:0022402~cell cycle process	11	1.46×10^{-4}
	GO:0005819~spindle	7	5.61×10^{-4}
	GO:0000278~mitotic cell cycle	9	8.25×10^{-4}
	GO:0022403~cell cycle phase	9	1.93×10^{-3}
	GO:0007049~cell cycle	11	2.74×10^{-3}
	GO:0015630~microtubule cytoskeleton	8	1.20×10^{-1}
	GO:0044430~cytoskeletal part	8	3.21
	GO:0005856~cytoskeleton	9	6.62

ES: enrichment score per cluster calculated by DAVID; FDR: False Discovery Rate.

Our results show that EBV infection is not as determinant as MSI-high status. Nevertheless, the presence of this virus in GC samples was associated with an immune T-cell inflamed phenotype, in line with current literature [4,6,8].

2.4. MSS/MSI Phenotype Classification Was the Major Molecular Classifier in GC

Given that MSI and EBV status were part of the molecular classification for GC proposed by TCGA [4], we next assessed the differential expression profile of our GC cases taking into account both molecular classifications. We detected 166 DE-genes associated with biological annotations such as interleukin-8-like chemokine, signal peptide and chemotaxis (Table 6).

Table 6. FDR-ranked top 10 biological terms significantly enriched in the set of 166 DE-genes when comparing the expression profile for 499 genes between MSS vs. MSI-high and EBV+ vs. EBV− GC cases.

Biological Term	Count	FDR
IPR001811:Small chemokine, interleukin-8-like	10	6.17×10^{-8}
signal peptide	58	1.97×10^{-7}
GO:0008009~chemokine activity	10	2.18×10^{-7}
GO:0006935~chemotaxis	15	3.16×10^{-7}
GO:0042330~taxis	15	3.16×10^{-7}
disulfide bond	53	3.22×10^{-7}
GO:0042379~chemokine receptor binding	10	3.97×10^{-7}
SM00199:SCY	10	8.05×10^{-7}
disulfide bond	53	8.56×10^{-7}
GO:0045321~leukocyte activation	17	9.73×10^{-7}

Count: number of DE-genes associated with a given biological term; FDR: False Discovery Rate.

From the 166 DE-genes, 117 were upregulated and 49 downregulated DE-genes in MSS/EBV+ cases vs. MSI-high/EBV−genes. Next, we plotted the expression of these DE-genes for all 46 GC cases and observed that, despite adding both molecular classifiers, MSI-high and MSS cases remained well separated (Figure 5a). As observed before, two MSI-high/EBV− GC cases were clustered together with MSS cases (*cluster 5A*, Figure 5a, gray circles with asterisk and *cluster 3A*, Figure 3a, circles with cross). Nevertheless, with PCA, the same two cases were clustered closer to MSI-high/EBV− GC cases.

PCA separated two other MSI-high/EBV− cases, which were already loosely clustered in cluster 5B (Figure 5, gray circles with cross).

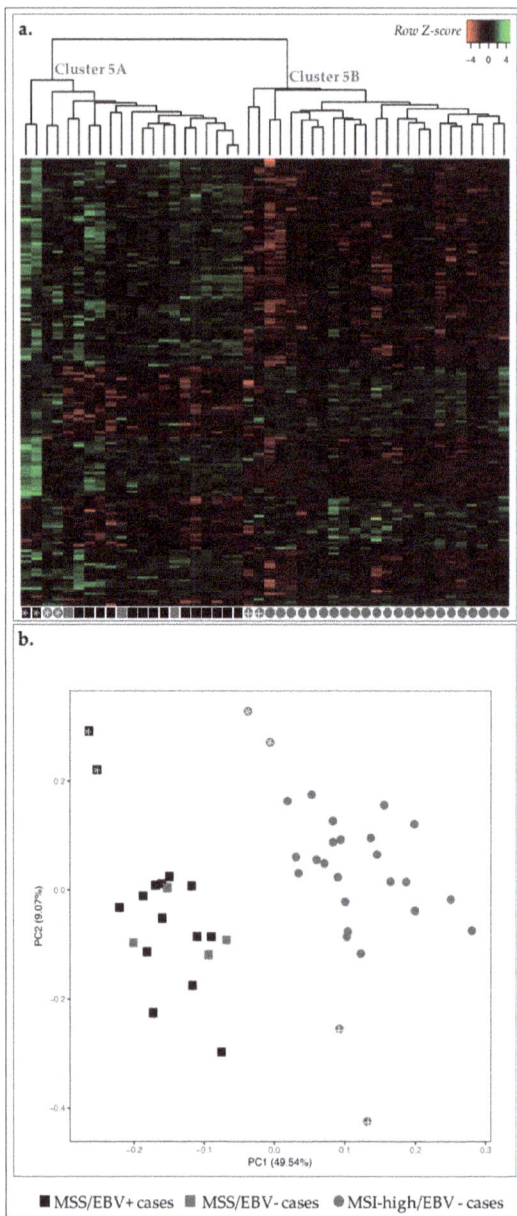

Figure 5. Expression profile of the 46 GC cases for 166 DE-genes between MSS/EBV+ and MSI-high/EBV− cases. (**a**) Heatmap for the expression of the 166 DE-genes (log 2 and Z-score scaled). Indicated are two main clusters: A and B. (**b**) PCA for principal components 1 and 2 for the 46 GC samples. Black squares correspond to MSS/EBV+ cases (*n* = 15), gray squares to MSS/EBV− cases (*n* = 4) and gray circles to MSI-high/EBV− cases (*n* = 27).

Separate annotation of up- and downregulated DE-genes in MSS/EBV+ cases revealed significant enrichment for five annotation clusters for upregulated genes: signal peptide and disulfide bond; chemotaxis and locomotion; leukocyte and T-cell activation; chemokines and chemokine activity, and; actin fibers (Table 7). Downregulated genes were separated in two clusters: cell cycle and mitosis, and cytoskeleton.

Table 7. Functional annotation clustering results for the 166 DE-genes derived from the comparison of MSS/EBV+ cases vs. MSI-high/EBV− cases. Notice that some terms among clusters are not significantly enriched (FDR > 0.05).

Cluster ID	Term	Count	FDR
	Upregulated DE-genes in MSS/EBV+ cases ($n = 117$)		
Cluster 1: ES = 12.5	disulfide bond	47	1.12×10^{-10}
	disulfide bond	47	3.06×10^{-10}
	signal	49	7.15×10^{-10}
	signal peptide	49	1.03×10^{-9}
Cluster 2: ES = 9.6	GO:0042330~taxis	14	2.32×10^{-8}
	GO:0006935~chemotaxis	14	2.32×10^{-8}
	GO:0007626~locomotory behavior	16	1.58×10^{-7}
	GO:0007610~behavior	16	2.31×10^{-4}
Cluster 3: ES = 8.3	GO:0045321~leukocyte activation	14	4.01×10^{-6}
	GO:0046649~lymphocyte activation	13	4.72×10^{-6}
	GO:0042110~T-cell activation	11	7.75×10^{-6}
	GO:0001775~cell activation	14	3.11×10^{-5}
Cluster 4: ES = 6.8	IPR001811:Small chemokine, interleukin-8-like	9	9.74×10^{-8}
	GO:0008009~chemokine activity	9	3.30×10^{-7}
	GO:0042379~chemokine receptor binding	9	5.62×10^{-7}
	SM00199:SCY	9	1.34×10^{-6}
	cytokine	9	5.94×10^{-3}
	109.Chemokine_families	9	4.48×10^{-3}
	hsa04062:Chemokine signaling pathway	11	1.87×10^{-2}
	GO:0005125~cytokine activity	9	2.77×10^{-2}
	hsa04060:Cytokine-cytokine receptor interaction	11	3.23×10^{-1}
Cluster 5: ES = 4.6	GO:0001725~stress fiber	5	2.38×10^{-2}
	GO:0032432~actin filament bundle	5	3.31×10^{-2}
	GO:0042641~actomyosin	5	3.87×10^{-2}
	Downregulated DE-genes in MSS/EBV+ cases ($n = 49$)		
Cluster 1: ES = 9.9	GO:0000278~mitotic cell cycle	14	2.51×10^{-8}
	GO:0000280~nuclear division	12	2.79×10^{-8}
	GO:0007067~mitosis	12	2.79×10^{-8}
	GO:0000087~M phase of mitotic cell cycle	12	3.39×10^{-8}
	GO:0048285~organelle fission	12	4.30×10^{-8}
	GO:0022403~cell cycle phase	14	1.02×10^{-7}
	GO:0000279~M phase	13	1.15×10^{-7}
	mitosis	10	3.25×10^{-7}
	cell division	11	3.84×10^{-7}
	cell cycle	12	5.83×10^{-6}
	GO:0051301~cell division	11	1.15×10^{-5}
Cluster 2: ES = 3.5	GO:0005819~spindle	7	4.12×10^{-3}
	GO:0015630~microtubule cytoskeleton	9	1.60×10^{-1}
	GO:0005856~cytoskeleton	11	5.27
	GO:0044430~cytoskeletal part	9	5.64

ES: enrichment score per cluster calculated by DAVID; FDR: False Discovery Rate.

These results were comparable to those previously observed when considering the molecular classifiers independently. To understand whether this was due to common set of DE-genes across analyses, we next compared the DE-genes obtained for each comparison: MSS with MSI-high cases; EBV+ with EBV− cases and; MSS/EBV+ with MSI-high/EBV− cases.

Most DE-genes were shared by the three analyses (*n* = 133, Figure 6), thus justifying the similar biological annotation enrichments obtained. Unlike EBV−-based classification, many DE-genes derived specifically from the MSI-high/MSS-based classification and became lost when combining both molecular subtypes (*n* = 34, Figure 6). Functional enrichment of this particular set of DE-genes, although without any FDR-significant results, pointed toward enrichment in extracellular matrix terms. Altogether, our results pinpointed MSI-high/MSS phenotype as the major molecular classifier in our GC cohort, independently of EBV− *tatus* classification.

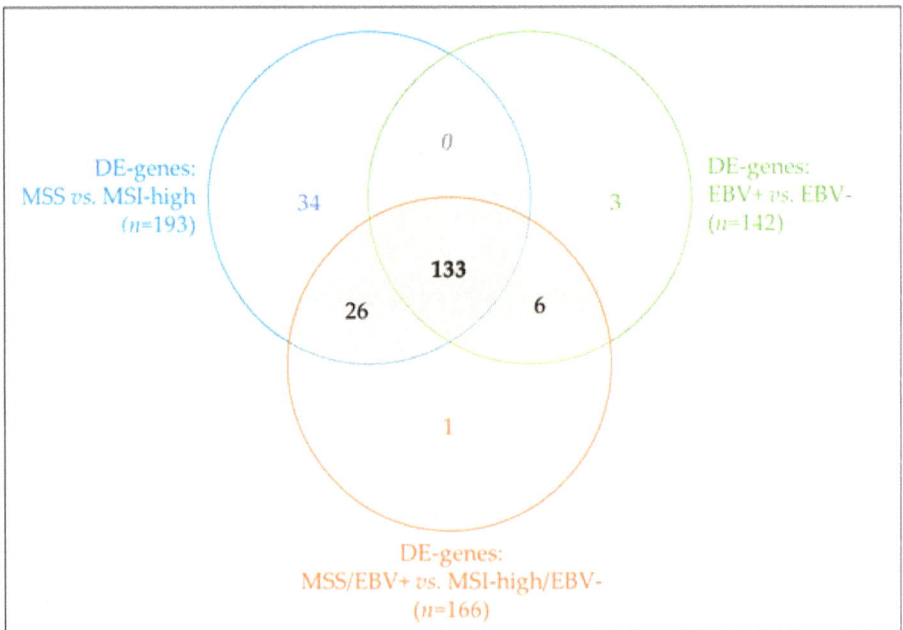

Figure 6. Venn diagram for shared (or not) DE-genes across the three analyses performed.

2.5. PD-L1 and PD-1 Displayed Opposite mRNA Expression Patterns and Were Differently Associated with GC Molecular Subtypes and Morphological Features

In GC, several clinical trials have been targeting immune checkpoint regulators, such as CTLA4, PD-1, PDL1 and VISTA/Dies1 [26]. Given the observed associations between immune response terms and MSS/EBV+ cases, we further assessed the mRNA expression of these immune checkpoint regulators across all cases from the 3 GC groups represented in our series (15 MSS/EBV+, 4 MSS/EBV− and 27 MSI-high/EBV−, Figure 7). CTLA4, PD-1 and VISTA/Dies1, but not PD-L1 mRNA expression was significantly enriched in MSS/EBV+ cases (Figure 7a). Therefore, we analyzed PD-L1 protein expression in cancer cells and in the immune cells infiltrating the tumor microenvironment (TME) to understand this difference. In cancer epithelial cells, PD-L1 protein expression did not differ between GC groups (Figure 7b). However, in the immune cells of the TME, MSI-high/EBV− cases often presented low expression of PD-L1, while MSS/EBV+ showed variable PD-L1 expression across all categories, from low to high (Figure 7c, Fisher's Exact Test *p*-value = 7.71×10^{-3})

These results prompted us to re-analyze the mRNA expression of the four immune checkpoint regulators on a case-by-case manner. While *CTLA4* and *VISTA/Dies1* followed the expression pattern of *PD-1*, *PD-L1* varied in an inverse manner in a large set of cases: for example, GC cases with highest expression of *PD-L1* displayed the lowest expression of *PD-1* (Figure 7d).

To validate this observation, we assessed the number of GC cases for each of the four PD-L1/PD-1 co-expression scenarios observed: (1) high expression of *PD-L1* and low expression of *PD-1* (*PD-L1*^{high}/*PD-1*^{low}, $n = 12$); (2) low expression of *PD-L1* and high expression of *PD-1* (*PD-L1*^{low}/*PD-1*^{high}, $n = 12$); (3) low expression for both (*PD-L1*^{low}/*PD-1*^{low}, $n = 14$) and; (4) high expression for both (*PD-L1*^{high}/*PD-1*^{high}, $n = 8$, Figure 7d,e). We observed that most MSS/EBV+ cases were either *PD-L1*^{low}/*PD-1*^{high} or *PD-L1*^{high}/*PD-1*^{high} ($n = 7$ and 6, respectively, Figure 7e), while most MSI-high/EBV− cases were *PD-L1*^{high}/*PD-1*^{low} or *PD-L1*^{low}/*PD-1*^{low} ($n = 23$, Figure 7e) (Fisher's Exact test, $p = 1.46 \times 10^{-5}$).

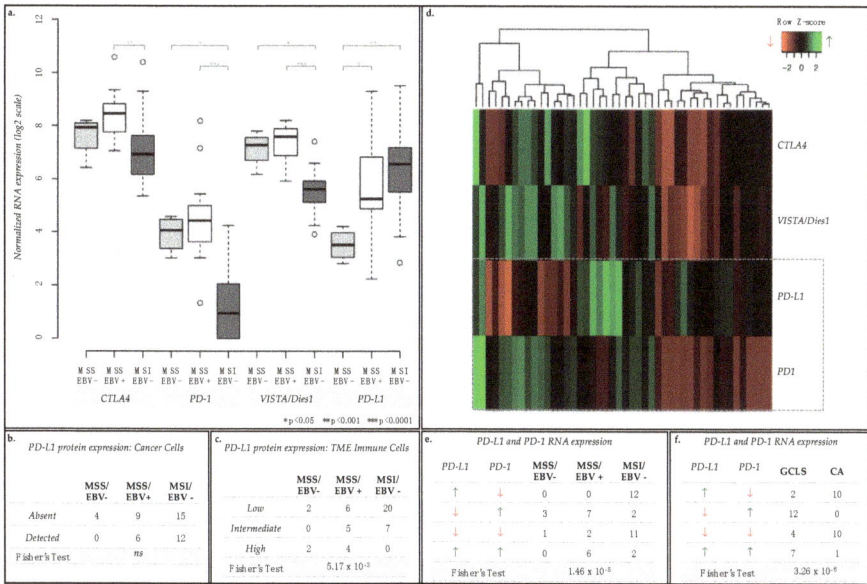

Figure 7. mRNA expression of immune checkpoint regulators *CTLA4*, *PD-1*, *VISTA/Dies1* and *PD-L1* and protein expression of PD-L1. (**a**) Boxplot for the normalized mRNA expression in log2 scale of *CTLA4*, *PD-1*, *VISTA/Dies1* and *PD-L1*. (**b**,**c**) Contingency tables for PD-L1 protein expression evaluated by in cancer cells (**b**, absent or detected) and in immune cells of the TME (**c**, low, intermediate, or high expression level). (**d**) Heatmap for the mRNA expression of each of the immune checkpoints assessed per case. (**e**,**f**) Contingency tables for combined *PD-L1* and *PD-1* mRNA expression for GC cases separated by MSI status and EBV infection (**e**) or by morphological characteristics (gastric cancer with lymphoid stroma, GCLS, or conventional-type adenocarcinoma, CA) (**f**). Green upward arrows for higher mRNA expression and red downward arrows for lower mRNA expression, as presented in the heatmap.

These significant results led us to further characterize our GC cohort for morphological characteristics by histopathological analysis. As a significant fraction of cases displayed a prominent lymphoid infiltration in the tumor stroma, showing the morphological features of GCLS, we stratified the GC series into GCLSs ($n = 25$) and conventional-type adenocarcinomas (CA), i.e., GC cases not presenting the morphological features of GCLS ($n = 21$). While most GCLS cases presented a *PD-L1*^{low}/*PD-1*^{high} or *PD-L1*^{high}/*PD-1*^{high} ($n = 12 + 7$, respectively, Figure 7f), CA cases either displayed a $PD\text{-}L1^{high}/PD\text{-}1^{low}$ or $PD\text{-}L1^{low}/PD\text{-}1^{low}$ (n = 10 + 10, respectively, Figure 7f). By combining this morphological characterization with the previously described molecular subtypes (Table 8), we observed that: (1) 20/21 MSI-high/EBV− CA cases presented a $PD\text{-}L1^{high}/PD\text{-}1^{low}$ or a $PD\text{-}L1^{low}/PD\text{-}1^{low}$ expression pattern; (2) 13/15 MSS/EBV+/GCLS cases presented either a $PD\text{-}L1^{low}/PD\text{-}1^{high}$ or a $PD\text{-}L1^{high}/PD\text{-}1^{high}$ expression pattern; (3) 3/4 MSS/EBV−/GCLS cases presented a $PD\text{-}L1^{low}/PD\text{-}1^{high}$ co-expression pattern.

Table 8. Contingency table for the number of MSS/EBV− or MSS/EBV+ or MSI/EBV− cases with morphological features of GCLS or CA for the four $PD\text{-}L1/PD\text{-}1$ mRNA expression scenarios.

mRNA Expression		MSS/EBV− (n = 4)		MSS/EBV+ (n = 15)		MSI/EBV− (n = 27)	
PD-L1	PD-1	CA (n = 0)	GCLS (n = 4)	CA (n = 0)	GCLS (n = 15)	CA (n = 21)	GCLS (n = 6)
↗	↙	0	0	0	0	10	2
↙	↗	0	3	0	7	0	2
↙	↙	0	1	0	2	10	1
↗	↗	0	0	0	6	1	1
			Fisher's Exact Test: $p = 3.71 \times 10^{-6}$				

The most important observation was that 19/25 GCLS cases displayed high $PD\text{-}1$ mRNA expression, independently of $PD\text{-}L1$ expression (12/19—low $PD\text{-}L1$; 7/19—high PD-L1). We then analyzed the expression of the other GC immunotherapy targets in the subset of GCLS: $Dies1/VISTA$ and $CTLA4$. From the 12 GCLS cases with high $PD\text{-}1$ and low $PD\text{-}L1$ mRNA expression, 10 displayed high $Dies1/VISTA$ mRNA expression (n = 7 + 3, Figure 8) and 8 high $CTLA4$ mRNA expression (n = 7 + 1, Figure 8). From the remaining seven GCLS cases with high $PD\text{-}1$ and $PD\text{-}L1$ mRNA expression, all displayed high $Dies1/VISTA$ and/or $CTLA4$ mRNA expression (Figure 8).

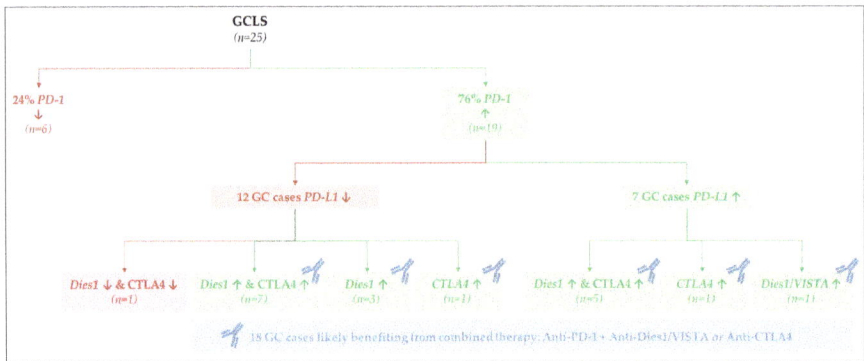

Figure 8. mRNA co-expression patterns for $PD\text{-}1$, $PD\text{-}L1$, $Dies1/VISTA$ and $CTLA4$ in GCLS cases.

Altogether, this gene-oriented analysis showed that $PD\text{-}L1$ and $PD\text{-}1$ exhibit particular co-expression patterns in an MSS/MSI-high and EBV infection-dependent manner. Moreover, our results suggest that the evaluation of the tumor immune infiltrate by histopathological analysis strengthened the stratification of GC cases and helped identifying more homogenous biological subgroups in terms of co-expression of immune checkpoint regulators.

3. Discussion

In this study, we explored the transcriptomic profile of EBV+ and MSI-high GC, using a Nanostring CodeSet with 499 genes involved in oncogenic signaling, immune response and molecular gene expression signatures. This small gene expression panel could segregate GCs of our cohort according to MSI-high status and, to a lesser extent, EBV infection, and was sufficient to reproduce the taxonomy developed by TCGA.

EBV infection and MSI-high status represent two alternative pathways of gastric carcinogenesis and two mutually exclusive GC molecular subtypes [11,12,27]. Herein, we confirmed that all EBV+ cases showed an MSS phenotype, and vice versa, that all MSI-high cases were negative for EBV infection.

When we focused on determining clusters of biologically-related annotation terms, underlying the DE-genes found for the two GC molecular subtypes, we found that MSI-high tumors showed an enrichment in genes related to DNA replication and mitotic cell cycle, as previously reported [4,5]. MSI-high status leads to the accumulation of numerous frameshift mutations throughout the genome [28] and may determine the inactivation of key tumor suppressor genes, including those involved in DNA damage repair, cell cycle control and apoptotic signaling [29]. Accordingly, as demonstrated in the MSI-high colorectal cancer model [30], mutations providing proliferative and survival advantage are selected during MSI-high GC initiation and/or progression, conferring a proliferative state. In contrast, EBV+ tumors showed a downregulation of genes involved in mitotic pathways.

By functional annotation of genes discriminating EBV+ tumors, we identified a gene signature involved in immune pathways, confirming the data already reported in the literature [4,6,8,31,32]. The immune signature was enriched for genes related to T-cell differentiation, cytotoxic signaling, pro-inflammatory cytokines/chemokines, leukocyte migration and genes of the immune checkpoint inhibitors pathways. These features reflect the immunogenicity of EBV infection and provide evidence of the biological significance of immune cell infiltration in EBV+ tumors [33]. Accordingly, the DE-genes downregulated in MSI-high cases, hence upregulated in MSS cases, were also found to be associated with immune response and cell migration. Therefore, in this study we demonstrated, using unbiased bioinformatics analyses, that the transcriptomic landscape of GCs with EBV+ and MSI-high phenotypes is different, associating each molecular entity with enrichment of different biological terms, i.e., mitotic activity and immune response. In this study, gene expression analysis was performed through the Nanostring Technology Platform, which has shown excellent robustness and sensitivity for the analysis of formalin-fixed paraffin-embedded (FFPE) samples [34]. Moreover, several authors have shown the reproducibility of the results obtained in GC tissues through Nanostring technology, using distinct molecular platforms [23,34]. Importantly, our results were able to confirm the transcriptomic data obtained in TCGA study, thus further contributing for the validation of the Nanostring CodeSet. In future studies, it would be interesting to confirm the enrichment of mitotic pathways in MSI GC cohorts, by investigating mitotic activity/index through histopathological analysis, as demonstrated already in the colorectal cancer model [30,35].

We also investigated the expression of molecules involved in immune checkpoint inhibitors pathways and current targets for immunotherapy in GC [26]. By assessing PD-L1 protein expression by IHC, the current predictive biomarker used for selecting GC patients eligible for Pembrolizumab immunotherapy [16], we found that PD-L1 protein expression, evaluated in cancer cells, showed no significant differences between the two molecular subgroups. However, when we evaluated PD-L1 expression in immune cells of the TME, most MSI-high/EBV— cases presented low expression, when compared to MSS/EBV+ tumors. This result shows the value of evaluating protein expression in tissue sections to improve knowledge of topographic distribution of molecular markers.

We also analyzed *PD-1*, *CTLA4* and *Dies1/VISTA* mRNA expression and observed that all were significantly enriched in MSS/EBV+ cases, in comparison with MSI-high/EBV— cases. This result highlighted the high correlation of *PD-1*, *CTLA4* and *Dies1/VISTA* increased mRNA expression with EBV+ cases, but not with EBV— cases. However, as we analyzed *PD-L1* mRNA expression, we did not observe any significant difference between the two molecular subgroups. This result prompted us to analyze the co-expression of *PD-1* and *PD-L1* at the mRNA level, the two most promising biomarkers for GC immunotherapy. Studies have shown that patients with mRNA co-expression of *PD-1/PD-L1* were those with better prognosis [36]. However, few GC cases in our cohort presented expression of both markers simultaneously and, interestingly, most were GCLS cases positive for EBV infection. Nevertheless, it has been shown that patients treated with anti-PD-1 therapy respond well even in the absence of PD-L1 expression [37], a fact that may reflect the different co-expression patterns observed in our cohort.

Taking all these observations into account, we further explored the pattern of co-expression of *PD-1* with *Dies1/VISTA* and *CTLA4*. In fact, combination immunotherapies, targeting simultaneously PD-1 and Dies1/VISTA or CTLA4 are being explored as new strategies for the treatment of GC [38,39]. We observed that from the 19 *PD-1* high-expressing GCLS cases, 18 cases also displayed high *Dies1/VISTA* and/or *CTLA4* mRNA expression. This observation suggests that the recognition of GCLS morphological features may contribute, in >70% cases, to the selection of patients who would benefit from a combination immunotherapy, targeting PD-1 and either Dies1/VISTA or CTLA4 (Figure 8). The results herein described raise the hypothesis that Dies1/VISTA and CTLA4 may be the silent PD-1 partners in GC, explaining the good response observed in patients harboring PD-L1-negative tumors, treated with anti-PD-1 therapy [18–20,37]. Overall, our results support that most GCLS patients will benefit from anti-PD-1 therapy combined with either anti-Dies1/VISTA or anti-CTLA4 (Figure 8). This novel data is worth further studies. To evaluate, in different GC cohorts, protein expression of multiple immunotherapy targets, besides PD-L1, would be crucial to integrate gene and protein expression data, as well to explore the topographic distribution (i.e., cancer cells versus TME immune cells) of different biomarkers. Of notice, Dies1/VISTA expression has already been assessed in a large GC series, and its expression was mostly detected in >80% of TME immune cells [26].

Our study also revealed that, beyond MSS/MSI-high and EBV infection, the morphological entity GCLS was strongly associated with PD-1 high expression. In fact, ~80% of all GCLS presented high *PD-1* mRNA expression (Figure 8).

Altogether, our data demonstrated that a small transcriptomic panel can separate MSI/EBV− from MSS/EBV+ GC cases, and this may have clinical utility. Also, our analysis demonstrates that EBV+ GCs with GCLS morphological features is the biological subgroup that would more likely respond to immunotherapy, as they present higher *PD-1* expression, the key immunotherapy target in GC, together with *Dies1/VISTA* and *CTLA4*. These observations support the ongoing GC clinical trials and highlight GCLS as a useful feature to stratify patients for targeted immunotherapies.

4. Materials and Methods

4.1. Case Series

Tissue samples were obtained retrospectively from 46 patients with GC who had undergone gastrectomy as primary treatment at Centro Hospitalar São João (Porto, Portugal). For mRNA extraction, frozen tissue was available from 23 cases, whereas FFPE tissue was used in the remaining 23 cases. The series was enriched with GC cases harboring EBV infection (*n* = 15) and MSI-high status (*n* = 27), whereas the remaining four cases were EBV− and MSS. EBV infection and MSI status were investigated as described below. Histopathological analysis was performed on H&E sections and the tumors were classified as GCLS or CA, based on the abundance of the lymphoid infiltrate.

4.2. EBV In Situ Hybridization

The presence of EBV infection was studied by chromogenic *in situ* hybridization (ISH) for EBV− encoded RNA (EBER-ISH, INFORM EBER probe, Ventana Medical Systems, Tucson, AZ, USA). One 3 μm section was processed in the automatic Ventana Benchmark Ultra platform with enzymatic digestion (ISH protease) and the iViewBlue detection kit.

4.3. PCR/Fragment Analysis for MSI Status

Genomic DNA was extracted from frozen or FFPE tissues (four sections, each 10 μm thick), using QIAamp DNA Mini Kit (Qiagen, Valencia, CA, USA), in accordance with the manufacturer's instructions. DNA purity and quantification were assessed using the NanoDrop 2000 UV-Vis spectrophotometer (NanoDrop products, Wilmington, DE, USA). Five mononucleotide markers (BAT-25, BAT-26, NR-24, NR-21 and NR-27) were used as a pentaplex panel to determine MSI status (Multiplex PCR, Qiagen, Valencia, CA, USA). Tumors with instability involving at least two of the five *loci* were classified as MSI.

4.4. Gene Expression Profiling by Nanostring nCounter Assay

Total RNA was extracted from frozen or FFPE tissues (four sections, each 10 μm thick), using miRNeasy Mini Kit (Qiagen, Valencia, CA, USA), in accordance with the manufacturer's instructions. High tumor content of the samples was ensured by morphological evaluation of mirror H&E sections of frozen samples and by microdissection of tumor areas in sections from FFPE blocks. For Nanostring nCounter assay, we used a custom-designed panel comprising 474 genes previously published [23] and additional genes associated with immune response (*CCL22, CCR7, CD3D, CD3E, CD3G, CD8A, CD8B, CD19, CD20, CD45, CD68, CXCL10, CXCL11, FOXP3, GZMA, GZMB, IL4, IL13, PD-1, PD-L1, TNFA, VISTA/Dies1*). Nanostring probe hybridization was performed as a service at Genome Institute of Singapore. Raw counts obtained for each sample were normalized using nSolver software version 3.0 (NanoString Technologies). We performed: (1) background subtraction using eight negative control probes included in the Nanostring CodeSet; (2) positive control normalization using six positive control probes also included in the Nanostring CodeSet; (3) housekeeping normalization using the standard method in the software and five independent housekeeping genes included in the Nanostring CodeSet. Normalized log2-scaled counts were used for to construct heatmaps, dendrograms and to perform PCA described in this study, using the R environment and the packages "ggplot2" and "ggfortify" [40–43]. Next, each sample was identified concerning its MSS/MSI-high phenotype and/or EBV infection status to perform comparison analysis using also the nSolver software (NanoString Technologies). Calculated ratios and FDR was used to define the set of up/downregulated DE-genes considering the comparison performed: genes with ratio above 1.5 and FDR < 0.05 were classified as differentially expressed upregulated genes; genes with ratio below 0.67 and FDR < 0.05 were classified as differentially expressed downregulated genes.

4.5. PD-L1 Immunohistochemistry

Staining for PD-L1 was performed in FFPE 3 μm sections with a rabbit monoclonal antibody (clone E1L3N, 1:1000; Cell Signaling Technology) on the automatic Ventana Benchmark Ultra platform, using the OptiView Universal DAB detection kit and the OptiView Amplification kit from the same manufacturer. PD-L1 immunoexpression was evaluated semi-quantitatively for tumor epithelial and stromal immune cells, according to the immunoreactivity scoring system (IRS) described by Boger et al. [44]. PD-L1 expression in tumor epithelial cells was dichotomized as positive (detected) or negative (absent) by an immunoreactivity score (IRS) of 2. PD-L1 expression in immune cells of the TME was defined as low (1–5% of positive cells), intermediate (6–20% of positive cells) or high (>20% of positive cells).

4.6. Functional Annotation and Statistical Analysis

Functional annotation was performed using the online tool DAVID 6.7 [24,25]. In particular, we have used the option 'Functional Annotation Clustering' using always the stringency 'high' and the option 'Functional Annotation Chart'. Selected clusters and/or biological terms were considered enriched and reported in this study if presenting an FDR < 0.05. Normalized log2-scaled counts for the genes *CTLA4, PD-1, VISTA/Dies1* and *PD-L1* was collected from nSolver software (NanoString

Technologies), as previously described. Boxplots were plotted using R [40] and represented *p*-values derived from a Wilcoxon test (Mann-Whitney) also performed using R and all samples (including outliers). After building a contingency table for the number of cases in each detailed condition, a Fisher's exact test was performed using R. This test was selected rather than the chi-square test, due to the low number of samples available in our cohort.

5. Conclusions

In this study, we have shown that the expression profile of GC cases for the assessed 499 genes was strongly correlated with the established molecular subtypes currently used for GC molecular stratification. Altogether, our results have clearly associated: (1) MSI-high/EBV− GC cases with mitosis and cell cycle biological terms; (2) MSS/EBV+ GC cases with immune response mediated by T-cells. Importantly, we have also shown that the MSI status is a much more relevant molecular classifier than EBV infection. We have also revealed that *PD-L1* and *PD-1* have opposite mRNA expression patterns in GC, in correlation with MSI phenotype, EBV status and prominent immune infiltrate, as revealed by the GCLS morphological feature, a highly relevant finding as both genes are nowadays actively pursued as targets for immunotherapy in GC. Moreover, our study has shown that Dies1/VISTA and CTLA4 are highly expressed in the majority of EBV+ and GCLS cases, strengthening the relevance of clinical trials using antibodies raised against these two proteins in combination with the promising anti-PD-1 therapy.

Author Contributions: I.G. participated in the concept, design, and planning of the study, selected the cohort, performed/participated in all described experimental procedures, participated in the classification of cases and staining patterns, co-designed and participated in the interpretation of the bioinformatic analyses and co-wrote the manuscript. J.C. co-designed and participated in the interpretation of the bioinformatic analyses and co-wrote the manuscript. D.M. performed the RNA extraction from GC cases. D.L., A.R.M. and M.F. participated in the bioinformatic analyses. C.O. participated in the concept, design, and planning of the study, co-designed the bioinformatic analyses and reviewed the manuscript. F.C. participated in the concept, design or planning of the study, co-designed the bioinformatic analyses, participated in the classification of cases and staining patterns and reviewed the manuscript. P.O. participated in the study design, co-designed, performed and interpreted all bioinformatics analyses and co-wrote the manuscript.

Funding: This work was supported by Fundo Europeu de Desenvolvimento Regional (FEDER) through the Operational Programme for Competitiveness Factors (COMPETE), Norte Portugal Regional Programme—NORTE 2020 (through the PORTUGAL 2020 Partnership Agreement), and National Funds through the Portuguese Foundation for Science and Technology (FCT), under the projects: DOCnet—NORTE-01-0145-FEDER-000003; Advancing Cancer Research: from basic knowledge to applicationNORTE-01-0145-FEDER-000029; GenomePT—POCI-01-0145-FEDER-022184 (ROTEIRO/0044/2013); post-doctoral grants: SFRH/BPD/86543/2012 (JC); SFRH/BPD/89764/2012 (PO).

Conflicts of Interest: The authors declare no conflict of interest.

Int. J. Mol. Sci. **2018**, *19*, 2079

Abbreviations

CA	Conventional-type Adenocarcinoma
DE	Differentially Expressed
EBV	Epstein-Barr Virus
ES	Enrichment Score
FDR	False Discovery Rate
GC	Gastric Cancer
GCLS	Gastric Cancer with Lymphoid Stroma
IFNγ	Interferon gamma
IHC	Immunohistochemistry
MSI-high	Microsatellite unstable
MSS	Microsatellite stable
PD-1	Program Death 1
PD-L1	Program Death Ligand 1
TCGA	The Cancer Genome Atlas
TME	Tumor Microenvironment

References

1. Gullo, I.; Carneiro, F.; Oliveira, C.; Almeida, G.M. Heterogeneity in Gastric Cancer: From Pure Morphology to Molecular Classifications. *Pathobiology* **2018**, *85*, 50–63. [CrossRef] [PubMed]
2. Yuen, S.T.; Leung, S.Y. Genomics Study of Gastric Cancer and Its Molecular Subtypes. *Adv. Exp. Med. Biol.* **2016**, *908*, 419–439. [CrossRef] [PubMed]
3. Baraniskin, A.; Van Laethem, J.L.; Wyrwicz, L.; Guller, U.; Wasan, H.S.; Matysiak-Budnik, T.; Gruenberger, T.; Ducreux, M.; Carneiro, F.; Van Cutsem, E.; et al. Clinical relevance of molecular diagnostics in gastrointestinal (GI) cancer: European Society of Digestive Oncology (ESDO) expert discussion and recommendations from the 17th European Society for Medical Oncology (ESMO)/World Congress on Gastrointestinal Cancer, Barcelona. *Eur. J. Cancer* **2017**, *86*, 305–317. [CrossRef] [PubMed]
4. TCGA. Comprehensive molecular characterization of gastric adenocarcinoma. *Nature* **2014**, *513*, 202–209. [CrossRef]
5. Cristescu, R.; Lee, J.; Nebozhyn, M.; Kim, K.M.; Ting, J.C.; Wong, S.S.; Liu, J.; Yue, Y.G.; Wang, J.; Yu, K.; et al. Molecular analysis of gastric cancer identifies subtypes associated with distinct clinical outcomes. *Nat. Med.* **2015**, *21*, 449–456. [CrossRef] [PubMed]
6. Sohn, B.H.; Hwang, J.E.; Jang, H.J.; Lee, H.S.; Oh, S.C.; Shim, J.J.; Lee, K.W.; Kim, E.H.; Yim, S.Y.; Lee, S.H.; et al. Clinical Significance of Four Molecular Subtypes of Gastric Cancer Identified by The Cancer Genome Atlas Project. Clinical cancer research. *Off. J. Am. Assoc. Cancer Res.* **2017**. [CrossRef] [PubMed]
7. Oliveira, C.; Seruca, R.; Seixas, M.; Sobrinho-Simões, M. The Clinicopathological Features of Gastric Carcinomas with Microsatellite Instability May Be Mediated by Mutations of Different "Target Genes": A Study of the TGFβ RII, IGFII R.; and BAX Genes. *Am. J. Pathol.* **1998**, *153*, 1211–1219. [CrossRef]
8. Derks, S.; Liao, X.; Chiaravalli, A.M.; Xu, X.; Camargo, M.C.; Solcia, E.; Sessa, F.; Fleitas, T.; Freeman, G.J.; Rodig, S.J.; et al. Abundant PD-L1 expression in Epstein-Barr Virus-infected gastric cancers. *Oncotarget* **2016**, *7*, 32925–32932. [CrossRef] [PubMed]
9. Park, C.; Cho, J.; Lee, J.; Kang, S.Y.; An, J.Y.; Choi, M.G.; Lee, J.H.; Sohn, T.S.; Bae, J.M.; Kim, S.; et al. Host immune response index in gastric cancer identified by comprehensive analyses of tumor immunity. *Oncoimmunology* **2017**, *6*, e1356150. [CrossRef] [PubMed]
10. Solcia, E.; Klersy, C.; Mastracci, L.; Alberizzi, P.; Candusso, M.E.; Diegoli, M.; Tava, F.; Riboni, R.; Manca, R.; Luinetti, O. A combined histologic and molecular approach identifies three groups of gastric cancer with different prognosis. *Virchows Arch.* **2009**, *455*, 197–211. [CrossRef] [PubMed]
11. Grogg, K.L.; Lohse, C.M.; Pankratz, V.S.; Halling, K.C.; Smyrk, T.C. Lymphocyte-rich gastric cancer: Associations with Epstein-Barr virus, microsatellite instability, histology, and survival. *Mod. Pathol.* **2003**, *16*, 641–651. [CrossRef] [PubMed]

12. Hissong, E.; Ramrattan, G.; Zhang, P.; Zhou, X.K.; Young, G.; Klimstra, D.S.; Shia, J.; Fernandes, H.; Yantiss, R.K. Gastric Carcinomas With Lymphoid Stroma: An Evaluation of the Histopathologic and Molecular Features. *Am. J. Surg. Pathol.* **2018**, *42*, 453–462. [CrossRef] [PubMed]

13. Gullo, I.; Oliveira, P.; Athelogou, M.; Gonçalves, G.; Pinto, M.L.; Carvalho, J.; Valente, A.; Pinheiro, H.; Andrade, S.; Almeida, G.M.; et al. New insights into the inflamed tumor immune microenvironment of Gastric Cancer with Lymphoid Stroma: From morphology and digital analysis to gene expression. *Gastric Cancer* **2018**. [CrossRef] [PubMed]

14. Bosman, F.T.; Carneiro, F.; Hruban, R.H.; Theise, N.D. *WHO Classification of Tumours of the Digestive System*, 4th ed.; IARC: Lyon, France, 2010.

15. Fuchs, C.S.; Doi, T.; Jang, R.W.-J.; Muro, K.; Satoh, T.; Machado, M.; Sun, W.; Jalal, S.I.; Shah, M.A.; Metges, J.-P.; et al. KEYNOTE-059 cohort 1: Efficacy and safety of pembrolizumab (pembro) monotherapy in patients with previously treated advanced gastric cancer. *J. Clin. Oncol.* **2017**, *35*, 4003. [CrossRef]

16. FDA Approves Merck's KEYTRUDA® (pembrolizumab) for Previously Treated Patients with Recurrent Locally Advanced or Metastatic Gastric or Gastroesophageal Junction Cancer Whose Tumors Express PD-L1 (CPS Greater Than or Equal to 1). Merck. Available online: http://investors.merck.com/home/default.aspx (accessed on 17 July 2018).

17. FDA Grants Accelerated Approval to Pembrolizumab for Tissue/Site Agnostic Indication. Available online: https://www.fda.gov/drugs/informationondrugs/approveddrugs/ucm560040.htm (accessed on 18 January 2018).

18. Muro, K.; Chung, H.C.; Shankaran, V.; Geva, R.; Catenacci, D.; Gupta, S.; Eder, J.P.; Golan, T.; Le, D.T.; Burtness, B.; et al. Pembrolizumab for patients with PD-L1-positive advanced gastric cancer (KEYNOTE-012): A multicentre, open-label, phase 1b trial. *Lancet Oncol.* **2016**, *17*, 717–726. [CrossRef]

19. Kang, Y.K.; Boku, N.; Satoh, T.; Ryu, M.H.; Chao, Y.; Kato, K.; Chung, H.C.; Chen, J.S.; Muro, K.; Kang, W.K.; et al. Nivolumab in patients with advanced gastric or gastro-oesophageal junction cancer refractory to, or intolerant of, at least two previous chemotherapy regimens (ONO-4538-12, ATTRACTION-2): A randomised, double-blind, placebo-controlled, phase 3 trial. *Lancet* **2017**, *390*, 2461–2471. [CrossRef]

20. Fuchs, C.S.; Doi, T.; Jang, R.W.; Muro, K.; Satoh, T.; Machado, M.; Sun, W.; Jalal, S.I.; Shah, M.A.; Metges, J.P.; et al. Safety and Efficacy of Pembrolizumab Monotherapy in Patients With Previously Treated Advanced Gastric and Gastroesophageal Junction Cancer: Phase 2 Clinical KEYNOTE-059 Trial. *JAMA Oncol.* **2018**, *4*, e180013. [CrossRef] [PubMed]

21. Ayers, M.; Lunceford, J.; Nebozhyn, M.; Murphy, E.; Loboda, A.; Kaufman, D.R.; Albright, A.; Cheng, J.D.; Kang, S.P.; Shankaran, V.; et al. IFN-gamma-related mRNA profile predicts clinical response to PD-1 blockade. *J. Clin. Investig.* **2017**, *127*, 2930–2940. [CrossRef] [PubMed]

22. Chen, D.S.; Mellman, I. Elements of cancer immunity and the cancer-immune set point. *Nature* **2017**, *541*, 321–330. [CrossRef] [PubMed]

23. Das, K.; Chan, X.B.; Epstein, D.; Teh, B.T.; Kim, K.-M.; Kim, S.T.; Park, S.H.; Kang, W.K.; Rozen, S.; Lee, J.; et al. NanoString expression profiling identifies candidate biomarkers of RAD001 response in metastatic gastric cancer. *ESMO Open* **2016**, *1*, e000009. [CrossRef] [PubMed]

24. Huang da, W.; Sherman, B.T.; Lempicki, R.A. Systematic and integrative analysis of large gene lists using DAVID bioinformatics resources. *Nat. Protoc.* **2009**, *4*, 44–57. [CrossRef] [PubMed]

25. Huang da, W.; Sherman, B.T.; Lempicki, R.A. Bioinformatics enrichment tools: Paths toward the comprehensive functional analysis of large gene lists. *Nucleic Acids Res.* **2009**, *37*, 1–13. [CrossRef] [PubMed]

26. Boger, C.; Behrens, H.M.; Kruger, S.; Rocken, C. The novel negative checkpoint regulator VISTA is expressed in gastric carcinoma and associated with PD-L1/PD-1: A future perspective for a combined gastric cancer therapy? *Oncoimmunology* **2017**, *6*, e1293215. [CrossRef] [PubMed]

27. Chiaravalli, A.M.; Cornaggia, M.; Furlan, D.; Capella, C.; Fiocca, R.; Tagliabue, G.; Klersy, C.; Solcia, E. The role of histological investigation in prognostic evaluation of advanced gastric cancer. Analysis of histological structure and molecular changes compared with invasive pattern and stage. *Virchows Arch.* **2001**, *439*, 158–169. [CrossRef] [PubMed]

28. Velho, S.; Fernandes, M.S.; Leite, M.; Figueiredo, C.; Seruca, R. Causes and consequences of microsatellite instability in gastric carcinogenesis. *World J. Gastroenterol.* **2014**, *20*, 16433–16442. [CrossRef] [PubMed]

29. Riquelme, I.; Saavedra, K.; Espinoza, J.A.; Weber, H.; Garcia, P.; Nervi, B.; Garrido, M.; Corvalan, A.H.; Roa, J.C.; Bizama, C. Molecular classification of gastric cancer: Towards a pathway-driven targeted therapy. *Oncotarget* **2015**, *6*, 24750–24779. [CrossRef] [PubMed]

30. Michael-Robinson, J.M.; Reid, L.E.; Purdie, D.M.; Biemer-Huttmann, A.E.; Walsh, M.D.; Pandeya, N.; Simms, L.A.; Young, J.P.; Leggett, B.A.; Jass, J.R.; et al. Proliferation, apoptosis, and survival in high-level microsatellite instability sporadic colorectal cancer. Clinical cancer research. *Off. J. Am. Assoc. Cancer Res.* **2001**, *7*, 2347–2356.

31. Shinozaki-Ushiku, A.; Kunita, A.; Fukayama, M. Update on Epstein-Barr virus and gastric cancer (review). *Int. J. Oncol.* **2015**, *46*, 1421–1434. [CrossRef] [PubMed]

32. Kim, S.Y.; Park, C.; Kim, H.J.; Park, J.; Hwang, J.; Kim, J.I.; Choi, M.G.; Kim, S.; Kim, K.M.; Kang, M.S. Deregulation of immune response genes in patients with Epstein-Barr virus-associated gastric cancer and outcomes. *Gastroenterology* **2015**, *148*, 137–147.e9. [CrossRef] [PubMed]

33. Strong, M.J.; Xu, G.; Coco, J.; Baribault, C.; Vinay, D.S.; Lacey, M.R.; Strong, A.L.; Lehman, T.A.; Seddon, M.B.; Lin, Z.; et al. Differences in gastric carcinoma microenvironment stratify according to EBV infection intensity: Implications for possible immune adjuvant therapy. *PLoS Pathog.* **2013**, *9*, e1003341. [CrossRef] [PubMed]

34. Veldman-Jones, M.H.; Brant, R.; Rooney, C.; Geh, C.; Emery, H.; Harbron, C.G.; Wappett, M.; Sharpe, A.; Dymond, M.; Barrett, J.C.; et al. Evaluating Robustness and Sensitivity of the NanoString Technologies nCounter Platform to Enable Multiplexed Gene Expression Analysis of Clinical Samples. *Cancer Res.* **2015**, *75*, 2587–2593. [CrossRef] [PubMed]

35. Takagi, S.; Kumagai, S.; Kinouchi, Y.; Hiwatashi, N.; Nagashima, F.; Takahashi, S.; Shimosegawa, T. High Ki-67 labeling index in human colorectal cancer with microsatellite instability. *Anticancer Res.* **2002**, *22*, 3241–3244. [PubMed]

36. Wu, Y.; Cao, D.; Qu, L.; Cao, X.; Jia, Z.; Zhao, T.; Wang, Q.; Jiang, J. PD-1 and PD-L1 co-expression predicts favorable prognosis in gastric cancer. *Oncotarget* **2017**, *8*, 64066–64082. [CrossRef] [PubMed]

37. Tie, Y.; Ma, X.; Zhu, C.; Mao, Y.; Shen, K.; Wei, X.; Chen, Y.; Zheng, H. Safety and efficacy of nivolumab in the treatment of cancers: A meta-analysis of 27 prospective clinical trials. *Int. J. Cancer* **2017**, *140*, 948–958. [CrossRef] [PubMed]

38. Goode, E.F.; Smyth, E.C. Immunotherapy for Gastroesophageal Cancer. *J. Clin. Med.* **2016**, *5*, 84. [CrossRef] [PubMed]

39. Janjigian, Y.Y.; Bendell, J.C.; Calvo, E.; Kim, J.W.; Ascierto, P.A.; Sharma, P.; Ott, P.A.; Bono, P.; Jaeger, D.; Evans, T.R.J.; et al. CheckMate-032: Phase, I./II, open-label study of safety and activity of nivolumab (nivo) alone or with ipilimumab (ipi) in advanced and metastatic (A/M) gastric cancer (GC). *J. Clin. Oncol.* **2016**, *34*, 4010. [CrossRef]

40. R Development Core Team. *R: A Language and Environment for Statistical Computing. R Foundation for Statistical Computing*; R Core Team: Vienna, Austria, 2008.

41. Wickham, H. *Ggplot2: Elegant Graphics for Data Analysis*; Springer: Berlin, Germany, 2009.

42. Tang, Y.; Horikoshi, M.; Li, W. Ggfortify: Unified Interface to Visualize Statistical. *R J.* **2016**, *8*, 474–485.

43. Horikoshi, M.; Tang, Y. Ggfortify: Data Visualization Tools for Statistical Analysis Results. Available online: https://CRAN.R-project.org/package=ggfortify (accessed on 17 July 2018).

44. Boger, C.; Behrens, H.M.; Mathiak, M.; Kruger, S.; Kalthoff, H.; Rocken, C. PD-L1 is an independent prognostic predictor in gastric cancer of Western patients. *Oncotarget* **2016**, *7*, 24269–24283. [CrossRef] [PubMed]

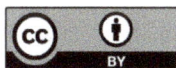

International Journal of
Molecular Sciences

MDPI

Review

Immunotherapy for Gastric Cancer: Time for a Personalized Approach?

Riccardo Dolcetti [1,*], **Valli De Re** [2,*] and **Vincenzo Canzonieri** [3]

1   University of Queensland Diamantina Institute, Translational Research Institute, 37 Kent Str, Woolloongabba, 4102 QLD, Australia
2   Immunopathology and Tumor Biomarkers Unit/Bio-proteomics Facility, Department of Translational Research and Advanced Tumor Diagnostics CRO National Cancer Institute, 33081 Aviano, Italy
3   Pathology Department of Translational Research and Advanced Tumor Diagnostics, CRO National Cancer Institute, 33081 Aviano, Italy; vcanzonieri@cro.it
*   Correspondence: r.dolcetti@uq.edu.au (R.D.); vdere@cro.it (V.D.R.); Tel.: +61-(0)7-344-36953 (R.D.); +39-0434-659672 (V.D.R.); Fax: +61-(0)7-3443-6966 (R.D.); +39-0434-659196 (V.D.R.)

Received: 30 April 2018; Accepted: 24 May 2018; Published: 29 May 2018

Abstract: Over the last decade, our understanding of the mechanisms underlying immune modulation has greatly improved, allowing for the development of multiple therapeutic approaches that are revolutionizing the treatment of cancer. Immunotherapy for gastric cancer (GC) is still in the early phases but is rapidly evolving. Recently, multi-platform molecular analyses of GC have proposed a new classification of this heterogeneous group of tumors, highlighting subset-specific features that may more reliably inform therapeutic choices, including the use of new immunotherapeutic drugs. The clinical benefit and improved survival observed in GC patients treated with immunotherapeutic strategies and their combination with conventional therapies highlighted the importance of the immune environment surrounding the tumor. A thorough investigation of the tumor microenvironment and the complex and dynamic interaction between immune cells and tumor cells is a fundamental requirement for the rational design of novel and more effective immunotherapeutic approaches. This review summarizes the pre-clinical and clinical results obtained so far with immunomodulatory and immunotherapeutic treatments for GC and discusses the novel combination strategies that are being investigated to improve the personalization and efficacy of GC immunotherapy.

Keywords: gastric cancer; immunotherapy; immune checkpoint; chimeric antigen receptor; cancer vaccine; adoptive immunotherapy; Epstein–Barr virus; microsatellite instability; tumor microenvironment

1. Introduction

Gastric carcinoma (GC) is the third most common cause of cancer deaths worldwide with a median overall survival (OS) time for patients diagnosed in a metastatic stage still less than one year [1]. A high proportion of patients diagnosed with GC (≈65%) present with inoperable or metastatic disease, and the survival rate of GC patients decreases dramatically as the tumor stage increases (Table 1). Surgical resection is the primary choice of treatment, with limited resection in stage T1N0; preoperative chemotherapy and surgery, followed by post-operative adjuvant chemo/radiotherapy in stages >T1N0 (advanced tumor); and palliative chemotherapy (supportive care, double, triple regimens ± targeted therapy) in metastatic disease (metastatic tumor) (Table 1). Currently, in non-metastatic advanced GC (>T1N0), the best available systemic therapy combinations only yield a median progression-free survival (PFS) time of 5 to 7 months and a median OS in the range of 8 to 11 months.

Table 1. Tumor stage and associated survival rate.

Tumor Stage	TNM Classification	Survival Rate (%, 5 Years)	Treatment
1	T1-2, N0-1, M0	69	Surgical resection
2	T1-4a, N0-3a, M0	43	Preoperative chemotherapy and surgery followed by post-operative adjuvant chemo/radio-therapy
3	T1-4b, N1-3b, M0	28	
4	Tx, Nx, M0	9	Palliative chemotherapy ± targeted therapy

TNM Classification of malignant tumors [2]. T: size of the primary tumor; N: lymph node involvement; M: metastasis.

Recently, immunotherapy has emerged as one of the most promising strategies in cancer treatment, with outstanding results in several tumor types [3–5]. The clinical successes of immune checkpoint inhibitors have revolutionized cancer treatment, clearly indicating that targeting the host's immune system rather than the tumor may be more effective than conventional therapies. Although encouraging, the results obtained so far in GC patients have, however, still been unsatisfactory, and the majority of novel immunotherapies in this setting are still in the early phases of clinical investigation [6,7]. The most promising response rates obtained so far by this class of immunotherapeutic drugs were induced by pembrolizumab monotherapy, targeting programmed death 1 (PD-1) cells in pre-treated patients with advanced GC [8]. Now, ongoing randomized clinical trials are conducted to assess pembrolizumab's safety and efficacy in earlier lines of therapy and in combination with chemotherapy for patients with advanced adenocarcinomas of the gastroesophageal junction (GEJ) [9]. Several complex factors are limiting the development of effective immunotherapeutic strategies for GC, including the heterogeneous immunogenicity among and within tumor subtypes and the different and still poorly defined immunosuppressive mechanisms that may hamper effective control of the tumor by host immune cells. In the recently proposed molecular Cancer Genome Atlas (TCGA) GC classification, the *PD-L1* gene was found to be amplified more commonly in Epstein–Barr virus (EBV)-positive and microsatellite instable (MSI)-high GC subtypes with respect to the other subtypes [10,11]. Nonetheless, clinical responses were also observed both in PD-L1- and EBV-negative patients, again highlighting the complexity of the mechanisms underlying the responses to immune checkpoint blockade. Thus, at the clinical level, it is not clear why some patients respond to certain immunotherapies and others do not. Therefore, there are no validated biomarkers allowing reliable discrimination of responders from non-responders. A deeper genetic and immunologic characterization of GC is required to guide patient selection and identify those who could benefit from immune intervention in monotherapy, or more likely, within combination schedules.

2. Immunosurveillance and Immunoescape

The critical role of host immunity in controlling cancer development and progression is now well recognized [12]. Data accumulated so far are consistent in indicating that our immune system is able to prevent cancer development through a process termed immune surveillance [12]. This complex process functions through a mechanism of "immunoediting", which consists of three sequential phases: (1) the elimination phase, in which growing tumors are effectively recognized and cleared by the synergic actions of innate and adaptive immune responses that also recognize remodeling of stroma and changes in the microenvironment; (2) The equilibrium phase, during which, antigen presenting cells, tumor cells and CD8+ T cells remain in a state of dynamic balance and the surviving tumor cells remain quiescent under the pressure of immune cells. In this long phase, the immune system of the host sculpts the immunogenicity of genetically unstable tumor clones, allowing for the selection of resistant tumor cells, thus leading to (3) the escape phase, favored by regulatory (Treg) cells and immunosuppressive cytokines, including transforming growth factor-β (TGF-β), Tumor Necrosis factor (TNF)-α, and Interleukin (IL)-10 [12].

Dying cancer cells may express and release tumor-specific and tumor-associated antigens that can be taken up and processed by tissue resident dendritic cells, which then maturate in professional antigen-presenting cells in the presence of an appropriate microenvironment, usually enriched in activator molecules, the so-called danger-associated molecular patterns (DAMPs) [12]. Induction of effective anti-cancer immunity generally requires that mature antigen presenting cells efficiently present tumor antigens in the form of peptides to CD8[+] T lymphocytes through major histocompatibility complex (MHC) Class I molecules and to CD4[+] T lymphocytes through MHC Class II molecules. The immunogenicity of tumor antigens varies considerably, the strongest tumor antigens being those provided by non-self or mutated proteins, such as those encoded by viruses or generated by somatic mutations occurring in expressed genes. These latter antigens, the so-called neo-antigens, are generally unique for each individual tumor, thus providing the rationale for personalized immunotherapy. For efficient activation of the CD8[+] T cells, three different signals are required: T-cell receptor signalling activation after recognition of antigenic peptides in the context of MHC Class I molecules, co-stimulatory molecules, and cytokines provided by professional antigen presenting cells [12]. After activation, T lymphocytes proliferate, infiltrate the tumor, promote the recruitment of other immune cells, and directly kill the cancer cells through the release of cytokines, perforin and granzymes [12]. Incomplete T-cell activation in response to suboptimal amounts of IL-2 or the absence of co-stimulatory signals usually results in T-cell anergy. Another important phenomenon negatively affecting the efficacy of antitumor immune responses is the induction of T-cell exhaustion promoted by the complex network of immunosuppressive cells and cytokines that characterize the tumor microenvironment [13]. T cell exhaustion is a state of altered functionality of these cells, which progressively lose their proliferation, cytokine production, and cytotoxic capabilities. Evidence accumulated so far clearly indicates that exhausted T cells up-regulate the expression of inhibitory receptors, including programmed cell death protein 1 (PD-1), cytotoxic T lymphocyte antigen-4 (CTLA-4), lymphocyte activation gene 3 (LAG-3), T cell immunoglobulin and mucin domain containing-3 (TIM-3), B and T lymphocyte attenuator (BTLA), and T cell immunoreceptor with Ig and ITIM domains (TIGIT) [13,14].

The tumor microenvironment may also impair anti-tumor immunity by promoting the polarization of infiltrating immune cells towards less cytotoxic and pro-inflammatory subsets of T cells (e.g., TH2, TH17 and Treg cells). In GC, the tumor-associated macrophages (TAMs) constitute one of the most abundant immune cell populations present in the tumor microenvironment. These cells can exert anti-tumor activities, or have pro-tumorigenic effects supporting cancer initiation and malignant progression according to differentiation patterns into M1 or M2 subtypes [15]. M1 TAMs exert anti-tumor effects through the release of pro-inflammatory cytokines (IL-1, IL-6, IL-23, TNF-α), whereas M2 TAMs may drive local immune suppression by producing IL-10 and TGF-β. Indeed, TAM infiltration has been shown to functionally inhibit T cells in GC [16,17] and may be a marker of poor prognosis [18,19]. Myeloid-derived suppressor cells (MDSCs) are a heterogeneous population of immature myeloid cells able to inhibit both innate and adaptive immune responses against tumors [20]. These cells are characterized by the ability display have unique features according to the different environments to which they are recruited. The various suppressive properties and functions displayed by MDSCs include increased arginase-1 (Arg-1) and inducible nitric oxide synthase activities, elevated production of nitric oxide and reactive oxygen species, and secretion of various pro-inflammatory cytokines [21]. It has been demonstrated that GC patients have increased numbers of MDSCs in the blood compared with healthy individuals, and this increase was associated with poor clinical outcomes [22]. Another major component of the immune suppressive tumor microenvironment is represented by Treg cells, which may inhibit cytotoxic lymphocytes and/or helper T-cell activity as well as natural killer (NK) cells. Physiologically, Treg cell function is critical to maintain immunological tolerance to self-antigens and suppress excessive immune responses that could potentially be deleterious to the host. Tregs have also been identified as the major regulatory component of the adaptive immune response in *H. pylori*-related inflammation, GC and bacterial persistence [23] as well as in EBV-related GC [24]. A recent study demonstrated that Foxp3⁺CD4⁺ICOS⁺ effector Tregs (eTregs), which has highly suppressive functions, was more abundant in late stage GCs [25]. These tumor infiltrating Tregs exhibited the ability to produce IL-10, but not IFN-γ, TNF-α, or IL-17 and to inhibit the proliferation of responder CD8⁺ T cells.

The presence of tumor infiltrating lymphocytes (TILs) can be detected in various cancers, including GC. Nevertheless, the considerable variability in the number, types and spatial distribution of infiltrates suggests that some tumor types are more immunogenic than others. Indeed, tumors with a low burden of neo-antigens generated by somatic mutations are considered poorly immunogenic and usually show limited or a total absence of infiltration by TILs (immune-desert tumors). The absence of intra-tumoral lymphoid infiltrate may also be due to defects intrinsic to the multi-step T-cell trafficking and homing cascade, a phenomenon that may significantly contribute to immunotherapy resistance [26].

Evidence accumulated so far indicates that TILs may have an important role in influencing the clinical course of various tumors, also including GC [27]. A higher density of both intra-tumoral cytotoxic CD8⁺ TILs and regulatory FoxP3⁺ Treg cells is associated with good prognosis, and this is particularly true for MSI GC, including those that are *H. pylori*- or EBV-positive [24,28]. A recent meta-analysis of 31 observational studies including 4,185 GC patients investigated the significance of the prognostic role of specific T-cell subsets, focusing on overall survival and disease-free survival [29]. In particular, the study concluded that the numbers of CD8⁺, FOXP3⁺, CD3⁺, CD57⁺, CD20⁺, CD45RO⁺, Granzyme B⁺ and T-bet⁺ infiltrating lymphocytes were significantly associated with improved survival ($p < 0.05$). Notably, the amount of CD3⁺ TILs in the intra-tumoral compartment was the most significant prognostic marker (pooled Hazard ratio, HR = 0.52; 95% CI = 0.43–0.63; $p < 0.001$). B-cell activation may also influence tumor prognosis, by producing antibodies against tumor antigens and by activating of a specific B-cell subset (i.e., Breg) that secrete anti-inflammatory mediators (e.g., IL-10) and convert T cells to regulatory T cells (Treg), thus attenuating anti-tumor immune responses [30]. It has been demonstrated that in vivo primed and in vitro activated B cells have showed therapeutic efficacy in adoptive immunotherapy protocols [31,32]. Notably, effector B cells were shown to directly kill tumor cells [32]. On the other hand, resting B cells can promote the development or malignant progression of cancer [33,34].

3. Immune-Based Therapies

3.1. Adoptive Cell Immunotherapy

The tumor-killing properties of T cells and natural killer (NK) cells provide opportunities to treat cancer. Tumor infiltrating lymphocytes (TILs) and NK cells may have predictive and prognostic relevance in GC [35–39]. Adoptive cell therapies may harness this potential with different modalities. The main strategy involves the isolation of immune cells from a cancer patient, their subsequent genetic modification or treatment to enhance their activity to specifically recognize and kill tumor cells. After adequate ex vivo expansion, these immune cell populations are re-infused into the patient [40]. This process is applicable to most of cancer patients who are unable to mount an effective anti-cancer immunity, and therefore, probably also unable to respond to immune checkpoint inhibitors. There are several different strategies of adoptive cell therapy being used for cancer treatment, most of them have been or are being investigated in the clinical setting for their potential efficacy in GC patients.

In this setting, MHC Class I-restricted T cells specifically recognizing GC antigens can be successfully isolated from primary tumors, metastatic lymph nodes and ascites from GC patients [41]. However, the limited proportion (about 40%) of biopsies yielding satisfactory T cell populations and the time (about 6 weeks) required to generate adequate numbers of cells for infusion have limited the applicability of approaches using TIL cells [35]. Alternative modalities to generate tumor-specific immune cells have been investigated to overcome these limitations, including the use of cytotoxic T-cell lines generated from the spleen of GC patients [42] or the expansion and re-infusion of T lymphocytes taken directly from a patient's blood after they have received a cancer vaccine. Indeed, it has been shown that "priming" rare tumor antigen specific T cells first, with active immunization, is associated with more effective expansion of tumor-specific T cells, which can be obtained in greater numbers for therapeutic infusion [35].

The use of in vitro expanded allogeneic NK cells, which have cytotoxic function and the potential to exert antibody-dependent cellular cytotoxicity (ADCC), appears particularly promising for cancer immunotherapy. Compared to autologous NK cells, allogeneic NK cells are more suitable for quality control and large-scale production and have the advantage of not being inhibited by self-histocompatibility antigens, unlike T cells. To expand ex vivo NK cells (over 1000-fold expansion), peripheral blood mononuclear cells of healthy donors or patients are co-cultured in the presence of irradiated K562 leukemia cells that have been modified to express membrane-bound IL-15 and 4-1BB ligands in the presence of IL-2 and IL-15 cytokines in the culture media [43]. However, clinical-grade NK cells at sufficiently high numbers represents a great challenge; therefore, alternative methods to obtain sufficient functional NK cells have been investigated [44–46]. Cytotoxic cell lines have been also established from patients with clonal NK-cell lymphoma, and one of them, the NK-92 cell line, has been infused into patients with advanced cancer and showed clinical benefit with minimal side effects [29]. The use of an established NK cell line offers several advantages compared to the use of in vitro expanded NK-cells. Notably, a NK-cell line does not cause graft versus host rejection, and thus can safely be used in allogeneic settings. Based on these considerations, researchers are now exploring the use of engineered NK cells, including the NK-92 cell line, for the treatment of various haematological and non-haematological malignancies. The first chimeric antigen receptor (CAR)-expressing NK-92 cells were generated almost 15 years ago [47]. These cells demonstrated high efficacy against Human Epidermal Growth Factor Receptor 2 (HER2)-positive breast and ovarian cancer cells both in vitro and in vivo [48]. The therapeutic efficacy of this HER2-CAR NK-92 cells has been tested in established mouse models of orthotopic human glioblastoma, renal cell and breast carcinoma [49]. Results of these studies demonstrated specific homing of the NK cells to the tumor sites, a reduction in the number of metastases and significant tumor regression, indicating that this could constitute a promising therapeutic approach for HER2+ GC.

Another adoptive cell therapy approach is based on the exploitation of the immunotherapeutic properties of a heterogeneous population of immune effector cells: the cytokine-induced killer cells (CIK). These cells can be obtained by treating peripheral blood lymphocytes with interferon-γ (IFN-γ), a monoclonal antibody against CD3 and an interleukin (IL)-2 [50]. CIK cells are mainly expansions of $CD3^+CD8^+CD56^-$ negative cells to terminally differentiated CD56-positive natural killer (NK) T cells. These cells have the peculiar capacity of recognising tumor cells both in the presence and in the absence of antibodies and MHC; thus, they can also recognise tumor cells that are missing MHC molecules on their surfaces. The cytotoxicity of CIKs is mediated by perforin release and is dependent on the interaction between killer cell lectin like receptor K1 (NKG2D) and NKG2D ligands. Moreover, in vivo CIK cells can also regulate and increase host cellular immune function through the secretion of several cytokines and chemokines. Available evidence indicates that combination therapy with chemotherapy and CIK generally improves the progression-free survival (PFS) and overall survival (OS) times of patients with cancer, including GC (Table 2). Some chemotherapies (e.g., doxorubicin, mitoxantrone, oxaliplatin and cyclophosphamide) may add positive immune effects by fostering $CD8^+$ T-cell infiltration into the tumor and promoting the release of tumor antigens through the induction of immunogenic death of tumor cells [51]. Two meta-analyses considering relevant clinical trials concluded that CIK cell therapy significantly increases the 5-year OS rate of GC patients compared to conventional chemotherapy, thus providing statistical evidence to support the activation of large-scale clinical trials with CIK cell therapy [52,53]. Interestingly, the percentage of lymphocyte subsets ($CD3^+$, $CD4^+$ and $CD3^-CD56^+$, $CD3^+CD56^+$; $p < 0.01$) and the levels of IL-12 and IFN-γ, which reflect immune function, were significantly increased ($p < 0.05$) after the CIK/DC-CIK therapy [53]. A particularly attractive perspective for the clinical exploitation of CIK cells is their combination with monoclonal antibodies [54]. Indeed, pre-clinical evidence has been provided indicating that CIK cells combined with a monoclonal antibody against epidermal growth factor receptor (EGFR) enhance the antitumor ability of CIK cells both in vitro and in vivo [55].

In summary, the overall data reported so far indicates that autologous immune cell administration with adjuvant chemotherapy is associated with better prognosis for patients with GC compared to those treated with chemotherapy only [34]. Some examples are reported in Table 2. Nevertheless, current approaches of adoptive cell-based immunotherapy need to be improved to make clinical application more feasible. In this respect, it has been shown that T/NK cell-mediated anti-tumor activity may be suppressed by tumor or stromal cells via inhibitory soluble factors/cytokines or through the engagement of inhibitory immune checkpoint molecules. These findings strongly suggested that blocking inhibitory regulators of T/NK cells might be an attractive and promising strategy to increase the efficacy of T/NK cell-based tumor immunotherapy [56].

Table 2. Adoptive cell immunotherapy for gastric carcinoma (GC).

Type of Treatment	Setting	Primary End-Point	References
Autologous tumor infiltrating lymphocytes (TILs) combined with rIL-2	advanced GC ($n = 23$)	13% CR 21.7% PR	[57]
Autologous peripheral blood lymphocytes activated by anti-CD3 antibody and interleukin (IL)-2 + chemotherapy	GC with a life expectancy >12 weeks ($n = 84$)	OS in patients that had received surgery was prolonged after EAAL immunotherapy	[58]
Ex vivo expanded natural killer (NK) in co-culture with K562			[43]
NK expansion using recombinant human fibronectin fragment (FN-CH296) + target-based chemotherapy	unresectable, locally advanced, and/or metastatic GC ($n = 3$)	phase I trial, good tolerability	[44]
Expanded NK with OK432, IL-2, and modified FN-CH296	unresectable, locally advanced and/or metastatic GC ($n = 3$)	phase I well tolerated with no severe adverse events	[45]
NK-92 cell line	advanced solid tumors	only pre-clinical studies	[29]
Autologous cytokine-induced killer cells (CIK)	post-operative locally advanced GC ($n = 151$)	5-year OS 46.8 vs. 31.4% intestinal type ($p = 0.045$), 5-year DFS 28.3 versus 10.4% ($p = 0.044$)	[59]
Autologous CIK + chemotherapy	post-operative locally advanced GC ($n = 95$)	DFS and OS were longer in pts with higher major histocompatibility complex (MHC)-I-related gene A (MICA)	[58]
Autologous CIK + chemotherapy	post-operative locally advanced GC ($n = 156$)	longer OS	[60]
Autologous CIK + chemotherapy	GC stage II-III ($n = 226$)	longer DFS and OS	[61]
Autologous CIK + oxaliplatin	post-operative stage II-III GC ($n = 167$)	higher 5-year OS rate (56.6% vs. 26.8%, $p = 0.014$) and progression-free survival (PFS) rate (49.1% vs. 24.1%, $p = 0.026$)	[62]
Autologous CIK + FolFox4	post-operative GC ($n = 51$)	reduced GC recurrence rates and enhanced survival rates	[63]

EAAL: expanded activated autologous lymphocytes; DFS: Disease-free survival.

3.2. Engineered Cells for Adoptive Immunotherapy

To broaden the applicability and enhance the efficacy of adoptive cell therapy that could potentially lead to the elimination of the tumor cells, techniques have been recently developed to introduce antitumor antigen receptors into normal T cells that could be then used for therapy. The specificity of T cells can be redirected towards tumor cells by the use of viral vectors, allowing the expression of CARs specific for tumor antigens [64,65]. The T-cell receptor (TCR) recognition process requires antigen presentation via the major histocompatibility (MHC) complex. However, a significant proportion of tumors down-regulate MHC expression to escape immune surveillance. Engineering T lymphocytes with chimeric antigen receptors (CAR) and combining B cell receptor-derived and T cell receptor domains, has the advantage of bypassing the need for MHC interaction and costimulatory molecules. The extracellular portion of CAR-T cells is a ligand-binding domain composed of a B cell receptor-derived single-chain variable fragment, whereas the signalling domain is composed of CD3ζ and one or more intracellular costimulatory domains (Figure 1).

The adoptive transfer of CAR-T cells has so far demonstrated promising antitumor effects in advanced hematologic malignancies, but only limited benefits in patients with solid tumors. This may be due to the heterogeneous tumor antigen expression, immunosuppressive networks in the tumor microenvironment, the suboptimal trafficking of T cells into solid tumors and the lack of effective costimulatory signals required for CAR-T persistence after infusion [64–66]. In pre-clinical models of GC, treatment with CAR-T cells specific for the HER2 oncoprotein as well as the use of a bifunctional αHER2(Ag1)/CD3 (Ag2) RNA-engineered CAR-T-like human T cells, induced a marked regression of the tumor and prolonged the survival of tumor-bearing mice [67,68]. Of note, in addition to classical CAR-T cells, CAR T-like constructs also able to secrete soluble forms of the CAR receptor were able not only to directly kill HER2+ GC, but also to transfer this ability to bystander T cells [68]. Another HER2-targeting CAR-T constructs harboring T-costimulatory molecules (i.e., 4-1BB, CD3ζ, exhibited a considerably enhanced tumor inhibition ability and was able to promote long-term survival and T-cell homing to GC xenotransplanted mice [69]. CAR-T cells were also shown to eliminate patient-derived GC stem-like cells, an important effect to search for and implement, to enhance the possibility of eradicating tumor cells [50]. A phase I/II clinical study (NCT02713984) involving patients with several HER2-expressing tumor types, including GC, and treatment with HER2-targeting CAR-T cells is ongoing. Another therapeutic target antigen for GC is the Human Carcinoembryonic Antigen (CEA), an oncofetal glycoprotein overexpressed in gastrointestinal carcinomas. With the aim of enhancing the antitumor activity and in vivo persistence of CAR-T cells, CAR-T were engineered with a construct, combining CEA with a fusion protein of IL-2. In comparison with free IL-2, the combination of CAR-T cells with IL-2 significantly enhanced the antitumor activity against human GC cell line MKN-45 cells [70]. Several phase I studies are investigating the safety and therapeutic efficacy of CAR T cells redirected towards different GC antigenic targets, including CEA, MUC1 (mucins lining the apical surface of epithelial cells in GC) and EpCAM (an epithelial cell adhesion/activating molecule) (Table 3).

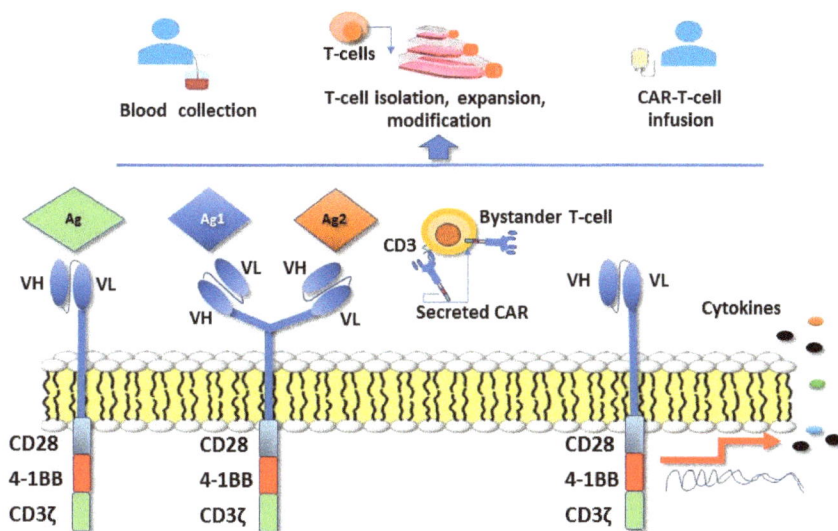

Figure 1. Chimeric antigen receptor (CAR)-T cell therapy T cells are isolated from blood of the patient or a donor, activated, and genetically engineered to express the CAR construct. Engineered CAR-T cells are then reinfused into the patient. The extracellular portion of CAR-T cells is a ligand-binding domain composed of a B cell receptor-derived single-chain variable fragment (VH-VL), whereas the T-cell receptor molecule signalling domain is composed of CD3 molecules and a ζ-chain (zeta chain) and one or more intracellular costimulatory domains required for T-cell stimulation (i.e., CD28 and 4-1BB or CD137). CAR-T cells can also be engineered to recognize two different antigens (dual specificity CAR-T cells). In addition to classical CAR-T cells, new CAR T-like constructs are also able to secrete soluble forms of the CAR receptor. The secreted CAR construct was demonstrated to be able not only to directly kill HER2+ GC, but also to transfer this ability to bystander T cells. More recent approaches have been based on the use of CAR-T cells genetically modified to express CARs along with a gene cassette driving the expression of cytokines (red arrow) that enhance T-cell activity.

Despite the efficacy shown by CAR-T-cell therapy in some clinical settings, this novel treatment strategy may be burdened by unique acute toxicities, which can be severe or even fatal [71]. Cytokine-release syndrome (CRS) is the most frequently observed adverse event, which can range in severity from low-grade constitutional symptoms to a high-grade syndrome associated with life-threatening multi-organ dysfunction. Only rarely, severe CRS can evolve into fulminant haemophagocytic lymphohistiocytosis. Neurotoxicity, defined as CAR-T-cell-related encephalopathy syndrome, is the second most frequent adverse event, and can occur concurrently with or after CRS. Considering that antigens on cancer cells may be also expressed on normal cells, on target off-tumor toxicity can occur upon stimulation of T cells following the binding of CARs to their antigens on the normal cells/tissues. Life-threatening on target off-tumor toxicity may particularly occur in cases in which the target antigen is expressed in vital tissues such as the respiratory system. This fatal occurrence was reported in a patient with metastatic colorectal cancer following the administration of ERBB2 CAR-Ts where low expression of ERBB2 on respiratory normal epithelial cells led to acute pulmonary manifestation and the patient's death 5 days after the injection of CAR-Ts [72]. New strategies such as designing CAR-Ts with limited life-span or "on-switch CARs" are under investigation to ameliorate the toxicity of CAR-T.

Table 3. Engineered adoptive T/NK cells—CAR-T cells.

Type of Treatment	Setting	Type of Study/Trial	Reference/Trial No.
CAR T cell therapy targeting human epidermal growth factor receptor 2 (HER2)	HER2+ GC	pre-clinical studies	[67,69]
CAR-T-like T cells targeting HER2	HER2+ GC	pre-clinical study	[68]
CAR targeting HER2+	HER2-positive solid tumors (breast cancer, ovarian cancer, lung cancer, GC, colorectal cancer, glioma, pancreatic cancer)	ongoing phase I studies	NCT02713984
CAR targeting the carcinoembryonic antigen (CEA)	GC CEA-positive	ongoing phase I studies	NCT02349724 NCT02850536 NCT02416466
CAR targeting Human Mucin-1 (MUC1)	GC MUC1-positive	ongoing phase I	NCT02617134
CAR targeting the epithelial cell adhesion molecule (EpCAM)	GC EpCAM-positive	ongoing phase I studies	NCT02725125 NCT03013712

3.3. Immune Checkpoint Inhibitors/Immune Modulatory Pathways

Immune checkpoint therapy exploits the function of molecules that physiologically regulate and balance immune responses by inhibiting T-cell activation or, alternatively, by activating stimulatory pathways with the final result to maintain homeostasis and avoid tissue damages due to excessive immune activation. In the field of cancer immunotherapy, these treatments are designed to release or enhance pre-existing anti-cancer immune responses. Indeed, tumor cells may induce T-cell suppressive signalling to successfully evade immune-mediated tumour eradication, a phenomenon called adaptive immune resistance. The inhibitory signals suppressing T-cell activation are mediated by a variety of "immune-checkpoint" molecules (inhibitory ligands and their cognate receptors), including the CD28/cytotoxic T-lymphocyte antigen 4 (CTLA-4) axis, and PD-L1/PD-1 pathway, which have emerged as promising targets. Other checkpoint molecules, such as TIM3, B7H3, VISTA, LAG3, and TIGIT, are currently being evaluated as potential targets for cancer immunotherapy [73] (Figure 2). Pathways involving these regulatory molecules are crucial for maintaining the tolerance against self-antigens and modulating the duration and amplitude of immune responses against non-self or mutated tumor antigens in order to avoid tissue damage. When these negative regulatory proteins are blocked, the inhibition of immune effectors is released, and these cells regain their ability to become activated and kill tumour cells. The binding of the PD-1 receptor expressed at the surface of T cells with its cognate ligands, PD-L1 and PD-L2, results in the inhibition of T-cell effector function and decreased cytotoxic activity within the tumor bed. This is consistent with the notion that antibodies targeting the PD-1/PD-L1 axis require the presence of tumor-specific T lymphocytes to be effective. On the other hand, the ubiquitous CTLA-4 has non-overlapping suppressive effects on antitumor immunity, being preferentially involved in controlling the earlier phases of the immune response (priming), primarily in lymphoid organs. These effects occurring at different sites and during different phases of the immune response support the rationale to combine the CTLA-4 blockade with antibodies targeting the PD-1/PD-L1 axis.

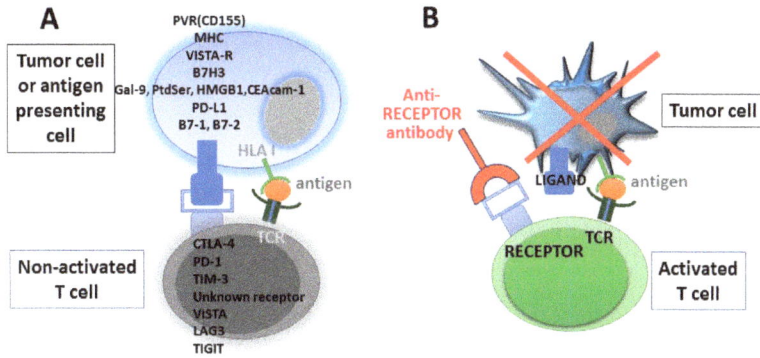

Figure 2. Blocking the immune checkpoint restores the ability of tumor-specific T lymphocytes to kill tumor cells. Antibodies/agents against receptors on T cells (i.e., CTLA-4, PD-1, etc.), and/or their relative ligands (i.e., B7, PDL-1, etc.) on antigen presenting cells or tumor cells re-activate pre-existing anti-tumor T cells that can induce tumor cell killing. Recognition of the human leukocyte antigen (HLA) Class I/peptide antigen complex by the T-cell receptor present on T cells is required to induce tumor cell killing; (**A**) Inhibitory receptor/ligand interaction is not blocked and the tumor cell is not killed; (**B**) the immune checkpoint receptor is blocked by an inhibitory antibody and the T-cell is re-activated and is thus able to kill tumor cells. PVR: poliovirus Receptor; MHC: Major Histocompatibility Complex; VISTA: V-domain Ig suppressor of T cell activation; VISTA-R: VISTA Receptor; Gal-9: Galectin-9; PtdSer: Phosphatidylserine; HMGB1: High Mobility Group Box 1; CEAcam-1: Carcinoembryonic antigen-related cell adhesion molecule 1; PD-L1: Programmed death-ligand 1; CTLA-4: Cytotoxic T-Lymphocyte Antigen 4; PD-1: PD-L1: Programmed death 1; TIM-3: T cell immunoglobulin and mucin domain 3; LAG-3: Lymphocyte-activation protein 3; TIGIT: T-cell immunoreceptor with Ig and ITIM domains.

With regard to GC, data collected so far indicate that PD-L1 is expressed in about 65% of GC tissues and CTLA-4 is expressed in 86% of cases, whereas these molecules are undetectable in normal gastric mucosa of healthy individuals [74–76]. Notably, positive tumour cell staining for PD-L1 or CTLA-4 has been associated with an inferior OS in GC patients and TILs express PD-1, PD-L1, and CTLA-4 molecules at a significantly higher level compared to the T cells of the peripheral blood [77]. A recent meta-analysis carried out on 15 studies, including 3291 GC patients, confirmed that the expression level of PD-L1 in tumour cells significantly correlates with a worse OS. In addition, a subgroup analysis showed that GC patients with deeper tumor infiltration, positive lymph node metastasis, positive venous invasion, Epstein–Barr virus (EBV) infection, or GC showing microsatellite instability (MSI) are more likely to express PD-L1. These findings suggest that GC patients, specifically those with EBV+ and MSI tumors, may be preferred candidates for PD-1-targeting therapies [78]. A FISH analysis demonstrated amplification of the gene encoding for PD-L1 in 11% of EBV+ cases, suggesting that this genetic change may be associated with, or even promote, the clonal evolution and malignant progression of EBV and GC [79]. The expression of PD-L1 by T/NK lymphocytes infiltrating GC may be also of potential prognostic relevance. Functional studies carried out in vitro revealed that blocking PD-1/PD-L1 signalling markedly enhanced cytokine production and cytotoxic activity while inhibiting NK cell apoptosis. Intriguingly, treatment with a PD-1 blocking antibody significantly inhibited the growth of xenografts in nude mice, an effect that was completely abrogated by NK depletion [80].

Like the alternative immune checkpoint molecule, VISTA appears particularly attractive as a potential therapeutic target. VISTA is a type I membrane protein expressed predominantly in myeloid, granulocytic and T cells. Although the ligands for VISTA are not yet known, available evidence indicates that VISTA may serve both as a ligand (for antigen presenting cells) and as a receptor (for T cells), and that VISTA suppresses T-cell activation, a function that could be independent of PD-1/PD-L1 signalling [81] an analysis of a cohort of 464 therapy-naive GC samples and 14 corresponding liver metastases disclosed that VISTA expression in tumor cells was detected in 41 GCs (8.8%) and two corresponding liver metastases (14.3%), but no significant correlation with patient outcome was observed [82].

TIM-3 is a member of the TNF family and a negative regulator of CD4$^+$ helper 1 and CD8$^+$ cytotoxic T cells. [83]. It has been reported that the expression of TIM-3 defines a subpopulation of specific PD-1$^+$ exhausted CD8$^+$ T cells with a low production of IFN-γ, TNF-α and IL-2, thus providing a rationale for combining immunotherapy targeting both TIM-3 and PD-1 inhibitory molecules [84,85].

The anti-CTLA-4 ipilimumab antibody and the anti-PD-1 antibodies, pembrolizumab and nivolumab, were first approved by the US Food and Drug Administration (FDA) for the treatment of patients with metastatic melanomas in 2011 and 2014, respectively. However, data accumulated so far indicates that while anti CTLA-4 antibodies yielded only partially satisfactory results, PD-1/PD-L1 inhibitors show more promising results (Table 4). Interestingly, patients with a post-treatment CEA antigen proliferative response had a median survival time of 17.1 months compared with 4.7 months for non-responders to the anti-CTLA-4, tremelimumab ($p = 0.004$), suggesting a rationale for combinations of CTLA-4 blockade with vaccines targeting GC antigens in the future [86]. Moreover, the efficacy of immunotherapies targeting the PD-1/PD-L1 in different solid tumours stimulated the activation of combination studies with other active targeted biologic agents or immune modulating treatments. Indeed, several clinical trials using new antibodies targeting the PD-1/PD-L1 axis in combination with other immunotherapies are ongoing (Table 4). The rationale supporting the combination of different immunotherapeutic agents is supported by several pre-clinical data which indicate that targeting only one of the complex steps required for the generation of effective anti-tumor immune responses is often insufficient. Moreover, taking into account the ability of several chemotherapeutic drugs to induce immunogenic cell death, therapeutic approaches combining immunotherapy and chemotherapy are also being actively investigated (Table 4).

Combination therapies with immune checkpoint inhibitors have also targeted the subset of HER2-overexpressing tumors which almost invariably become resistant to trastuzumab-containing regimens and progress. Pre-clinical evidence supports the rationale for combining trastuzumab and inhibitors of the PD-1/PD-L1 axis. In fact, it has been demonstrated that HER-2 inhibition can promote T-cell activation and trafficking, enhance IFNγ production by NK cells and boost antibody-dependent cellular cytotoxicity which may efficiently synergize with inhibition of the PD-1/PD-L1 pathway [87]. A phase Ib/II, open-label, dose-escalation study is investigating the novel anti-HER2 mAb, margetuximab, in combination with pembrolizumab in patients with advanced HER2-amplified GC who are refractory to standard trastuzumab-based combination chemotherapy (NCT02689284) [88]. A variety of other combinations is being investigated in which, on the backbone of inhibitors of the PD-1/PD-L1 axis, other drugs target additional nodes in the cancer immunity cycle [89]. The latter include agents inhibiting other immune checkpoints (TIM3, LAG3), T-cell costimulatory agonist antibodies (GITR, OX40, 4-1BB), enzymatic inhibitors (IDO-1), as well as radiation and other cytotoxic drugs. In addition, the combination of nivolumab and GS-5745, a matrix metalloproteinase 9 inhibitor, is also being investigated in patients with unresectable or recurrent GC/GEJ adenocarcinoma (NCT02864381). Combination with radiotherapy, although still poorly explored in the setting of GC, represents another promising therapeutic opportunity. Indeed, single dose and fractionated radiotherapy has been found to upregulate tumor PD-L1 expression in various pre-clinical models but also promotes the immunogenicity of tumor cells through the generation of new antigens or enhanced exposure or release of existing tumor antigens. Therefore, concomitant treatment with anti-PD1 antibodies may overcome the immune suppression activity mediated by PD-L1 that is up-regulated by radiotherapy, thus allowing for the generation of more effective anti-tumor immune responses that may lead to long-term tumor control [90]. Clinical trials involving GC patients are ongoing, including studies combining pembrolizumab with palliative radiotherapy in the metastatic setting, as well as with neoadjuvant chemoradiotherapy for GEJ and gastric cardia cancers in earlier stage resettable disease (NCT02730546) [91].

Table 4. Immune checkpoint inhibitors.

Type of Treatment	Setting	Primary End-Point	Reference/Trial No.
Tremelimumab (IgG2 anti B7 ligand of CTLA-4)	metastatic gastric and esophageal carcinomas (n = 18)	phase II, OS similar to conventional therapy	[86]
Tremelimumab + Durvalumab	GC/gastroesophageal junction (GEJ) (n = 135)	phase Ib/II, ongoing	NCT02340975
Ipilimumab (IgG1κ anti CTL-4)	unresectable locally advanced/metastatic GC/GEJ (n = 143)	phase II, OS similar to conventional therapy	[92]
Ipilimumab + Nivolumab (Anti-PD-1)	GC/GEJ pre-operative setting and nivolumab combined with chemo-radiation	phase Ib, ongoing	NCT03044613
Pembrolizumab (IgG4 anti PD-1)	recurrent or metastatic GC/GEJ (n = 39)	phase Ib, 22% partial response, toxicity manageable	[93]
	PD-L1+ advanced solid tumors including GC/GEJ (n = 23)	phase Ib, 30% Overall response rate (ORR), median 15 months, better response in patients with high interferon (IFN)-γ gene signature	[94]
	recurrent or metastatic GC/GEJ, 2 line (n = 259)	phase II improved ORR (12%), progression-free survival (PFS) 2 months, and OS 6 months	[95]
	recurrent or metastatic GC/GEJ ≥1% PD-L1+, 1 line	phase II. improved ORR (26%), PFS 3 months, and OS not reach in GC with ≥1% expression of PD-L1	[95]
Pembrolizumab + chemotherapy	recurrent or metastatic GC/GEJ	phase II. improved ORR (60%), PFS 7 months, and OS 14 months	[95]
	recurrent or metastatic GC/GEJ	phase III ongoing	[96]
Pembrolizumab + Ramucirumab (anti VEGFR2)	locally advanced and unresectable or metastatic GC and other tumors (n = 155)	phase I, study ongoing	[97]
Pembrolizumab + Margetuximab (anti HER2)	advanced and metastatic GC/GEJ HER2+ (n =72)	phase I, dose escalation, safety, efficacy. Study ongoing	[88]
neoadjuvant Pembrolizumab + chemo/radiotherapy	resectable, locally advanced GEJ or GC of cardia (n = 68)	phase Ib/II, side effects and best way to give the treatment. Study ongoing	[91]
Nivolumab (IgG4 anti PD-1)	recurrent or metastatic GC/GEJ (n = 160)	phase I/II, ORR 24% Nivolumab and Ipilimumab vs 12% Nivolumab in monotherapy with lower toxicity	[98]
Nivolumab + Ipilimumab	unresectable advanced or recurrent gastric or GEJ cancer, refractory to, or intolerant of, two or more prior chemotherapy regimens, only patients from Asian countries	phase III, improved OS (26.6% at 1 year, median 5.32 months), PFS (1.61 months). ORR 11.2%	[99]
Avelumab (IgG1 anti PD-L1)	advanced or metastatic previously treated solid tumors, including GC/GEJ	phase Ia, dose escalation trial, acceptable toxicity	[100]
	3 line recurrent or metastatic GC/GEJ (n = 371)	phase III, Avelumab + best supportive care (BSC) vs BSC ± chemotherapy, study on going at the moment, it did not improve overall survival (OS)	[101]
	unresectable, locally advanced or metastatic GC	Avelumab vs continuation of first-line chemotherapy	[102]
Durvalumab (IgG1κ anti PD-L1)	2/3 line metastatic GC	phase Ib/II Durvalumab or Durvalumab + Tremelimumab vs Tremelimumab alone. study is ongoing	[103]

Table 4. *Cont.*

Type of Treatment	Setting	Primary End-Point	Reference/Trial No.
Durvalumab + Ramucirumab (anti VEGFR2)	refractory GC/GEJ (*n* = 114)	phase Ia/Ib. Safety and efficacy	[104]
Durvalumab + Indoleamine 2,3-dioxygenase (IDO) Inhibitor	selected advanced solid tumors (*n* = 192)	phase I/II safety, tolerability, and efficacy. study ongoing	NCT02318277
Atezolizumab (IgG1κ anti PD-L1)	locally advanced or metastatic solid tumors including GC (*n* = 661)	phase I. Dose escalation Study of the safety and pharmacokinetics. Study is ongoing	NCT01375842
Atezolizumab + IDO inhibitor	locally advanced, recurrent, or metastatic incurable solid tumors including GC (*n* = 158)	phase I. Dose limiting toxicity, adverse events. study is ongoing	NCT02471846
Atezolizumab + FLOT (docetaxel, oxaliplatin, and fluorouracil /leucovorin) chemotherapy	locally advanced unresectable or metastatic GC/GEJ (*n* = 357)	phase Ib/II	NCT03281369
Atezolizumab + Ramucirumab + chemotherapy	GC/GEJ (*n* = 295)	phase II, Atezolizumab + FLOT vs. FLOT. study is ongoing	NCT03421288

3.4. Agonistic Antibodies for Costimulatory Receptors

The generation of therapeutically effective immune responses requires not only relieving the inhibition of negative regulatory pathways but also promoting T cell activation. T cell costimulation through receptors, like OX40, 4-1BB or ICOS, provides a potent activation signal that actively promotes the expansion and proliferation of killer CD8 and helper CD4 T cells [105–107]. Studies carried out in pre-clinical models have demonstrated that treatment with OX40 agonists, including both anti-OX40 mAb and OX40L-Fc fusion proteins, results in tumor regression [105]. These effects are mainly due to the ability of OX40 ligands to promote the survival and expansion of CD8 and conventional, non-regulatory CD4 T cells. On the other hand, it is still unclear whether OX40 activation promotes or inhibits Treg cell responses, as available data in this respect are not univocal [105]. A murine IgG monoclonal agonistic antibody against OX40 was investigated in a phase I clinical trial in 30 patients with metastatic solid malignancies. The treatment was overall tolerable, and six patients achieved stable disease, whereas no partial response was observed [108]. Several phase I clinical trials are currently ongoing with agonistic monoclonal antibodies targeting OX40 as a single therapy or in combination with checkpoint inhibitors [105].

4-1BB (CD137) is an inducible costimulatory receptor expressed by T cells, NK cells, and antigen presenting cells. Activation of 4-1BB by its ligand stimulates the proliferation and activation of T and NK cells [106] Considering that activation of NK cells results in enhanced antibody-dependent cell-mediated cytoxicity (ADCC), treatment with anti-41BB agonists not only increases immune-mediated antitumor activity but may also enhance the therapeutic efficacy of monoclonal antibodies, such as rituximab and trastuzumab, that function through ADCC mechanisms [109]. Gonistic 4-1BB antibodies have demonstrated potent anti-cancer efficacy in murine models and, on the basis of promising pre-clinical findings [110], several clinical trials have been initiated using the utomilumab and urelumab antibodies, mainly in patients with advanced solid tumors.

Inducible costimulator (ICOS) is a T cell costimulatory molecule belonging to the CD28/CTLA-4 family, which promotes the proliferation and cytokine production, mainly of CD4 T lymphocytes [111]. Up-regulation of ICOS is frequently found in activated T lymphocytes, particularly in patients treated with anti-CTLA4 antibodies, and its expression is regarded as a biomarker that is indicative of the binding of an anti-CTLA4 antibody to its cognate target [112]. Notably, the combination of ICOS agonist antibodies with CTLA4 blockade results in strong synergistic effects due to the marked up-regulation of ICOS expression of ICOS after anti-CTLA4 therapy [111]. JTX-2011, GSK3359609 and MEDI-570 are ICOS agonistic monoclonal antibodies that are currently being investigated in phase I/II clinical trials as monotherapies or in combination with checkpoint inhibitors, mainly in patients with advanced solid malignancies.

3.5. Safety Issues Related to the Use of Checkpoint Inhibitors

Overall, checkpoint inhibitors are generally better tolerated than chemotherapy regimens administered to patients with GC. Generally, the profiles of side effects that occur with different anti–PD-1/PD-L1 inhibitors are broadly similar [113]. About 10–20% of GC patients treated with anti-PD-1/PD-L1 monotherapy have adverse grade ≥ 3 events, including fatigue, anemia, and elevated alanine and aspartate aminotransferase levels. Checkpoint inhibitor therapy may also induce immune-related AEs (irAEs) that may affect rheumatic, gastrointestinal, skin, pulmonary, endocrine, neurological, hepatic, cardiac, and renal tissues [114]. In patients with GC, pneumonitis and colitis are the most common grade ≥ 3 irAEs. Usually, higher rates of treatment-related adverse events are observed in patients treated with anti–CTLA-4 antibodies and combination regimens as compared with anti-PD-1/PD-L1 monotherapies [114]. Although these adverse events are clinically manageable in most cases, long-term sequelae and deaths have been reported in a small proportion of patients [114], pointing to the need to adequately educate healthcare professionals and patients, perform close monitoring, and activate multidisciplinary collaborations to effectively manage these adverse events.

3.6. Cancer Vaccines

The therapeutic potential of cancer vaccines is due to their ability to activate and boost anti-tumor immune responses. Dendritic cells (DCs), the critical target of all cancer vaccines, are professional antigen presenting cells that play a pivotal role in orchestrating and coordinating anti-tumor immune responses, and are able to activate NK cells, B lymphocytes, and naïve and memory T cells by presenting tumor antigen/MHC complexes. In GC patients, higher numbers of DCs infiltrating the tumor have been associated with lower lymph node metastases and better patient survival [115]. Several strategies have been used to load DCs with tumor antigen as a vaccine, such as (i) synthetic peptide pulsed on DCs, (ii) DCs engineered with plasmid DNA, RNA, or viruses, (iii) tumor cell lysate (e.g. RNA, whole cell, phagosomes) mixed with immature DCs, (iv) DCs fused with whole tumor cells via PEG or electroporation. The most widely used vaccines are based on DCs pulsed with MHC-restricted peptides derived from known tumor-associated antigens, although the use of DCs in the clinical setting is limited by the short life span of these cells in vivo. The tumor-associated antigens targeted so far by vaccines for GC patients are melanoma-associated antigen (MAGE) A3 [116,117], HER2($_{p369}$) peptide [116], gastrin-17 diphtheria toxoid (G17DT) [118,119], URLC10 or VEGFR1 epitopes [120] and heat shock protein gp96 [121]; adjuvant BCG (Bacillus Calmette–Guérin) was also tested with chemotherapy [122] (Table 5). To personalize the choice of peptides to be used as vaccines in individual GC patients, pre-vaccination peripheral blood mononuclear cells of each patients were tested for their reactivity in vitro to the repertoire of each MHC peptide, and only the reactive peptides were administered in vivo [120]. Delayed-type hypersensitivity (DTH) to the vaccinated peptides was observed in some patients, whereas increased cellular and humoral immune responses to the vaccinated peptides were observed in others, with a concomitant prolonged survival [123]. Recently, encouraging clinical results were obtained using HLA-A24-restricted vascular endothelial growth factor receptor 1 (VEGFR1)-1084 and VEGFR2-169 peptides, combined with S-1 and cisplatin chemotherapy [120]. Most patients (82%) showed the induction of VEGFR1-specific cytotoxic T lymphocyte responses, twelve patients (55%) showed partial responses and 10 had stable disease after two cycles of the therapy. Notably, patients showing VEGFR-specific T-cell responses had a significant higher OS and time to progression (TTP), indicating that cancer vaccination combined with standard chemotherapy warrants further analysis as a promising strategy for the treatment of advanced GC [124]. To enhance GC vaccine efficacy, antigenic formulations targeting multiple antigens are being explored. In this direction, a cocktail vaccine including multiple peptides (DEPDC1, FOXM1, KIF20, URLC10, and VEGFR1) combined with S-1 chemotherapy was administered as a post-operative adjuvant therapy in a series of pathologically stage III advanced GC patients [125,126]. The treatment was well tolerated, and an optimal relative dose was achieved, paving the way for further studies aiming at assessing the efficacy of this therapeutic strategy an alternative approach to target multiple antigens is the fusion of DCs with whole tumor gastric cells to generate DC-tumor hybrids, e.g., by the electrofusion technique. These hybrid cells have the advantage of combining the potent antigen presenting capacity of DCs with the availability of the full repertoire of antigens expressed by tumor cells [127,128]. To circumvent the disadvantage of the limited availability of viable autologous tumor cells for the fusion, allogeneic GC cells may be used instead of autologous GC cells (cross-priming antigens) Therefore, it is not necessary to match the HLA haplotype between patients and allogeneic tumor cells used to generate the fusion. Although DC-tumor hybrids are safe and have induced efficient antitumor immune responses in early clinical trials, limited positive clinical responses have been reported in GC, with better results occurring with the use of costimulation with IL-12 [129] and the use of the of combination of TLR2 and TLR4 agonists [130].

Table 5. Vaccines.

Type of Vaccine	Setting	Primary End-Point	Reference
DC pulsed with melanoma-associated antigen (MAGE) A3 peptides	MAGE-3-expressing advanced GC (*n* = 12)	phase I, safe and exhibits antitumor effects in some patients	[117]
HER2$_{(p369)}$ peptide	advanced or recurrent GC HER2+ (*n* = 9)	phase I, tumor specific T-cell response	[116]
BCG (Bacillus Calmette–Guérin) + chemotherapy	radically resected stage III/IV GC	prolonged 10-year OS (47.1%) as compared to mono-chemotherapy (30%) or surgery alone (15.2%)	[122]
gastrin-17 diphtheria toxoid (G17DT) + chemotherapy	metastatic GC/GEJ (*n* = 94)	phase II, longer TTP and OS in responders	[118]
URLC10 or VEGFR1 Epitopes	chemotherapy-resistant advanced GC (*n* = 14)	phase I, tumor specific T cell responses	[120,124]
heat shock protein GP96 + oxaliplatinum	GC (*n* = 45)	phase II, 81.9% 2-year OS	[121]
OTSGC-A24 (5 HLA-A24-restricted peptides DEPDC1, FOXM1, KIF20, URLC10, and VEGFR1)	inoperable/unresectable, metastatic GC, 2 line therapy or greater (*n* = 23)	favourable results for safety and immune reactivity	[126]

4. Concluding Remarks and Future Perspectives

Over the last decade, our understanding of the mechanisms underlying immune modulation has greatly improved, allowing for the development of multiple therapeutic approaches that are revolutionizing the treatment of cancer. Immunotherapy for GC is still in the early phase but is rapidly evolving. The challenges moving forward are to put much effort into biologic and immunologic exploration in GC setting to fine-tune and tailor, more precisely, the various available or emerging immunotherapeutic approaches. In the near future, it will be necessary to design large prospective trials to validate reliable predictive factors, allowing for the selection of GC patients with the highest chance of benefitting from immunotherapy.

Author Contributions: R.D., V.C. and V.D.R. contributed to the writing and editing of this review.

Acknowledgments: This work was supported by 5x1000_2010_MdS. The funder had no role in study design, data collection and analysis, decision to publish, or preparation of the manuscript.

Conflicts of Interest: The authors declare no conflict of interest.

References

1. Bilici, A. Treatment options in patients with metastatic gastric cancer: Current status and future perspectives. *World J. Gastroenterol.* **2014**, *20*, 3905–3915. [CrossRef] [PubMed]
2. Brierley, J.D.; Gospodarowicz, M.K.; Wittekind, C. *TNM Classification of Malignant Tumors*, 8th ed.; John Wiley & Sons, Inc.: Chichester, UK; Hoboken, NJ, USA, 2017.
3. Larkin, J.; Chiarion-Sileni, V.; Gonzalez, R.; Grob, J.J.; Cowey, C.L.; Lao, C.D.; Schadendorf, D.; Dummer, R.; Smylie, M.; Rutkowski, P.; et al. Combined nivolumab and ipilimumab or monotherapy in untreated melanoma. *N. Engl. J. Med.* **2015**, *373*, 23–34. [CrossRef] [PubMed]
4. Motzer, R.J.; Escudier, B.; McDermott, D.F.; George, S.; Hammers, H.J.; Srinivas, S.; Tykodi, S.S.; Sosman, J.A.; Procopio, G.; Plimack, E.R.; et al. Nivolumab versus everolimus in advanced renal-cell carcinoma. *N. Engl. J. Med.* **2015**, *373*, 1803–1813. [CrossRef] [PubMed]
5. Reck, M.; Rodriguez-Abreu, D.; Robinson, A.G.; Hui, R.; Csoszi, T.; Fulop, A.; Gottfried, M.; Peled, N.; Tafreshi, A.; Cuffe, S.; et al. Pembrolizumab versus chemotherapy for PD-L1-positive non-small-cell lung cancer. *N. Engl. J. Med.* **2016**, *375*, 1823–1833. [CrossRef] [PubMed]
6. Bonotto, M.; Garattini, S.K.; Basile, D.; Ongaro, E.; Fanotto, V.; Cattaneo, M.; Cortiula, F.; Iacono, D.; Cardellino, G.G.; Pella, N.; et al. Immunotherapy for gastric cancers: Emerging role and future perspectives. *Expert Rev. Clin. Pharmacol.* **2017**, *10*, 609–619. [CrossRef] [PubMed]

7. Procaccio, L.; Schirripa, M.; Fassan, M.; Vecchione, L.; Bergamo, F.; Prete, A.A.; Intini, R.; Manai, C.; Dadduzio, V.; Boscolo, A.; et al. Immunotherapy in gastrointestinal cancers. *Biomed. Res. Int.* **2017**, *3*, 4346576. [CrossRef] [PubMed]

8. Fuchs, C.S.; Doi, T.; Jang, R.W.; Muro, K.; Satoh, T.; Machado, M.; Sun, W.; Jalal, S.I.; Shah, M.A.; Metges, J.P.; et al. Safety and efficacy of pembrolizumab monotherapy in patients with previously treated advanced gastric and gastroesophageal junction cancer: Phase 2 Clinical KEYNOTE-059 Trial. *JAMA Oncol.* **2018**, *4*, e180013. [CrossRef] [PubMed]

9. National Institutes of Health. Study of Pembrolizumab (MK-3475) as First-Line Monotherapy and Combination Therapy for Treatment of Advanced Gastric or Gastroesophageal Junction Adenocarcinoma (MK-3475-062/KEYNOTE-062). Available online: https://clinicaltrials.gov/ct2/show/NCT02494583 (accessed on 10 July 2015).

10. Cancer Genome Atlas Research Network. Comprehensive molecular characterization of gastric adenocarcinoma. *Nature* **2014**, *513*, 202–209. [CrossRef]

11. Derks, S.; Liao, X.; Chiaravalli, A.M.; Xu, X.; Camargo, M.C.; Solcia, E.; Sessa, F.; Fleitas, T.; Freeman, G.J.; Rodig, S.J.; et al. Abundant PD-L1 expression in Epstein–Barr Virus-infected gastric cancers. *Oncotarget* **2016**, *7*, 32925–32932. [CrossRef] [PubMed]

12. Finn, O.J. A believer's overview of cancer immunosurveillance and immunotherapy. *J. Immunol.* **2018**, *200*, 385–391. [CrossRef] [PubMed]

13. Davoodzadeh, G.M.; Kardar, G.A.; Saeedi, Y.; Heydari, S.; Garssen, J.; Falak, R. Exhaustion of T lymphocytes in the tumor microenvironment: Significance and effective mechanisms. *Cell. Immunol.* **2017**, *322*, 1–14. [CrossRef] [PubMed]

14. Wherry, E.J. T cell exhaustion. *Nat. Immunol.* **2011**, *12*, 492–499. [CrossRef] [PubMed]

15. Murray, P.J.; Allen, J.E.; Biswas, S.K.; Fisher, E.A.; Gilroy, D.W.; Goerdt, S.; Gordon, S.; Hamilton, J.A.; Ivashkiv, L.B.; Lawrence, T.; et al. Macrophage activation and polarization: Nomenclature and experimental guidelines. *Immunity* **2014**, *41*, 14–20. [CrossRef] [PubMed]

16. Ishigami, S.; Natsugoe, S.; Tokuda, K.; Nakajo, A.; Okumura, H.; Matsumoto, M.; Miyazono, F.; Hokita, S.; Aikou, T. Tumor-associated macrophage (TAM) infiltration in gastric cancer. *Anticancer Res.* **2003**, *23*, 4079–4083. [PubMed]

17. Mitchem, J.B.; Brennan, D.J.; Knolhoff, B.L.; Belt, B.A.; Zhu, Y.; Sanford, D.E.; Belaygorod, L.; Carpenter, D.; Collins, L.; Piwnica-Worms, D.; et al. Targeting tumor-infiltrating macrophages decreases tumor-initiating cells, relieves immunosuppression, and improves chemotherapeutic responses. *Cancer Res.* **2013**, *73*, 1128–1141. [CrossRef] [PubMed]

18. Park, J.Y.; Sung, J.Y.; Lee, J.; Park, Y.K.; Kim, Y.W.; Kim, G.Y.; Won, K.Y.; Lim, S.J. Polarized CD163+ tumor-associated macrophages are associated with increased angiogenesis and CXCL12 expression in gastric cancer. *Clin. Res. Hepatol. Gastroenterol.* **2016**, *40*, 357–365. [CrossRef] [PubMed]

19. Wu, M.H.; Lee, W.J.; Hua, K.T.; Kuo, M.L.; Lin, M.T. Macrophage infiltration induces gastric cancer invasiveness by activating the β-catenin pathway. *PLoS ONE* **2015**, *10*, e0134122. [CrossRef] [PubMed]

20. Bronte, V.; Brandau, S.; Chen, S.H.; Colombo, M.P.; Frey, A.B.; Greten, T.F.; Mandruzzato, S.; Murray, P.J.; Ochoa, A.; Ostrand-Rosenberg, S.; et al. Recommendations for myeloid-derived suppressor cell nomenclature and characterization standards. *Nat. Commun.* **2016**, *7*, 12150. [CrossRef] [PubMed]

21. Ben-Meir, K.; Twaik, N.; Baniyash, M. Plasticity and biological diversity of myeloid derived suppressor cells. *Curr. Opin. Immunol.* **2018**, *51*, 154–161. [CrossRef] [PubMed]

22. Choi, B.D.; Gedeon, P.C.; Herndon, J.E.; Archer, G.E.; Reap, E.A.; Sanchez-Perez, L.; Mitchell, D.A.; Bigner, D.D.; Sampson, J.H. Human regulatory T cells kill tumor cells through granzyme-dependent cytotoxicity upon retargeting with a bispecific antibody. *Cancer Immunol. Res.* **2013**, *1*, 163–167. [CrossRef] [PubMed]

23. Kandulski, A.; Malfertheiner, P.; Wex, T. Role of regulatory T-cells in *H. pylori*-induced gastritis and gastric cancer. *Anticancer Res.* **2010**, *30*, 1093–1103. [PubMed]

24. Kang, B.W.; Seo, A.N.; Yoon, S.; Bae, H.I.; Jeon, S.W.; Kwon, O.K.; Chung, H.Y.; Yu, W.; Kang, H.; Kim, J.G. Prognostic value of tumor-infiltrating lymphocytes in Epstein–Barr virus-associated gastric cancer. *Ann. Oncol.* **2016**, *27*, 494–501. [CrossRef] [PubMed]

25. Nagase, H.; Takeoka, T.; Urakawa, S.; Morimoto-Okazawa, A.; Kawashima, A.; Iwahori, K.; Takiguchi, S.; Nishikawa, H.; Sato, E.; Sakaguchi, S.; et al. ICOS⁺ Foxp3⁺ TILs in gastric cancer are prognostic markers and effector regulatory T cells associated with *Helicobacter pylori*. *Int. J. Cancer* **2017**, *140*, 686–695. [CrossRef] [PubMed]

26. Sackstein, R.; Schatton, T.; Barthel, S.R. T-lymphocyte homing: An underappreciated yet critical hurdle for successful cancer immunotherapy. *Lab. Investig.* **2017**, *97*, 669–697. [CrossRef] [PubMed]

27. Badalamenti, G.; Fanale, D.; Incorvaia, L.; Barraco, N.; Listì, A.; Maragliano, R.; Vincenzi, B.; Calò, V.; Iovanna, J.L.; Bazan, V.; et al. Role of tumor-infiltrating lymphocytes in patients with solid tumors: Can a drop dig a stone? *Cell. Immunol.* **2018**. [CrossRef] [PubMed]

28. Kim, K.J.; Lee, K.S.; Cho, H.J.; Kim, Y.H.; Yang, H.K.; Kim, W.H.; Kang, G.H. Prognostic implications of tumor-infiltrating FoxP3+ regulatory T cells and CD8+ cytotoxic T cells in microsatellite-unstable gastric cancers. *Hum. Pathol.* **2014**, *45*, 285–293. [CrossRef] [PubMed]

29. Klingemann, H.; Boissel, L.; Toneguzzo, F. Natural killer cells for immunotherapy—Advantages of the NK-92 cell line over blood NK cells. *Front. Immunol.* **2016**, *7*, 91. [CrossRef] [PubMed]

30. Sarvaria, A.; Madrigal, J.A.; Saudemont, A. B cell regulation in cancer and anti-tumor immunity. *Cell. Mol. Immunol.* **2017**, *14*, 662–674. [CrossRef] [PubMed]

31. Li, Q.; Teitz-Tennenbaum, S.; Donald, E.J.; Li, M.; Chang, A.E. In vivo sensitized and in vitro activated B cells mediate tumor regression in cancer adoptive immunotherapy. *J. Immunol.* **2009**, *183*, 3195–3203. [CrossRef] [PubMed]

32. Li, Q.; Lao, X.; Pan, Q.; Ning, N.; Yet, J.; Xu, Y.; Li, S.; Chang, A.E. Adoptive transfer of tumor reactive B cells confers host T-cell immunity and tumor regression. *Clin. Cancer Res.* **2011**, *17*, 4987–4995. [CrossRef] [PubMed]

33. Perricone, M.A.; Smith, K.A.; Claussen, K.A.; Plog, M.S.; Hempel, D.M.; Roberts, B.L.; St George, J.A.; Kaplan, J.M. Enhanced efficacy of melanoma vaccines in the absence of B lymphocytes. *J. Immunother.* **2004**, *27*, 273–281. [CrossRef] [PubMed]

34. Shah, S.; Divekar, A.A.; Hilchey, S.P.; Cho, H.M.; Newman, C.L.; Shin, S.U.; Nechustan, H.; Challita-Eid, P.M.; Segal, B.M.; Yi, K.H.; et al. Increased rejection of primary tumors in mice lacking B cells: Inhibition of anti-tumor CTL and TH1 cytokine responses by B cells. *Int. J. Cancer* **2005**, *117*, 574–586. [CrossRef] [PubMed]

35. Kang, B.W.; Kim, J.G.; Lee, I.H.; Bae, H.I.; Seo, A.N. Clinical significance of tumor-infiltrating lymphocytes for gastric cancer in the era of immunology. *World J. Gastrointest. Oncol.* **2017**, *9*, 293–299. [CrossRef] [PubMed]

36. Ishigami, S.; Natsugoe, S.; Tokuda, K.; Nakajo, A.; Xiangming, C.; Iwashige, H.; Aridome, K.; Hokita, S.; Aikou, T. Clinical impact of intratumoral natural killer cell and dendritic cell infiltration in gastric cancer. *Cancer Lett.* **2000**, *159*, 103–108. [CrossRef]

37. Malmberg, K.J.; Carlsten, M.; Bjorklund, A.; Sohlberg, E.; Bryceson, Y.T.; Ljunggren, H.G. Natural killer cell-mediated immunosurveillance of human cancer. *Semin. Immunol.* **2017**, *31*, 20–29. [CrossRef] [PubMed]

38. Rosso, D.; Rigueiro, M.P.; Kassab, P.; Ilias, E.J.; Castro, O.A.; Novo, N.F.; Lourenco, L.G. Correlation of natural killer cells with the prognosis of gastric adenocarcinoma. *Arq. Bras. Cir. Dig.* **2012**, *25*, 114–117. [CrossRef] [PubMed]

39. Saito, H.; Takaya, S.; Osaki, T.; Ikeguchi, M. Increased apoptosis and elevated FAS expression in circulating natural killer cells in gastric cancer patients. *Gastric. Cancer* **2013**, *16*, 473–479. [CrossRef] [PubMed]

40. Yang, J.C.; Rosenberg, S.A. Adoptive T-Cell Therapy for Cancer. *Adv. Immunol.* **2016**, *130*, 279–294. [CrossRef] [PubMed]

41. Kono, K.; Ichihara, F.; Iizuka, H.; Sekikawa, T.; Matsumoto, Y. Differences in the recognition of tumor-specific CD8+ T cells derived from solid tumor, metastatic lymph nodes and ascites in patients with gastric cancer. *Int. J. Cancer* **1997**, *71*, 978–981. [CrossRef]

42. Fujie, T.; Tanaka, F.; Tahara, K.; Li, J.; Tanaka, S.; Mori, M.; Ueo, H.; Takesako, K.; Akiyoshi, T. Generation of specific antitumor reactivity by the stimulation of spleen cells from gastric cancer patients with MAGE-3 synthetic peptide. *Cancer Immunol. Immunother.* **1999**, *48*, 189–194. [CrossRef] [PubMed]

43. Voskens, C.J.; Watanabe, R.; Rollins, S.; Campana, D.; Hasumi, K.; Mann, D.L. Ex-vivo expanded human NK cells express activating receptors that mediate cytotoxicity of allogeneic and autologous cancer cell lines by direct recognition and antibody directed cellular cytotoxicity. *J. Exp. Clin. Cancer Res.* **2010**, *29*, 134. [CrossRef] [PubMed]
44. Ishikawa, T.; Okayama, T.; Sakamoto, N.; Ideno, M.; Oka, K.; Enoki, T.; Mineno, J.; Yoshida, N.; Katada, K.; Kamada, K.; et al. Phase I clinical trial of adoptive transfer of expanded natural killer cells in combination with IgG1 antibody in patients with gastric or colorectal cancer. *Int. J. Cancer* **2018**, *142*, 2599–2609. [CrossRef] [PubMed]
45. Sakamoto, N.; Ishikawa, T.; Kokura, S.; Okayama, T.; Oka, K.; Ideno, M.; Sakai, F.; Kato, A.; Tanabe, M.; Enoki, T.; et al. Phase I clinical trial of autologous NK cell therapy using novel expansion method in patients with advanced digestive cancer. *J. Transl. Med.* **2015**, *13*, 277. [CrossRef] [PubMed]
46. Kloss, S.; Oberschmidt, O.; Morgan, M.; Dahlke, J.; Arseniev, L.; Huppert, V.; Granzin, M.; Gardlowski, T.; Matthies, N.; Soltenborn, S.; et al. Optimization of human NK cell manufacturing: Fully automated separation, improved ex vivo expansion using IL-21 with autologous feeder cells, and generation of anti-CD123-CAR-expressing effector cells. *Hum. Gene Ther.* **2017**, *28*, 897–913. [CrossRef] [PubMed]
47. Uherek, C.; Tonn, T.; Uherek, B.; Becker, S.; Schnierle, B.; Klingemann, H.G.; Wels, W. Retargeting of natural killer-cell cytolytic activity to ErbB2-expressing cancer cells results in efficient and selective tumor cell destruction. *Blood* **2002**, *100*, 1265–1273. [PubMed]
48. Schonfeld, K.; Sahm, C.; Zhang, C.; Naundorf, S.; Brendel, C.; Odendahl, M.; Nowakowska, P.; Bonig, H.; Kohl, U.; Kloess, S.; et al. Selective inhibition of tumor growth by clonal NK cells expressing an ErbB2/HER2-specific chimeric antigen receptor. *Mol. Ther.* **2015**, *23*, 330–338. [CrossRef] [PubMed]
49. Zhang, C.; Burger, M.C.; Jennewein, L.; Genssler, S.; Schonfeld, K.; Zeiner, P.; Hattingen, E.; Harter, P.N.; Mittelbronn, M.; Tonn, T.; et al. ErbB2/HER2-specific NK cells for targeted therapy of glioblastoma. *J. Natl. Cancer Inst.* **2015**, *108*, 375. [CrossRef] [PubMed]
50. Guo, Y.; Han, W. Cytokine-induced killer (CIK) cells: From basic research to clinical translation. *Chin. J. Cancer* **2015**, *34*, 99–107. [CrossRef] [PubMed]
51. Pfirschke, C.; Engblom, C.; Rickelt, S.; Cortez-Retamozo, V.; Garris, C.; Pucci, F.; Yamazaki, T.; Poirier-Colame, V.; Newton, A.; Redouane, Y.; et al. Immunogenic chemotherapy sensitizes tumors to checkpoint blockade therapy. *Immunity* **2016**, *44*, 343–354. [CrossRef] [PubMed]
52. Liu, K.; Song, G.; Hu, X.; Zhou, Y.; Li, Y.; Chen, Q.; Feng, G. A positive role of cytokine-induced killer cell therapy on gastric cancer therapy in a Chinese population: A systematic meta-analysis. *Med. Sci. Monit.* **2015**, *21*, 3363–3370. [CrossRef] [PubMed]
53. Mu, Y.; Zhou, C.H.; Chen, S.F.; Ding, J.; Zhang, Y.X.; Yang, Y.P.; Wang, W.H. Effectiveness and safety of chemotherapy combined with cytokine-induced killer cell/dendritic cell-cytokine-induced killer cell therapy for treatment of gastric cancer in China: A systematic review and meta-analysis. *Cytotherapy* **2016**, *18*, 1162–1177. [CrossRef] [PubMed]
54. Introna, M.; Correnti, F. Innovative clinical perspectives for CIK cells in cancer patients. *Int. J. Mol. Sci.* **2018**, *19*, 358. [CrossRef] [PubMed]
55. Zhang, L.; Zhao, G.; Hou, Y.; Zhang, J.; Hu, J.; Zhang, K. The experimental study on the treatment of cytokine-induced killer cells combined with EGFR monoclonal antibody against gastric cancer. *Cancer Biother. Radiopharm.* **2014**, *29*, 99–107. [CrossRef] [PubMed]
56. Del Zotto, G.; Marcenaro, E.; Vacca, P.; Sivori, S.; Pende, D.; Della, C.M.; Moretta, F.; Ingegnere, T.; Mingari, M.C.; Moretta, A.; et al. Markers and function of human NK cells in normal and pathological conditions. *Cytometry B Clin. Cytom.* **2017**, *92*, 100–114. [CrossRef] [PubMed]
57. Xu, X.; Xu, L.; Ding, S.; Wu, M.; Tang, Z.; Fu, W.; Ni, Q. Treatment of 23 patients with advanced gastric cancer by intravenously transfer of autologous tumor-infiltrating lymphocytes combined with rIL-2. *Chin. Med. Sci. J.* **1995**, *10*, 185–187. [PubMed]
58. Zhang, G.Q.; Zhao, H.; Wu, J.Y.; Li, J.Y.; Yan, X.; Wang, G.; Wu, L.L.; Zhang, X.G.; Shao, Y.; Wang, Y.; et al. Prolonged overall survival in gastric cancer patients after adoptive immunotherapy. *World J. Gastroenterol.* **2015**, *21*, 2777–2785. [CrossRef] [PubMed]
59. Shi, L.; Zhou, Q.; Wu, J.; Ji, M.; Li, G.; Jiang, J.; Wu, C. Efficacy of adjuvant immunotherapy with cytokine-induced killer cells in patients with locally advanced gastric cancer. *Cancer Immunol. Immunother.* **2012**, *61*, 2251–2259. [CrossRef] [PubMed]

60. Jiang, J.T.; Shen, Y.P.; Wu, C.P.; Zhu, Y.B.; Wei, W.X.; Chen, L.J.; Zheng, X.; Sun, J.; Lu, B.F.; Zhang, X.G. Increasing the frequency of CIK cells adoptive immunotherapy may decrease risk of death in gastric cancer patients. *World J. Gastroenterol.* **2010**, *16*, 6155–6162. [CrossRef] [PubMed]

61. Chen, Y.; Guo, Z.Q.; Shi, C.M.; Zhou, Z.F.; Ye, Y.B.; Chen, Q. Efficacy of adjuvant chemotherapy combined with immunotherapy with cytokine-induced killer cells for gastric cancer after d2 gastrectomy. *Int. J. Clin. Exp. Med.* **2015**, *8*, 7728–7736. [PubMed]

62. Zhao, H.; Fan, Y.; Li, H.; Yu, J.; Liu, L.; Cao, S.; Ren, B.; Yan, F.; Ren, X. Immunotherapy with cytokine-induced killer cells as an adjuvant treatment for advanced gastric carcinoma: A retrospective study of 165 patients. *Cancer Biother. Radiopharm.* **2013**, *28*, 303–309. [CrossRef] [PubMed]

63. Liu, H.; Song, J.; Yang, Z.; Zhang, X. Effects of cytokine-induced killer cell treatment combined with FolFox4 on the recurrence and survival rates for gastric cancer following surgery. *Exp. Ther. Med.* **2013**, *6*, 953–956. [CrossRef] [PubMed]

64. Mirzaei, H.R.; Rodriguez, A.; Shepphird, J.; Brown, C.E.; Badie, B. Chimeric antigen receptors T cell therapy in solid tumor: Challenges and clinical APPLICATIONS. *Front. Immunol.* **2017**, *8*, 1850. [CrossRef] [PubMed]

65. Fesnak, A.D.; June, C.H.; Levine, B.L. Engineered T cells: The promise and challenges of cancer immunotherapy. *Nat. Rev. Cancer* **2016**, *16*, 566–581. [CrossRef] [PubMed]

66. Feng, K.; Liu, Y.; Guo, Y.; Qiu, J.; Wu, Z.; Dai, H.; Yang, Q.; Wang, Y.; Han, W. Phase I study of chimeric antigen receptor modified T cells in treating HER2-positive advanced biliary tract cancers and pancreatic cancers. *Protein Cell* **2017**, 1–10. [CrossRef] [PubMed]

67. Han, Y.; Liu, C.; Li, G.; Li, J.; Lv, X.; Shi, H.; Liu, J.; Liu, S.; Yan, P.; Wang, S.; et al. Antitumor effects and persistence of a novel HER2 CAR T cells directed to gastric cancer in preclinical models. *Am. J. Cancer Res.* **2018**, *8*, 106–119. [PubMed]

68. Luo, F.; Qian, J.; Yang, J.; Deng, Y.; Zheng, X.; Liu, J.; Chu, Y. Bifunctional αHER2/CD3 RNA-engineered CART-like human T cells specifically eliminate HER2+ gastric cancer. *Cell Res.* **2016**, *26*, 850–853. [CrossRef] [PubMed]

69. Song, Y.; Tong, C.; Wang, Y.; Gao, Y.; Dai, H.; Guo, Y.; Zhao, X.; Wang, Y.; Wang, Z.; Han, W.; et al. Effective and persistent antitumor activity of HER2-directed CAR-T cells against gastric cancer cells in vitro and xenotransplanted tumors in vivo. *Protein Cell* **2017**, 1–12. [CrossRef] [PubMed]

70. Shibaguchi, H.; Luo, N.; Shirasu, N.; Kuroki, M.; Kuroki, M. Enhancement of antitumor activity by using a fully human gene encoding a single-chain fragmented antibody specific for carcinoembryonic antigen. *Onco Targets Ther.* **2017**, *10*, 3979–3990. [CrossRef] [PubMed]

71. Neelapu, S.S.; Tummala, S.; Kebriaei, P.; Wierda, W.; Gutierrez, C.; Locke, F.L.; Komanduri, K.V.; Lin, Y.; Jain, N.; Daver, N.; et al. Chimeric antigen receptor T-cell therapy—Assessment and management of toxicities. *Nat. Rev. Clin. Oncol.* **2018**, *15*, 47–62. [CrossRef] [PubMed]

72. Morgan, R.A.; Yang, J.C.; Kitano, M.; Dudley, M.E.; Laurencot, C.M.; Rosenberg, S.A. Case report of a serious adverse event following the administration of T cells transduced with a chimeric antigen receptor recognizing ERBB2. *Mol. Ther.* **2010**, *18*, 843–851. [CrossRef] [PubMed]

73. Sharma, P.; Allison, J.P. Immune checkpoint targeting in cancer therapy: Toward combination strategies with curative potential. *Cell* **2015**, *161*, 205–214. [CrossRef] [PubMed]

74. Tran, P.N.; Sarkissian, S.; Chao, J.; Klempner, S.J. PD-1 and PD-L1 as emerging therapeutic targets in gastric cancer: Current evidence. *Gastrointest. Cancer* **2017**, *7*, 1–11. [CrossRef] [PubMed]

75. Boger, C.; Behrens, H.M.; Mathiak, M.; Kruger, S.; Kalthoff, H.; Rocken, C. PD-L1 is an independent prognostic predictor in gastric cancer of Western patients. *Oncotarget* **2016**, *7*, 24269–24283. [CrossRef] [PubMed]

76. Kim, J.W.; Nam, K.H.; Ahn, S.H.; Park, D.J.; Kim, H.H.; Kim, S.H.; Chang, H.; Lee, J.O.; Kim, Y.J.; Lee, H.S.; et al. Prognostic implications of immunosuppressive protein expression in tumors as well as immune cell infiltration within the tumor microenvironment in gastric cancer. *Gastric Cancer* **2016**, *19*, 42–52. [CrossRef] [PubMed]

77. Schlosser, H.A.; Drebber, U.; Kloth, M.; Thelen, M.; Rothschild, S.I.; Haase, S.; Garcia-Marquez, M.; Wennhold, K.; Berlth, F.; Urbanski, A.; et al. Immune checkpoints programmed death 1 ligand 1 and cytotoxic T lymphocyte associated molecule 4 in gastric adenocarcinoma. *Oncoimmunology* **2015**, *5*, e1100789. [CrossRef] [PubMed]

78. Gu, L.; Chen, M.; Guo, D.; Zhu, H.; Zhang, W.; Pan, J.; Zhong, X.; Li, X.; Qian, H.; Wang, X. PD-L1 and gastric cancer prognosis: A systematic review and meta-analysis. *PLoS ONE* **2017**, *12*, e0182692. [CrossRef] [PubMed]

79. Saito, R.; Abe, H.; Kunita, A.; Yamashita, H.; Seto, Y.; Fukayama, M. Overexpression and gene amplification of PD-L1 in cancer cells and PD-L1+ immune cells in Epstein–Barr virus-associated gastric cancer: The prognostic implications. *Mod. Pathol.* **2017**, *30*, 427–439. [CrossRef] [PubMed]

80. Liu, Y.; Cheng, Y.; Xu, Y.; Wang, Z.; Du, X.; Li, C.; Peng, J.; Gao, L.; Liang, X.; Ma, C. Increased expression of programmed cell death protein 1 on NK cells inhibits NK-cell-mediated anti-tumor function and indicates poor prognosis in digestive cancers. *Oncogene* **2017**, *36*, 6143–6153. [CrossRef] [PubMed]

81. Nowak, E.C.; Lines, J.L.; Varn, F.S.; Deng, J.; Sarde, A.; Mabaera, R.; Kuta, A.; Le, M.I.; Cheng, C.; Noelle, R.J. Immunoregulatory functions of VISTA. *Immunol. Rev.* **2017**, *276*, 66–79. [CrossRef] [PubMed]

82. Boger, C.; Behrens, H.M.; Kruger, S.; Rocken, C. The novel negative checkpoint regulator VISTA is expressed in gastric carcinoma and associated with PD-L1/PD-1: A future perspective for a combined gastric cancer therapy? *Oncoimmunology* **2017**, *6*, e1293215. [CrossRef] [PubMed]

83. Du, W.; Yang, M.; Turner, A.; Xu, C.; Ferris, R.L.; Huang, J.; Kane, L.P.; Lu, B. TIM-3 as a target for cancer immunotherapy and mechanisms of action. *Int. J. Mol. Sci.* **2017**, *18*, 645. [CrossRef] [PubMed]

84. Takano, S.; Saito, H.; Ikeguchi, M an increased number of PD-1+ and Tim-3+ CD8+ T cells is involved in immune evasion in gastric cancer. *Surg. Today* **2016**, *46*, 1341–1347. [CrossRef] [PubMed]

85. Lu, X.; Yang, L.; Yao, D.; Wu, X.; Li, J.; Liu, X.; Deng, L.; Huang, C.; Wang, Y.; Li, D.; et al. Tumor antigen-specific CD8+ T cells are negatively regulated by PD-1 and Tim-3 in human gastric cancer. *Cell. Immunol.* **2017**, *313*, 43–51. [CrossRef] [PubMed]

86. Ralph, C.; Elkord, E.; Burt, D.J.; O'Dwyer, J.F.; Austin, E.B.; Stern, P.L.; Hawkins, R.E.; T histlethwaite, F.C. Modulation of lymphocyte regulation for cancer therapy: A phase II trial of tremelimumab in advanced gastric and esophageal adenocarcinoma. *Clin. Cancer Res.* **2010**, *16*, 1662–1672. [CrossRef] [PubMed]

87. Vanneman, M.; Dranoff, G. Combining immunotherapy and targeted therapies in cancer treatment. *Nat. Rev. Cancer* **2012**, *12*, 237–251. [CrossRef] [PubMed]

88. Catenacci, D.V.; Kim, S.S.; Gold, P.J.; Philip, P.A.; Enzinger, P.C.; Coffie, J.; Schmidt, E.V.; Baldwin, M.; Nordstrom, J.L.; Bonvini, E.; et al. A phase 1b/2, open label, dose-escalation study of margetuximab (M) in combination with pembrolizumab (P) in patients with relapsed/refractory advanced HER2+ gastroesophageal (GEJ) junction or gastric (G) cancer. *J. Clin. Oncol.* **2018**, *35*, TPS219. [CrossRef]

89. Chen, D.S.; Mellman, I. Oncology meets immunology: The cancer-immunity cycle. *Immunity* **2013**, *39*, 1–10. [CrossRef] [PubMed]

90. Ngwa, W.; Irabor, O.C.; Schoenfeld, J.D.; Hesser, J.; Demaria, S.; Formenti, S.C. Using immunotherapy to boost the abscopal effect. *Nat. Rev. Cancer* **2018**. [CrossRef] [PubMed]

91. Chao, J.; Chen, Y.; Frankel, P.H.; Chung, V.M.; Lim, D.; Li, D.; Fakih, M.; Lee, P.P. Combining pembrolizumab and palliative radiotherapy in gastroesophageal cancer to enhance antitumor T-cell response and augment the abscopal effect. *J. Clin. Oncol.* **2018**, *35*, TPS220. [CrossRef]

92. Bang, Y.J.; Cho, J.Y.; Kim, Y.H.; Kim, J.W.; Di, B.M.; Ajani, J.A.; Yamaguchi, K.; Balogh, A.; Sanchez, T.; Moehler, M. Efficacy of sequential ipilimumab monotherapy versus best supportive care for unresectable locally advanced/metastatic gastric or gastroesophageal junction cancer. *Clin. Cancer Res.* **2017**, *23*, 5671–5678. [CrossRef] [PubMed]

93. Muro, K.; Chung, H.C.; Shankaran, V.; Geva, R.; Catenacci, D.; Gupta, S.; Eder, J.P.; Golan, T.; Le, D.T.; Burtness, B.; et al. Pembrolizumab for patients with PD-L1-positive advanced gastric cancer (KEYNOTE-012): A multicentre, open-label, phase 1b trial. *Lancet Oncol.* **2016**, *17*, 717–726. [CrossRef]

94. Doi, T.; Piha-Paul, S.A.; Jalal, S.I.; Saraf, S.; Lunceford, J.; Koshiji, M.; Bennouna, J. Safety and antitumor activity of the anti-programmed death-1 antibody pembrolizumab in patients with advanced esophageal carcinoma. *J. Clin. Oncol.* **2018**, *36*, 61–67. [CrossRef] [PubMed]

95. Wainberg, Z.A.; Jalal, S.; Muro, K.; Yoon, H.H.; Garrido, M.; Golan, T.; Doi, T.; Catenacci, D.V.; Geva, R.; Ku, G.; et al. Oesophageal cancer gastric cancer cancer immunology and immunotherapy. In Proceedings of the ESMO 2017 Congress, Annals of Oncology, Madrid, Spain, 8–12 September 2018; Volume 28, pp. v605–v649.

96. Ohtsu, A.; Tabernero, J.; Bang, Y.; Fuchs, C.S.; Sun, L.; Wang, Z.; Csiki, I.; Koshiji, M.; Cutsem, E.V. Pembrolizumab (MK-3475) versus paclitaxel as second-line therapy for advanced gastric or gastroesophageal junction (GEJ) adenocarcinoma: Phase 3 KEYNOTE-061 study. *J. Clin. Oncol.* **2018**, *34*, TPS183. [CrossRef]

97. Chau, I.; Bendell, J.C.; Calvo, E.; Santana-Davila, R.; Ahnert, J.R.; Penel, N.; Arkenau, H.; Yang, Y.; Rege, J.; Mi, G.; et al. Interim safety and clinical activity in patients (pts) with advanced gastric or gastroesophageal junction (G/GEJ) adenocarcinoma from a multicohort phase 1 study of ramucirumab (R) plus pembrolizumab (P). *J. Clin. Oncol.* **2018**, *35*, 102. [CrossRef]

98. Janjigian, Y.Y.; Ott, P.A.; Calvo, E.; Kim, J.W.; Ascierto, P.A.; Sharma, P.; Peltola, K.J.; Jaeger, D.; Jeffry Evans, T.R.; De Braud, F.G.; et al. Nivolumab ± ipilimumab in pts with advanced (adv)/metastatic chemotherapy-refractory (CTx-R) gastric (G), esophageal (E), or gastroesophageal junction (GEJ) cancer: CheckMate 032 study. *J. Clin. Oncol.* **2018**, *35*, 4014.

99. Kang, Y.K.; Boku, N.; Satoh, T.; Ryu, M.H.; Chao, Y.; Kato, K.; Chung, H.C.; Chen, J.S.; Muro, K.; Kang, W.K.; et al. Nivolumab in patients with advanced gastric or gastro-oesophageal junction cancer refractory to, or intolerant of, at least two previous chemotherapy regimens (ONO-4538-12, ATTRACTION-2): A randomised, double-blind, placebo-controlled, phase 3 trial. *Lancet* **2017**, *390*, 2461–2471. [CrossRef]

100. Heery, C.R.; O'Sullivan-Coyne, G.; Madan, R.A.; Cordes, L.; Rajan, A.; Rauckhorst, M.; Lamping, E.; Oyelakin, I.; Marte, J.L.; Lepone, L.M.; et al. Avelumab for metastatic or locally advanced previously treated solid tumours (JAVELIN Solid Tumor): A phase 1a, multicohort, dose-escalation trial. *Lancet Oncol.* **2017**, *18*, 587–598. [CrossRef]

101. Bang, Y.Y.; Wyrwicz, L.; Park, Y.L.; Ryu, M.; Muntean, A.; Gomez-Martin, C.; Guimbaud, R.; Ciardiello, F.; Boku, N.; Van Cutsem, E.; et al. Avelumab (MSB0010718C.; anti-PD-L1) + best supportive care (BSC) vs BSC ± chemotherapy as third-line treatment for patients with unresectable, recurrent, or metastatic gastric cancer: The phase 3 JAVELIN Gastric 300 trial. *J. Clin. Oncol.* **2018**, *34*, TPS4135.

102. Marcus, H.; Moehler, M.H.; Taïeb, J.; Gurtler, J.S.; Xiong, H.; Zhang, J.; Cuillerot, J.; Boku, N. Maintenance therapy with avelumab (MSB0010718C.; anti-PD-L1) vs continuation of first-line chemotherapy in patients with unresectable, locally advanced or metastatic gastric cancer: The phase 3 JAVELIN Gastric 100 trial. *J. Clin. Oncol.* **2018**, *34*, TPS4134.

103. Kelly, R.J.; Chung, K.; Gu, Y.; Steele, K.E.; Rebelatto, M.C.; Robbins, P.B.; Tavakkoli, F.; Karakunnel, J.J.; Lai, D.W.; Almhanna, K. Phase Ib/II study to evaluate the safety and antitumor activity of durvalumab (MEDI4736) and tremelimumab as monotherapy or in combination, in patients with recurrent or metastatic gastric/gastroesophageal junction adenocarcinoma. *J. Immunother. Cancer* **2018**, *3*, P157. [CrossRef]

104. Bang, Y.J.; Golan, T.; Lin, C.; Kang, Y.; Wainberg, Z.A.; Wasserstrom, H.; Jin, J.; Mi, G.; McNeely, S.; Laing, N.; et al. Interim safety and clinical activity in patients with locally advanced and unresectable or metastatic gastric or gastroesophageal junction (G/GEJ) adenocarcinoma from a multicohort phase I study of ramucirumab plus durvalumab. *J. Clin. Oncol.* **2018**, *36*, 92.

105. Linch, S.N.; McNamara, M.J.; Redmond, W.L. OX40 Agonists and combination immunotherapy: Putting the pedal to the metal. *Front. Oncol.* **2015**, *5*, 34. [CrossRef] [PubMed]

106. Chester, C.; Sanmamed, M.F.; Wang, J.; Melero, I. Immunotherapy targeting 4-1BB: Mechanistic rationale, clinical results, and future strategies. *Blood* **2018**, *131*, 49–57. [CrossRef] [PubMed]

107. Burugu, S.; Dancsok, A.R.; Nielsen, T.O. Emerging targets in cancer immunotherapy. *Semin. Cancer Biol.* **2017**, 10–17. [CrossRef] [PubMed]

108. Curti, B.D.; Kovacsovics-Bankowski, M.; Morris, N.; Walker, E.; Chisholm, L.; Floyd, K.; Walker, J.; Gonzalez, I.; Meeuwsen, T.; Fox, B.A.; et al. OX40 is a potent immune-stimulating target in late-stage cancer patients. *Cancer Res.* **2013**, *73*, 7189–7198. [CrossRef] [PubMed]

109. Chester, C.; Ambulkar, S.; Kohrt, H.E. 4-1BB agonism: Adding the accelerator to cancer immunotherapy. *Cancer Immunol. Immunother.* **2016**, *65*, 1243–1248. [CrossRef] [PubMed]

110. Takeda, K.; Kojima, Y.; Uno, T.; Hayakawa, Y.; Teng, M.W.; Yoshizawa, H.; Yagita, H.; Gejyo, F.; Okumura, K.; Smyth, M.J. Combination therapy of established tumors by antibodies targeting immune activating and suppressing molecules. *J. Immunol.* **2010**, *184*, 5493–5501. [CrossRef] [PubMed]

111. Sanmamed, M.F.; Pastor, F.; Rodriguez, A.; Perez-Gracia, J.L.; Rodriguez-Ruiz, M.E.; Jure-Kunkel, M.; Melero, I. Agonists of co-stimulation in cancer immunotherapy directed against CD137, OX40, GITR, CD27, CD28, and ICOS. *Semin. Oncol.* **2015**, *42*, 640–655. [CrossRef] [PubMed]

112. Fan, X.; Quezada, S.A.; Sepulveda, M.A.; Sharma, P.; Allison, J.P. Engagement of the ICOS pathway markedly enhances efficacy of CTLA-4 blockade in cancer immunotherapy. *J. Exp. Med.* **2014**, *211*, 715–725. [CrossRef] [PubMed]

113. Taieb, J.; Moehler, M.; Boku, N.; Ajani, J.A.; Yanez, R.E.; Ryu, M.H.; Guenther, S.; Chand, V.; Bang, Y.J. Evolution of checkpoint inhibitors for the treatment of metastatic gastric cancers: Current status and future perspectives. *Cancer Treat. Rev.* **2018**, *66*, 104–113. [CrossRef] [PubMed]

114. Kottschade, L.A. Incidence and management of immune-related adverse events in patients undergoing treatment with immune checkpoint inhibitors. *Curr. Oncol. Rep.* **2018**, *20*, 24. [CrossRef] [PubMed]

115. Niccolai, E.; Taddei, A.; Prisco, D.; Amedei, A. Gastric cancer and the epoch of immunotherapy approaches. *World J. Gastroenterol.* **2015**, *21*, 5778–5793. [CrossRef] [PubMed]

116. Kono, K.; Takahashi, A.; Sugai, H.; Fujii, H.; Choudhury, A.R.; Kiessling, R.; Matsumoto, Y. Dendritic cells pulsed with HER-2/neu-derived peptides can induce specific T-cell responses in patients with gastric cancer. *Clin. Cancer Res.* **2002**, *8*, 3394–3400. [PubMed]

117. Sadanaga, N.; Nagashima, H.; Mashino, K.; Tahara, K.; Yamaguchi, H.; Ohta, M.; Fujie, T.; Tanaka, F.; Inoue, H.; Takesako, K.; et al. Dendritic cell vaccination with MAGE peptide is a novel therapeutic approach for gastrointestinal carcinomas. *Clin. Cancer Res.* **2001**, *7*, 2277–2284. [PubMed]

118. Ajani, J.A.; Hecht, J.R.; Ho, L.; Baker, J.; Oortgiesen, M.; Eduljee, A.; Michaeli, D an open-label, multinational, multicenter study of G17DT vaccination combined with cisplatin and 5-fluorouracil in patients with untreated, advanced gastric or gastroesophageal cancer: The GC4 study. *Cancer* **2006**, *106*, 1908–1916. [CrossRef] [PubMed]

119. He, Q.; Gao, H.; Gao, M.; Qi, S.; Yang, K.; Zhang, Y.; Wang, J. Immunogenicity and safety of a novel tetanus toxoid-conjugated anti-gastrin vaccine in BALB/c mice. *Vaccine* **2018**, *36*, 847–852. [CrossRef] [PubMed]

120. Higashihara, Y.; Kato, J.; Nagahara, A.; Izumi, K.; Konishi, M.; Kodani, T.; Serizawa, N.; Osada, T.; Watanabe, S. Phase I clinical trial of peptide vaccination with URLC10 and VEGFR1 epitope peptides in patients with advanced gastric cancer. *Int. J. Oncol.* **2014**, *44*, 662–668. [CrossRef] [PubMed]

121. Zhang, K.; Peng, Z.; Huang, X.; Qiao, Z.; Wang, X.; Wang, N.; Xi, H.; Cui, J.; Gao, Y.; Huang, X.; et al. Phase II trial of adjuvant immunotherapy with autologous tumor-derived Gp96 vaccination in patients with gastric CANCER. *J. Cancer* **2017**, *8*, 1826–1832. [CrossRef] [PubMed]

122. Popiela, T.; Kulig, J.; Czupryna, A.; Szczepanik, A.M.; Zembala, M. Efficiency of adjuvant immunochemotherapy following curative resection in patients with locally advanced gastric cancer. *Gastric Cancer* **2004**, *7*, 240–245. [CrossRef] [PubMed]

123. Sato, Y.; Shomura, H.; Maeda, Y.; Mine, T.; Une, Y.; Akasaka, Y.; Kondo, M.; Takahashi, S.; Shinohara, T.; Katagiri, K.; et al. Immunological evaluation of peptide vaccination for patients with gastric cancer based on pre-existing cellular response to peptide. *Cancer Sci.* **2003**, *94*, 802–808. [CrossRef] [PubMed]

124. Masuzawa, T.; Fujiwara, Y.; Okada, K.; Nakamura, A.; Takiguchi, S.; Nakajima, K.; Miyata, H.; Yamasaki, M.; Kurokawa, Y.; Osawa, R.; et al. Phase I/II study of S-1 plus cisplatin combined with peptide vaccines for human vascular endothelial growth factor receptor 1 and 2 in patients with advanced gastric cancer. *Int. J. Oncol.* **2012**, *41*, 1297–1304. [CrossRef] [PubMed]

125. Fujiwara, Y.; Sugimura, K.; Miyata, H.; Omori, T.; Nakano, H.; Mochizuki, C.; Shimizu, K.; Saito, H.; Ashida, K.; Honjyo, S.; et al. A pilot study of post-operative adjuvant vaccine for advanced gastric cancer. *Yonago Acta Med.* **2017**, *60*, 101–105. [PubMed]

126. Sundar, R.; Rha, S.Y.; Yamaue, H.; Katsuda, M.; Kono, K.; Kim, H.S.; Kim, C.; Mimura, K.; Kua, L.F.; Yong, W.P. A phase I/Ib study of OTSGC-A24 combined peptide vaccine in advanced gastric cancer. *BMC Cancer* **2018**, *18*, 332. [CrossRef] [PubMed]

127. Koido, S. Dendritic-tumor fusion cell-based cancer vaccines. *Int. J. Mol. Sci.* **2016**, *17*, 828. [CrossRef] [PubMed]

128. Takakura, K.; Kajihara, M.; Ito, Z.; Ohkusa, T.; Gong, J.; Koido, S. Dendritic-tumor fusion cells in cancer immunotherapy. *Discov. Med.* **2015**, *19*, 169–174. [PubMed]

Int. J. Mol. Sci. **2018**, *19*, 1602

129. Lasek, W.; Zagozdzon, R.; Jakobisiak, M. Interleukin 12: Still a promising candidate for tumor immunotherapy? *Cancer Immunol. Immunother.* **2014**, *63*, 419–435. [CrossRef] [PubMed]

130. Koido, S.; Homma, S.; Okamoto, M.; Namiki, Y.; Takakura, K.; Takahara, A.; Odahara, S.; Tsukinaga, S.; Yukawa, T.; Mitobe, J.; et al. Combined TLR2/4-activated dendritic/tumor cell fusions induce augmented cytotoxic T lymphocytes. *PLoS ONE* **2013**, *8*, e59280. [CrossRef] [PubMed]

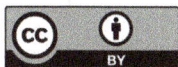

International Journal of
Molecular Sciences

MDPI

Review

Inhibition of the CCL5/CCR5 Axis against the Progression of Gastric Cancer

Donatella Aldinucci * and Naike Casagrande

Department of Molecular Oncology, CRO Aviano National Cancer Institute, via F. Gallini 2, I-33081 Aviano, Italy; naike.casagrande@libero.it
* Correspondence: daldinucci@cro.it

Received: 26 April 2018; Accepted: 14 May 2018; Published: 16 May 2018

Abstract: Despite the progress made in molecular and clinical research, patients with advanced-stage gastric cancer (GC) have a bad prognosis and very low survival rates. Furthermore, it is challenging to find the complex molecular mechanisms that are involved in the development of GC, its progression, and its resistance to therapy. The interactions of chemokines, also known as chemotactic cytokines, with their receptors regulate immune and inflammatory responses. However, updated research demonstrates that cancer cells subvert the normal chemokine role, transforming them into fundamental constituents of the tumor microenvironment (TME) with tumor-promoting effects. C-C chemokine ligand 5 (CCL5) is a chemotactic cytokine, and its expression and secretion are regulated in T cells. C-C chemokine receptor type 5 (CCR5) is expressed in T cells, macrophages, other leukocytes, and certain types of cancer cells. The interaction between CCL5 and CCR5 plays an active role in recruiting leukocytes into target sites. This review summarizes recent information on the role of the CCL5 chemokine and its receptor CCR5 in GC cell proliferation, metastasis formation, and in the building of an immunosuppressive TME. Moreover, it highlights the development of new therapeutic strategies to inhibit the CCL5/CCR5 axis in different ways and their possible clinical relevance in the treatment of GC.

Keywords: CCL5; CCR5; gastric cancer; tumor microenvironment; invasion; CCR5 antagonists

---

1. Introduction

Several research findings suggest that unresolved pathogen infections and chronic inflammation promote tumor development. Hence, inflammation has become another hallmark of cancer [1–3]. Indeed, inflammatory cellular effectors and cytokines within the tumor microenvironment (TME) can promote an antitumor immune response or support tumor pathogenesis [3–5]. Thus, the new challenge is to find drugs or drug combinations that are capable of counteracting the pro-tumorigenic effects of the TME or its formation [6].

Tumor cells can promote the formation of an immunosuppressive/protective TME by recruiting and then "educating" monocytes, myeloid cells, or T cells to become immunosuppressive tumor-associated macrophages (M2-TAM) [7], myeloid-derived suppressor cells (MDSC), T-regulatory cells (T-reg) [8], and mesenchymal stromal cells (MSCs) [9] capable of suppressing T and natural killer cells (NK) responses [10]. Consistently, the presence of inflammatory cells and high amounts of inflammatory mediators (e.g., cytokines, chemokines, enzymes) in the primary tumor is often associated with a bad prognosis and an increased capability to form metastasis [4,11,12].

Tumor cells and the TME can communicate through direct contact and/or through paracrine signals [6], including cytokines and chemokines, which are considered to be key orchestrators not only in inflammation and immune surveillance, but also in cancer progression [13,14] since they can act as survival/growth factors [15,16], improve angiogenesis [17], affect tumor immunity, and influence therapeutic outcomes in patients [18].

A variety of chemokines and chemokine receptors has been detected in neoplastic tissues [1,6]. We will focus our attention primarily on the C-C chemokine ligand 5 (CCL5), also known as RANTES (Regulated upon Activation, Normal T cell Expressed, and Secreted), and its receptor, C-C chemokine receptor type 5 (CCR5). CCL5 belongs to the C-C chemokine family whose members also include CCL3(MIP-1α) and CCL4(MIP-1β) [19]. CCL5, a target gene of nuclear factor kappa-light-chain-enhancer of activated B cells (NF-κB) [20,21], is expressed by T lymphocytes, macrophages, platelets, synovial fibroblasts, tubular epithelium, and certain types of tumor cells [19].

CCL5 induces the recruitment of different leukocyte types, including T cells, monocytes/macrophages, eosinophils, and basophils to sites of injury and infection. In collaboration with IL-2 and IFN-γ which are released by T cells, CCL5 induces the activation and proliferation of particular NK cells to generate C-C chemokine-activated killer cells [19].

CCL5 activity is mediated mainly by binding to CCR5, but also to CCR1 and CCR3 [19]. CCR4 [20,22] and CD44 are auxiliary receptors for CCL5 [22,23]. CCR5 is a promiscuous receptor that binds with high affinity CCL5, CCL3, and CCL4. CCR5 is the major co-receptor for HIV cell entry [24], and this property has significantly boosted the research on CCR5 antagonists/inhibitors [25].

2. The CCL5/CCR5 Axis in Cancer: General Mechanisms

2.1. CCL5–CCR5 Interactions May Favor Tumor Development in Multiple Ways

2.1.1. Proliferation

CCL5 can increase cancer cell growth [15,18,26,27]. It stimulates cell proliferation by inducing the mammalian target of rapamycin (mTOR) pathway followed by a rapid upregulation of cyclin D1, c-Myc, and Dad-1 expression, or by enhancing glucose uptake with increased ATP production and glycolysis [28]. CCL5 may act indirectly by recruiting the TME, monocytes/macrophages, or fibroblasts that, in turn, may promote and sustain tumor cell survival/proliferation [14,29].

2.1.2. Immunosuppression

Tumor-associated macrophage (TAM)s are a heterogeneous population of myeloid cells that contribute to immunosuppression, favoring the establishment and persistence of solid tumors as well as metastatic dissemination. The immunosuppressive effect of TAMs stems from their enzymatic activities and their production of anti-inflammatory cytokines, such as indoleamine 2,3-dioxygenase (IDO), interleukin-10 (IL-10), and transforming growth factor β (TGF-β), which have inhibitory effects on tumoricidal lymphocytes and expand T-reg populations [30]. Consistently, Halama et al. found that blocking the CCR5/CCL5 axis with the CCR5 antagonist Maraviroc (MVC) in functional organoids derived from metastatic colorectal cancer (CRC) patients, determined a macrophage repolarization with anti-tumoral effects. Myeloid-derived suppressor cells (MDSCs) are a heterogeneous population of myeloid cells that can limit productive immune responses against tumors [31]. Targeting the autocrine CCL5/CCR5 axis with MVC was found to reprogram the MDSCs and reinvigorate the antitumor immunity [32].

2.1.3. Angiogenesis

Angiogenesis is a prerequisite for tumor growth and invasion [33]. CCL5 exerts proangiogenic effects by promoting endothelial cell migration, spreading, neovessel formation, and vascular endothelial growth factor (VEGF) secretion. Moreover, tumor cells, upon CCL5 stimulation, can produce VEGF or, by secreting CCL5, may recruit CCR5-expressing TAMs [19,34]. In turn, by secreting VEGF, TAMs can induce angiogenesis [18,30,35]. Thus, targeting tumor-promoting TAMs, which are now considered to be the major players in the regulation of tumor angiogenesis, may represent an attractive new therapeutic strategy.

2.1.4. Migration (Metastasis Formation)

The binding of chemokines to their G-protein-coupled receptors (GPCRs) activates a series of downstream effects that facilitate receptor internalization and signal transduction, leading to integrin activation (adhesion) and polarization of the actin cytoskeleton [36]. The consequences are directional sensing, cell polarization, accumulation of the small GTPases Rac and Cdc42 and of PI3K at the leading edge, actin polymerization, and F-actin formation. These changes cause actomyosin contraction, tail retraction, and, finally, cell migration [36]. More specifically, in lung cancer, CCL5 contributes to the activation of the $\alpha v \beta 3$ integrin and to cell migration through PI3K/Akt, which in turn activates IKKalpha/beta and NF-κB [37]. In ovarian cancer, CCL5 can induce matrix metalloproteinases-9 (MMP-9) secretion by monocytes, which, by degrading the matrix, allows for tumor cell extravasation [38]. In prostate cancer, CCL5 promotes invasion by increasing the secretion of both MMP-2 and -9 and by activating extracellular signal–regulated kinases (ERK) and Rac signaling [39]. In osteosarcoma, CCL5/CCR5 interactions act via MEK, ERK, and then NF-κB, resulting in the activation of $\alpha v \beta 3$ integrin [40].

A schematic representation of the consequences of the CCL5/CCR5 interactions in cancer is shown in Figure 1.

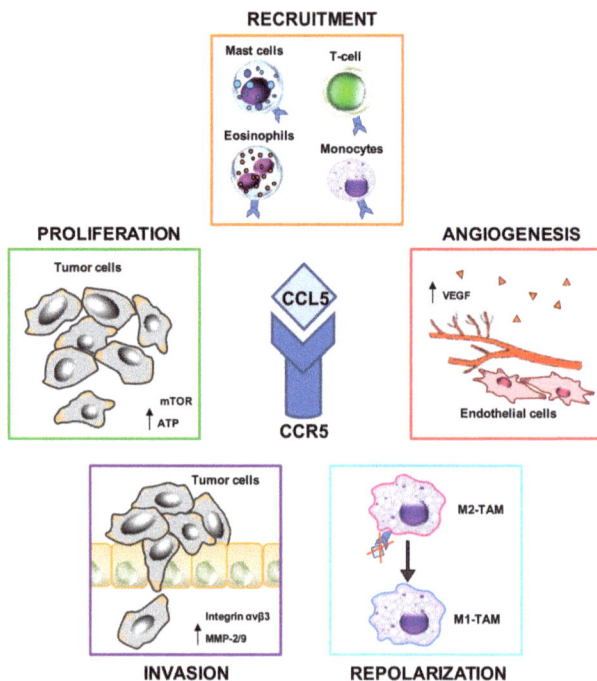

Figure 1. Effects of the C-C chemokine ligand 5 (CCL5) and C-C chemokine receptor type 5 (CCR5) interactions on cancer. CCL5 secreted by tumor cells or by cancer-associated fibroblasts (CAFs) recruits monocytes, T cells, eosinophils, and mast cells in the tumor microenvironment (TME). CCL5 induces tumor cell proliferation via the mammalian target of rapamycin (mTOR) pathway and increases ATP production, enhances tumor cell migration/invasion through $\alpha v \beta 3$ integrin activation and matrix metalloproteinases-2/9 (MMP-2/9) upregulation, promotes angiogenesis by inducing vascular endothelial growth factor (VEGF) secretion; targeting the CCR5/CCL5 axis reprograms the immunosuppressive M2-tumor-associated macrophage (TAM) to anti-tumoral M1-TAM. Thin arrow, up-regulation; bold arrow, repolarization; red cross, inhibition.

3. Possible Clinical Applications: CCL5 and CCR5 as Therapeutic Targets

One of the strategies in cancer therapy is to counteract the formation of a pro-tumorigenic and immunosuppressive TME. There is evidence suggesting possible clinical applications of drugs that are capable of inhibiting the CCR5/CCL5 axis or decreasing CCL5 production/secretion by tumor cells or by the TME [18].

Moreover, CCL5 levels, as well as their changes in liquid biopsy samples, could potentially be useful to monitor or predict disease progress and treatment outcomes. Clinical evidence has revealed that elevated levels of tissue or plasma CCL5 are markers of an unfavorable outcome in patients with breast [41–44], cervical [45], prostate [26], ovarian [46], gastric [47,48], colorectal [49], or pancreatic cancer [50].

3.1. Inhibition of CCL5–CCR5 Interactions

Finding new therapies for cancer patients is necessary, however the discovery of safe and efficacious drugs remains expensive and time-consuming [51,52]. Thus, several non-oncology drugs have been successfully repurposed for cancer [52], including the CCR5 antagonists TAK-779, Anibamine, and, especially, MVC [18,53].

MVC is a U.S. Food and Drug Administration (FDA)-approved CCR5 antagonist, which is highly selective and well tolerated, originally developed for HIV patients as a viral entry blocking inhibitor. Recently, it has demonstrated its potential to treat different types of cancer (Table 1).

Table 1. CCL5/CCR5 axis inhibitors used in preclinical studies and clinical trials (cancer and HIV).

Compound	Mechanism/Molecule	Cancer-Related Studies	References
Maraviroc Selzentry, Celsentri, UK-427857 (Pfizer) Approved by US FDA in 2007 for the treatment of HIV patients.	CCR5 antagonist	Enhanced cell killing mediated by DNA-damaging chemotherapeutic agents in breast cancer.	[54]
		Reprogrammed immunosuppressive myeloid cells and reinvigorated antitumor immunity.	[32]
		Repolarized TAMs. Objective clinical responses in advanced colorectal cancer patients with liver metastases (Phase I trial).	[53]
		Decreased migration of CCR5+ regulatory T cells, reduced breast cancer growth in the lungs.	[55]
Vicriviroc SCH 417690, SCH-D (Merck)	Pyrimidine CCR5 entry inhibitor of HIV-1	Enhanced cell killing mediated by DNA-damaging chemotherapeutic agents in breast cancer.	[54]
		Inhibited invasiveness and metastatic potential in preclinical models of breast cancer.	[56]
TAK-779 (Takeda)	CCR5 antagonist, nonpeptide, quaternary ammonium derivative	Failed to protect from developing liver metastases in mice.	[57]
		Reduced T-regs infiltration and tumor growth in a pancreatic cancer mouse model.	[58]
Met-CCL5 Met-RANTES	CCR5 inhibitor, competitive chemokine receptor blocker	Decreased mammary tumor cell invasion and activation of matrix metalloproteinases induced by mesenchymal stem cell-derived CCL9 and CCL5.	[59]
		Decreased breast tumor growth, infiltrating macrophages, increased stromal development and necrosis in mice.	[60]

Table 1. *Cont.*

Compound	Mechanism/Molecule	Cancer-Related Studies	References
OTR4120 and OTR4131	GAG mimetics, inhibit CCL5 binding to GAG	Strongly inhibited CCL5-induced migration and invasion of hepatocellular carcinoma.	[61]
Anibamine	CCR5 antagonist, natural product	Inhibited the proliferation of ovarian cancer cell lines, showing reduced cytotoxicity.	[62]
		Inhibited prostate cancer cell growth, adhesion, and invasion. Reduced tumor growth in mice.	[63]
DT-13	Steroidal saponin of dwarf lilyturf tuber	Inhibited gastric cancer cell migration by downregulation of both CCR5 and CCL5 expression.	[64]
		Inhibited breast cancer cell proliferation, adhesion, and migration and lung metastasis in vivo by reducing VEGF, CCR5, HIF-1α.	[65]
Aplaviroc (GlaxoSmithKline)	CCR5 entry inhibitor	Developed for the treatment of HIV infection. Studies of Aplaviroc were discontinued because of liver toxicity.	[66]
GSK706769 (GlaxoSmithKline)	CCR5 antagonist	2008 Completed phase I trial for HIV treatment.	https://adisinsight.springer.com/drugs/800023238
INCB009471 (Incyte Corporation)	CCR5 inhibitor	Phase of Development: II (discontinued). HIV treatment.	https://aidsinfo.nih.gov/drugs/print/516/incb-9471/0/1/professional
Cenicriviroc TBR-652, TAK-652 (Takeda)	Inhibitor of CCR2 and CCR5 receptors	Completed study in a Phase IIb clinical trial for HIV treatment.	https://www.clinicaltrials.gov/ct2/show/NCT01338883

In breast cancer, MVC decreased the migration of CCR5$^+$ regulatory T cells, reduced metastatic breast cancer growth in the lungs [55,67], and enhanced cell killing mediated by DNA-damaging chemotherapeutic agents [54]. In human colon cancer, it reduced the accumulation of fibroblasts in the tumor [68]. Recently, Halama et al. [53] demonstrated that T cells at the invasive margins of human CRC liver metastases produced CCL5 which had tumor-promoting effects and was responsible for the functional reprogramming/education of immunosuppressive TAMs toward a pro-tumorigenic phenotype. In a phase I trial in patients with liver metastases of advanced refractory CRC, MVC confirmed antitumoral potency [53], since treatment with the drug was associated with mitigation of tumor-promoting inflammation within the tumor tissue and objective tumor responses [53].

TAK-779, a quaternary ammonium derivative, is a non-peptide CCR5 antagonist with a small molecular weight, that binds exclusively to CCR5. It inhibited HIV infection and CCL5-induced proliferation and invasion of prostate cancer cells (PCa) [18].

Anibamine is the first natural product reported as a CCR5 antagonist. It produced significant inhibition of both PCa and ovarian (OVCAR-3) cancer cell line proliferation and suppressed adhesion, invasion, and tumor growth in mice [62,63].

A detailed list of inhibitors of the CCL5/CCR5 axis used in preclinical studies and clinical trials in cancer and HIV patients is shown in Table 1.

3.2. Inhibition of CCL5 Secretion

The inhibition of CCL5 secretion by cancer cells or by TME may represent an additional system to affect tumor progression [18]. In classical Hodgkin lymphoma, the PI3Kδ-specific inhibitors GS-1101 [17] and Auranofin [69] and the NF-κB inhibitor dehydroxymethylepoxyquinomicin (DHMEQ) [70] not only were cytotoxic, but also decreased CCL5 secretion by cancer cells, leading to a reduced capability to recruit peripheral blood mononuclear cells (PBMCs) [69].

Another therapeutic modality that deserves some consideration deals with the possibility to counteract the cross talk mediated by the CCL5/CCR5 axis between cancer cells and MSCs.

Breast cancer cells stimulated de novo secretion of the chemokine CCL5 from mesenchymal stem cells, which then acted in a paracrine fashion on the cancer cells to enhance their motility, invasion, and metastasis [71]. Zoledronic acid (ZA) [72], as well as PEGylated nanoparticles (NPs) encapsulating ZA [73], decreased both CCL5 and IL-6 secretion by MSCs, suggesting that ZA may exert antitumor activity by affecting the ability of MSCs to interact with breast cancer cells.

Along this line, we recently found that the epidermal growth factor receptor (EGFR) tyrosine kinase inhibitor, gefitinib decreased the capability of supernatants from PCa cells to increase CCL5 secretion by MSCs [74].

Overall, decreasing cancer cells or TME secretion of CCL5 using anticancer drugs may affect both tumor cell proliferation and/or the formation of a protective/immunosuppressive TME.

4. Gastric Cancer and Its TME

Gastric cancer (GC) is the fifth most common cancer worldwide [75]. The precise pathogenesis of GC remains unclear. It has been correlated to many factors, such as eating habits, environmental factors, hereditary predisposition, chronic gastritis, gastric polyps, gastric mucosa abnormal hyperplasia, and *Helicobacter pylori* (*H. pylori*) infection. At diagnosis, over 50% of patients present locally advanced or metastatic GC and consequently are ineligible for curative surgery. When surgery is not possible, chemotherapy is often given to reduce tumors, but with low benefit to patients. Therefore, to improve GC treatment, it is fundamental that we find the molecular events that are responsible for the development and progression of this malignancy [76,77].

Inflammation plays a decisive role at different stages of tumor development, including initiation, promotion, malignant conversion, invasion, and metastasis [1,2,77–80]. *H. pylori*, a microaerophilic gram-negative bacterium that colonizes the gastric mucosa of 50% of the human population, plays a predominant role in the etiology of GC [81]. Its carcinogenic potential is driven by the interplay between bacterial virulence factors and the host's immune responses that allow *H. pylori* to switch between commensalism and pathogenicity. The result is chronic inflammation, with the production of cytokines/chemokines and cell proliferation, which increases the risk of DNA damage and, consequently, tumorigenesis [81]. According to the strong association between infections with *H. pylori* and neoplastic transformation in the human stomach, *H. pylori* has been classified as a class I carcinogen by the World Health Organisation in 1994, representing the strongest known risk factor for GC [81,82]. While many virulence factors of *H. pylori* have been described, the CagA (cytotoxin-associated gene A) toxin, which is translocated into gastric epithelial cells via a bacterial secretion system, appears to be the most specific for the development of a pathological phenotype. Infection with *H. pylori*, a potent activator of NF-κB in gastric epithelial cells, increases CCL5 [47,81–83] and induces the expression of a variety of genes, including IL-1, IL-6, IL-8, IL-10, TNF-α, VEGF, cyclooxygenase-2 (COX-2), inducible nitric oxide synthase (iNOS), cell cycle regulators, the matrix metalloproteinases (MMP)-2, MMP-7, MMP-9, and also adhesion molecules [82,84].

The chronic inflammatory state of the stomach, caused by *H. pylori* infection as well as the production of inflammatory mediators, cytokines, and chemokines, such as CCL5 within gastric tissues, plays an important role in the initiation and progression of GC. Furthermore, in GC, tumor cell survival, growth, proliferation, and metastasis are promoted by the interaction with the TME [84]. The TME of GC is composed of many different types of cells, including TAMs, lymphocytes, cancer-associated fibroblasts (CAFs), and endothelial cells [84].

4.1. Macrophages (TAMs)

Monocytes from the peripheral blood are recruited in the TME and differentiate into TAMs in response to chemokines, including CCL5, and growth factors produced by stromal and tumor cells [30]. In GC, TAMs can improve genetic instability, promote cancer stem cells [85], increase metastasis, and contribute to the formation of an immunosuppressive TME by inhibiting T cell activation [86,87]. Thus, inhibition of monocytes/macrophage recruitment and/or survival in tumors or their immunosuppressive reprogramming may also represent a new therapeutic option for GC. Indeed, TAM levels into GC tumor tissue directly correlate with tumor vascularity [84] and the strength of tumor invasion, nodal status, and clinical stage [84,87].

4.2. Regulatory T Cells (T-Regs)

T-regs are functionally immunosuppressive subsets of T cells, and play an important role in immunological self-tolerance [88]. T-reg (FOXp3[+]) cells have been identified as regulatory components of the adaptive immune response and are associated with *H. pylori*-related inflammation and bacterial persistence [89]. The frequency of T-regs among tumor infiltrating lymphocytes (TILs) derived from tumor-draining regional lymph nodes or peripheral blood lymphocytes is higher in GC than in normal gastric tissue [84,89]. Patients with a higher proportion of T-regs showed poorer survival rates than those with a lower proportion. Interestingly, after patients underwent curative resection for GC, the proportion of T-regs decreased and came back to levels comparable to those for normal, healthy donors [89]. Thus, naturally occurring Foxp3[+] T-regs may be induced to migrate from the peripheral blood to the tumor sites by the chemokines CCL17, CCL22, and CCL5 and then increase in number by tumor-related factors to create a favorable environment for tumor growth [89].

4.3. Cancer-Associated Fibroblasts (CAFs)

CAFs are important components of various types of tumors, including GC [90,91]. During tumorigenesis and progression, CAFs play critical roles in tumor invasion and metastasis via a series of functions, i.e., extracellular matrix deposition, metabolism reprogramming, and chemoresistance [90,91]. CAFs may modulate several aspects of tumor biological behavior in GC, including the ability to proliferate, metastasize, and invade. Additionally, CAFs increase the infiltration of immune cells into GC stroma and increase the rate of angiogenesis by secreting VEGF [92].

4.4. Endothelial Cells (Angiogenesis)

Angiogenesis is the result of an imbalance between positive and negative angiogenic factors released by tumor and host cells into the TME. In GC, angiogenesis is promoted by *H. pylori* [93], high numbers of CAFs [77,92], and TAMs [94,95]. In addition, both GC tumor and stromal cells produce various angiogenic factors, including VEGF, IL-8, and platelet-derived endothelial cell growth factor (PD-ECGF). Tumor angiogenesis plays an essential role in growth, invasion, and metastatic spread of GC [96], indicating that pharmacologic blockade of angiogenesis is a promising new therapy, and that the real-time assessment of the vasculature status is a promising approach to predict the efficacy of the treatments and improve the clinical management of patients with GC [97]. Indeed, high levels of angiogenic factors in serum and tumors are associated with worse outcomes in GC patients. VEGF-A, the most extensively studied angiogenic factor, appears to be a useful biomarker for disease progression and remission, but not for diagnosis [96].

5. The CCL5/CCR5 Axis in GC Development and/or Progression

GC is a common gastrointestinal tumor characterized by rapid lesion development and poor prognosis. Diagnosis of GC is difficult because most patients are asymptomatic in the early stages of disease, which leads to a delay in treatment [81]. Therefore, early diagnosis of GC is essential, and cytokines detection is now regarded as a potential diagnostic tool.

Existing literature highlights the fundamental role of CCL5 in GC progression. GC patients have significantly higher serum CCL5 levels compared with control groups [47,98]. The overall survival of patients with CCL5 levels higher than 71 pg/mL was found to be significantly lower than that of patients with less CCL5 [47,99]. Higher CCL5 levels were associated with lower histological differentiation, higher depth of tumor invasion, more frequent lymph nodes involvement, and advanced tumor stage [99]. More recently, a retrospective analysis of 105 patients with GC demonstrated that increased CCL5 serum levels correlated with more advanced T and N stages, poorly- or undifferentiated histological types, peritoneal metastasis, higher rates of residual tumor, and shorter survival [100].

Patients in the high CCL5 group also had stronger CCL5 immunohistochemistry (IHC) staining in tumor tissues [47,98] and in metastatic lymph nodes [101]. Thus, high CCL5 serum levels, along with strong IHC (CCL5) staining and poorly- or undifferentiated cancer, may be used to predict peritoneal dissemination and a poorer prognosis [100].

A novel prognostic gene expression risk score, including the expression of CCL5, CTNNB1, EXOSC3, LZTR1, and clinical parameters, was recently established and validated for perioperative chemotherapy treatment of GC [102]. CCL5 was also included among genomic markers that could be useful predictors of chemotherapy efficacy for better prognosis and survival outcomes in GC [103]. High expression of the *CCL5* and *CXCL12* genes in Lauren's diffuse type of GC and increased expression of ADAMTS1, CXCL12, and *CCL19* genes were found in peritoneal metastasis, suggesting their involvement in tumor progression [103].

Human GC cell lines characterized by a high metastatic potential have increased CCL5 expression levels [104]. In vitro studies demonstrated that supernatants from highly metastatic GC cell lines increased CCL5 expression in PBMCs. In turn, GC cells cultured with PBMCs had higher invasion properties, and this process was inhibited by neutralizing anti-CCL5 antibodies [105].

Sugasawa et al. [106] demonstrated that CCL5 is expressed by TILs (CD4+ rather than CD8+ cells) and CCR5 is expressed by GC cells. CD4+ cells, but not CD8+ cells, cocultured with GC cells (MKN45 and KATO III cell lines) remarkably enhanced CCL5 production in a direct cell–cell contact manner [106]. Treatment of GC cells with CCL5 increased the proliferation and cocultivation of CCL5-treated GC cells, and PBMCs decreased the proportion of CD8+ cells but not CD4+ cells, suggesting a Fas-FasL-mediated apoptosis in CD8+ cells. In immunodeficient mice coinjected with KATO III and PBMCs, neutralization of CCL5 decreased tumor growth, suggesting that GC cells may induce CD4+ T cells to secrete the tumor-promoting CCL5 and may inhibit the anticancer activity of CD8+ cells [106].

CAFs represent the prominent stromal cellular components in the GC TME [92,107]. The Krüppel-like factor (KLF) KLF5 is a DNA-binding transcriptional regulator that is involved in the tumor-initiating properties of cancer stem-like cells, migration, and drug resistance [108]. In GC patients, high levels of KLF5 in CAFs were closely associated with clinical pathological features such as tumor size, invasion depth, cell grade, and lymph node metastasis, as well as poor prognosis [109]. Yang T et al. demonstrated that the upregulation of KLF5 in CAFs promoted tumor growth, migration, and invasion of GC cells in vitro and in vivo. The major factor contributing to these effects was the increased secretion of CCL5 due to KFL5 in CAFs. Moreover, they found that CCR5 expression in GC cells was activated by CCL5 produced by CAFs. Since the downregulation of KLF5 in CAFs inhibited GC cell progression, KLF5 and/or the CCL5/CCR5 axis may represent promising targets for the treatment of GC [109].

Monocytes/macrophages, which are crucial drivers of tumor progression, express the CCR5 receptor [30]. Consistently, a significant positive correlation was found between the expression of CCL5 and CD68 (macrophage marker) in GC tissues [85]. High levels of CCL5 and CD68 are associated with tumor size, degree of tumor invasion, lymphatic metastasis, pathological grading, and tumor thrombus, but are unrelated to patient age and gender [85].

In addition, Ding et al. also [98] found that CCL5 and CD68 expression are positively correlated, were highly expressed in GC tissues, and were associated with the depth of invasion, lymph node metastasis, TNM staging, and tumor differentiation. In vitro experiments demonstrated that the co-cultivation of GC cells with THP-1 used as a model for monocytes/macrophages, increased CCL5, MMP2, and MMP9 in THP-1 cells [98] and increased proliferation, clone-forming ability, and movement/migration in GC cells (also enhanced by exogenous CCL5) [98]. Thus, the authors suggested that, by secreting CCL5, TAMs promote GC cell proliferation, invasion, and metastasis.

In conclusion, CCL5 may represent a marker of GC staging, disease progression, and a new therapeutic target [98].

6. Possible Clinical Applications of MVC in GC

The CCL5/CCR5 axis is a potential therapeutic target in different cancer types. Since several studies have demonstrated its involvement in GC progression [48,101,106,110], counteracting the pro-tumorigenic effects of the CCL5/CCR5 axis with CCR5-antagonists, such as MVC [53,111], or alternatively, with drugs that are capable to of decreasing CCL5 secretion [69] may be a new therapeutic options for GC treatment.

By using anti-CCL5 antibodies, Cao et al. [92] reverted chemotaxis of GC cells induced by protein extracts from GC lymph nodes harboring metastasis, suggesting that CCL5 and CCR5 contribute to the migration of GC cells from primary to metastatic sites.

In another study, Mencarelli et al. demonstrated that MKN45, MKN74, and KATOIII GC cell lines at different stages of differentiation expressed both CCR5 and CCL5 and that MVC reduced tumor cell migration induced by CCL5 and adhesion to the explanted murine peritoneum [110]. MVC treatment decreased tumor xenograft growth of MKN45 GC cells and the extent of peritoneal disease and increased mice survival. Thus, the CCR5/CCR5-ligand axis seems to be involved in GC cell dissemination, suggesting anticancer potential of CCR5 antagonists [110].

Consistently, DT-13, a saponin of dwarf lilyturf tuber (Table 1), was found to inhibit BGC-823 and HGC-27 GC cell lines migration through downregulation of both CCR5 and CCL5 expression [64].

More recently, using CCR5 antagonists, Wang et al. demonstrated the involvement of CCL5/CCR5 signaling in the cross-talk between GC cells and TAMs leading to tumor growth [112], providing an additional link between inflammation and GC. Chronic inflammation can promote tumor progression via aberrant DNA methylation, an epigenetic modification [113] in neoplastic cells. DNA methylation is catalyzed by enzymes of the DNA methyltransferase (DNMT) family, including DNMT1, the major DNMT in adult cells, highly expressed in GC [114]. Gelsolin (GSN) is an actin-binding protein that controls actin filament assembly and disassembly. Its expression is downregulated in many cancers, including GC tissues, which suggests that it has a potential role in tumor suppression [112]. GSN staining in gastric tumors revealed high GSN expression in early-stage GC compared with advanced-stage tumors [112]. GSN decrease was mediated by DNMT1 promoter methylation and low GSN levels, associated with high DNMT1, and predicted poor survival in GC.

Wang et al. [112] found that TAMs infiltration in GC tissues correlated with high DNMT1 expression. Consistently, co-culture experiments demonstrated that M2-like macrophages suppressed GSN expression in GC cells by upregulating DNMT1. Using anti-CCL5 neutralizing antibodies and the CCR5 antagonist MVC, Wang et al. [112] demonstrated that co-cultivation of GC cells with macrophages increased the secretion of several cytokines, but only CCL5 (secreted by M2-like macrophages) stimulated DNMT1 expression. Moreover, treatment with 5-AZA, a potent DNMT1 inhibitor, or with the CCR5-antagonist MVC slowed GC tumor xenograft growth, revealing the antitumor effects of DNMT1 suppression by the inhibition of CCR5 engagement in GC. Thus, MVC, which is capable of disrupting CCL5/CCR5 interactions, may represent a new potential therapeutic option to counteract TAM-induced tumorigenesis [112].

A schematic view of the CCL5 functions in GC and possible clinical applications of MVC are shown in Figure 2.

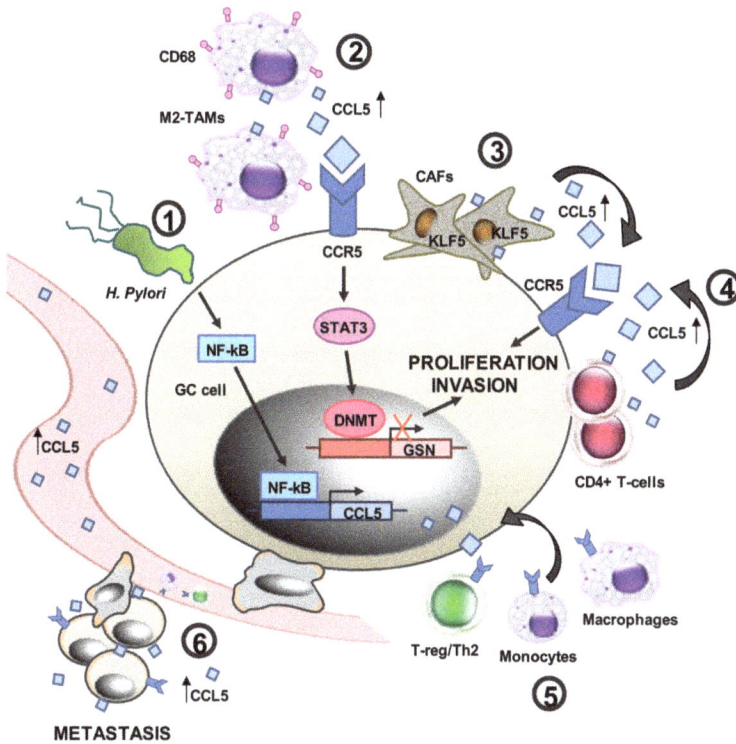

Figure 2. A schematic representation of the proposed role of CCL5 in gastric cancer (GC). (**1**) By activating nuclear factor kappa-light-chain-enhancer of activated B cells (NF-κB), Helicobacter pylori may induce CCL5 expression in GC cells. (**2**) By secreting CCL5, M2-TAMs may activate signal transducer and activator of transcription 3 (STAT3) and DNA methyltransferase (DNMT) and inhibit gelsolin (GSN) expression, leading to enhanced GC cancer cell proliferation and invasion/metastasis formation. CCL5 up-regulation (**3**) Krüppel-like factors 5 (KLF5) overexpression in CAFs enhances the secretion of CCL5, which induces GC cell invasion and proliferation. (**4**) By secreting CCL5, CD4+ tumor-associated lymphocytes (TILs) may enhance GC cell proliferation and invasion. (**5**) By secreting CCL5, GC cells may recruit T-regulatory cells (T-regs), monocytes, and macrophages in the TME. (**6**) Increased CCL5 in GC metastatic tissues and serum may enhance GC cell invasion. Thin up-arrow, CCL5 up-regulation; red cross, inhibition; curved arrow, binding of CCL5 to CCR5 (3, 4); curved arrow, cell migration to GC cells (5).

7. Conclusions

Collectively, several studies suggest that the CCL5/CCR5 axis is associated with GC progression due to increased growth and metastasis formation, though we cannot rule out a role of CCL5 also in the formation of an immunosuppressive TME [32,53]. Our current knowledge leads us to suggest the CCL5/CCR5 axis as a potential therapeutic target in GC.

Author Contributions: N.C. wrote the manuscript, D.A. wrote and revised the manuscript.

Acknowledgments: This work was supported by grant IG 15844 from the Italian Association for Cancer Research (D.A.) and 5X1000CRO-2011.

Conflicts of Interest: The authors declare no conflict of interest.

Int. J. Mol. Sci. **2018**, *19*, 1477

References

1. Mantovani, A. Molecular pathways linking inflammation and cancer. *Curr. Mol. Med.* **2010**, *10*, 369–373. [CrossRef] [PubMed]
2. Hanahan, D.; Coussens, L.M. Accessories to the crime: Functions of cells recruited to the tumor microenvironment. *Cancer Cell* **2012**, *21*, 309–322. [CrossRef] [PubMed]
3. Kershaw, M.H.; Westwood, J.A.; Darcy, P.K. Gene-engineered T cells for cancer therapy. *Nat. Rev. Cancer* **2013**, *13*, 525–541. [CrossRef] [PubMed]
4. Shalapour, S.; Karin, M. Immunity, inflammation, and cancer: An eternal fight between good and evil. *J. Clin. Investig.* **2015**, *125*, 3347–3355. [CrossRef] [PubMed]
5. Shrihari, T.G. Dual role of inflammatory mediators in cancer. *Ecancermedicalscience* **2017**, *11*, 721. [CrossRef] [PubMed]
6. Jain, R.K. Normalizing tumor microenvironment to treat cancer: Bench to bedside to biomarkers. *J. Clin. Oncol.* **2013**, *31*, 2205–2218. [CrossRef] [PubMed]
7. Cook, J.; Hagemann, T. Tumour-associated macrophages and cancer. *Curr. Opin. Pharmacol.* **2013**, *13*, 595–601. [CrossRef] [PubMed]
8. Chang, L.Y.; Lin, Y.C.; Mahalingam, J.; Huang, C.T.; Chen, T.W.; Kang, C.W.; Peng, H.M.; Chu, Y.Y.; Chiang, J.M.; Dutta, A.; et al. Tumor-derived chemokine CCL5 enhances TGF-beta-mediated killing of CD8(+) T cells in colon cancer by T-regulatory cells. *Cancer Res.* **2012**, *72*, 1092–1102. [CrossRef] [PubMed]
9. Yang, X.; Hou, J.; Han, Z.; Wang, Y.; Hao, C.; Wei, L.; Shi, Y. One cell, multiple roles: Contribution of mesenchymal stem cells to tumor development in tumor microenvironment. *Cell Biosci.* **2013**, *3*, 5. [CrossRef] [PubMed]
10. Schlecker, E.; Stojanovic, A.; Eisen, C.; Quack, C.; Falk, C.S.; Umansky, V.; Cerwenka, A. Tumor-infiltrating monocytic myeloid-derived suppressor cells mediate CCR5-dependent recruitment of regulatory T cells favoring tumor growth. *J. Immunol.* **2012**, *189*, 5602–5611. [CrossRef] [PubMed]
11. Allavena, P.; Germano, G.; Marchesi, F.; Mantovani, A. Chemokines in cancer related inflammation. *Exp. Cell Res.* **2011**, *317*, 664–673. [CrossRef] [PubMed]
12. Rajput, S.; Wilber, A. Roles of inflammation in cancer initiation, progression, and metastasis. *Front. Biosci.* **2010**, *2*, 176–183.
13. Balkwill, F.R. The chemokine system and cancer. *J. Pathol.* **2012**, *226*, 148–157. [CrossRef] [PubMed]
14. Nagarsheth, N.; Wicha, M.S.; Zou, W. Chemokines in the cancer microenvironment and their relevance in cancer immunotherapy. *Nat. Rev. Immunol.* **2017**, *17*, 559–572. [CrossRef] [PubMed]
15. Aldinucci, D.; Lorenzon, D.; Cattaruzza, L.; Pinto, A.; Gloghini, A.; Carbone, A.; Colombatti, A. Expression of CCR5 receptors on Reed-Sternberg cells and Hodgkin lymphoma cell lines: Involvement of CCL5/Rantes in tumor cell growth and microenvironmental interactions. *Int. J. Cancer* **2008**, *122*, 769–776. [CrossRef] [PubMed]
16. Aldinucci, D.; Celegato, M.; Casagrande, N. Microenvironmental interactions in classical Hodgkin lymphoma and their role in promoting tumor growth, immune escape and drug resistance. *Cancer Lett.* **2016**, *380*, 243–252. [CrossRef] [PubMed]
17. Meadows, S.A.; Vega, F.; Kashishian, A.; Johnson, D.; Diehl, V.; Miller, L.L.; Younes, A.; Lannutti, B.J. PI3Kdelta inhibitor, GS-1101 (CAL-101), attenuates pathway signaling, induces apoptosis, and overcomes signals from the microenvironment in cellular models of Hodgkin lymphoma. *Blood* **2012**, *119*, 1897–1900. [CrossRef] [PubMed]
18. Aldinucci, D.; Colombatti, A. The inflammatory chemokine CCL5 and cancer progression. *Mediat. Inflamm.* **2014**, *2014*, 292376. [CrossRef] [PubMed]
19. Soria, G.; Ben-Baruch, A. The inflammatory chemokines CCL2 and CCL5 in breast cancer. *Cancer Lett.* **2008**, *267*, 271–285. [CrossRef] [PubMed]
20. Appay, V.; Rowland-Jones, S.L. RANTES: A versatile and controversial chemokine. *Trends Immunol.* **2001**, *22*, 83–87. [CrossRef]
21. Aldinucci, D.; Gloghini, A.; Pinto, A.; Colombatti, A.; Carbone, A. The role of CD40/CD40L and interferon regulatory factor 4 in Hodgkin lymphoma microenvironment. *Leuk. Lymphoma* **2012**, *53*, 195–201. [CrossRef] [PubMed]

22. Udi, J.; Schuler, J.; Wider, D.; Ihorst, G.; Catusse, J.; Waldschmidt, J.; Schnerch, D.; Follo, M.; Wasch, R.; Engelhardt, M. Potent in vitro and in vivo activity of sorafenib in multiple myeloma: Induction of cell death, CD138-downregulation and inhibition of migration through actin depolymerization. *Br. J. Haematol.* **2013**, *161*, 104–116. [CrossRef] [PubMed]

23. Roscic-Mrkic, B.; Fischer, M.; Leemann, C.; Manrique, A.; Gordon, C.J.; Moore, J.P.; Proudfoot, A.E.; Trkola, A. RANTES (CCL5) uses the proteoglycan CD44 as an auxiliary receptor to mediate cellular activation signals and HIV-1 enhancement. *Blood* **2003**, *102*, 1169–1177. [CrossRef] [PubMed]

24. Oppermann, M. Chemokine receptor CCR5: Insights into structure, function, and regulation. *Cell. Signal.* **2004**, *16*, 1201–1210. [CrossRef] [PubMed]

25. Kim, M.B.; Giesler, K.E.; Tahirovic, Y.A.; Truax, V.M.; Liotta, D.C.; Wilson, L.J. CCR5 receptor antagonists in preclinical to phase II clinical development for treatment of HIV. *Expert Opin. Investig. Drugs* **2016**, *25*, 1377–1392. [CrossRef] [PubMed]

26. Vaday, G.G.; Peehl, D.M.; Kadam, P.A.; Lawrence, D.M. Expression of CCL5 (RANTES) and CCR5 in prostate cancer. *Prostate* **2006**, *66*, 124–134. [CrossRef] [PubMed]

27. Murooka, T.T.; Rahbar, R.; Fish, E.N. CCL5 promotes proliferation of MCF-7 cells through mTOR-dependent mRNA translation. *Biochem. Biophys. Res. Commun.* **2009**, *387*, 381–386. [CrossRef] [PubMed]

28. Gao, D.F.; Fish, E.N. 89: A role for CCL5 in breast cancer cell metabolism. *Cytokine* **2013**, *63*, 264. [CrossRef]

29. Relation, T.; Dominici, M.; Horwitz, E.M. Concise Review: An (Im)Penetrable Shield: How the Tumor Microenvironment Protects Cancer Stem Cells. *Stem Cells* **2017**, *35*, 1123–1130. [CrossRef] [PubMed]

30. Mantovani, A.; Marchesi, F.; Malesci, A.; Laghi, L.; Allavena, P. Tumour-associated macrophages as treatment targets in oncology. *Nat. Rev. Clin. Oncol.* **2017**, *14*, 399–416. [CrossRef] [PubMed]

31. Bronte, V.; Brandau, S.; Chen, S.H.; Colombo, M.P.; Frey, A.B.; Greten, T.F.; Mandruzzato, S.; Murray, P.J.; Ochoa, A.; Ostrand-Rosenberg, S.; et al. Recommendations for myeloid-derived suppressor cell nomenclature and characterization standards. *Nat. Commun.* **2016**, *7*, 12150. [CrossRef] [PubMed]

32. Ban, Y.; Mai, J.; Li, X.; Mitchell-Flack, M.; Zhang, T.; Zhang, L.; Chouchane, L.; Ferrari, M.; Shen, H.; Ma, X. Targeting autocrine CCL5-CCR5 axis reprograms immunosuppressive myeloid cells and reinvigorates antitumor immunity. *Cancer Res.* **2017**, *77*, 2857–2868. [CrossRef] [PubMed]

33. Quail, D.F.; Joyce, J.A. Microenvironmental regulation of tumor progression and metastasis. *Nat. Med.* **2013**, *19*, 1423–1437. [CrossRef] [PubMed]

34. Ben-Baruch, A. The Tumor-Promoting Flow of Cells Into, Within and Out of the Tumor Site: Regulation by the Inflammatory Axis of TNFalpha and Chemokines. *Cancer Microenviron.* **2012**, *5*, 151–164. [CrossRef] [PubMed]

35. Wang, S.W.; Liu, S.C.; Sun, H.L.; Huang, T.Y.; Chan, C.H.; Yang, C.Y.; Yeh, H.I.; Huang, Y.L.; Chou, W.Y.; Lin, Y.M.; et al. CCL5/CCR5 axis induces vascular endothelial growth factor-mediated tumor angiogenesis in human osteosarcoma microenvironment. *Carcinogenesis* **2015**, *36*, 104–114. [CrossRef] [PubMed]

36. Ridley, A.J.; Schwartz, M.A.; Burridge, K.; Firtel, R.A.; Ginsberg, M.H.; Borisy, G.; Parsons, J.T.; Horwitz, A.R. Cell migration: Integrating signals from front to back. *Science* **2003**, *302*, 1704–1709. [CrossRef] [PubMed]

37. Huang, C.Y.; Fong, Y.C.; Lee, C.Y.; Chen, M.Y.; Tsai, H.C.; Hsu, H.C.; Tang, C.H. CCL5 increases lung cancer migration via PI3K, Akt and NF-kappaB pathways. *Biochem. Pharmacol.* **2009**, *77*, 794–803. [CrossRef] [PubMed]

38. Long, H.; Xie, R.; Xiang, T.; Zhao, Z.; Lin, S.; Liang, Z.; Chen, Z.; Zhu, B. Autocrine CCL5 signaling promotes invasion and migration of CD133+ ovarian cancer stem-like cells via NF-kappaB-mediated MMP-9 upregulation. *Stem Cells* **2012**, *30*, 2309–2319. [CrossRef] [PubMed]

39. Kato, T.; Fujita, Y.; Nakane, K.; Mizutani, K.; Terazawa, R.; Ehara, H.; Kanimoto, Y.; Kojima, T.; Nozawa, Y.; Deguchi, T.; et al. CCR1/CCL5 interaction promotes invasion of taxane-resistant PC3 prostate cancer cells by increasing secretion of MMPs 2/9 and by activating ERK and Rac signaling. *Cytokine* **2013**, *64*, 251–257. [CrossRef] [PubMed]

40. Wang, S.W.; Wu, H.H.; Liu, S.C.; Wang, P.C.; Ou, W.C.; Chou, W.Y.; Shen, Y.S.; Tang, C.H. CCL5 and CCR5 interaction promotes cell motility in human osteosarcoma. *PLoS ONE* **2012**, *7*, e35101. [CrossRef] [PubMed]

41. Gonzalez, R.M.; Daly, D.S.; Tan, R.; Marks, J.R.; Zangar, R.C. Plasma biomarker profiles differ depending on breast cancer subtype but RANTES is consistently increased. *Cancer Epidemiol. Biomark. Prev.* **2011**, *20*, 1543–1551. [CrossRef] [PubMed]

42. Smeets, A.; Brouwers, B.; Hatse, S.; Laenen, A.; Paridaens, N.; Floris, G.; Vildiers, H.; Christiaens, M.R. Circulating CCL5 Levels in Patients with Breast Cancer: Is There a Correlation with Lymph Node Metastasis? *ISRN Immunol.* **2013**, *10*, 1–5. [CrossRef]

43. Dehqanzada, Z.A.; Storrer, C.E.; Hueman, M.T.; Foley, R.J.; Harris, K.A.; Jama, Y.H.; Shriver, C.D.; Ponniah, S.; Peoples, G.E. Assessing serum cytokine profiles in breast cancer patients receiving a HER2/neu vaccine using Luminex technology. *Oncol. Rep.* **2007**, *17*, 687–694. [CrossRef] [PubMed]

44. Yaal-Hahoshen, N.; Shina, S.; Leider-Trejo, L.; Barnea, I.; Shabtai, E.L.; Azenshtein, E.; Greenberg, I.; Keydar, I.; Ben-Baruch, A. The chemokine CCL5 as a potential prognostic factor predicting disease progression in stage II breast cancer patients. *Clin. Cancer Res.* **2006**, *12*, 4474–4480. [CrossRef] [PubMed]

45. Niwa, Y.; Akamatsu, H.; Niwa, H.; Sumi, H.; Ozaki, Y.; Abe, A. Correlation of tissue and plasma RANTES levels with disease course in patients with breast or cervical cancer. *Clin. Cancer Res.* **2001**, *7*, 285–289. [PubMed]

46. Tsukishiro, S.; Suzumori, N.; Nishikawa, H.; Arakawa, A.; Suzumori, K. Elevated serum RANTES levels in patients with ovarian cancer correlate with the extent of the disorder. *Gynecol. Oncol.* **2006**, *102*, 542–545. [CrossRef] [PubMed]

47. Sima, A.R.; Sima, H.R.; Rafatpanah, H.; Hosseinnezhad, H.; Ghaffarzadehgan, K.; Valizadeh, N.; Mehrabi, B.M.; Hakimi, H.R.; Masoom, A.; Noorbakhsh, A.; et al. Serum chemokine ligand 5 (CCL5/RANTES) level might be utilized as a predictive marker of tumor behavior and disease prognosis in patients with gastric adenocarcinoma. *J. Gastrointest. Cancer* **2014**, *45*, 476–480. [CrossRef] [PubMed]

48. Sugasawa, H.; Ichikura, T.; Tsujimoto, H.; Kinoshita, M.; Morita, D.; Ono, S.; Chochi, K.; Tsuda, H.; Seki, S.; Mochizuki, H. Prognostic significance of expression of CCL5/RANTES receptors in patients with gastric cancer. *J. Surg. Oncol.* **2008**, *97*, 445–450. [CrossRef] [PubMed]

49. Suenaga, M.; Mashima, T.; Kawata, N.; Wakatsuki, T.; Horiike, Y.; Matsusaka, S.; Dan, S.; Shinozaki, E.; Seimiya, H.; Mizunuma, N.; et al. Serum VEGF-A and CCL5 levels as candidate biomarkers for efficacy and toxicity of regorafenib in patients with metastatic colorectal cancer. *Oncotarget* **2016**, *7*, 34811–34823. [CrossRef] [PubMed]

50. Duell, E.J.; Casella, D.P.; Burk, R.D.; Kelsey, K.T.; Holly, E.A. Inflammation, genetic polymorphisms in proinflammatory genes TNF-A, RANTES, and CCR5, and risk of pancreatic adenocarcinoma. *Cancer Epidemiol. Biomark. Prev.* **2006**, *15*, 726–731. [CrossRef] [PubMed]

51. Bertolini, F.; Sukhatme, V.P.; Bouche, G. Drug repurposing in oncology—Patient and health systems opportunities. *Nat. Rev. Clin. Oncol.* **2015**, *12*, 732–742. [CrossRef] [PubMed]

52. Weir, S.J.; DeGennaro, L.J.; Austin, C.P. Repurposing approved and abandoned drugs for the treatment and prevention of cancer through public-private partnership. *Cancer Res.* **2012**, *72*, 1055–1058. [CrossRef] [PubMed]

53. Halama, N.; Zoernig, I.; Berthel, A.; Kahlert, C.; Klupp, F.; Suarez-Carmona, M.; Suetterlin, T.; Brand, K.; Krauss, J.; Lasitschka, F.; et al. Tumoral Immune Cell Exploitation in Colorectal Cancer Metastases Can Be Targeted Effectively by Anti-CCR5 Therapy in Cancer Patients. *Cancer Cell* **2016**, *29*, 587–601. [CrossRef] [PubMed]

54. Jiao, X.; Velasco-Velazquez, M.A.; Wang, M.; Li, Z.; Rui, H.; Peck, A.R.; Korkola, J.E.; Chen, X.; Xu, S.; DuHadaway, J.B.; et al. CCR5 governs DNA damage and breast cancer stem cell expansion. *Cancer Res.* **2018**. [CrossRef] [PubMed]

55. Halvorsen, E.C.; Hamilton, M.J.; Young, A.; Wadsworth, B.J.; LePard, N.E.; Lee, H.N.; Firmino, N.; Collier, J.L.; Bennewith, K.L. Maraviroc decreases CCL8-mediated migration of CCR5(+) regulatory T cells and reduces metastatic tumor growth in the lungs. *Oncoimmunology* **2016**, *5*, e1150398. [CrossRef] [PubMed]

56. Velasco-Velazquez, M.; Pestell, R.G. The CCL5/CCR5 axis promotes metastasis in basal breast cancer. *Oncoimmunology* **2013**, *2*, e23660. [CrossRef] [PubMed]

57. Cambien, B.; Richard-Fiardo, P.; Karimdjee, B.F.; Martini, V.; Ferrua, B.; Pitard, B.; Schmid-Antomarchi, H.; Schmid-Alliana, A. CCL5 neutralization restricts cancer growth and potentiates the targeting of PDGFRbeta in colorectal carcinoma. *PLoS ONE* **2011**, *6*, e28842. [CrossRef] [PubMed]

58. Tan, M.C.; Goedegebuure, P.S.; Belt, B.A.; Flaherty, B.; Sankpal, N.; Gillanders, W.E.; Eberlein, T.J.; Hsieh, C.S.; Linehan, D.C. Disruption of CCR5-dependent homing of regulatory T cells inhibits tumor growth in a murine model of pancreatic cancer. *J. Immunol.* **2009**, *182*, 1746–1755. [CrossRef] [PubMed]

59. Swamydas, M.; Ricci, K.; Rego, S.L.; Dreau, D. Mesenchymal stem cell-derived CCL-9 and CCL-5 promote mammary tumor cell invasion and the activation of matrix metalloproteinases. *Cell Adhes. Migr.* **2013**, *7*, 315–324. [CrossRef] [PubMed]
60. Robinson, S.C.; Scott, K.A.; Wilson, J.L.; Thompson, R.G.; Proudfoot, A.E.; Balkwill, F.R. A chemokine receptor antagonist inhibits experimental breast tumor growth. *Cancer Res.* **2003**, *63*, 8360–8365. [PubMed]
61. Sutton, A.; Friand, V.; Papy-Garcia, D.; Dagouassat, M.; Martin, L.; Vassy, R.; Haddad, O.; Sainte-Catherine, O.; Kraemer, M.; Saffar, L.; et al. Glycosaminoglycans and their synthetic mimetics inhibit RANTES-induced migration and invasion of human hepatoma cells. *Mol. Cancer Ther.* **2007**, *6*, 2948–2958. [CrossRef] [PubMed]
62. Zhang, Y.; Arnatt, C.K.; Zhang, F.; Wang, J.; Haney, K.M.; Fang, X. The potential role of anibamine, a natural product CCR5 antagonist, and its analogues as leads toward development of anti-ovarian cancer agents. *Bioorg. Med. Chem. Lett.* **2012**, *22*, 5093–5097. [CrossRef] [PubMed]
63. Zhang, X.; Haney, K.M.; Richardson, A.C.; Wilson, E.; Gewirtz, D.A.; Ware, J.L.; Zehner, Z.E.; Zhang, Y. Anibamine, a natural product CCR5 antagonist, as a novel lead for the development of anti-prostate cancer agents. *Bioorg. Med. Chem. Lett.* **2010**, *20*, 4627–4630. [CrossRef] [PubMed]
64. Lin, S.S.; Fan, W.; Sun, L.; Li, F.F.; Zhao, R.P.; Zhang, L.Y.; Yu, B.Y.; Yuan, S.T. The saponin DT-13 inhibits gastric cancer cell migration through down-regulation of CCR5-CCL5 axis. *Chin. J. Nat. Med.* **2014**, *12*, 833–840. [CrossRef]
65. Ren-Ping, Z.; Sen-Sen, L.; Yuan, S.T.; Yu, B.Y.; Bai, X.S.; Sun, L.; Zhang, L.Y. DT-13, a saponin of dwarf lilyturf tuber, exhibits anti-cancer activity by down-regulating C-C chemokine receptor type 5 and vascular endothelial growth factor in MDA-MB-435 cells. *Chin. J. Nat. Med.* **2014**, *12*, 24–29. [CrossRef]
66. Nichols, W.G.; Steel, H.M.; Bonny, T.; Adkison, K.; Curtis, L.; Millard, J.; Kabeya, K.; Clumeck, N. Hepatotoxicity observed in clinical trials of aplaviroc (GW873140). *Antimicrob. Agents Chemother.* **2008**, *52*, 858–865. [CrossRef] [PubMed]
67. Velasco-Velazquez, M.; Jiao, X.; De La Fuente, M.; Pestell, T.G.; Ertel, A.; Lisanti, M.P.; Pestell, R.G. CCR5 antagonist blocks metastasis of basal breast cancer cells. *Cancer Res.* **2012**, *72*, 3839–3850. [CrossRef] [PubMed]
68. Tanabe, Y.; Sasaki, S.; Mukaida, N.; Baba, T. Blockade of the chemokine receptor, CCR5, reduces the growth of orthotopically injected colon cancer cells via limiting cancer-associated fibroblast accumulation. *Oncotarget* **2016**, *7*, 48335–48345. [CrossRef] [PubMed]
69. Celegato, M.; Borghese, C.; Casagrande, N.; Mongiat, M.; Kahle, X.U.; Paulitti, A.; Spina, M.; Colombatti, A.; Aldinucci, D. Preclinical activity of the repurposed drug Auranofin in classical Hodgkin lymphoma. *Blood* **2015**, *126*, 1394–1397. [CrossRef] [PubMed]
70. Celegato, M.; Borghese, C.; Umezawa, K.; Casagrande, N.; Colombatti, A.; Carbone, A.; Aldinucci, D. The NF-kappaB inhibitor DHMEQ decreases survival factors, overcomes the protective activity of microenvironment and synergizes with chemotherapy agents in classical Hodgkin lymphoma. *Cancer Lett.* **2014**, *349*, 26–34. [CrossRef] [PubMed]
71. Karnoub, A.E.; Dash, A.B.; Vo, A.P.; Sullivan, A.; Brooks, M.W.; Bell, G.W.; Richardson, A.L.; Polyak, K.; Tubo, R.; Weinberg, R.A. Mesenchymal stem cells within tumour stroma promote breast cancer metastasis. *Nature* **2007**, *449*, 557–563. [CrossRef] [PubMed]
72. Gallo, M.; De Luca, A.; Lamura, L.; Normanno, N. Zoledronic acid blocks the interaction between mesenchymal stem cells and breast cancer cells: Implications for adjuvant therapy of breast cancer. *Ann. Oncol.* **2012**, *23*, 597–604. [CrossRef] [PubMed]
73. Borghese, C.; Casagrande, N.; Pivetta, E.; Colombatti, A.; Boccellino, M.; Amler, E.; Normanno, N.; Caraglia, M.; De Rosa, G.; Aldinucci, D. Self-assembling nanoparticles encapsulating zoledronic acid inhibit mesenchymal stromal cells differentiation, migration and secretion of proangiogenic factors and their interactions with prostate cancer cells. *Oncotarget* **2017**, *8*, 42926–42938. [CrossRef] [PubMed]
74. Borghese, C.; Cattaruzza, L.; Pivetta, E.; Normanno, N.; De Luca, A.; Mazzucato, M.; Celegato, M.; Colombatti, A.; Aldinucci, D. Gefitinib inhibits the cross-talk between mesenchymal stem cells and prostate cancer cells leading to tumor cell proliferation and inhibition of docetaxel activity. *J. Cell. Biochem.* **2013**, *114*, 1135–1144. [CrossRef] [PubMed]
75. Torre, L.A.; Siegel, R.L.; Ward, E.M.; Jemal, A. Global Cancer Incidence and Mortality Rates and Trends—An Update. *Cancer Epidemiol. Biomark. Prev.* **2016**, *25*, 16–27. [CrossRef] [PubMed]

76. Song, H.; Zhu, J.; Lu, D. Molecular-targeted first-line therapy for advanced gastric cancer. *Cochrane Database Syst. Rev.* **2016**, *7*, CD011461. [CrossRef] [PubMed]

77. Bergfeld, S.A.; DeClerck, Y.A. Bone marrow-derived mesenchymal stem cells and the tumor microenvironment. *Cancer Metastasis Rev.* **2010**, *29*, 249–261. [CrossRef] [PubMed]

78. Marelli, G.; Sica, A.; Vannucci, L.; Allavena, P. Inflammation as target in cancer therapy. *Curr. Opin. Pharmacol.* **2017**, *35*, 57–65. [CrossRef] [PubMed]

79. Crusz, S.M.; Balkwill, F.R. Inflammation and cancer: Advances and new agents. *Nat. Rev. Clin. Oncol.* **2015**, *12*, 584–596. [CrossRef] [PubMed]

80. Echizen, K.; Oshima, H.; Nakayama, M.; Oshima, M. The inflammatory microenvironment that promotes gastrointestinal cancer development and invasion. *Adv. Biol. Regul.* **2018**, S2212–S4926. [CrossRef] [PubMed]

81. Sonnenberg, W.R. Gastrointestinal Malignancies. *Prim. Care* **2017**, *44*, 721–732. [CrossRef] [PubMed]

82. Ferreira, R.M.; Machado, J.C.; Figueiredo, C. Clinical relevance of *Helicobacter pylori* vacA and cagA genotypes in gastric carcinoma. *Best Pract. Res. Clin. Gastroenterol.* **2014**, *28*, 1003–1015. [CrossRef] [PubMed]

83. Gambhir, S.; Vyas, D.; Hollis, M.; Aekka, A.; Vyas, A. Nuclear factor kappa B role in inflammation associated gastrointestinal malignancies. *World J. Gastroenterol.* **2015**, *21*, 3174–3183. [CrossRef] [PubMed]

84. Chung, H.W.; Lim, J.B. Role of the tumor microenvironment in the pathogenesis of gastric carcinoma. *World J. Gastroenterol.* **2014**, *20*, 1667–1680. [CrossRef] [PubMed]

85. Han, X.; Qu, B. Expression of chemotactic factor CCL5 in gastric cancer tissue and its correlation with macrophage marker CD86. *Biomed. Res.* **2017**, *28*, 6388–6391.

86. Mills, C.D.; Lenz, L.L.; Harris, R.A. A Breakthrough: Macrophage-Directed Cancer Immunotherapy. *Cancer Res.* **2016**, *76*, 513–516. [CrossRef] [PubMed]

87. Shiao, S.L.; Chu, G.C.; Chung, L.W. Regulation of prostate cancer progression by the tumor microenvironment. *Cancer Lett.* **2016**, *380*, 340–348. [CrossRef] [PubMed]

88. Frydrychowicz, M.; Boruczkowski, M.; Kolecka-Bednarczyk, A.; Dworacki, G. The Dual Role of Treg in Cancer. *Scand. J. Immunol.* **2017**, *86*, 436–443. [CrossRef] [PubMed]

89. Nagase, H.; Takeoka, T.; Urakawa, S.; Morimoto-Okazawa, A.; Kawashima, A.; Iwahori, K.; Takiguchi, S.; Nishikawa, H.; Sato, E.; Sakaguchi, S.; et al. ICOS(+) Foxp3(+) TILs in gastric cancer are prognostic markers and effector regulatory T cells associated with *Helicobacter pylori*. *Int. J. Cancer* **2017**, *140*, 686–695. [CrossRef] [PubMed]

90. Yan, Y.; Wang, R.; Guan, W.; Qiao, M.; Wang, L. Roles of microRNAs in cancer associated fibroblasts of gastric cancer. *Pathol. Res. Pract.* **2017**, *213*, 730–736. [CrossRef] [PubMed]

91. Yan, Y.; Wang, L.F.; Wang, R.F. Role of cancer-associated fibroblasts in invasion and metastasis of gastric cancer. *World J. Gastroenterol.* **2015**, *21*, 9717–9726. [CrossRef] [PubMed]

92. Zhang, Q.; Peng, C. Cancer-associated fibroblasts regulate the biological behavior of cancer cells and stroma in gastric cancer. *Oncol. Lett.* **2018**, *15*, 691–698. [CrossRef] [PubMed]

93. Liu, N.; Zhou, N.; Chai, N.; Liu, X.; Jiang, H.; Wu, Q.; Li, Q. *Helicobacter pylori* promotes angiogenesis depending on Wnt/beta-catenin-mediated vascular endothelial growth factor via the cyclooxygenase-2 pathway in gastric cancer. *BMC Cancer* **2016**, *16*, 321–2351. [CrossRef] [PubMed]

94. Sammarco, G.; Gadaleta, C.D.; Zuccala, V.; Albayrak, E.; Patruno, R.; Milella, P.; Sacco, R.; Ammendola, M.; Ranieri, G. Tumor-Associated Macrophages and Mast Cells Positive to Tryptase Are Correlated with Angiogenesis in Surgically-Treated Gastric Cancer Patients. *Int. J. Mol. Sci.* **2018**, *19*, 1176. [CrossRef] [PubMed]

95. Dirkx, A.E.; Oude Egbrink, M.G.; Wagstaff, J.; Griffioen, A.W. Monocyte/macrophage infiltration in tumors: Modulators of angiogenesis. *J. Leukoc. Biol.* **2006**, *80*, 1183–1196. [CrossRef] [PubMed]

96. Macedo, F.; Ladeira, K.; Longatto-Filho, A.; Martins, S.F. Gastric Cancer and Angiogenesis: Is VEGF a Useful Biomarker to Assess Progression and Remission? *J. Gastric Cancer* **2017**, *17*, 1–10. [CrossRef] [PubMed]

97. Spessotto, P.; Fornasarig, M.; Pivetta, E.; Maiero, S.; Magris, R.; Mongiat, M.; Canzonieri, V.; De Paoli, P.; De Paoli, A.; Buonadonna, A.; et al. Probe-based confocal laser endomicroscopy for in vivo evaluation of the tumor vasculature in gastric and rectal carcinomas. *Sci. Rep.* **2017**, *7*, 9819–10963. [CrossRef] [PubMed]

98. Ding, H.; Zhao, L.; Dai, S.; Li, L.; Wang, F.; Shan, B. CCL5 secreted by tumor associated macrophages may be a new target in treatment of gastric cancer. *Biomed. Pharmacother.* **2016**, *77*, 142–149. [CrossRef] [PubMed]

99. Kim, H.K.; Song, K.S.; Park, Y.S.; Kang, Y.H.; Lee, Y.J.; Lee, K.R.; Kim, H.K.; Ryu, K.W.; Bae, J.M.; Kim, S. Elevated levels of circulating platelet microparticles, VEGF, IL-6 and RANTES in patients with gastric cancer: Possible role of a metastasis predictor. *Eur. J. Cancer* **2003**, *39*, 184–191. [CrossRef]

100. Wang, T.; Wei, Y.; Tian, L.; Song, H.; Ma, Y.; Yao, Q.; Feng, M.; Wang, Y.; Gao, M.; Xue, Y. C-C motif chemokine ligand 5 (CCL5) levels in gastric cancer patient sera predict occult peritoneal metastasis and a poorer prognosis. *Int. J. Surg.* **2016**, *32*, 136–142. [CrossRef] [PubMed]

101. Cao, Z.; Xu, X.; Luo, X.; Li, L.; Huang, B.; Li, X.; Tao, D.; Hu, J.; Gong, J. Role of RANTES and its receptor in gastric cancer metastasis. *J. Huazhong Univ. Sci. Technol. Med. Sci.* **2011**, *31*, 342–347. [CrossRef] [PubMed]

102. Bauer, L.; Hapfelmeier, A.; Blank, S.; Reiche, M.; Slotta-Huspenina, J.; Jesinghaus, M.; Novotny, A.; Schmidt, T.; Grosser, B.; Kohlruss, M.; et al. A novel pretherapeutic gene expression based risk score for treatment guidance in gastric cancer. *Ann. Oncol.* **2017**, *29*, 127–132. [CrossRef] [PubMed]

103. Das, K.; Taguri, M.; Imamura, H.; Sugimoto, N.; Nishikawa, K.; Yoshida, K.; Tan, P.; Tsuburaya, A. Genomic predictors of chemotherapy efficacy in advanced or recurrent gastric cancer in the GC0301/TOP002 phase III clinical trial. *Cancer Lett.* **2018**, *412*, 208–215. [CrossRef] [PubMed]

104. Fukui, R.; Nishimori, H.; Hata, F.; Yasoshima, T.; Ohno, K.; Nomura, H.; Yanai, Y.; Tanaka, H.; Kamiguchi, K.; Denno, R.; et al. Metastases-related genes in the classification of liver and peritoneal metastasis in human gastric cancer. *J. Surg. Res.* **2005**, *129*, 94–100. [CrossRef] [PubMed]

105. Okita, K.; Furuhata, T.; Kimura, Y.; Kawakami, M.; Yamaguchi, K.; Tsuruma, T.; Zembutsu, H.; Hirata, K. The interplay between gastric cancer cell lines and PBMCs mediated by the CC chemokine RANTES plays an important role in tumor progression. *J. Exp. Clin. Cancer Res.* **2005**, *24*, 439–446. [PubMed]

106. Sugasawa, H.; Ichikura, T.; Kinoshita, M.; Ono, S.; Majima, T.; Tsujimoto, H.; Chochi, K.; Hiroi, S.; Takayama, E.; Saitoh, D.; et al. Gastric cancer cells exploit CD4+ cell-derived CCL5 for their growth and prevention of CD8+ cell-involved tumor elimination. *Int. J. Cancer* **2008**, *122*, 2535–2541. [CrossRef] [PubMed]

107. Albini, A.; Bruno, A.; Gallo, C.; Pajardi, G.; Noonan, D.M.; Dallaglio, K. Cancer stem cells and the tumor microenvironment: Interplay in tumor heterogeneity. *Connect. Tissue Res.* **2015**, *56*, 414–425. [CrossRef] [PubMed]

108. Farrugia, M.K.; Vanderbilt, D.B.; Salkeni, M.A.; Ruppert, J.M. Kruppel-like Pluripotency Factors as Modulators of Cancer Cell Therapeutic Responses. *Cancer Res.* **2016**, *76*, 1677–1682. [CrossRef] [PubMed]

109. Yang, T.; Chen, M.; Yang, X.; Zhang, X.; Zhang, Z.; Sun, Y.; Xu, B.; Hua, J.; He, Z.; Song, Z. Down-regulation of KLF5 in cancer-associated fibroblasts inhibit gastric cancer cells progression by CCL5/CCR5 axis. *Cancer Biol. Ther.* **2017**, *18*, 806–815. [CrossRef] [PubMed]

110. Mencarelli, A.; Graziosi, L.; Renga, B.; Cipriani, S.; D'Amore, C.; Francisci, D.; Bruno, A.; Baldelli, F.; Donini, A.; Fiorucci, S. CCR5 Antagonism by Maraviroc Reduces the Potential for Gastric Cancer Cell Dissemination. *Transl. Oncol.* **2013**, *6*, 784–793. [CrossRef] [PubMed]

111. Bronte, V.; Bria, E. Interfering with CCL5/CCR5 at the Tumor-Stroma Interface. *Cancer Cell* **2016**, *29*, 437–439. [CrossRef] [PubMed]

112. Wang, H.C.; Chen, C.W.; Yang, C.L.; Tsai, I.M.; Hou, Y.C.; Chen, C.J.; Shan, Y.S. Tumor-Associated Macrophages Promote Epigenetic Silencing of Gelsolin through DNA Methyltransferase 1 in Gastric Cancer Cells. *Cancer Immunol. Res.* **2017**, *5*, 885–897. [CrossRef] [PubMed]

113. Sharma, S.; Kelly, T.K.; Jones, P.A. Epigenetics in cancer. *Carcinogenesis* **2010**, *31*, 27–36. [CrossRef] [PubMed]

114. Mutze, K.; Langer, R.; Schumacher, F.; Becker, K.; Ott, K.; Novotny, A.; Hapfelmeier, A.; Hofler, H.; Keller, G. DNA methyltransferase 1 as a predictive biomarker and potential therapeutic target for chemotherapy in gastric cancer. *Eur. J. Cancer* **2011**, *47*, 1817–1825. [CrossRef] [PubMed]

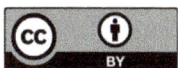

International Journal of
Molecular Sciences

MDPI

Review

Matrix-Assisted Laser Desorption/Ionisation Mass Spectrometry Imaging in the Study of Gastric Cancer: A Mini Review

Andrew Smith [†], Isabella Piga [†], Manuel Galli [†], Martina Stella [†], Vanna Denti, Marina Del Puppo and Fulvio Magni *

Department of Medicine and Surgery, University of Milano-Bicocca, Clinical Proteomics and Metabolomics Unit, 20854 Vedano al Lambro, Italy; andrew.smith@unimib.it (A.S.); isabella.piga@unimib.it (I.P.); m.galli27@campus.unimib.it (M.G.); m.stella12@campus.unimib.it (M.S.); v.denti@campus.unimib.it (V.D.); marina.delpuppo@unimib.it (M.D.P.)
* Correspondence: fulvio.magni@unimib.it; Tel.: +39-02-6448-8213
† These authors contributed equally to this work.

Received: 31 October 2017; Accepted: 28 November 2017; Published: 1 December 2017

Abstract: Gastric cancer (GC) is one of the leading causes of cancer-related deaths worldwide and the disease outcome commonly depends upon the tumour stage at the time of diagnosis. However, this cancer can often be asymptomatic during the early stages and remain undetected until the later stages of tumour development, having a significant impact on patient prognosis. However, our comprehension of the mechanisms underlying the development of gastric malignancies is still lacking. For these reasons, the search for new diagnostic and prognostic markers for gastric cancer is an ongoing pursuit. Modern mass spectrometry imaging (MSI) techniques, in particular matrix-assisted laser desorption/ionisation (MALDI), have emerged as a plausible tool in clinical pathology as a whole. More specifically, MALDI-MSI is being increasingly employed in the study of gastric cancer and has already elucidated some important disease checkpoints that may help us to better understand the molecular mechanisms underpinning this aggressive cancer. Here we report the state of the art of MALDI-MSI approaches, ranging from sample preparation to statistical analysis, and provide a complete review of the key findings that have been reported in the literature thus far.

Keywords: gastric cancer; MALDI imaging; proteomics; metabolomics; lipidomics

1. Introduction

Gastric cancer (GC) develops from the lining of the stomach and is the fifth most common malignancy worldwide [1]. The prognosis of patients with this cancer is related to tumour extent; often early stages of the disease can be asymptomatic, and consequently late diagnosis in advanced stages makes treatment less likely to succeed and reduces patients' chances of survival. The general prognosis is in fact rather grim for gastric cancer patients, with less than 25% of patients surviving at the five-year time-point following diagnosis [2]. Given the high morbidity and mortality rate, the study of GC represents a pressing area of clinical research and much work is ongoing. However, our comprehension of the mechanisms underlying the development of gastric malignancies is still lacking. Given the breadth of modern analytical instrumentation now at our disposal, the detection of early diagnostic biomarkers of GC may not be a distant hope and such findings could be used to elucidate potential pathways for tailored therapeutic treatment.

Mass spectrometry (MS)-based techniques have become some of the most prevalently employed analytical strategies for the detection and identification of endogenous biomolecules in tissue. The application of these techniques is now commonplace in clinical research [3–5] and the mass spectrometric detection of pathologically significant molecules has already shown promise in the study of gastric cancer, providing greater insights into the molecular aspects of the disease and aiding in the identification of candidate biomarkers [6]. Furthermore, the emergence of modern mass spectrometry imaging (MSI) techniques has further revolutionised this area of research. Using MSI, the chemical specificity of MS can be combined with the imaging capabilities offered by optical microscopy in order to simultaneously detect the distribution of hundreds, if not thousands, of biomolecules directly in situ, making it an ideal discovery method for new potential biomarkers for gastric cancer.

Matrix-assisted laser desorption/ionisation (MALDI) remains the most widely applied MSI technique owing to its capability to analyse a wide range of analyte classes (xenobiotics, metabolites, lipids, and proteins) [5]. In particular, the MS-imaging of proteins has been readily performed given their significant role in a large number of pathways involved in defective cellular signalling cascades. Therefore, the ability to spatially resolve the localisation of a number of proteins within the same section of pathological tissue can enable the detection of pathological processes, and, ultimately, define biomarker candidates. Additionally, it has also become increasingly common for the distribution of lipids and metabolites to be recorded by MALDI-MSI, owing in particular to their ease of analysis. Furthermore, there is an ever-increasing body of evidence to suggest that these small molecules play a significant role in biological systems and, as such, are heavily involved in disease pathogenesis. Finally, MALDI-MSI is now readily used to monitor the distribution of xenobiotics and their metabolites within tissue, establishing itself as an invaluable tool in drug distribution studies [7].

In this review, we provide a concise overview of the methodological aspects of MALDI-MSI and summarise how the technique has been used to advance gastric cancer research for the purpose of biomarker detection and monitoring treatment response.

2. Matrix-Assisted Laser Desorption/Ionisation-Mass Spectrometry Imaging (MALDI-MSI) in a Nutshell

MALDI-MSI applied to thin mammalian tissue sections was formally introduced in 1997 and its use has increased exponentially in recent years [8]. The technique relies on the use of a MALDI matrix, which consists of small organic molecules that are designed to absorb the energy of a pulsed laser beam. These molecules commonly possess a suitable chromophore, usually in the form of an aromatic core, and it is this property of the matrix that facilitates the absorption of the UV laser energy. When this matrix is applied to the surface of a sample, it promotes the formation of a ubiquitous layer of co-crystals, which incorporates both matrix and analyte molecules in its network. When the laser beam is applied to the surface of the sample, the absorbed energy leads to rapid desorption of both the matrix and analyte crystals and subsequent "soft" ionisation [3].

Typical MALDI-MSI analysis is most commonly performed on tissue sections that have been sectioned and mounted onto electrically conductive glass slides, such as those coated with indium tin oxide (ITO) [9]. For protein, lipid, xenobiotics and metabolite imaging, the analysis is most commonly performed using fresh-frozen (FF) tissue [10,11].

Regarding the imaging of drugs and products of drug metabolism, MALDI-MSI has been readily used within the pharmaceutical community for the purpose of drug discovery and development [12]. The monitoring of the spatial distribution of drugs and their metabolites in order to evaluate a drug's absorption properties, as well as the characterisation of a drug's delivery and penetration in a target organ, represent some examples of how MALDI-MSI tools have been successfully applied in this field [13,14]. In addition to qualitative MALDI-MSI approaches, the ability to obtain absolute quantitative information by MALDI-MSI for drug analysis, by applying internal standards, has recently been further investigated [15,16].

In the case of protein imaging, formalin-fixed paraffin-embedded (FFPE) tissue is now also readily employed [17]. FFPE tissue accounts for a large percentage of the patient samples collected and stored in medical centres [18] and thus represents a potential gold mine of information for histopathological studies involving MALDI-MSI. It also facilitates multi-centric studies using tissue specimens from numerous tissue banks [19,20]. However, the sample preparation for protein imaging of FFPE tissue is more complex and requires an antigen retrieval step followed by tryptic digestion prior to MALDI-MSI analysis. Metabolite imaging has also been conducted on FFPE tissue [21]; however, it has been less extensively investigated with respect to proteins. Finally, a number of groups have focused on the analysis of N-glycans in tissue [22,23], demonstrating that it is possible to monitor the distribution of both N-glycans and proteins within the same tissue section [23]. The potential to monitor N-glycans, one of the most common post-translational modifications, may significantly advance MALDI-MSI investigations in gastric cancer given their fundamental role in many cellular processes and their establishment as clinical biomarkers [23]. A general overview of the MALDI-MSI sample preparation and analysis workflow is given in Figure 1.

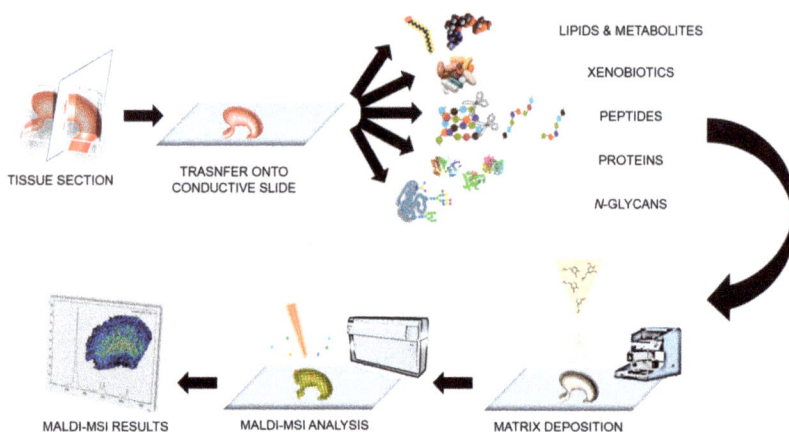

Figure 1. Illustration of the workflow for the matrix-assisted laser desorption/ionisation-mass spectrometry imaging (MALDI-MSI) analysis.

2.1. Sample Preparation

Particular attention to detail must be paid during the collection of FF tissue, as negligence during the sample collection can lead to degradation and delocalisation of the analytes of interest. The method most commonly employed during collection is snap-freezing using liquid nitrogen; however, this procedure can damage tissue morphology if it cools at different rates. This can be overcome to some degree by lightly wrapping the tissue in aluminium in order for it to cool at a more uniform rate [24]. Alternatively, Goodwin et al. recommend the use of ethanol or isopropanol solutions at temperatures of $\leq -70\,^{\circ}\mathrm{C}$ [25]. Once snap-frozen, FF tissue sections can be maintained at $-80\,^{\circ}\mathrm{C}$ for up to a year without evidence of degradation [3,24,26]. Prior to matrix application, tissue washes are also performed in order to remove any molecules that may interfere with the ionisation of the target analytes, including any compounds used during the sectioning procedure. Standard protocols for protein MS-imaging recommend washing the tissue sequentially in increasing concentrations of ethanol, whilst, for example in tissue with a high lipidomic content, washing this tissue with chloroform or xylene can improve protein detection [24,25,27]. Conversely, different washing protocols should be used if the intended analytes are not proteins, e.g., ethanol (70%) with the addition of ammonium acetate ($\mathrm{NH_4Ac}$) is recommended for the desalting of tissue prior to lipidomic analysis [28].

Regarding FFPE tissue, metabolite MS-imaging requires tissue immersion in xylene, or a similar organic solvent, in order to remove any paraffin [21]. Protein MS-imaging, however, requires a more complex procedure [4,29,30]. Following paraffin removal, tissue rehydration is then performed prior to antigen retrieval. The antigen retrieval step is generally performed at $97\,^{\circ}\mathrm{C}$ whilst immersed in a buffer solution that most commonly contains either Tris-HCl or citric acid [31–33], and is required in order to break the methylene bridges that have formed between amino acids during the fixation process. Whilst enzymatic digestion is conventionally performed in solution for proteomic investigations, here the spatial integrity of the proteins is required, and thus the procedure is performed in situ. However, the hydrophobic nature of certain proteins renders them proteolytically resistant to digestion and ultimately limits the peptide yield when performed in this manner. The addition of detergents to the trypsin solution can improve solubilisation by unfolding the proteins, increasing the number of possible enzymatic cleavage sites. A number of detergents have been shown to be compatible with MALDI-MSI analysis, such as *N*-Octanoyl-*N*-methylglucamin (MEGA-8) and RapiGest SF (Waters Corporation, Manchester, UK) [34,35], and significantly improved peptide yield as well as signal intensity, facilitating a greater number of peptide identifications whilst using a bottom-up approach. Alternatively, enzymatic digestion can be performed using *N*-glycosidase F (PNGase F) in order to visualise the distribution of *N*-glycans that are associated with different pathological states of tissue [23].

Matrix deposition plays a crucial role in MALDI-MSI experiments and can limit the true spatial resolution that can be achieved. The general aim of the co-crystallisation process is to maximise analyte extraction whilst at the same time limiting the degree of lateral diffusion, which is equally important to the choice of matrix [9]. Wet matrix deposition methods, involving the use of automated spotters [36] and, in particular, sprayers [37], are particularly efficient for the extraction of proteins and peptides and commonly lead to the formation of crystals of between 10 and 50 μm in diameter. On the other hand, solvent-free matrix deposition involving sublimation has surged in popularity for the analysis of lipids and metabolites due to its ability to deposit a uniform coating of fine matrix crystals that are only a few microns in diameter [38]. Therefore, sublimation represents a highly cost-effective approach to matrix deposition that is both reproducible and compatible with high spatial resolution MALDI-MSI [9]. In contrast to sublimation methods that deposit dry matrix onto the surface of the tissue section, microscope glass slides can also be pre-coated with a MALDI matrix prior to tissue mounting [39]. This has also been shown to be a high-throughput approach that can be effective for the analysis of both proteins [39] and low molecular weight compounds, such as lipids and metabolites [40].

Depending on the target analyte of choice, a number of different matrices can be used. For example, DHB (2,5-Dihydroxybenzoic acid), sinapinic acid (SA; 3,5-dimethoxy-4-hydroxycinnamic acid) and α-CHCA (α-cyano-4-hydroxycinnamic acid) are the most common matrices of choice for the extraction of low molecular weight proteins, peptides, and lipids (1–20 kDa) [41]. However, the addition of hexafluoroisopropanol (1,1,1,3,3,3-hexaluoro-2-propanol) and 2,2,2-trifluoroethanol to the matrix solution [42], along with the use of detectors designed for the detection of higher molecular weight analytes, has been shown to enhance the potential to detect higher molecular weight proteins whilst using SA (up to 110 kDa) [43]. Alternatively, ferulic acid (3-(4-hydroxy-3-methoxy-phenyl)-prop-2-enoic acid) may also be used for the extraction of high molecular weight proteins (up to 140 kDa) [44]. Additionally, ionic matrices such as CHCA/aniline (CHCA/ANI) and CHCA/*N*,*N*-dimethylaniline (CHCA/DANI) have been employed to obtain a more ubiquitous matrix layer and enhance the detection of protein signals [45]. For metabolite imaging, 9-aminoacridine (9AA) is often employed and the mass spectrometer is set in negative-ion mode [46]. In view of the rapid evolution in mass spectrometric instrumentation, the search for novel matrices and matrix deposition protocols has also come to the fore. For example, Garate et al. demonstrated the use of MBT (2-mercaptobenzothiazole) and DAN (2,5-diaminonaphthalene) as MALDI matrices that produced very small crystals and were not a limiting factor during the acquisition of MALDI-MS images with pixel sizes as low as 5 μm [47].

2.2. Instrumental Advancements

MALDI mass spectrometry instrumentation has rapidly evolved in recent years, offering ever more mass resolution and increased sensitivity. In fact, state-of-the-art MALDI-MS instrumentation enables the generation of individual spectra with intensities measured at 25,000–50,000 *m*/*z*-bins for

ToF MS and even greater than 1,000,000 m/z-bins for Fourier-transform ion cyclotron resonance (FTICR) MS measurements [48]. These advancements have enabled more comprehensive analysis and the better resolution of species with similar m/z values. In fact, modern MALDI-FTICR-MS instrumentation, as well as MALDI linear ion trap (Orbitrap), can enable the unequivocal identification of certain analytes (particularly for small molecular weight compounds such as lipids, drugs and metabolites) based on their accurate mass alone [49,50]. Furthermore, the addition of a separate dimension, the drift time, to quadrupole-ToF and ion mobility instrumentation can overcome the inability of MALDI-ToF instruments to differentiate isobaric ions, enabling the detection of a higher number of peaks [51]. Notwithstanding this rapid evolution, several technical issues related to MALDI-MSI still need to be improved, such as spatial resolution and sensitivity. However, next-generation instruments are beginning to address these limiting factors [52], not only improving spatial resolution and sensitivity, but also increasing the spectral acquisition rate as well as minimising pixel-to-pixel variability, facilitating higher quality and more robust analysis. Continuing in this vein, MALDI-MSI will be able to not only analyse single cells, but also potentially delve deeper and analyse at a subcellular level, enabling the intra-cellular proteome to be investigated. Furthermore, it will also be possible to routinely generate three-dimensional MALDI-MS images in order to obtain a snapshot of the pathological state of an entire organ by combining MALDI-MS images of consecutive tissue sections and reconstructing a three-dimensional representation using the appropriate (and currently available) software [53–55].

2.3. Statistical Analysis and Data Elaboration

MALDI-MSI records the presence and relative abundance of a great variety of molecules on tissue, allowing the localisation and spatial distribution of such molecules to be visualised. For each pixel of the digitalised tissue image, a mass spectrum is acquired, generating a so-called "data cube" (Figure 2A), a tensor in which the two spatial dimensions (x and y axes) of the digitalised tissue section are combined with a third dimension consisting of the mass-to-charge ratio (m/z) of the molecules present within the tissue section. Depending on the spatial resolution and the number of data points (sampling rate) per spectrum, a MALDI-MSI dataset can be of several gigabytes, even terabytes. Therefore, efficient statistical methods for data mining must be employed in order to extract information from the spectral data [56].

Before proceeding with the statistical analysis, however, a series of pre-processing steps are required in order to remove the analytical variability connected with the chemical impurities present in the samples and the electronic nature of the mass spectrometric instrumentation [57,58]. These steps adequately prepare the MS data for statistical analysis and enhance the biological information present within the data (Figure 2B) [59]. Smoothing, performed by employing algorithms such as the Savitzky–Golay filter and the moving average window, aims at discarding the fluctuations in the spectrum mainly due to the electronic nature of the mass spectrometer: this process enhances and eases the peak detection phase, since false positive peaks corresponding to electrical noise are discarded. Baseline subtraction, performed by algorithms such as TopHat, iterative convolution and convex hull, ensures that the spectra all lie on the x-axis and all the peak intensities are estimated from the x-axis itself. Normalisation multiplies the intensity of the data points of the spectra by a scaling factor in order to bring the intensity scale (merely related with the analogue-digital conversion of the signal) within the same range and therefore make analyses more reproducible [60]: the total ion count (TIC) method divides the spectrum intensities by the sum of all the intensity values for that spectrum; the root mean square (RMS) method divides the spectrum intensities by the square root of the sum of the intensity values for that spectrum squared; the median method divides the spectrum intensities by the median intensity of that spectrum. Finally, peak picking extracts the information regarding the peaks present within the mass spectrum, in the form of m/z and intensity pair values. After peak maxima have been aligned to each other in order to account for fluctuations in the peak values among the spectra of the dataset related with the peak picking process, the data can be submitted to statistical analysis. Mostly, machine learning algorithms are employed for statistical analysis of the data cube, and, depending on the data provided and on the aim of the data mining process, unsupervised or supervised approaches are carried out (Figure 2C,D) [61].

Unsupervised learning takes unlabelled data as input, i.e., data in which the outcome is not known; by the exploitation of the intrinsic information present in the data, clustering operations are performed in order to highlight hidden structures and/or patterns within the data and are achieved by estimating the similarities among data observations [62]. However, these approaches can also be used in a partially supervised manner, in such a way that the outcome of each observation is preserved during the unsupervised analysis but not taken into account by the algorithm, which performs its operations blind.

Examples of the unsupervised methods for statistical analysis that have been applied in the case of MALDI-MSI gastric cancer datasets are hierarchical clustering analysis (HCA), principal component analysis (PCA) and t-distributed stochastic neighbour embedding (t-SNE). Hierarchical clustering analysis (HCA) estimates the pairwise distance among data observations and generates a dendrogram, in which the observations are grouped under the same nodes based on their similarity to each other [62]. In mass spectrometry imaging, data observations correspond to individual spectra and pixels are associated with spectra; therefore, pixels corresponding to spectra under the same node can be coloured in the same way, generating an unsupervised segmentation tissue image, which can highlight areas of interest on a molecular basis without a priori knowledge regarding the presence of such areas in the tissue section [63]. Therefore, the MSI approach has the potential to aid the diagnostic process by bringing areas of tissue to the attention of the pathologist and highlighting the molecular alterations, even if they do not correlate with cyto-morphological features. Principal component analysis (PCA) is a mathematical technique that aims at reducing data dimensionality whilst preserving the information present within the data [64]. PCA provides an overview of the entire spectral dataset by generating new variables (called principal components, PC) from the linear combination of the spectral features (i.e., peaks): since the PCs are generated orthogonally to one another, no redundancy among the new variables is present and PCs are sorted according to the amount of variance that is retained from the original dataset. This is done in such a way that an overview of almost all the information present within the data can be obtained by looking at the first principal components. The output of a PCA consists of a score chart and a loadings plot: the former places data observations in a 2D or 3D graph according to the score of the PCs, allowing the degree of similarity among the spectra to be evaluated according to their distribution/clustering in the chart; the latter, by resembling the distribution of the former, allows us to evaluate which feature contributes more significantly in driving the distribution/clustering of data observations in the score chart. By combining the two plots, not only is it possible to determine whether the data is capable of discriminating among different classes, but also putative signals of interest can be highlighted for further investigation. t-SNE is a non-linear dimensionality reduction technique that aims at reducing the number of dimensions to two or three in such a way that a 2D or 3D visualisation is easily computed [65]: each n-dimensional data point is mapped to a two- or three-dimensional point in such a way that similar observations correspond to close points in the mapped space. While PCA generates new variables by computing a linear combination of features, t-SNE retains all the features as they are in order to perform the computations. In the case of spectral datasets, t-SNE can be applied by employing either all the individual peaks or only the spectral data points.

On the other hand, supervised learning aims at employing algorithms, referred to as classifiers, which learn from labelled data, i.e., data in which the outcome is known, in order to exploit known features (which correspond to peaks in the mass spectrometry imaging dataset) to make predictions about new, unknown data, resembling the classification problem [66]. The first phase, the training phase, allows classifiers to build the mathematical formula by taking labelled data as input and discriminate among the provided categories via different techniques: for example, support vector machines (SVMs) fit a hyperplane, with the additional aid of kernel functions, to maximise the distance between the closest data observations belonging to different classes [67]; random forests (RF) build a decision tree in which thresholds of feature values determine whether the observation belongs to a class or to another [68]. The following phase is the validation phase, in which the performances of the classifiers are evaluated by the predictions made in a partition of the same training set (cross validation) or in an externally labelled dataset (external validation). The discrepancy between the predicted class and the actual class yields the performance parameters of the model, such as sensitivity (TPR), specificity (TNR), positive predictive value (PPV) and negative predictive value (NPV). Finally, the classifier can be employed for making predictions regarding new data, which can also be weighed according to the performance parameters evaluated in the previous phases. In MSI, an on-tissue classification can be obtained, by generating a MS segmentation image resembling the classification by colouring pixels according to the predicted class.

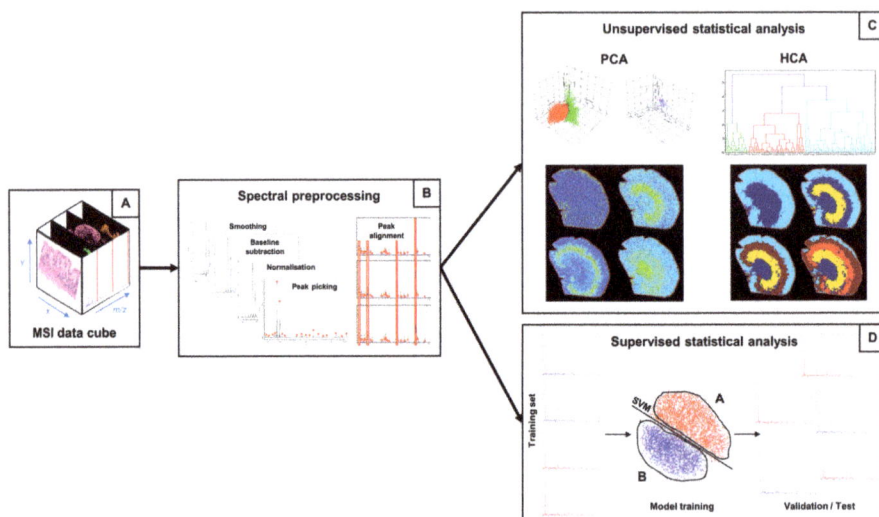

Figure 2. A schematic overview of the MSI data elaboration workflow. (**A**) Data cube; (**B**) the series of spectra pre-processing steps; (**C**) unsupervised and (**D**) supervised statistical analysis performed on a spectra dataset. MSI, mass spectrometry imaging; PCA, principal component analysis; HCA, hierarchical clustering analysis; SVM, support vector machine.

3. Applications in Gastric Cancer

Gastric cancer is a complex, heterogeneous and aggressive disease that represents the third leading cause of cancer-related deaths worldwide [1]. Unfortunately, patients are frequently diagnosed at advanced stages, when the survival outcome is poor [69]. Thus, the discovery of novel drug targets and treatment strategies for patients with advanced GC is the most challenging task in clinical practice.

Recent genomic studies have discovered mutations in the GTPase, Ras homolog family member A (RHOA), that are associated with a poor clinical prognosis in patients with diffuse-type gastric cancers [70,71]. The RHOA signalling pathway activates RHO-associated protein kinases 1 and 2 (ROCK 1/2), which regulate cell contractility, and thus migration and growth may play a role in cancer development [72]. Hisenkamp et al. recently demonstrated that MALDI-MSI could be used to determine the distribution of the drug fasudil to the tumour and surrounding tissues, and to evaluate the pharmacological inhibition of ROCK 1/2 and its effectiveness against gastric cancer in mice [73]. In particular, this study revealed that the parent drug, fasudil, distributed into the stomach and was converted to its active metabolite, hydroxyfasudil. Furthermore, the distribution of the drug in tumorous and non-tumorous tissue was not homogeneous. Fasudil signal intensities were higher in columnar epithelia of the gastric corpus and in parts in the squamous epithelia of the forestomach [73]. There was no obvious enrichment of fasudil or hydroxyfasudil in the tumour areas compared with the non-malignant regions of the stomach. Nevertheless, a significant amount of the drug and its metabolite was able to distribute to the gastrointestinal tumour, suggesting that the drug reached the target organ of interest without being selective for tumour cells [73]. In this analysis, several ion signals were elevated in the tumour region compared to stromal tissue. One signal in particular was then identified as potassium-adducted phophatidylcholine [PC(34:1) + K]$^+$ (m/z 798.541) using FTICR-MS/MS [73]. Similarly, MALDI-MSI has been used to simultaneously map differences in the lipid distribution between gastric cancer lesions and non-neoplastic mucosa whilst preserving the morphological integrity of the analysed tissue. Interestingly, the lipid ion at m/z 798.5 has been detected in another MALDI-imaging study by Uehara et al., revealing that it was overexpressed in cancer tissue compared to the adjacent non neoplastic mucosa [74]. On the contrary, the intensity of the lipid signal at m/z 496.3, identified as the proton-adducted lysophosphatidylcholine (LPC) (16:0), was low in cancer lesions [74].

A recent study based on the integrated strategy of MALDI-MSI and immunohistochemical assays investigated the association of cancer progression and the effects of de novo lipogenesis [75]. In fact, it has been reported that high lipogenic activity is one hallmark of tumour cells [76]. In particular, MALDI-FTICR-MSI has been used to analyse lipid localisation in six types of cancer tissue, including 19 samples of gastric cancer (adenocarcinoma), and the results highlighted that the levels of lipids with monounsaturated acyl chains were increased in the cancer microenvironment compared with the adjacent normal tissue, whereas polyunsaturated lipids were decreased in the cancerous area [75].

In addition, MALDI-MSI in negative ion mode has the ability to visualise small molecule metabolites (typically < 500 Da), which are important cellular components closely linked with tumour development and progression [77]. Guo et al. developed an electric field matrix-assisted scanning spraying matrix coating system to deposit matrix on tissue with crystal sizes of <10 μm [78]. The method enabled the in situ detection of cancer-related small molecule metabolites and to visualise their distribution by MALDI-FTICR mass spectrometry imaging on snap-frozen tissues from five gastric cancer patients. It was found that the lipids octadecenoic acid and lysophosphatidylethanolamine (18:1), as well as phosphorylated nucleosides, were significantly upregulated in cancerous areas compared with the adjacent noncancerous areas [78]. On the other hand, nucleosides and N-acetylneuraminic acid were significantly decreased in the cancerous area [78].

The poor prognosis of gastric cancer is due to a lack of reliable tumour markers that may improve early-stage diagnosis of cancer. Recently, proteomic approaches using MALDI-MSI techniques have been adopted in order to better understand the pathology and to search for novel diagnostic and therapeutic targets through the characterisation of the proteome profile of a malignant lesion with respect to the non-tumour area.

Deininger et al. employed hierarchical cluster analysis along with principal component analysis in order to uncover proteomic differences in gastric cancer tissue and non-neoplastic stomach mucosa [79]. They demonstrated that histological differences could also be detected on the sole basis of different protein and peptide profiles, thus confirming the reliability of the approach. Furthermore, it was also proposed that MALDI-MSI may be capable of highlighting phenotypic tumour heterogeneity, which cannot be uncovered by using traditional histology [79].

A recent MALDI-MSI study detected seven tumour-specific proteins that predicted unfavourable disease outcome in a cohort of 63 patients with intestinal gastric cancer [80]. Three proteins were identified and successfully validated by immunohistochemistry on an independent set of 118 samples. A protein previously unknown to be implicated in gastric cancer, cysteine-rich intestinal protein 1 (CRIP1), which plays a key role in tumour behaviour, was confirmed to be an independent prognostic factor for gastric cancer. Furthermore, human neutrophil peptide-1 (HNP-1) and S100 calcium binding protein A6 (S100A6) were found to be able to further classify patients with gastric cancer disease at stage I from patients at more advanced stages [80]. Human neutrophil peptides (HNPs) are expressed in neutrophil granules of the innate immune system and are found to be highly expressed in a variety of cancers [81–83]. Interestingly, the protein detected at m/z 3445 (HNP-1) was overexpressed in cancer tissue, confirming the observation of two other MALDI-MSI studies on gastric cancer [84,85], and another that performed MALDI-MS profiling [86]. Besides HNP-1, Cheng et al. demonstrated that HNPs α-defensin 2 and 3 were also overexpressed in gastric cancer tissues and the distribution of HNPs 1–3 overlapped in cancerous tissues, with high abundance in the lamina propria [85]. Similarly, the calcium-binding protein S100A6 was highly expressed in gastric cancer lesions and has also been identified by MALDI-MSI as a potential marker for tumour development of Barrett's adenocarcinoma [87], known to develop more rapidly than any other gastrointestinal malignancy. Another protein signal, at m/z 4156, has been observed in the cancer area of intestinal-type gastric cancer and oesophageal adenocarcinoma [84,87], and its role in carcinogenesis and drug resistance was highlighted [88]. Moreover, MALDI-MSI of fresh-frozen Barrett's adenocarcinoma samples revealed the prognostic role of cytochrome c oxidase subunit 7A2 (COX7A2) and transgelin-2 (TAGLN2) concerning the disease-free survival, whereas the expression of the protein ion at m/z 11,185, identified as S100 calcium binding protein A10 (S100A10), was an independent prognostic factor [87]. Morita et al. introduced an easy-to-use method for the detection of histological type-specific proteins using a MALDI-MSI approach and 12 FFPE tissue microarrays (TMA) from well, moderately, and poorly differentiated gastric carcinoma samples [89]. Among the detected signals, 54 were classified as signals specific to cancer, with statistically significant differences between adenocarcinoma and normal tissues being observed. The tryptic peptide at m/z 1325.6 was specifically increased in the poorly differentiated cancer tissue and was identified as histone H4 [89]. Recently, Munteanu et al. employed MALDI-MSI for the in situ analysis of a histone deacetylase inhibitor, the hydroxamic acid panobinostat (LBH-589), focusing on its pharmacodynamic effects in order to visualise the spatiotemporal distribution of acetylated histones and the tumour-selective pharmacodynamic responses in a mouse model of gastrointestinal cancer [90]. Following LBH-589 administration, the nonacetylated (0 Ac) histone H4 was decreased, whereas the acetylated (Ac) H4 states (2 to 4 Ac) were markedly increased in the tumour regions [90].

The MALDI imaging approach in combination with two classification models (support vector machine and random forest) has been promisingly used for gastric cancer tumour classification as well as for the classification of the human epidermal growth factor receptor 2 (HER2/neu) status prediction in gastric cancer [91,92]. Meding et al. were able to classify both the training set and the test set of gastric cancer and Barrett's adenocarcinoma primary tumour entities with high accuracy [91]. The training set could be classified nearly perfectly, whereas the classification of the test set yielded an accuracy above 94% for Barrett's cancer and above 88% for gastric cancer with both classifiers [91]. Balluff et al. demonstrated that the HER2/neu status of gastric cancer could be predicted by specific protein patterns originating from breast cancer, with accuracies above 90% independent of the prediction method [92].

Thus far, intratumor heterogeneity is an unresolved factor that influences the evolution of cancer and adversely affects patient outcome. Phenotypically distinct gastric cancer subpopulations have been investigated by MALDI imaging in combination with advanced clustering methods and t-SNE [65,84]. In particular, extensive heterogeneity was noted within and between individual tumour samples. Both studies highlighted two proteins, at m/z 3445 (HNP-1) and m/z 14021 (histone H2A), respectively, which were found to be involved in the prognostic signature of the subpopulations [65,84].

Among the post-translational modifications, glycosylation is the most abundant and complex, and alterations in the glycosylation of gastric cancer cells have an impact on gastric carcinogenesis and cancer progression [93,94]. Kunzke et al. investigated in situ native-glycans (*N*-glycans) in 106 primary resected FFPE human gastric cancer tissues by MALDI-MSI in order to understand the underlying molecular mechanisms and discover the clinical implications of glycosylation in gastric cancer [95]. The study pointed out the presence of a glycosaminoglycan fragment (HexNAc-HexA-HexNAc) in tumour stroma regions, an independent prognostic factor for gastric cancer patients [95].

4. Concluding Remarks

In the context of gastric cancer, the application of MALDI-MSI is still in its relative infancy. However, there is already sufficient evidence in the literature to suggest that MALDI-MSI can play a crucial role in uncovering the molecular pathways implicated in the development of this particularly deadly cancer.

This approach has already detected molecular alterations associated with gastric cancer at the proteomic, lipidomic, and metabolomic level, and can also monitor the distribution and xenoboiotic metabolism of prospective therapeutic agents such as fasudil. On the basis of these findings, the potential of MALDI-MSI is evident and, by combining these findings using integrative omics approaches, we can improve our understanding of gastric cancer at numerous molecular levels and assist in the clinical management of patients. Whilst this final goal is not imminent, and cannot be achieved using a single approach, MALDI-MSI can certainly make a significant contribution to this pursuit. Nevertheless, the potential of MALDI-MSI for obtaining findings able to contribute to the diagnosis, prognosis, and understanding of numerous diseases, most specifically cancer, is expected to grow in the future as this technology advances.

Acknowledgments: This work was supported by grants from the MIUR: FIRB 2007 (RBRN07BMCT_11), FAR 2013–2016; and in part by Fondazione Gigi & Pupa Ferrari Onlus.

Conflicts of Interest: The authors declare no conflict of interest.

Abbreviations

FF	Fresh-frozen
FFPE	Formalin-fixed paraffin-embedded
FTICR	Fourier transform ion cyclotron resonance
GC	Gastric cancer
HCA	Hierarchical clustering analysis
HER2/neu	Human epidermal growth factor receptor 2
HNP	Human neutrophil peptide
MALDI	Matrix-assisted laser desorption/ionisation
MSI	Mass spectrometry imaging
PCA	Principal component analysis
ROCK 1/2	RHO-associated protein kinase 1 and 2
ToF	Time of flight
t-SNE	t-Distributed stochastic neighbour embedding

References

1. Ferlay, J.; Soerjomataram, I.; Dikshit, R.; Eser, S.; Mathers, C.; Rebelo, M.; Parkin, D.M.; Forman, D.; Bray, F. Cancer incidence and mortality worldwide: Sources, methods and major patterns in GLOBOCAN 2012: Globocan 2012. *Int. J. Cancer* **2015**, *136*, E359–E386. [CrossRef] [PubMed]
2. Aichler, M. Proteomic and metabolic prediction of response to therapy in gastric cancer. *World J. Gastroenterol.* **2014**, *20*, 13648–13657. [CrossRef] [PubMed]
3. Chugtai, K.; Heeren, R. Mass spectrometric imaging for biomedical tissue analysis. *Chem. Rev.* **2010**, *110*, 3237–3277. [CrossRef] [PubMed]
4. Casadonte, R.; Longuespée, R.; Kriegsmann, J.; Kriegsmann, M. MALDI IMS and Cancer Tissue Microarrays. In *Advances in Cancer Research*; Elsevier: Amsterdam, The Netherlands, 2017; Volume 134, pp. 173–200, ISBN 978-0-12-805249-5.
5. Kriegsmann, J.; Kriegsmann, M.; Casadonte, R. MALDI TOF imaging mass spectrometry in clinical pathology: A valuable tool for cancer diagnostics. *Int. J. Oncol.* **2015**, *46*, 893–906. [CrossRef] [PubMed]
6. Kang, C.; Lee, Y.; Lee, J.E. Recent advances in mass spectrometry-based proteomics of gastric cancer. *World J. Gastroenterol.* **2016**, *22*, 8283–8293. [CrossRef] [PubMed]

7. Aichler, M.; Walch, A. MALDI Imaging mass spectrometry: Current frontiers and perspectives in pathology research and practice. *Lab. Investig.* **2015**, *95*, 422–431. [CrossRef] [PubMed]

8. Caprioli, R.M.; Farmer, T.B.; Gile, J. Molecular Imaging of Biological Samples: Localization of Peptides and Proteins Using MALDI-TOF MS. *Anal. Chem.* **1997**, *69*, 4751–4760. [CrossRef] [PubMed]

9. Baker, T.C.; Han, J.; Borchers, C.H. Recent advancements in matrix-assisted laser desorption/ionization mass spectrometry imaging. *Curr. Opin. Biotechnol.* **2017**, *43*, 62–69. [CrossRef] [PubMed]

10. Goodwin, R.J.A.; Nilsson, A.; Borg, D.; Langridge-Smith, P.R.R.; Harrison, D.J.; Mackay, C.L.; Iverson, S.L.; Andrén, P.E. Conductive carbon tape used for support and mounting of both whole animal and fragile heat-treated tissue sections for MALDI MS imaging and quantitation. *J. Proteom.* **2012**, *75*, 4912–4920. [CrossRef] [PubMed]

11. Nilsson, A.; Goodwin, R.J.A.; Shariatgorji, M.; Vallianatou, T.; Webborn, P.J.H.; Andrén, P.E. Mass Spectrometry Imaging in Drug Development. *Anal. Chem.* **2015**, *87*, 1437–1455. [CrossRef] [PubMed]

12. Greer, T.; Sturm, R.; Li, L. Mass spectrometry imaging for drugs and metabolites. *J. Proteom.* **2011**, *74*, 2617–2631. [CrossRef] [PubMed]

13. Giordano, S.; Morosi, L.; Veglianese, P.; Licandro, S.A.; Frapolli, R.; Zucchetti, M.; Cappelletti, G.; Falciola, L.; Pifferi, V.; Visentin, S.; et al. 3D Mass Spectrometry Imaging Reveals a very Heterogeneous Drug Distribution in Tumors. *Sci. Rep.* **2016**, *6*. [CrossRef] [PubMed]

14. Thompson, C.G.; Bokhart, M.T.; Sykes, C.; Adamson, L.; Fedoriw, Y.; Luciw, P.A.; Muddiman, D.C.; Kashuba, A.D.M.; Rosen, E.P. Mass Spectrometry Imaging Reveals Heterogeneous Efavirenz Distribution within Putative HIV Reservoirs. *Antimicrob. Agents Chemother.* **2015**, *59*, 2944–2948. [CrossRef] [PubMed]

15. Chumbley, C.W.; Reyzer, M.L.; Allen, J.L.; Marriner, G.A.; Via, L.E.; Barry, C.E.; Caprioli, R.M. Absolute Quantitative MALDI Imaging Mass Spectrometry: A Case of Rifampicin in Liver Tissues. *Anal. Chem.* **2016**, *88*, 2392–2398. [CrossRef] [PubMed]

16. Groseclose, M.R.; Castellino, S. A Mimetic Tissue Model for the Quantification of Drug Distributions by MALDI Imaging Mass Spectrometry. *Anal. Chem.* **2013**, *85*, 10099–10106. [CrossRef] [PubMed]

17. Longuespée, R.; Casadonte, R.; Kriegsmann, M.; Pottier, C.; Picard de Muller, G.; Delvenne, P.; Kriegsmann, J.; De Pauw, E. MALDI mass spectrometry imaging: A cutting-edge tool for fundamental and clinical histopathology. *Proteom. Clin. Appl.* **2016**, *10*, 701–719. [CrossRef] [PubMed]

18. Stauber, J.; MacAleese, L.; Franck, J.; Claude, E.; Snel, M.; Kaletas, B.K.; Wiel, I.M.V.D.; Wisztorski, M.; Fournier, I.; Heeren, R.M.A. On-tissue protein identification and imaging by MALDI-ion mobility mass spectrometry. *J. Am. Soc. Mass Spectrom.* **2010**, *21*, 338–347. [CrossRef] [PubMed]

19. De Sio, G.; Smith, A.J.; Galli, M.; Garancini, M.; Chinello, C.; Bono, F.; Pagni, F.; Magni, F. A MALDI-Mass Spectrometry Imaging method applicable to different formalin-fixed paraffin-embedded human tissues. *Mol. Biosyst.* **2015**, *11*, 1507–1514. [CrossRef] [PubMed]

20. Gorzolka, K.; Walch, A. MALDI mass spectrometry imaging of formalin-fixed paraffin-embedded tissues in clinical research. *Histol. Histopathol.* **2014**, *29*, 1365–1376. [CrossRef] [PubMed]

21. Ly, A.; Buck, A.; Balluff, B.; Sun, N.; Gorzolka, K.; Feuchtinger, A.; Janssen, K.-P.; Kuppen, P.J.K.; van de Velde, C.J.H.; Weirich, G.; et al. High-mass-resolution MALDI mass spectrometry imaging of metabolites from formalin-fixed paraffin-embedded tissue. *Nat. Protoc.* **2016**, *11*, 1428–1443. [CrossRef] [PubMed]

22. Briggs, M.T.; Ho, Y.Y.; Kaur, G.; Oehler, M.K.; Everest-Dass, A.V.; Packer, N.H.; Hoffmann, P. *N*-Glycan matrix-assisted laser desorption/ionization mass spectrometry imaging protocol for formalin-fixed paraffin-embedded tissues. *Rapid Commun. Mass Spectrom.* **2017**, *31*, 825–841. [CrossRef] [PubMed]

23. Heijs, B.; Holst, S.; Briaire-de Bruijn, I.H.; van Pelt, G.W.; de Ru, A.H.; van Veelen, P.A.; Drake, R.R.; Mehta, A.S.; Mesker, W.E.; Tollenaar, R.A.; et al. Multimodal Mass Spectrometry Imaging of *N*-Glycans and Proteins from the Same Tissue Section. *Anal. Chem.* **2016**, *88*, 7745–7753. [CrossRef] [PubMed]

24. Schwartz, S.A.; Reyzer, M.L.; Caprioli, R.M. Direct tissue analysis using matrix-assisted laser desorption/ionization mass spectrometry: Practical aspects of sample preparation. *J. Mass Spectrom.* **2003**, *38*, 699–708. [CrossRef] [PubMed]

25. Goodwin, R.J.A.; Pennington, S.R.; Pitt, A.R. Protein and peptides in pictures: Imaging with MALDI mass spectrometry. *Proteomics* **2008**, *8*, 3785–3800. [CrossRef] [PubMed]

26. Patel, E. Fresh Frozen Versus Formalin-Fixed Paraffin Embedded for Mass Spectrometry Imaging. *Methods Mol. Biol.* **2017**, *1618*, 7–14. [CrossRef] [PubMed]

27. Lemaire, R.; Wisztorski, M.; Desmons, A.; Tabet, J.C.; Day, R.; Salzet, M.; Fournier, I. MALDI-MS direct tissue analysis of proteins: Improving signal sensitivity using organic treatments. *Anal. Chem.* **2006**, *78*, 7145–7153. [CrossRef] [PubMed]

28. Wang, H.-Y.J.; Liu, C.B.; Wu, H.-W. A simple desalting method for direct MALDI mass spectrometry profiling of tissue lipids. *J. Lipid Res.* **2011**, *52*, 840–849. [CrossRef] [PubMed]

29. Thomas, A.; Chaurand, P. Advances in tissue section preparation for MALDI imaging MS. *Bioanalysis* **2014**, *6*, 967–982. [CrossRef] [PubMed]

30. Goodwin, R.J.A. Sample preparation for mass spectrometry imaging: Small mistakes can lead to big consequences. *J. Proteom.* **2012**, *75*, 4893–4911. [CrossRef] [PubMed]

31. Boskamp, T.; Lachmund, D.; Oetjen, J.; Cordero Hernandez, Y.; Trede, D.; Maass, P.; Casadonte, R.; Kriegsmann, J.; Warth, A.; Dienemann, H.; et al. A new classification method for MALDI imaging mass spectrometry data acquired on formalin-fixed paraffin-embedded tissue samples. *Biochim. Biophys. Acta* **2017**, *1865*, 916–926. [CrossRef] [PubMed]

32. Groseclose, M.R.; Massion, P.P.; Chaurand, P.; Caprioli, R.M. High-throughput proteomic analysis of formalin-fixed paraffin-embedded tissue microarrays using MALDI imaging mass spectrometry. *Proteomics* **2008**, *8*, 3715–3724. [CrossRef] [PubMed]

33. Gustafsson, J.O.R.; Oehler, M.K.; McColl, S.R.; Hoffmann, P. Citric acid antigen retrieval (CAAR) for tryptic peptide imaging directly on archived formalin-fixed paraffin-embedded tissue. *J. Proteome Res.* **2010**, *9*, 4315–4328. [CrossRef] [PubMed]

34. Huang, H.Z.; Nichols, A.; Liu, D. Direct Identification and Quantification of Aspartyl Succinimide in an IgG2 mAb by RapiGest Assisted Digestion. *Anal. Chem.* **2009**, *81*, 1686–1692. [CrossRef] [PubMed]

35. Patel, E.; Clench, M.R.; West, A.; Marshall, P.S.; Marshall, N.; Francese, S. Alternative surfactants for improved efficiency of in situ tryptic proteolysis of fingermarks. *J. Am. Soc. Mass Spectrom.* **2015**, *26*, 862–872. [CrossRef] [PubMed]

36. Franck, J.; Arafah, K.; Barnes, A.; Wisztorski, M.; Salzet, M.; Fournier, I. Improving Tissue Preparation for Matrix-Assisted Laser Desorption Ionization Mass Spectrometry Imaging. Part 1: Using Microspotting. *Anal. Chem.* **2009**, *81*, 8193–8202. [CrossRef] [PubMed]

37. Beine, B.; Diehl, H.C.; Meyer, H.E.; Henkel, C. Tissue MALDI Mass Spectrometry Imaging (MALDI MSI) of Peptides. In *Proteomis in Systems Biology*; Reinders, J., Ed.; Springer: New York, NY, USA, 2016; Volume 1394, pp. 129–150, ISBN 978-1-4939-3339-6.

38. Hankin, J.A.; Barkley, R.M.; Murphy, R.C. Sublimation as a method of matrix application for mass spectrometric imaging. *J. Am. Soc. Mass Spectrom.* **2007**, *18*, 1646–1652. [CrossRef] [PubMed]

39. Yang, J.; Caprioli, R.M. Matrix pre-coated targets for high throughput MALDI imaging of proteins: Matrix pre-coated targets for MALDI imaging MS. *J. Mass Spectrom.* **2014**, *49*, 417–422. [CrossRef] [PubMed]

40. Grove, K.J.; Frappier, S.L.; Caprioli, R.M. Matrix Pre-Coated MALDI MS Targets for Small Molecule Imaging in Tissues. *J. Am. Soc. Mass Spectrom.* **2011**, *22*, 192–195. [CrossRef] [PubMed]

41. Kaletaş, B.K.; van der Wiel, I.M.; Stauber, J.; Dekker, L.J.; Güzel, C.; Kros, J.M.; Luider, T.M.; Heeren, R.M.A. Sample preparation issues for tissue imaging by imaging MS. *Proteomics* **2009**, *9*, 2622–2633. [CrossRef] [PubMed]

42. Franck, J.; Longuespée, R.; Wisztorski, M.; Van Remoortere, A.; Van Zeijl, R.; Deelder, A.; Salzet, M.; McDonnell, L.; Fournier, I. MALDI mass spectrometry imaging of proteins exceeding 30,000 daltons. *Med. Sci. Monit. Int. Med. J. Exp. Clin. Res.* **2010**, *16*, BR293–BR299.

43. Van Remoortere, A.; van Zeijl, R.J.M.; van den Oever, N.; Franck, J.; Longuespée, R.; Wisztorski, M.; Salzet, M.; Deelder, A.M.; Fournier, I.; McDonnell, L.A. MALDI imaging and profiling MS of higher mass proteins from tissue. *J. Am. Soc. Mass Spectrom.* **2010**, *21*, 1922–1929. [CrossRef] [PubMed]

44. Mainini, V.; Bovo, G.; Chinello, C.; Gianazza, E.; Grasso, M.; Cattoretti, G.; Magni, F. Detection of high molecular weight proteins by MALDI imaging mass spectrometry. *Mol. Biosyst.* **2013**, *9*, 1101. [CrossRef] [PubMed]

45. Calvano, C.D.; Carulli, S.; Palmisano, F. Aniline/α-cyano-4-hydroxycinnamic acid is a highly versatile ionic liquid for matrix-assisted laser desorption/ionization mass spectrometry. *Rapid Commun. Mass Spectrom.* **2009**, *23*, 1659–1668. [CrossRef] [PubMed]

46. Fagerer, S.; Nielsen, S.; Ibáñez, A.; Zenobi, R. Matrix-assisted laser desorption/ionization matrices for negative-mode metabolomics. *Eur. J. Mass Spectrom.* **2013**, *19*, 39. [CrossRef]

47. Garate, J.; Fernández, R.; Lage, S.; Bestard-Escalas, J.; Lopez, D.H.; Reigada, R.; Khorrami, S.; Ginard, D.; Reyes, J.; Amengual, I.; et al. Imaging mass spectrometry increased resolution using 2-mercaptobenzothiazole and 2,5-diaminonaphtalene matrices: Application to lipid distribution in human colon. *Anal. Bioanal. Chem.* **2015**, *407*, 4697–4708. [CrossRef] [PubMed]

48. Spraggins, J.M.; Rizzo, D.G.; Moore, J.L.; Noto, M.J.; Skaar, E.P.; Caprioli, R.M. Next-generation technologies for spatial proteomics: Integrating ultra-high speed MALDI-TOF and high mass resolution MALDI FTICR imaging mass spectrometry for protein analysis. *Proteomics* **2016**, *16*, 1678–1689. [CrossRef] [PubMed]

49. Cornett, D.S.; Frappier, S.L.; Caprioli, R.M. MALDI-FTICR imaging mass spectrometry of drugs and metabolites in tissue. *Anal. Chem.* **2008**, *80*, 5648–5653. [CrossRef] [PubMed]

50. Römpp, A.; Spengler, B. Mass spectrometry imaging with high resolution in mass and space. *Histochem. Cell Biol.* **2013**, *139*, 759–783. [CrossRef] [PubMed]

51. Kettling, H.; Vens-Cappell, S.; Soltwisch, J.; Pirkl, A.; Haier, J.; Müthing, J.; Dreisewerd, K. MALDI Mass Spectrometry Imaging of Bioactive Lipids in Mouse Brain with a Synapt G2-S Mass Spectrometer Operated at Elevated Pressure: Improving the Analytical Sensitivity and the Lateral Resolution to Ten Micrometers. *Anal. Chem.* **2014**, *86*, 7798–7805. [CrossRef] [PubMed]

52. Ogrinc Potočnik, N.; Porta, T.; Becker, M.; Heeren, R.M.A.; Ellis, S.R. Use of advantageous, volatile matrices enabled by next-generation high-speed matrix-assisted laser desorption/ionization time-of-flight imaging employing a scanning laser beam. *Rapid Commun. Mass Spectrom.* **2015**, *29*, 2195–2203. [CrossRef] [PubMed]

53. Oetjen, J.; Veselkov, K.; Watrous, J.; McKenzie, J.S.; Becker, M.; Hauberg-Lotte, L.; Kobarg, J.H.; Strittmatter, N.; Mróz, A.K.; Hoffmann, F.; et al. Benchmark datasets for 3D MALDI- and DESI-imaging mass spectrometry. *GigaScience* **2015**, *4*, 20. [CrossRef] [PubMed]

54. Patterson, N.H.; Doonan, R.J.; Daskalopoulou, S.S.; Dufresne, M.; Lenglet, S.; Montecucco, F.; Thomas, A.; Chaurand, P. Three-dimensional imaging MS of lipids in atherosclerotic plaques: Open-source methods for reconstruction and analysis. *Proteomics* **2016**, *16*, 1642–1651. [CrossRef] [PubMed]

55. Anderson, D.M.G.; Van de Plas, R.; Rose, K.L.; Hill, S.; Schey, K.L.; Solga, A.C.; Gutmann, D.H.; Caprioli, R.M. 3-D imaging mass spectrometry of protein distributions in mouse Neurofibromatosis 1 (NF1)-associated optic glioma. *J. Proteom.* **2016**, *149*, 77–84. [CrossRef] [PubMed]

56. Trede, D.; Kobarg, J.H.; Oetjen, J.; Thiele, H.; Maass, P.; Alexandrov, T. On the Importance of Mathematical Methods for Analysis of MALDI-Imaging Mass Spectrometry Data. *J. Integr. Bioinform.* **2012**, *9*, 1–11.

57. Ràfols, P.; Vilalta, D.; Brezmes, J.; Cañellas, N.; del Castillo, E.; Yanes, O.; Ramírez, N.; Correig, X. Signal preprocessing, multivariate analysis and software tools for MA(LDI)-TOF mass spectrometry imaging for biological applications. *Mass Spectrom. Rev.* **2016**, 1–26. [CrossRef] [PubMed]

58. Norris, J.L.; Cornett, D.S.; Mobley, J.A.; Andersson, M.; Seeley, E.H.; Chaurand, P.; Caprioli, R.M. Processing MALDI Mass Spectra to Improve Mass Spectral Direct Tissue Analysis. *Int. J. Mass Spectrom.* **2007**, *260*, 212–221. [CrossRef] [PubMed]

59. Galli, M.; Zoppis, I.; Smith, A.; Magni, F.; Mauri, G. Machine learning approaches in MALDI-MSI: Clinical applications. *Expert Rev. Proteom.* **2016**, *13*, 685–696. [CrossRef] [PubMed]

60. Deininger, S.-O.; Cornett, D.S.; Paape, R.; Becker, M.; Pineau, C.; Rauser, S.; Walch, A.; Wolski, E. Normalization in MALDI-TOF imaging datasets of proteins: Practical considerations. *Anal. Bioanal. Chem.* **2011**, *401*, 167–181. [CrossRef] [PubMed]

61. Jones, E.A.; Deininger, S.-O.; Hogendoorn, P.C.W.; Deelder, A.M.; McDonnell, L.A. Imaging mass spectrometry statistical analysis. *J. Proteom.* **2012**, *75*, 4962–4989. [CrossRef] [PubMed]

62. Murtagh, F.; Contreras, P. Algorithms for hierarchical clustering: An overview. *Wiley Interdiscip. Rev. Data Min. Knowl. Discov.* **2012**, *2*, 86–97. [CrossRef]

63. Alexandrov, T.; Becker, M.; Deininger, S.-O.; Ernst, G.; Wehder, L.; Grasmair, M.; von Eggeling, F.; Thiele, H.; Maass, P. Spatial Segmentation of Imaging Mass Spectrometry Data with Edge-Preserving Image Denoising and Clustering. *J. Proteome Res.* **2010**, *9*, 6535–6546. [CrossRef] [PubMed]

64. Jolliffe, I.T.; Cadima, J. Principal component analysis: A review and recent developments. *Philos. Trans. R. Soc. Math. Phys. Eng. Sci.* **2016**, *374*, 20150202. [CrossRef] [PubMed]

65. Abdelmoula, W.M.; Balluff, B.; Englert, S.; Dijkstra, J.; Reinders, M.J.T.; Walch, A.; McDonnell, L.A.; Lelieveldt, B.P.F. Data-driven identification of prognostic tumor subpopulations using spatially mapped t-SNE of mass spectrometry imaging data. *Proc. Natl. Acad. Sci. USA* **2016**, *113*, 12244–12249. [CrossRef] [PubMed]

66. Kotsiantis, S.B. Supervised Machine Learning: A Review of Classification Techniques. *Informatica* **2007**, *31*, 249–268.

67. Cristianini, N.; Shawe-Taylor, J. *An Introduction to Support Vector Machines and Other Kernel-Based Learning Methods*; Cambridge University Press: Cambridge, UK, 2000; ISBN 978-0-511-80138-9.

68. Breiman, L. Bagging predictors. *Mach. Learn.* **1996**, *24*, 123–140. [CrossRef]

69. Takahashi, T.; Saikawa, Y.; Kitagawa, Y. Gastric Cancer: Current Status of Diagnosis and Treatment. *Cancers* **2013**, *5*, 48–63. [CrossRef] [PubMed]

70. Kakiuchi, M.; Nishizawa, T.; Ueda, H.; Gotoh, K.; Tanaka, A.; Hayashi, A.; Yamamoto, S.; Tatsuno, K.; Katoh, H.; Watanabe, Y.; et al. Recurrent gain-of-function mutations of RHOA in diffuse-type gastric carcinoma. *Nat. Genet.* **2014**, *46*, 583–587. [CrossRef] [PubMed]

71. The Cancer Genome Atlas Research Network. Comprehensive molecular characterization of gastric adenocarcinoma. *Nature* **2014**, *513*, 202–209. [CrossRef]

72. Wei, L.; Surma, M.; Shi, S.; Lambert-Cheatham, N.; Shi, J. Novel Insights into the Roles of Rho Kinase in Cancer. *Arch. Immunol. Ther. Exp.* **2016**, *64*, 259–278. [CrossRef] [PubMed]

73. Hinsenkamp, I.; Schulz, S.; Roscher, M.; Suhr, A.-M.; Meyer, B.; Munteanu, B.; Fuchser, J.; Schoenberg, S.O.; Ebert, M.P.A.; Wängler, B.; et al. Inhibition of Rho-Associated Kinase 1/2 Attenuates Tumor Growth in Murine Gastric Cancer. *Neoplasia* **2016**, *18*, 500–511. [CrossRef] [PubMed]

74. Uehara, T.; Kikuchi, H.; Miyazaki, S.; Iino, I.; Setoguchi, T.; Hiramatsu, Y.; Ohta, M.; Kamiya, K.; Morita, Y.; Tanaka, H.; et al. Overexpression of Lysophosphatidylcholine Acyltransferase 1 and Concomitant Lipid Alterations in Gastric Cancer. *Ann. Surg. Oncol.* **2016**, *23*, 206–213. [CrossRef] [PubMed]

75. Guo, S.; Wang, Y.; Zhou, D.; Li, Z. Significantly increased monounsaturated lipids relative to polyunsaturated lipids in six types of cancer microenvironment are observed by mass spectrometry imaging. *Sci. Rep.* **2015**, *4*, 5959. [CrossRef] [PubMed]

76. Zaidi, N.; Lupien, L.; Kuemmerle, N.B.; Kinlaw, W.B.; Swinnen, J.V.; Smans, K. Lipogenesis and lipolysis: The pathways exploited by the cancer cells to acquire fatty acids. *Prog. Lipid Res.* **2013**, *52*, 585–589. [CrossRef] [PubMed]

77. Sullivan, L.B.; Gui, D.Y.; Heiden, M.G.V. Altered metabolite levels in cancer: Implications for tumour biology and cancer therapy. *Nat. Rev. Cancer* **2016**, *16*, 680–693. [CrossRef] [PubMed]

78. Guo, S.; Wang, Y.; Zhou, D.; Li, Z. Electric Field-Assisted Matrix Coating Method Enhances the Detection of Small Molecule Metabolites for Mass Spectrometry Imaging. *Anal. Chem.* **2015**, *87*, 5860–5865. [CrossRef] [PubMed]

79. Deininger, S.-O.; Ebert, M.P.; Fütterer, A.; Gerhard, M.; Röcken, C. MALDI Imaging Combined with Hierarchical Clustering as a New Tool for the Interpretation of Complex Human Cancers. *J. Proteome Res.* **2008**, *7*, 5230–5236. [CrossRef] [PubMed]

80. Balluff, B.; Rauser, S.; Meding, S.; Elsner, M.; Schöne, C.; Feuchtinger, A.; Schuhmacher, C.; Novotny, A.; Jütting, U.; Maccarrone, G.; et al. MALDI Imaging Identifies Prognostic Seven-Protein Signature of Novel Tissue Markers in Intestinal-Type Gastric Cancer. *Am. J. Pathol.* **2011**, *179*, 2720–2729. [CrossRef] [PubMed]

81. Gaspar, D.; Freire, J.M.; Pacheco, T.R.; Barata, J.T.; Castanho, M.A.R.B. Apoptotic human neutrophil peptide-1 anti-tumor activity revealed by cellular biomechanics. *Biochim. Biophys. Acta Mol. Cell Res.* **2015**, *1853*, 308–316. [CrossRef] [PubMed]

82. Kemik, O.; Kemik, A.; Sumer, A.; Begenik, H.; Purisa, S.; Tuzun, S. Human neutrophil peptides 1, 2 and 3 (HNP 1–3): Elevated serum levels in colorectal cancer and novel marker of lymphatic and hepatic metastasis. *Hum. Exp. Toxicol.* **2013**, *32*, 167–171. [CrossRef] [PubMed]

83. Lundy, F.T.; Orr, D.F.; Gallagher, J.R.; Maxwell, P.; Shaw, C.; Napier, S.S.; Gerald Cowan, C.; Lamey, P.-J.; Marley, J.J. Identification and overexpression of human neutrophil α-defensins (human neutrophil peptides 1, 2 and 3) in squamous cell carcinomas of the human tongue. *Oral Oncol.* **2004**, *40*, 139–144. [CrossRef]

84. Balluff, B.; Frese, C.K.; Maier, S.K.; Schöne, C.; Kuster, B.; Schmitt, M.; Aubele, M.; Höfler, H.; Deelder, A.M.; Heck, A.J.; et al. De novo discovery of phenotypic intratumour heterogeneity using imaging mass spectrometry. *J. Pathol.* **2015**, *235*, 3–13. [CrossRef] [PubMed]

85. Cheng, C.-C.; Chang, J.; Chen, L.-Y.; Ho, A.-S.; Ker-Jer, H.; Lee, S.-C.; Mai, F.-D.; Chang, C.-C. Human neutrophil peptides 1-3 as gastric cancer tissue markers measured by MALDI-imaging mass spectrometry: Implications for infiltrated neutrophils as a tumor target. *Dis. Markers* **2012**, *32*, 21–31. [CrossRef] [PubMed]

86. Kim, H.K.; Reyzer, M.L.; Choi, I.J.; Kim, C.G.; Kim, H.S.; Oshima, A.; Chertov, O.; Colantonio, S.; Fisher, R.J.; Allen, J.L.; et al. Gastric Cancer-Specific Protein Profile Identified Using Endoscopic Biopsy Samples via MALDI Mass Spectrometry. *J. Proteome Res.* **2010**, *9*, 4123–4130. [CrossRef] [PubMed]

87. Elsner, M.; Rauser, S.; Maier, S.; Schöne, C.; Balluff, B.; Meding, S.; Jung, G.; Nipp, M.; Sarioglu, H.; Maccarrone, G.; et al. MALDI imaging mass spectrometry reveals COX7A2, TAGLN2 and S100-A10 as novel prognostic markers in Barrett's adenocarcinoma. *J. Proteom.* **2012**, *75*, 4693–4704. [CrossRef] [PubMed]

88. Aichler, M.; Elsner, M.; Ludyga, N.; Feuchtinger, A.; Zangen, V.; Maier, S.K.; Balluff, B.; Schöne, C.; Hierber, L.; Braselmann, H.; et al. Clinical response to chemotherapy in oesophageal adenocarcinoma patients is linked to defects in mitochondria: Mitochondrial defects predict chemotherapy response. *J. Pathol.* **2013**, *230*, 410–419. [CrossRef] [PubMed]

89. Morita, Y.; Ikegami, K.; Goto-Inoue, N.; Hayasaka, T.; Zaima, N.; Tanaka, H.; Uehara, T.; Setoguchi, T.; Sakaguchi, T.; Igarashi, H.; et al. Imaging mass spectrometry of gastric carcinoma in formalin-fixed paraffin-embedded tissue microarray. *Cancer Sci.* **2010**, *101*, 267–273. [CrossRef] [PubMed]

90. Munteanu, B.; Meyer, B.; von Reitzenstein, C.; Burgermeister, E.; Bog, S.; Pahl, A.; Ebert, M.P.; Hopf, C. Label-Free in Situ Monitoring of Histone Deacetylase Drug Target Engagement by Matrix-Assisted Laser Desorption Ionization-Mass Spectrometry Biotyping and Imaging. *Anal. Chem.* **2014**, *86*, 4642–4647. [CrossRef] [PubMed]

91. Meding, S.; Nitsche, U.; Balluff, B.; Elsner, M.; Rauser, S.; Schöne, C.; Nipp, M.; Maak, M.; Feith, M.; Ebert, M.P.; et al. Tumor Classification of Six Common Cancer Types Based on Proteomic Profiling by MALDI Imaging. *J. Proteome Res.* **2012**, *11*, 1996–2003. [CrossRef] [PubMed]

92. Balluff, B.; Elsner, M.; Kowarsch, A.; Rauser, S.; Meding, S.; Schuhmacher, C.; Feith, M.; Herrmann, K.; Röcken, C.; Schmid, R.M.; et al. Classification of HER2/neu Status in Gastric Cancer Using a Breast-Cancer Derived Proteome Classifier. *J. Proteome Res.* **2010**, *9*, 6317–6322. [CrossRef] [PubMed]

93. Pinho, S.S.; Reis, C.A. Glycosylation in cancer: Mechanisms and clinical implications. *Nat. Rev. Cancer* **2015**, *15*, 540–555. [CrossRef] [PubMed]

94. Duarte, H.O.; Balmaña, M.; Mereiter, S.; Osório, H.; Gomes, J.; Reis, C.A. Gastric Cancer Cell Glycosylation as a Modulator of the ErbB2 Oncogenic Receptor. *Int. J. Mol. Sci.* **2017**, *18*, 2262. [CrossRef] [PubMed]

95. Kunzke, T.; Balluff, B.; Feuchtinger, A.; Buck, A.; Langer, R.; Luber, B.; Lordick, F.; Zitzelsberger, H.; Aichler, M.; Walch, A. Native glycan fragments detected by MALDI-FT-ICR mass spectrometry imaging impact gastric cancer biology and patient outcome. *Oncotarget* **2017**, *8*, 68012–68025. [CrossRef] [PubMed]

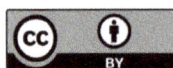

International Journal of
Molecular Sciences

MDPI

Article

Molecular Characterization of Gastric Epithelial Cells Using Flow Cytometry

Kevin A. Bockerstett, Chun Fung Wong, Sherri Koehm, Eric L. Ford and Richard J. DiPaolo *

Department of Molecular Microbiology and Immunology, Saint Louis University School of Medicine,
Saint Louis, MO 63104, USA; kevin.bockerstett@slu.edu (K.A.B.); johnny.wong@health.slu.edu (C.F.W.);
sherri.koehm@health.slu.edu (S.K.); eric.ford@health.slu.edu (E.L.F.)
* Correspondence: richard.dipaolo@health.slu.edu; Tel.: +1-(314)-977-8860; Fax: +1-(314)-977-8717

Received: 24 March 2018; Accepted: 4 April 2018; Published: 6 April 2018

Abstract: The ability to analyze individual epithelial cells in the gastric mucosa would provide important insight into gastric disease, including chronic gastritis and progression to gastric cancer. However, the successful isolation of viable gastric epithelial cells (parietal cells, neck cells, chief cells, and foveolar cells) from gastric glands has been limited due to difficulties in tissue processing. Furthermore, analysis and interpretation of gastric epithelial cell flow cytometry data has been difficult due to the varying sizes and light scatter properties of the different epithelial cells, high levels of autofluorescence, and poor cell viability. These studies were designed to develop a reliable method for isolating viable single cells from the corpus of stomachs and to optimize analyses examining epithelial cells from healthy and diseased stomach tissue by flow cytometry. We performed a two stage enzymatic digestion in which collagenase released individual gastric glands from the stromal tissue of the corpus, followed by a Dispase II digestion that dispersed these glands into greater than 1 $\times 10^6$ viable single cells per gastric corpus. Single cell suspensions were comprised of all major cell lineages found in the normal gastric glands. A method describing light scatter, size exclusion, doublet discrimination, viability staining, and fluorescently-conjugated antibodies and lectins was used to analyze individual epithelial cells and immune cells. This technique was capable of identifying parietal cells and revealed that gastric epithelial cells in the chronically inflamed mucosa significantly upregulated major histocompatibility complexes (MHC) I and II but not CD80 or CD86, which are costimulatory molecules involved in T cell activation. These studies describe a method for isolating viable single cells and a detailed description of flow cytometric analysis of cells from healthy and diseased stomachs. These studies begin to identify effects of chronic inflammation on individual gastric epithelial cells, a critical consideration for the study of gastric cancer.

Keywords: flow cytometry; gastric epithelium; autoimmune gastritis; atrophic gastritis

1. Introduction

Chronic atrophic gastritis is a common complication after infection with *Helicobacter pylori* and in individuals that develop autoimmune gastritis [1]. Chronic atrophic gastritis is a major risk factor for developing gastric cancer, which is the third most common cause of cancer-related deaths worldwide [2,3]. The pathophysiology of gastric cancer development has been well studied in several mouse models using primarily histopathological microscopy techniques [4]. While these are the standard techniques to analyze progression of pathologic changes in gastric epithelial tissue, there are difficulties in obtaining organ-wide surveys of epithelial cells. Proper statistical analysis would require the counting of numerous cells in many different areas of tissue [5]. With respect to these technical difficulties, flow cytometric analysis is ideal for measuring protein expression on individual gastric epithelial cells.

Flow cytometry relies on the identification of proteins using antibodies conjugated to fluorochromes that, when excited by incident light, emit fluorescence at distinct wavelengths. This enables identification of cell populations based on the wavelength of fluorescence detected [6]. Flow cytometry provides an organ-wide survey of protein expression that can be used to differentiate cell types, identify surface receptors, assess production of secreted protein products, determine activation state of transcription factors, and many other applications [7–10]. Flow cytometry analysis is used sparingly in the analysis of freshly isolated gastric epithelial cells partly due to the difficulties in tissue processing and data interpretation of highly autofluorescent populations [5,11–13].

The goal of this study was to provide a comprehensive methodology for single cell analysis of the complex gastric gland that is composed of parietal, chief, foveolar, and mucous neck cell types. This necessitated isolating individual cells from gastric corpus glands, staining for surface molecules, and gating that allows for analysis of gastric epithelial cells by flow cytometry. Generation of single cell suspension from the stomachs of BALB/c mice was assessed morphologically using cytospin preparations of gastric epithelial cells at various stages of digestion. Staining for antibodies against epithelial cell adhesion molecule (EpCAM) and cluster of differentiation (CD)45 were used to differentiate epithelial cells and hematopoietically derived immune cells, respectively. Analysis of gastric epithelial cells from control mice and from mice that develop autoimmune chronic atrophic gastritis (TxA23) allowed for a comparison of cells in the fundic mucosa under normal conditions and conditions of inflammatory gastric preneoplasia [14,15]. After generating single cell suspensions from cohorts of BALB/c and TxA23 mice, we used flow cytometry to: (1) Identify gastric epithelial cells; (2) identify immune cells in the gastric mucosa of mice with chronic atrophic gastritis; (3) identify parietal cells; and (4) demonstrate that inflammation causes a significant increase in major histocompatibility complex (MHC) molecules on the surface of gastric epithelial cells. The ability to isolate cells from the corpus mucosa, identify immune and epithelial cell populations using lineage specific markers, and analyze inflammation-induced changes by flow cytometry significantly enhances our ability to study the effects of chronic gastritis on the gastric epithelium in this model of gastric preneoplasia and others.

2. Results

2.1. Enzymatic Digestion Results in a Single Cell Suspension Comprised of Major Gastric Epithelial Cell Lineages

As flow cytometric analysis requires single cell suspensions, we sought to optimize a protocol that yielded high numbers of gastric epithelial single cells. We isolated gastric glands using collagenase and observed normal glandular structure by light microscopy following cytospin preparation (Figure 1A, left). Glands were then further digested into single cells using Dispase II and Cytospin preparations, confirming a majority of single cells present in solution (Figure 1A, right). We next isolated RNA from these single cell suspensions and assessed the major gastric epithelial cell lineages present using quantitative RT-PCR probes against parietal cells (*Atp4a*), chief cells (*Gif*), surface mucous cells (*Muc5ac*), and mucous neck cells (*Muc6*). This analysis determined that all of these major lineage transcripts were present, particularly *Atp4a* and *Gif*, which had crossing threshold (CT) values lower than that of the control target *Gapdh* (Figure 1B). Finally, we performed cell counting using Trypan blue exclusion and observed that these isolation methods yield on average over 1×10^6 viable cells (Figure 1C). Therefore, this epithelial cell isolation method generates single cell suspensions that contain major cell populations present in the stomach.

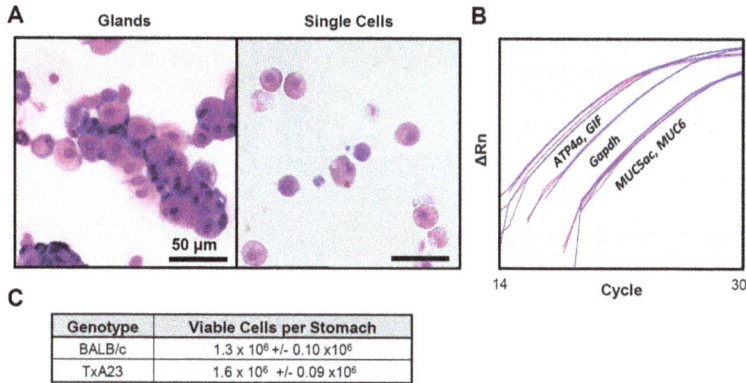

Figure 1. Isolating single cells from gastric corpus glands. (**A**) Representative cytospins of freshly isolated glands (left) and single cell suspensions generated from glands isolated from the corpus mucosa of stomach from mice (right). (**B**) qRT-PCR analysis of lineage markers for parietal cells (*Atp4a*), chief cells (*Gif*), surface mucous cells (*Muc5ac*), and mucous neck cells (*Muc6*). mRNA was isolated from gastric glands as seen in (**A**). (**C**) Table showing average viable cell number determined using Trypan blue exclusion from BALB/c and TxA23 mice. *n* = 3 mice per group.

2.2. Optimizing Flow Cytometric Analysis of Gastric Epithelial Cells

Gastric epithelial cells have proven to be difficult to analyze by flow cytometry, in part, due to the degree of cell-intrinsic autofluorescence and the tendency of epithelial cells to re-aggregate after isolation. To minimize autofluorescence and the improper analysis of cell doublets, we developed a strategy to: (1) Filter cells immediately before analysis, (2) exclude highly autofluorescent cell fragments according to size and internal complexity, (3) exclude aggregated cells according to the ratio of cell height to cell area, and (4) differentiate dead cells according to cell viability dye. The forward-scatter vs. side-scatter gate specifically excludes very small cell fragments and debris (Figure 2A, left). The single cell gate compares the height of a given event to its area, and events that fall along the central axis are single cells rather than aggregated multiplets (Figure 2A, center). Finally, dead cells are excluded using a viability dye, 7-aminoactinomycin D (AAD), that preferentially stains dying cells with porous membranes (Figure 2A, right). We then selected epithelial cells according to the expression of epithelial cell adhesion molecule (EpCAM/CD206). In the case of cells isolated from our mouse model of autoimmune gastritis, it is necessary to exclude infiltrating immune cells present in the sample using CD45 staining, a cellular protein expressed on all hematopoietically-derived cells (Figure 2B). These methods minimize autofluorescence and cell aggregation and provide a way to specifically analyze the effect of chronic inflammation on individual gastric epithelial cells while excluding hematopoietically derived immune cells. Finally, we wanted to use this methodology to identify a gastric epithelial cell lineage. *Dolichos biflorus* agglutinin (DBA) has been previously shown to be a parietal cell-specific staining reagent [16,17]. We performed immunocytochemistry on glands from BALB/c mice and stained them with Hoechst, DBA-fluorescein isothiocyanate (FITC), and anti-EpCAM antibodies and observed parietal cell specific staining (Figure 2C). We then adapted DBA staining to our flow cytometry analysis and observed a subset of EpCAM+cells that were also DBA+ (Figure 2D), demonstrating the ability to identify parietal cells using flow cytometry.

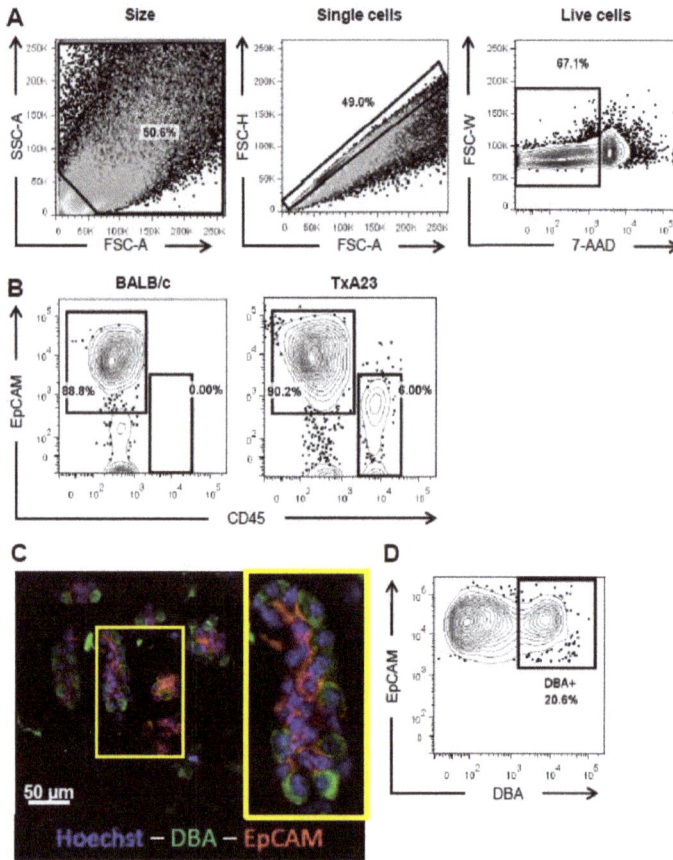

Figure 2. Gating strategy for analyzing gastric epithelial cells by flow cytometry. (**A**) A gate based of forward area and side scatter area is first established, these cells are then put through a forward scatter area and forward scatter height gate to identify single cells, finally, 7-AAD is used to separate live cells from dead/dying cells; (**B**) Representative flow plots of live single cells from healthy BALB/c and TxA23 mice stained with an epithelial cell marker (EpCAM) and an immune cell marker (CD45). Immune cells are undetectable in the gastric mucosa control mice, and present in TxA23 mice that have autoimmune gastritis; (**C**) Representative immunocytochemistry of glands isolated from a 2 month old BALB/c mouse and stained with hoechst (blue), parietal cell marker Dolichous bifluorous agglutinin (DBA, green), and anti-EpCAM (red) with a high magnification inset in yellow showing an individual gland; (**D**) A representative flow cytometry plot of live single cells from a BALB/c mouse stained with anti-EpCAM and DBA demonstrating a subset of EpCAM + DBA + parietal cells.

2.3. Gastric Epithelial Cells Upregulate MHC-I and MHC-II in Response to Chronic Inflammation

Cell lines and immunofluorescent staining of gastric mucosal tissue sections have been used to demonstrate that gastric epithelial cells respond to inflammatory stimuli such as interferon-γ by expressing MHC-II [18,19]. Preparation of single cell suspensions involves the use of proteases that could alter the detection of proteins expressed on the cell surface by flow cytometry. To determine if our methodology was capable of detecting MHC-I and MHC-II upregulation directly ex vivo from chronically inflamed mucosa we analyzed MHC-I and MHC-II on gastric epithelial cells (GECs) isolated from normal BALB/c stomachs and chronically inflamed TxA23 stomachs. Analysis revealed that MHC-I proteins were upregulated >150-fold on TxA23 GECs compared to BALB/c (mean fluorescence intensity: 260 ± 19.5 vs. $42,390 \pm 1783$). Furthermore, while MHC-II expression levels were undetectable on BALB/c GECs, expression levels were >1500 fold higher on GECs isolated from mice with autoimmune gastritis (mean fluorescence intensity: 12.6 ± 12.6 vs. $19,990 \pm 1682$) (Figure 3A–D). Immunofluorescent staining of corpus sections from BALB/c and TxA23 confirmed that MHC-II protein expression was much higher on epithelial cells in the chronically inflamed stomach (Figure 3E). Overall these studies indicate that this method is both sensitive and specific to inflammation-induced changes in the gastric epithelium and can be used for direct ex vivo analysis of gastric epithelial samples.

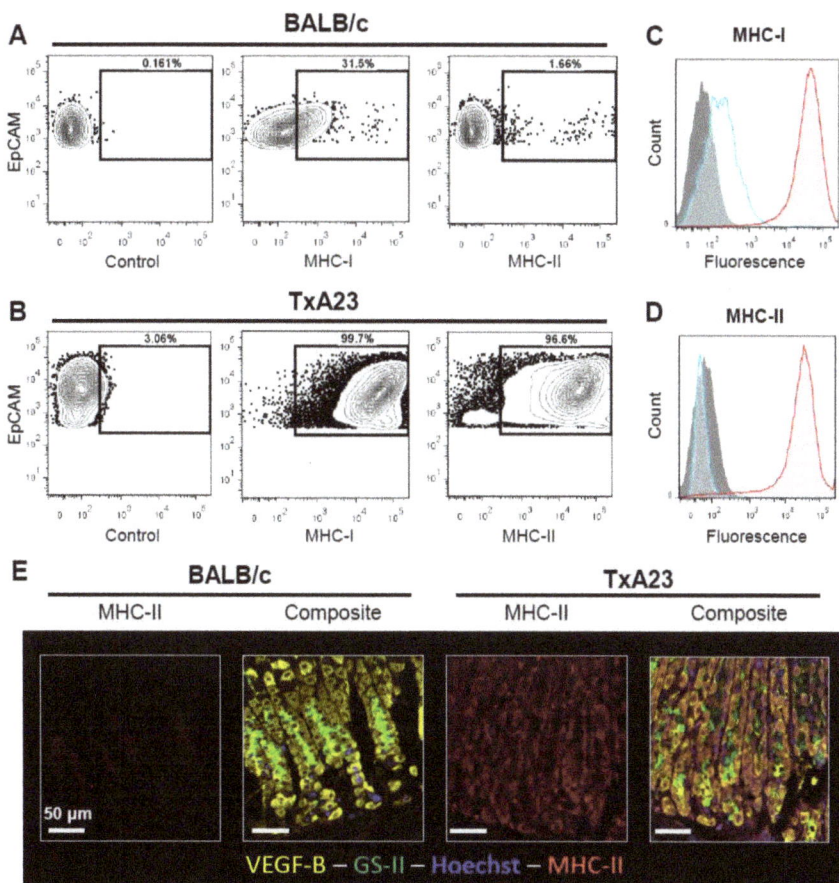

Figure 3. Gastric epithelial cells upregulate MHC-I and MHC-II in response to inflammation. (**A,B**) Representative flow plots of EpCAM+CD45-gated cells stained with antibodies to detect MHC-I or MHC-II surface proteins. Identical gating strategies show that MHC-I and MHC-II molecules are expressed at higher levels on gastric epithelial cells from mice with autoimmune gastritis (TxA23 mice). (**C,D**) Histograms showing the relative expression of MHC I and MHC II in BALB/c (blue) and TxA23 (red) mice. Data are representative of 2 experiments, 5 mice per group. (**E**) Representative images of gastric tissue sections from BALB/c and TxA23 mice stained with Hoechst (blue), VEGF-B (yellow), GS-II (green), and MHC-II (red).

3. Discussion

Microscopic analysis is standard in studies of the pathophysiology of gastric diseases. It allows for the qualitative assessment of disease phenotype and epithelial cell changes and, when coupled with techniques like immunofluorescence and immunohistochemistry, it also allows for comparisons of protein expression. However, quantitation of these data is time-consuming and highly dependent upon proper tissue preparation and sampling of many portions of the tissue in the case of focal disease processes. To assess gastric epithelial cell changes in our model of inflammation-induced gastric atrophy, TxA23, we have developed a reliable method for processing tissue and analyzing via flow cytometry that yields repeatable results.

Our method of tissue processing involves a two-step enzymatic digestion: first with collagenase to release the glands from the stromal tissue, followed by a digestion step with Dispase II that further separates glands into single cells. While previous publications have noted that enzyme digestion is harsh on cells and significantly effects viability, our use of this method generates an average of 1 million viable single cells per stomach (Figure 1C) [5]. Moreover, this digestion protocol requires no special equipment beyond a microtiter plate shaker placed at 37 degrees Celsius. We have also observed that gastric epithelial cells are very sensitive to centrifugation, with speeds above 50× gravity decreasing viability. This change in protocol could explain our improved cell yields despite the use of enzyme digestion. While previous studies have used various forms of enzymatic digestion, these publications reported additional steps involving mechanical disruption, microdissection, DNase incubation, or frequent media changes during digestion. However, we did not determine these additional steps to be necessary for successful isolation of viable single cells. [5,11,13] (Table 1).

Table 1. Comparison of Methods for Generating Single Cell Suspensions.

Reference	Disruption	Enzymes	Region	FACs Gating Description
Zavros et al.; 2000 [5]	Medimachine	Collagenase	Whole Stomach	No
Moore et al.; 2015 [11]	Medimachine	Dispase II	Corpus	No
Hinkle et al.; 2003 [13]	None	Pronase	Corpus	No
Bockerstett et al.; 2018	None	Collagenase + Dispase II	Corpus	Yes

Following single cell suspension, cells were stained with 7-AAD, a DNA-binding viability dye that efficiently discriminates between live and dead cells during flow cytometric analysis. Attempts to use fixable viability dyes that bind to free amines as a measure of cell viability proved difficult to interpret due to high background staining. This is possibly due to nonspecific staining of mucins, as 7-AAD binds to nucleic acid rather than protein substrates. Anti-EpCAM was also used to select only the epithelial cells, which is critical for distinguishing between immune and epithelial cells in models with significant inflammatory infiltrate. All staining was done in PBS supplemented with 0.5% bovine serum albumin and 2 mM ethylenediamineteraacetic acid (EDTA) to prevent aggregation of cells during staining. When analyzing, we first exclude cells by size and internal complexity using forward and side scatter of incident light. As GECs are much larger and more complex than typical lymphocytes, voltage levels for the forward-scatter and side-scatter detectors were adjusted accordingly. We then gated on viability dye negative, EpCAM positive cells for the remainder of the analysis. To verify the ability of this method to detect differential expression of surface markers, we stained epithelial cells with anti-major histocompatibility complex class I (MHC-I), which is present on most nucleated cells and compared it to the expression of MHC class II, which is a molecule typically limited to antigen presenting cells of the immune system. In normal BALB/c mice, we see typical expression of MHC-I and little to no expression of MHC-II on gastric epithelial cells. While antibodies against lineage markers of the gastric epithelium have been published as effective in differentiating the different cell types using flow cytometry [5,12,20], we found no staining conditions that were sufficiently specific to confidently distinguish between lineages using the published antibodies. However, we were able to identify parietal cells using the fluorescently conjugated DBA lectin that has been published in tissue staining as a parietal cell specific marker [16,17]. This is the first report of using flow cytometry to identify parietal cells according to staining with DBA. It should also be noted that use of a hematopoietic immune cell marker such as CD45 also allows for the analysis of infiltrating immune cells without interference from the more problematic epithelial cell populations, which has also been a focus of some groups [21]. We repeated these analyses using C57Bl6 mice, which are commonly used in mouse models of gastric cancer, and observed no difference in the efficacy of these cell isolation and FACs analysis methods.

It has been described that epithelial cells of the gastrointestinal tract, such as those of the small intestine, react to inflammatory stimuli by upregulating MHC-I and MHC-II and are even capable of presenting antigens to CD4+ T cells. It has also been shown that gastric epithelial cell lines exhibit this phenomenon and that MHC-II plays a role in the adherence of *Helicobacter pylori* to the gastric epithelium and induction of apoptosis by crosslinking of MHC-II molecules [18,19]. We wanted to use our method to perform a direct ex vivo analysis of inflammation-induced changes in MHC expression. To do this, we analyzed MHC-I and MHC-II expression on gastric epithelial cells of mice with chronic atrophic gastritis (TxA23) compared to normal gastric epithelium (BALB/c). We observed a significant upregulation in both MHC-I and MHC-II, which duplicates results seen by other groups using immunofluorescent staining. While we did not observe the expression of costimulatory molecules required for naïve T cell activation, MHC-II expression could implicate a role for gastric epithelial cells in reactivating infiltrating CD4 T cells during chronic inflammatory states, furthering disease progression by stimulating the production of more inflammatory cytokines. However, this requires further experimentation to determine unequivocally.

From these experiments we conclude that enzymatic digestion to single cells followed by flow cytometric analysis is an effective way to analyze large numbers of viable gastric epithelial cells, and that this method is useful for studying inflammatory changes in surface markers on gastric epithelial cells during chronic disease processes such as *Helicobacter* infection or autoimmune gastritis. It is anticipated that this method will enable valuable future studies in the gastric cancer field such as: analysis of immune activating or inhibitory receptors on gastric epithelial cells, changes in the expression of these receptors during inflammation, fluorescence activated cell sorting of gastric epithelial cell populations based on protein expression, and single cell RNA-SEQ analysis of gastric epithelium.

4. Methods

4.1. Mice

TxA23 mice express a transgenic T cell receptor specific for a peptide from H^+/K^+ ATPase alpha chain and spontaneously develop preneoplastic lesions such as parietal cell atrophy, mucous neck cell hyperplasia, and spasmolytic polypeptide expressing metaplasia [14,15,22,23]. BALB/c mice were purchased from Jackson Laboratories. All mice were maintained in our animal facility and cared for in accordance with institutional guidelines (Protocol 2600, Approved 6-07-2016 by the Saint Louis University Institutional Care and Use Committee).

4.2. Immunofluorescence/Immunohistochemistry

Stomachs were prepared, stained, and imaged using methods modified from Ramsey et al. [24]. The primary antibodies used for immunostaining were goat anti-VEGF-B (1:100 from Santa Cruz Biotechnology, Santa Cruz, CA, USA, sc-13083) and rat anti-mouse MHC-II (1:100 from BD Biosciences, San Jose, CA, USA, 556999). Secondary antibodies, nuclear labeling, and GS-II lectin labeling were as described.

4.3. Generation of Gastric Epithelial Single Cell Suspensions

Gastric glands were isolated from the corpus region of BALB/c and TxA23 mouse stomachs using collagenase (10 mg/mL from Sigma-Aldrich, St. Louis, MO, USA, C9891) in a digestion media comprised of advanced MEM (Gibco, Gaithersburg, MD, USA, 12492-013), 20 mM HEPES, 0.2% BSA (Millipore, Burlington, MA, USA, 810033), penicillin-streptomycin (Sigma-Aldrich, P7081), and 50 µg/mL gentamycin (Sigma-Aldrich, G-1914). The whole gastric corpus was separated from the forestomach, antrum, and esophagus and agitated at 600 rpm in collagenase for 30 min at 37 °C. Following digestion, remaining gastric serosa and connective tissue were removed from the glands. Glands were pelleted by centrifugation at $50 \times g$ gravity for 10 min and washed twice using DMEM/F12 (Sigma-Aldrich, D6421) supplemented with penicillin-streptomycin, gentamycin, and 0.5 mM 1,4-Dithiothreitol (DTT) (Sigma-Aldrich, GE17-1318-01). Glands were then digested into single cells by agitating at 600 rpm using Dispase II (Sigma-Aldrich, D4693) for 90 min at 37 °C. Following Dispase digestion, single cells were washed twice using flow cytometry staining buffer supplemented with 20 mM EDTA (Promega, Madison, WI, USA, V4231) and counted using Trypan blue exclusion. For Cytospins, glands and cells were stained using the Hema 3 Stat Pack (Fisher Scientific, Hampton, NH, USA, 123-869) and spun onto microscopy slides using the Cytospin 4 Cytocentrifuge (ThermoFisher, Waltham, MA, USA, A78300003). For immunocytochemistry, Cytospin preparations were fixed in 4% PFA for 10 min followed by permeabilization in 0.5% BSA/0.1% Triton X-100/ 2 mM EDTA and then stained according to immunofluorescent protocols listed above.

4.4. Quantitative Real Time PCR

Total RNA was prepared using RNeasy Mini Kit (Qiagen, Hilden, Germany, 74104). The quantity and quality of RNA was determined using a NanoDrop 2000 spectrophotometer (Thermo Scientific). cDNA copy of RNA isolated from cells was done according to the manufacturer's instruction (High Capacity cDNA Reverse Transcription Kit, Applied Biosystems, Foster City, CA, USA). Quantitative PCR was run on the 7500 Real-Time PCR System (Applied Biosystems). The following primer/probe sets were used: *Gapdh* (Mm99999915_g1), *Atp4a* (Mm00444417_m1), *Gif* (Mm00433596_m1), *Muc5ac* (Mm01276718_M1), *Muc6* (Mm00725165_m1).

4.5. Flow Cytometry

Cell surface staining was performed on gastric epithelial cells in staining buffer (PBS + 2% BSA) supplemented with 20 mM EDTA. Cells were kept on ice at all points during the staining procedure and analysis to prevent cell aggregation. Staining against surface antigens was performed using antibodies against Pan CD45 (BD Biosciences, San Jose, CA, USA 559864), EpCAM (eBioscience, San Diego, CA, USA, 47-5791-80), CD45.1 (BD Pharmigen, San Jose, CA, USA, 553776), MHC-I (BioLegend, San Diego, CA, USA, 125506), MHC-II (BD Biosciences, 557000). Following surface stain, cells were washed twice, passed through a 40 µm filter, and resuspended in staining buffer with 1 µL/mL 7-AAD (eBioscience, 00-6993-42) for dead cell exclusion. For identification of parietal cells, single cell suspensions were fixed in 4% PFA for 5 min at 37 degrees Celsius followed by permeabilization in 0.5% BSA/0.1% Triton X-100/2 mM EDTA for 30 min in the dark at room temperature on a plate shaker. *Dolichos biflorus* agglutinin conjugated to FITC (EYLabs, San Mateo, CA, USA, F-1201) was then added to cells at 1:500 and incubated for 1 h in the dark at room temperature. All flow cytometry was performed on a BD LSRII and analyzed using FlowJo (FlowJo, LLC, Ashland, OH, USA).

4.6. Statistical Analysis

Data are expressed as means of individual determinations ± standard error. Statistical analysis was performed by either the Mann-Whitney *U* Test, an unpaired Student's *t*-test, or a two-way ANOVA with Bonferroni post-tests (* $p < 0.05$; ** $p < 0.01$; *** $p < 0.001$) using GraphPad Prism 5 (GraphPad Software, La Jolla, USA).

Acknowledgments: The authors thank Joy Eslick for assistance with flow cytometry; Grant Kolar, Barbara Nagel, and Katie Phelps from the Saint Louis University Research Microscopy and Histology Core for generation of tissue sections; and the Saint Louis University Comparative Medicine department for assistance in maintaining mouse colonies. Richard J. DiPaolo and is supported by the AGA Funderburg Research Award, the American Cancer Society (RSG-12-171-01-LIB), the National Institutes of Health (NIH) National Institute of Diabetes and Digestive and Kidney Diseases (RO1 DK110406) and a grant from the Digestive Diseases Research Core Center of the Washington University School of Medicine NIDDK P30DK52574.

Author Contributions: Kevin A. Bockerstett: study concept and design, acquisition of data, analysis and interpretation of data, drafting of the manuscript; Chun Fung Wong: acquisition of data, analysis and interpretation of data; Sherri Koehm: technical support, acquisition of data, analysis and interpretation of data; Eric L. Ford: acquisition of data, technical support; Richard J. DiPaolo: study concept and design, revision of manuscript, interpretation of data, obtained funding.

Conflicts of Interest: The authors declare no conflict of interest.

References

1. Ohata, H.; Kitauchi, S.; Yoshimura, N.; Mugitani, K.; Iwane, M.; Nakamura, H.; Yoshikawa, A.; Yanaoka, K.; Arii, K.; Tamai, H.; et al. Progression of chronic atrophic gastritis associated with helicobacter pylori infection increases risk of gastric cancer. *Int. J. Cancer* **2004**, *109*, 138–143. [CrossRef] [PubMed]

2. Ferlay, J.; Soerjomataram, I.; Dikshit, R.; Eser, S.; Mathers, C.; Rebelo, M.; Parkin, D.M.; Forman, D.; Bray, F. Cancer incidence and mortality worldwide: Sources, methods and major patterns in globocan 2012. *Int. J. Cancer* **2015**, *136*, E359–E386. [CrossRef] [PubMed]

3. Landgren, A.M.; Landgren, O.; Gridley, G.; Dores, G.M.; Linet, M.S.; Morton, L.M. Autoimmune disease and subsequent risk of developing alimentary tract cancers among 4.5 million us male veterans. *Cancer* **2011**, *117*, 1163–1171. [CrossRef] [PubMed]

4. Correa, P. A human model of gastric carcinogenesis. *Cancer Res.* **1988**, *48*, 3554–3560. [PubMed]

5. Zavros, Y.; van Antwerp, M.; Merchant, J.L. Use of flow cytometry to quantify mouse gastric epithelial cell populations. *Dig. Dis. Sci.* **2000**, *45*, 1192–1199. [CrossRef] [PubMed]

6. Brown, M.; Wittwer, C. Flow cytometry: Principles and clinical applications in hematology. *Clin. Chem.* **2000**, *46*, 1221–1229. [PubMed]

7. Lyons, A.B.; Parish, C.R. Determination of lymphocyte division by flow cytometry. *J. Immunol. Methods* **1994**, *171*, 131–137. [CrossRef]

8. Jung, T.; Schauer, U.; Heusser, C.; Neumann, C.; Rieger, C. Detection of intracellular cytokines by flow cytometry. *J. Immunol. Methods* **1993**, *159*, 197–207. [CrossRef]

9. Riccardi, C.; Nicoletti, I. Analysis of apoptosis by propidium iodide staining and flow cytometry. *Nat. Protoc.* **2006**, *1*, 1458–1461. [CrossRef] [PubMed]

10. Krutzik, P.O.; Crane, J.M.; Clutter, M.R.; Nolan, G.P. High-content single-cell drug screening with phosphospecific flow cytometry. *Nat. Chem. Biol.* **2008**, *4*, 132–142. [CrossRef] [PubMed]

11. Moore, B.D.; Jin, R.U.; Osaki, L.; Romero-Gallo, J.; Noto, J.; Peek, R.M., Jr.; Mills, J.C. Identification of alanyl aminopeptidase (CD13) as a surface marker for isolation of mature gastric zymogenic chief cells. *Am. J. Physiol. Gastrointest. Liver Physiol.* **2015**, *309*, G955–G964. [CrossRef] [PubMed]

12. Bertaux-Skeirik, N.; Feng, R.; Schumacher, M.A.; Li, J.; Mahe, M.M.; Engevik, A.C.; Javier, J.E.; Peek, R.M., Jr.; Ottemann, K.; Orian-Rousseau, V.; et al. CD44 plays a functional role in helicobacter pylori-induced epithelial cell proliferation. *PLoS Pathog.* **2015**, *11*, e1004663. [CrossRef] [PubMed]

13. Hinkle, K.L.; Bane, G.C.; Jazayeri, A.; Samuelson, L.C. Enhanced calcium signaling and acid secretion in parietal cells isolated from gastrin-deficient mice. *Am. J. Physiol. Gastrointest. Liver Physiol.* **2003**, *284*, G145–G153. [CrossRef] [PubMed]

14. McHugh, R.S.; Shevach, E.M.; Margulies, D.H.; Natarajan, K. A t cell receptor transgenic model of severe, spontaneous organ-specific autoimmunity. *Eur. J. Immunol.* **2001**, *31*, 2094–2103. [CrossRef]

15. Nguyen, T.L.; Khurana, S.S.; Bellone, C.J.; Capoccia, B.J.; Sagartz, J.E.; Kesman, R.A., Jr.; Mills, J.C.; DiPaolo, R.J. Autoimmune gastritis mediated by CD4⁺ T cells promotes the development of gastric cancer. *Cancer Res.* **2013**, *73*, 2117–2126. [CrossRef] [PubMed]

16. Li, Q.; Karam, S.M.; Gordon, J.I. Diphtheria toxin-mediated ablation of parietal cells in the stomach of transgenic mice. *J. Biol. Chem.* **1996**, *271*, 3671–3676. [CrossRef] [PubMed]

17. Mills, J.C.; Syder, A.J.; Hong, C.V.; Guruge, J.L.; Raaii, F.; Gordon, J.I. A molecular profile of the mouse gastric parietal cell with and without exposure to helicobacter pylori. *Proc. Natl. Acad. Sci. USA* **2001**, *98*, 13687–13692. [CrossRef] [PubMed]

18. Fan, X.; Crowe, S.E.; Behar, S.; Gunasena, H.; Ye, G.; Haeberle, H.; van Houten, N.; Gourley, W.K.; Ernst, P.B.; Reyes, V.E. The effect of class II major histocompatibility complex expression on adherence of helicobacter pylori and induction of apoptosis in gastric epithelial cells: A mechanism for T helper cell type 1-mediated damage. *J. Exp. Med.* **1998**, *187*, 1659–1669. [CrossRef] [PubMed]

19. Fan, X.; Gunasena, H.; Cheng, Z.; Espejo, R.; Crowe, S.E.; Ernst, P.B.; Reyes, V.E. Helicobacter pylori urease binds to class ii mhc on gastric epithelial cells and induces their apoptosis. *J. Immunol.* **2000**, *165*, 1918–1924. [CrossRef] [PubMed]

20. Jain, R.N.; Al-Menhali, A.A.; Keeley, T.M.; Ren, J.; El-Zaatari, M.; Chen, X.; Merchant, J.L.; Ross, T.S.; Chew, C.S.; Samuelson, L.C. Hip1r is expressed in gastric parietal cells and is required for tubulovesicle formation and cell survival in mice. *J. Clin. Investig.* **2008**, *118*, 2459–2470. [CrossRef] [PubMed]

21. El-Zaatari, M.; Kao, J.Y.; Tessier, A.; Bai, L.; Hayes, M.M.; Fontaine, C.; Eaton, K.A.; Merchant, J.L. Gli1 deletion prevents helicobacter-induced gastric metaplasia and expansion of myeloid cell subsets. *PLoS ONE* **2013**, *8*, e58935. [CrossRef] [PubMed]

22. Nguyen, T.L.; Dipaolo, R.J. A new mouse model of inflammation and gastric cancer. *Oncoimmunology* **2013**, *2*, e25911. [CrossRef] [PubMed]

23. Nguyen, T.L.; Makhlouf, N.T.; Anthony, B.A.; Teague, R.M.; DiPaolo, R.J. In vitro induced regulatory t cells are unique from endogenous regulatory t cells and effective at suppressing late stages of ongoing autoimmunity. *PLoS ONE* **2014**, *9*, e104698. [CrossRef] [PubMed]

24. Ramsey, V.G.; Doherty, J.M.; Chen, C.C.; Stappenbeck, T.S.; Konieczny, S.F.; Mills, J.C. The maturation of mucus-secreting gastric epithelial progenitors into digestive-enzyme secreting zymogenic cells requires mist1. *Development* **2007**, *134*, 211–222. [CrossRef] [PubMed]

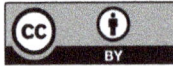

International Journal of
Molecular Sciences

MDPI

Review

Is There a Role for the Non-*Helicobacter pylori* Bacteria in the Risk of Developing Gastric Cancer?

Jackie Li and Guillermo I. Perez Perez *

Department of Medicine, New York University School of Medicine, New York, NY 10016, USA;
Jackie.Li@nyumc.org
* Correspondence: perezg02@med.nyu.edu; Tel.: +1-646-581-1339

Received: 4 April 2018; Accepted: 27 April 2018; Published: 3 May 2018

Abstract: *Helicobacter pylori* is the most abundant bacterium in the gastric epithelium, and its presence has been associated with the risk of developing gastric cancer. As of 15 years ago, no other bacteria were associated with gastric epithelial colonization; but thanks to new methodologies, many other non-*H. pylori* bacteria have been identified. It is possible that non-*H. pylori* may have a significant role in the development of gastric cancer. Here, we discuss the specific role of *H. pylori* as a potential trigger for events that may be conducive to gastric cancer, and consider whether or not the rest of the gastric microbiota represent an additional risk in the development of this disease.

Keywords: *H. pylori*; gastric microbiota; gastric cancer; pro-inflammation

1. Introduction

Helicobacter pylori was the first bacterium whose presence was associated with increased risk of developing any type of cancer, in this case gastric cancer [1,2]. This was an alarming finding in 1991, because *H. pylori* was, and continues to be, responsible for one of the most prevalent infections in humans globally [3]. However, it was demonstrated that only a minority of the subjects infected with *H. pylori* eventually developed gastric cancer [4]. *H. pylori* infected more than half of the world's population [3], but it is currently estimated that only between 1% and 3% of those infected individuals develop distal gastric cancer [5,6]. Furthermore, this risk is decreasing gradually with the decrease of *H. pylori* prevalence that has been occurring in the last 100 years [7,8]. This declining risk of developing gastric cancer varies by regions of the world, in which underdeveloped countries possess the larger number of cases for distal gastric cancer. Likewise, these same countries are where the prevalence of *H. pylori* is at its peak [9].

H. pylori is responsible for a series of histopathological changes in the gastric mucosa that are recognized as major factors in the development of gastric cancer. This particular series of histopathological changes that lead to gastric cancer are collectively known as Correa's model [10]. Correa's model was proposed several years before the discovery and isolation of *H. pylori*, and almost 15 years before the recognition of this organism as a risk factor for gastric cancer [1]. The model was developed exclusively based on histopathological observations related to the gradual progression from a normal gastric epithelium to gastric cancer [11]. Surprisingly, each of the histological changes proposed by Correa in his original paper were later confirmed with *H. pylori* findings, with the progression from a normal gastric mucosa prior to infection followed by chronic superficial gastritis, atrophic gastritis, intestinal metaplasia, dyspepsia and finally gastric carcinoma [12].

Recent progress in the identification of bacteria that colonize different body sites of the human host since birth, collectively named microbiota, has provided detailed insights into the numerous organisms present in the gut and a variety of other body sites, including the oral cavity, skin, lungs, etc. [13]. The human stomach is no exception, and we now know that in addition to *H. pylori*, many other organisms can be present, colonizing the stomach [14]. The relative abundance of bacteria other than *H. pylori* varies depending of the *H. pylori* status of the individual [14]. As a result of these findings, there are now major concerns of the role of bacteria other than *H. pylori* in the development of gastric cancer.

We discuss, in this review, the potential role of the human gastric microbiota in gastric carcinogenesis in the presence or absence of *H. pylori*. We also discuss which *H. pylori* traits contribute to increasing the risk of the development of gastric cancer and whether other members of the gastric microbiota possess similar capabilities.

2. Is *H. pylori* a Risk Factor or a True Carcinogen?

The first solid evidence of the association between *H. pylori* infection and gastric cancer was derived from three independent epidemiological studies published in 1991. All three studies reported elevated odds ratios for the development of gastric cancer in subjects who had tested positive for *H. pylori* more than 2 decades before the diagnosis of gastric cancer, when compared with subjects without *H. pylori* infection [15–17]. These types of studies have been repeated, and have confirmed the role of *H. pylori* as the most relevant risk factor in the development of gastric cancer [18].

The second type of evidence that implicates *H. pylori* as a risk factor in gastric pathology was obtained from animal models, including piglets, dogs and monkeys. Their normal gastric mucosa was challenged with *H. pylori*, and the development of active and chronic superficial gastritis, and in some cases atrophic gastritis, was confirmed to be associated with *H. pylori* colonization, but not with gastric cancer [19]. The first animal report of *H. pylori* inducing a progression from superficial gastritis to intestinal metaplasia (pre-malignant lesion) was with the use of the Mongolian gerbil model [20]. Some years later, using the same animal model it was confirmed that colonization with *H. pylori* can lead to the development of gastric cancer [21]. More recently, a report summarized the findings of several investigators who had developed a mouse model of gastric cancer in which *H. pylori* challenges were associated with the development of gastric cancer [22]. This model represents a major step forward in the study of *H. pylori* and its role in gastric cancer.

Another approach to documenting the role of *H. pylori* in gastric carcinogenesis is the use of in vitro models. Most of these studies have been dedicated to investigating the role of the major virulence factors of *H. pylori*, including the cytotoxin-associated gene pathogenicity island (CagPAI). It was discovered that *H. pylori* strains expressing the CagPAI are more virulent, and are more frequently isolated from patients with severe clinical outcomes of the infection, including peptic ulcer disease and gastric cancer. The CagPAI is a major chromosomal insertion, encoding around 34 genes, that can be acquired by horizontal transfer [23]. The demonstration that a subset of the CagPAI genes comprises a type IV secretion system was followed by multiple studies confirming the intimate interaction of the transferred CagA protein into the host cells [24]. As a result of these observations, it has been suggested that CagA may be the oncogenic factor in *H. pylori* [25]. It is important to mention that until now, there has not been a single study in vitro that has confirmed the mutagenic ability of *H. pylori* CagA, vacuolating cytotoxin (VacA), or any of its other components. Assessment of mutagenic activity of these factors using methods such as the Ames test is needed to confirm the role of CagA as a true oncogenic protein. The Ames test is a biological assay to assess mutagenic potential of individual compounds using bacteria to test its mutagenic activity. An in vivo experiment in a transgenic mouse model demonstrated that expression of CagA predominantly in the stomach was associated with epithelial hyperplasia, gastric polyps and adenocarcinoma. Systemic expression of CagA was associated with leukocytosis, leukemia and B cell lymphomas [26]. It is important to mention that such neoplastic effects mostly occur after 70 weeks of age, suggesting a chronic process. If *H. pylori* and its components have no direct mutagenic effects in gastric epithelial cells, how does *H. pylori* affect the gastric epithelium in order for it to be considered a major risk factor in gastric cancer development?

Int. J. Mol. Sci. **2018**, *19*, 1353

To answer this question, we need to revisit the Correa model. Colonization with *H. pylori* occurs early in life, and is maintained for decades or perhaps for the whole life of the colonized individual. The presence of *H. pylori* induces a superficial chronic gastritis influencing the balance between the rate of cellular loss and regeneration [27]. The chronic inflammation induced by *H. pylori* maintains a constant production of a cascade of cytokines, which attracts neutrophils that generate oxidative radicals that have the potential to damage the host DNA. Infection with *H. pylori* has been associated with a reduction in cell replication, and increase in apoptosis, autophagy induction, and endoplasmic reticulum and oxidative/nitrosative stress [28]. These innate immune responses are important to enhance cell survival and proliferation, but as a consequence of the chronic inflammation process due to *H. pylori*, there is a greater chance of acquiring potentially malignant characteristics, which may explain the relevance of this infection as a major risk factor in the development of gastric cancer [28]. This chronic, so-called pro-inflammatory, process appears to be a common denominator and initiator of several chronic diseases [29]. The pro-inflammatory conditions, in concert with the immune response, can lead to a necrotic state. In infections with hepatitis virus B and C, this has been linked to the development of liver cancer. This identical pathophysiological mechanism might be related to *H. pylori* infection and the development of gastric cancer.

Pro-inflammation is a key player in the chronic interaction between *H. pylori* and the host. The original study of El-Omar et al. [30] reported a strong association between pro-inflammatory cytokine polymorphisms and increase risk of developing *H. pylori*-associated gastric cancer. This study provides strong evidence for the influence of host genetic factors and the possibility that the immune necrotic state is relevant for the development of gastric cancer. In addition, these results indicate that an increased inflammatory response, particularly linked with an over-production of pro-inflammatory cytokines and mediators in the Th1 pathway, increase the odds ratio of *H. pylori*-positive individuals developing gastric cancer [31]. Several studies have reported an even greater risk of developing gastric cancer in individuals that are colonized with highly virulent *H. pylori* strains expressing CagA and VacA, and simultaneously carrying cytokine polymorphisms associated with pro-inflammation. Here, the odds ratio for developing gastric cancer increases more than 40-fold [32].

With the improvement of sequencing technology, it has been demonstrated that in addition to *H. pylori*, other bacteria also colonize the gastric mucosa [14]. An important medical question to ask is: What is the role of the non-*H. pylori* microbiota in the process of gastric carcinogenesis? Particularly, what role do these microorganisms play once *H. pylori* has produced gastric atrophy and intestinal metaplasia, and is no longer capable of colonizing the affected gastric mucosa?

3. Gastric Microbiota and its Influence on Gastric Carcinogenesis

The recent development of methods for the analysis of 16S rRNA data has provided a clear picture of the bacterial communities present in the human host [33]. Of particular relevance to the detected microbes for this review has been the characterization of the gastric microbiota in patients with and without *H. pylori* infection [34]. One interesting observation was the presence of *H. pylori* sequences in biopsy samples of subjects who had been identified as *H. pylori* negative by most conventional methods [35]. These results show that we now have a powerful and highly sensitive method for detecting bacteria present in very low numbers. However, Kim et al. have established that a key indicator of the biological relevance of detected microbes is the relative abundances of their sequences [35]. In the majority of studies in which subjects were reported negative for *H. pylori* by conventional methods, the sequence data demonstrated the relative abundances of *Helicobacter* to be <2.0%. The clinical relevance of these low-relative-abundance sequences of *H. pylori* remains unsolved. To assess the role of the gastric microbiota as a potential player in *H. pylori*-associated gastric cancer, and to determine the potential interactions between the gastric commensal bacteria and *H. pylori*, it is important to consider the relative abundance of these players, and what type of effect they could produce. In addition, we need to consider the presence of *H. pylori* and its impact on the gastric microbiota, as well as the selectivity that *H. pylori* has in colonizing the gastric epithelium, where any changes affecting the gastric mucosa may affect the ability of *H. pylori* to colonize the stomach.

Another relevant point that needs to be considered is the occurrence of dysbiosis in the gastric community. Most currently available studies report changes in the gastric microbiota in patients with gastric cancer compared to those without [6]. Because of the series of histological changes leading to gastric cancer, the assessment of variations in the gastric microbiota in cancer patients versus non-gastric cancer patients can be clearly predictive. The Correa model describes the histological changes that lead to the progression from a normal gastric mucosa to gastric cancer. The normal acidic pH of the stomach is no longer a main feature of patients with gastric cancer, and they are more likely to present achlorhydria, which is a condition that makes the stomach more permissible for colonization [36,37]. Therefore, the number and type of bacteria colonizing the stomachs of cancer patients will be different from those without cancer.

We need to remember that the chronic infection of *H. pylori* in the stomach induces several histopathological changes in the gastric epithelium. In particular, the early pre-malignant changes involving the presence of intestinal metaplasia may precipitate the elimination of *H. pylori* from the human stomach (Figure 1). We believe that those histological changes are critical in the gradual loss of *H. pylori* colonization and the replacement with other microbiota with the capabilities to colonize the modified gastric tissue.

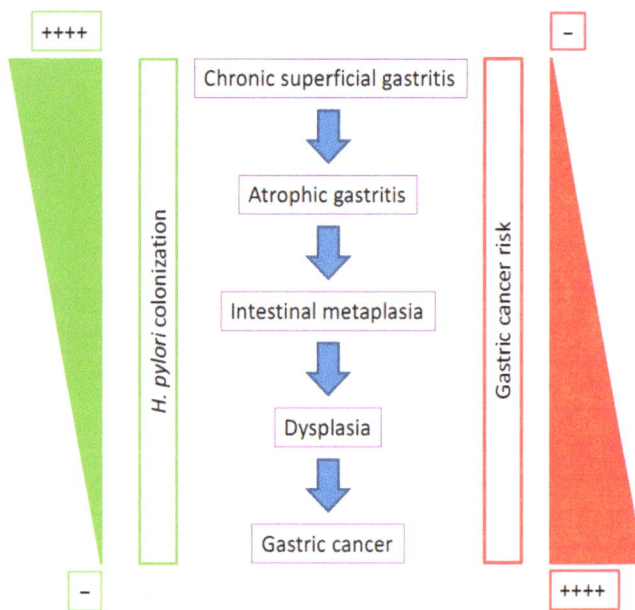

Figure 1. Opposite trends for *H. pylori* density and noncardia gastric cancer risk in relation to the histopathological changes in the human gastric mucosa.

Another important point in the study of the gastric microbiota and its association with *H. pylori* and gastric carcinogenesis is the nature of *H. pylori* colonization, which has a patchy distribution [11]. There are no systematic studies of the gastric microbiota that evaluate whether the presence and composition of the microbiota in the gastric epithelium is homogeneous, or whether it is patchy, like that of *H. pylori*. In order to evaluate this point, multiple gastric biopsies from the same individual need to be studied to determine the true distribution of the gastric microbiota. Furthermore, location of *H. pylori* colonization in the stomach may predict the clinical outcome [38]. It has been suggested that colonization of the antrum region of the stomach is linked with the development of duodenal ulcer. In contrast, the colonization of the body or corpus of the stomach has been associated with a higher risk of developing gastric ulcers and gastric cancer. This topographic distribution of the diseases associated with *H. pylori* may be related to the fact that the enzyme gastric HK-ATPase is found in the gastric parietal cells that are mostly located at the oxyntic gastric glands of the gastric body [39]. The distribution of the acid-producing cells mentioned above might explain why colonization with *H. pylori* of this specific stomach region is a major risk factor for the development of gastric cancer. Future studies aiming to evaluate the role of the gastric microbiota in the development of gastric cancer should specify from which region of the stomach the gastric biopsies are taken.

The relevance of the gastric microbiota in the development of gastric cancer has been confirmed using the transgenic insulin-gastrin mouse model. INS-GAS mice colonized with *H. pylori* alone have a delayed onset of gastric cancer when compared with mice infected with *H. pylori* harboring a gastric microbiota [40]. These results indicate that a gastric microbiota magnifies the effects of *H. pylori* in gastric carcinogenesis but does not necessarily have a direct role in carcinogenesis. *H. pylori* is the major trigger of the histopathological changes leading to gastric cancer and its presence influences the gastric microbiota. In addition, most of the effects related to the development of gastric cancer in *H. pylori* infection are exacerbated if the infected strain is CagA+. However, infection with *H. pylori* CagA+ strains has minor effects on the gastric microbiota, affecting alpha diversity, but not beta diversity or its relative abundance [41].

Most studies of the gastric microbiota have shown that the most dominant phyla are Proteobacteria, Firmicutes, Actinobacteria, Bacteroides, and Fusobacteria [39]. These same phyla are dominant in all the other sites of the human host [33]. This constant prevalence of the same microbes makes it difficult to identify major differences in the microbiota in patients with different clinical outcomes. However, even as some of the studies reported differences in the gastric microbiota between patients with gastritis and patients with gastric cancer [6], it is impossible to determine whether those differences are the cause or the effect of the changes in the gastric epithelium.

Only a few studies have investigated the changes in the gastric microbiota in the pre-malignant stages of gastric cancer (gastric atrophy and intestinal metaplasia) [6,42], or compared the composition of the gastric microbiota in cancer tissue versus non-cancer tissue from the same patient [43]. In the pre-malignant stages, the main finding is that *H. pylori* dominates the microbiota, making it difficult to observe relevant taxa differences between cancer and non-cancer tissue in the same patient.

There are no well-designed studies that implicate the participation of non-*H. pylori* gastric microbiota in the development of gastric cancer. However, in some regions of the world, despite the decline of *H. pylori* infections, increased incidence of gastric cancer has been reported [44,45]. Interestingly, most of these cases have been observed in young adults (<40 years) [46–48]. This new epidemiological data may suggest that changes in the gastric microbiota mainly associated with new standards of living, and not infection with *H. pylori*, could be implicated in this age-specific increase in gastric cancer [46]. There are some characteristics of these new cases of non-cardia cancer in young individuals that are different from the traditional non-cardia cancer of all individuals. There is a concordance in most of the reports that young subjects (<40 years) with non-cardia cancer had a more diffuse type than older subjects (>40 years) [46–49]. Furthermore, contrary to previous statistics in which gastric cancer affected males twice as frequently as females [48], non-cardia cancer in young subjects (<40 years) had an occurrence in women that was higher than or equal to that in men [46–48].

A possible explanation for the recent increase in gastric cancer in the USA is perhaps the large immigration of Hispanic populations that has occurred recently [49]. However, the incidence of gastric cancer in Hispanics cannot explain the increased incidence of gastric cancer in young individuals in all regions of the world. Another possibility is that changes in non-cardia cancer related to age and sex might be associated with an increased risk of developing autoimmune gastritis [46]. Autoimmune gastritis was associated with elderly women of Northern European ancestry, but has recently been recognized as a disease in all populations and ethnic groups [50], with a predominance in women and early-age onset, similar to the incidence of gastric cancer in young individuals. This disease could be an alternative explanation for the increased incidence of gastric cancer in young subjects (<40 years). However, autoimmune gastritis occurs in all populations and ethnic groups [51], and does not explain the specific increase of non-cardia cancer exclusively in the white non-Hispanic population in the US [46].

A recent Japanese study suggested the assessment of aberrant DNA methylation in gastric tissue as a means to determine risk of gastric cancer [52]. Hypermethylation of DNA sequences in specific genes, such as tumor suppressor genes, has been observed in the gastric mucosa of infected *H. pylori* subjects [28]. Therefore, identification of epigenetic markers for gastric cancer risk might be important for assessing gastric cancer risk. It is imperative to monitor older subjects who are *H. pylori* negative and living in high-prevalence areas of gastric cancer and *H. pylori* infection for potential development of gastric cancer. Two independent studies have recently reported the benefits of antibiotic treatment in reducing the development of gastric cancer particularly in older individuals [53,54]. Both studies found that early treatment had a significant reduction in the risk of developing gastric cancer. In addition, one of the studies found that the risk for gastric cancer gradually increases with increased number of eradication treatments in patients [54].

In conclusion, the published studies support the idea that the presence of *H. pylori* has a major effect on the composition and relative abundance of the gastric microbiota. In the absence of *H. pylori* the gastric microbiota likely contributes to the perpetuation of the inflammatory stimuli. The role of the microbiota as inflammation stimuli is particularly important in patients previously colonized by *H. pylori*. The pre-malignant changes in the gastric epithelium may favor the conditions for bacteria other than *H. pylori* to induce the inflammatory process related to cancer development. The term "point of no return" in the cascade of events that lead to gastric cancer has been associated with patients with intestinal metaplasia and dysplasia, independent of *H. pylori* status, who are at the highest risk of developing gastric cancer [28]. This phenomenon could explain why patients who become spontaneously negative for *H. pylori* continue on the pathway of gastric carcinogenesis.

Author Contributions: J.L. and G.I.P.P. made equal contributions to the design of this review. Both worked on creating the draft and substantively revised it. Both authors have approved the submitted version.

Conflicts of Interest: The authors declare no conflict of interest.

References

1. International Agency for Research on Cancer. IARC Monographs on the evaluation of carcinogenic risk to humans. In *Schistosomaotes, Liver Flukes and Helicobacter pylori*; IARC: Lyon, France, 1994; Volume 61, pp. 12–41.
2. European *Helicobacter pylori* study group. Current European concepts in the management of *Helicobacter pylori* infection—The Maastricht consensus report. *Gut* **1997**, *41*, 81–83.
3. Hooi, J.K.Y.; Lai, W.Y.; Suen, M.M.Y.; Underwood, F.E.; Tanyingoh, D.; Malfertheiner, P.; Graham, D.Y.; Wong, V.W.S.; Wu, J.C.Y.; Chan, F.K.L.; et al. Global prevalence of *Helicobacter pylori* infection: Systematic review and meta-analysis. *Gastroenterology* **2017**, *153*, 4204–4229. [CrossRef] [PubMed]
4. Peek, R.M.; Crabtree, J.E. *Helicobacter pylori* and gastric neoplasia. *J. Pathol.* **2006**, *208*, 2332–2348. [CrossRef] [PubMed]
5. Yakirevich, E.; Resnick, M.B. Pathology of gastric cancer and its precursor lesions. *Gastroenterol. Clin. N. Am.* **2013**, *42*, 2612–2684. [CrossRef] [PubMed]
6. Hsieh, Y.Y.; Tung, S.Y.; Pan, H.Y.; Yen, C.W.; Xu, H.W.; Lin, Y.J.; Deng, Y.F.; Hsu, W.T.; Wu, C.S.; Li, C. Increased abundance of *Clostridium* and *Fusobacterium* in gastric microbiota of patients with gastric cancer in Taiwan. *Sci. Rep.* **2018**, *8*, 158. [CrossRef] [PubMed]
7. Sonnenberg, A. Time trends of mortality from gastric cancer in Europe. *Dig. Dis. Sci.* **2011**, *56*, 1112–1118. [CrossRef] [PubMed]
8. Sonnenberg, A. Temporal trends and geographical variations of peptic ulcer disease. *Aliment. Pharmacol. Ther.* **1995**, *9* (Suppl. 2), 3–12. [PubMed]

9. Khalifa, M.M.; Sharaf, R.R.; Aziz, R.K. *Helicobacter pylori*: A poor man's gut pathogen? *Gut Pathog.* **2010**, *2*, 2. [CrossRef] [PubMed]

10. Correa, P.; Cuello, C.; Duque, E.; Burbano, L.C.; Garcia, F.T.; Bolanos, O.; Brown, C.; Haenszel, W. Gastric cancer in Colombia. III Natural history of precursor lesions. *J. Natl. Cancer Inst.* **1976**, *57*, 1027–1035. [CrossRef] [PubMed]

11. Correa, P. Human gastric carcinogenesis: A multistep and multifactorial process-First American Cancer Society Award lecture on Cancer Epidemiology and Prevention. *Cancer Res.* **1992**, *52*, 6735–6740. [PubMed]

12. Correa, P. *Helicobacter pylori* and gastric carcinogenesis. *Am. J. Surg. Pathol.* **1995**, *19* (Suppl. 1), S37–S43. [PubMed]

13. Relman, D.A. Microbiology: Learning about who we are. *Nature* **2012**, *486*, 1941–1995. [CrossRef] [PubMed]

14. Llorca, L.; Perez Perez, G.; Urruzuno, P.; Martinez, M.J.; Iizumi, T.; Gao, Z.; Shon, J.; Chung, J.; Cox, L.; Simon-Soro, A.; et al. Characterization of the gastric microbiota in a pediatric population according to *Helicobacter pylori* status. *Pediatr. Infect. Dis.* **2017**, *36*, 1731–1778. [CrossRef] [PubMed]

15. Forman, D.; Newell, D.G.; Fullerton, F.; Yarnell, J.W.; Stacey, A.R.; Wald, N.; Sitas, F. Association between infection of *Helicobacter pylori* and risk of gastric cancer: Evidence from a prospective investigation. *BMJ* **1991**, *302*, 1302–1305. [CrossRef] [PubMed]

16. Nomura, A.; Stemmermann, G.N.; Chyou, P.H.; Kato, I.; Perez Perez, G.I.; Blaser, M.J. *Helicobacter pylori* infection and gastric carcinoma among Japanese American in Hawaii. *N. Engl. J. Med.* **1991**, *325*, 1132–1136. [CrossRef] [PubMed]

17. Parsonnet, J.; Friedman, G.D.; Vandersteen, D.P.; Chang, Y.; Vogelman, J.H.; Orentreich, N.; Sibley, R.K. *Helicobacter pylori* infection and the risk of gastric carcinoma. *N. Engl. J. Med.* **1991**, *325*, 1127–1131. [CrossRef] [PubMed]

18. Huang, J.Q.; Hunt, R.H. The evolving epidemiology of *Helicobacter pylori* infection and gastric cancer. *Can. J. Gastroenterol.* **2003**, *17* (Suppl. B), 18B–20B. [CrossRef] [PubMed]

19. Sugiyama, T. development of gastric cancer associated with *Helicobacter pylori* infection. *Cancer Chemother. Pharmacol.* **2004**, *54* (Suppl. 1), S12–S20. [CrossRef] [PubMed]

20. Hirayama, F.; Takagi, S.; Kusuhara, H.; Iwao, E.; Yokoyama, Y.; Ikeda, Y. Induction of gastric ulcer and intestinal metaplasia in Mongolian gerbils infected with *Helicobacter pylori*. *J. Gastroenterol.* **1996**, *31*, 755–757. [CrossRef] [PubMed]

21. Hirayama, F.; Takagi, S.; Iwao, E.; Yokoyama, Y.; Haga, K.; Hanada, S. Development of poor differentiated adenocarcinoma and carcinoid due to long term *Helicobacter pylori* colonization in Mongolian gerbils. *J. Gastroenterol.* **1999**, *34*, 450–454. [CrossRef] [PubMed]

22. Poh, A.R.; O'Donoghue, R.J.J.; Ernst, M.; Putoczki, T.L. Mouse models for gastric cancer: Matching models to biological questions. *J. Gastroenterol. Hepatol.* **2016**, *31*, 1257–1272. [CrossRef] [PubMed]

23. Covacci, A.; Telford, J.L.; Del Giudice, G.; Parsonnet, J.; Rappuoli, R. *Helicobacter pylori* virulence and genetic geography. *Science* **1999**, *284*, 1328–1333. [CrossRef] [PubMed]

24. Higashi, H.; Tsutsumi, R.; Muto, S.; Sugiyama, T.; Azuma, T.; Asaka, M.; Hatekayama, M. SHP-2 tyrosine phosphatase as an intercellular target of *Helicobacter pylori* CagA protein. *Science* **2002**, *295*, 683–686. [CrossRef] [PubMed]

25. Zhang, C.; Powell, S.E.; Betel, D.; Shah, M.A. The gastric microbiome and its influence on gastric carcinogenesis. Current knowledge and ongoing research. *Hematol. Oncol. Clin. N. Am.* **2017**, *31*, 389–408. [CrossRef] [PubMed]

26. Ohnishi, N.; Yuasa, H.; Tanaka, S.; Sawa, H.; Miura, M.; Matsui, A.; Higashi, H.; Musashi, M.; Iwabuchi, K.; Suzuki, M.; et al. Transgenic expression of *Helicobacter pylori* CagA induces gastrointestinal and hematopoietic neoplasms in mouse. *Proc. Natl. Acad. Sci. USA* **2008**, *105*, 1003–1008. [CrossRef] [PubMed]

27. Sugiyama, T.; Asaka, M. *Helicobacter pylori* infection and gastric cancer. *Med. Electron Microsc.* **2004**, *37*, 149–157. [CrossRef] [PubMed]

28. Diaz, P.; Valenzuela Valderrama, M.; Bravo, J.; Quest, A.F.G. *Helicobacter pylori* and gastric cancer: Adaptive cellular mechanisms involved in diasese progression. *Front. Microbiol.* **2018**, *9*, 5. [CrossRef] [PubMed]

29. Esch, T.; Stefano, G.B. Proinflammation: A common denominator or initiator of different pathophysiological disease processes. *Med. Sci. Monit.* **2002**, *8*, HY1–HY9. [PubMed]

30. El-Omar, E.M.; Carrington, M.; Chow, W.; McColl, K.E.; Bream, J.H.; Young, H.A.; Herrera, J.; Lissowska, J.; Yuan, C.C.; Rothman, N.; et al. Interleukin-1 polymorphisms associated with increased risk of gastric cancer. *Nature* **2000**, *404*, 398–402. [CrossRef] [PubMed]

31. El-Omar, E.M. The importance of interleukin 1β in *Helicobacter pylori* associated disease. *Gut* **2001**, *48*, 743–747. [CrossRef] [PubMed]

32. Figueiredo, C.; Machado, J.C.; Pharoah, P.; Seruca, R.; Sousa, S.; Carvalho, R.; Capelinha, A.F.; Quint, W.; Caldas, C.; van Doorn, L.J.; et al. *Helicobacter pylori* and interleukin 1 genotyping: An opportunity to identify high-risk individuals for gastric carcinoma. *J. Natl. Cancer Inst.* **2002**, *94*, 1680–1687. [CrossRef] [PubMed]

33. Cho, I.; Blaser, M.J. The human microbiome at the interface of health and disease. *Nat. Rev. Genet.* **2012**, *3*, 260–270. [CrossRef] [PubMed]

34. Espinoza, J.L.; Matsumoto, A.; Tanaka, H.; Matsumura, I. Gastric microbiota: An emerging player in *Helicobacter pylori*-induced gastric malignancies. *Cancer Lett.* **2018**, *414*, 147–152. [CrossRef] [PubMed]

35. Kim, J.; Kim, N.; Jo, H.J.; Park, J.H.; Nam, R.H.; Seok, Y.J.; Kim, Y.R.; Kim, J.S.; Kim, J.M.; Kim, J.M.; et al. An appropriate cutoff value for determining the colonization of *Helicobacter pylori* by pyrosequencing method: Comparison with conventional methods. *Helicobacter* **2015**, *20*, 370–380. [CrossRef] [PubMed]

36. Parson, B.N.; Ijaz, U.; D'Amore, R.; Burkitt, M.D.; Eccles, R.; Lenzi, L.; Duckworth, C.A.; Moore, A.R.; Tiszlavicz, L.; Varro, A.; et al. Comparison of the human gastric microbiota in hypochlorhydria states arising as results of *Helicobacter pylori*-induced atrophic gastritis, autoimmune atrophic gastritis and proton pump inhibitor use. *PLoS Pathog.* **2017**. [CrossRef] [PubMed]

37. Thorell, K.; Bengtsson-Palme, J.; Liu, O.H.; Palacios Gonzales, R.V.; Nookaew, I.; Rabeneck, L.; Paszat, L.; Graham, D.Y.; Nielsen, J.; Lundin, S.B.; et al. In vivo analysis of the viable microbiota and *Helicobacter pylori* transcriptome in gastric infection and early stages of carcinogenesis. *Infect. Immun.* **2017**, *85*, e00031-17. [CrossRef] [PubMed]

38. Shanks, A.M.; El-Omar, E.M. *Helicobacter pylori* infection, host genetics and gastric cancer. *J. Dig. Dis.* **2009**, *10*, 157–164. [CrossRef] [PubMed]

39. Shon, S.H.; Kim, N.; Jo, H.J.; Kim, J.; Park, J.H.; Nam, R.H.; Seok, Y.-J.; Kim, Y.-R.; Lee, D.H. Analysis of gastric body microbiota by pyrosequencing : Possible role of bacteria other than *Helicobacter pylori* in the gastric carcinogenesis. *J. Cancer Prev.* **2017**, *22*, 115–125. [CrossRef]

40. Lofgren, J.L.; Whary, M.T.; Ge, Z.; Muthupalani, S.; Taylor, N.S.; Mobley, M.; Potter, A.; Varro, A.; Elbach, D.; Suerbaum, S.; et al. Lack of commensal flora in *Helicobacter pylori*-infected INS-GAS mice reduces gastritis and delays intraepithelial neoplasia. *Gastroenterology* **2011**, *140*, 210–220. [CrossRef] [PubMed]

41. Klymiuk, I.; Bilgilier, C.; Stadlmann, A.; Thannesberger, J.; Kastner, M.T.; Hogenauer, C.; Puspok, A.; Biowski-Frotz, S.; Schrutka-Kolbl, C.; Thallinger, G.G.; et al. The human gastric microbiome is predicated upon infection with *Helicobacter pylori*. *Front. Microbiol.* **2017**, *8*, 2508. [CrossRef] [PubMed]

42. Ferreira, R.M.; Pereira-Marques, J.; Pinto-Ribero, I.; Costa, J.L.; Carneiro, F.; Machado, J.C.; Figueiredo, C. Gastric microbial community profiling reveals a dysbiotic cancer-associated microbiota. *Gut* **2018**, *67*, 226–236. [CrossRef] [PubMed]

43. Coker, O.O.; Dai, Z.; Nie, Y.; Zhao, G.; Cao, L.; Nakatsu, G.; Wu, W.K.; Wong, S.H.; Chen, Z.; Sung, J.J.Y.; et al. Mucosal Microbiome dysbiosis in gastric carcinogenesis. *Gut* **2017**, in press. [CrossRef] [PubMed]

44. Zhou, F.; Shi, J.; Fang, C.; Zou, X.; Huang, O. Gastric carcinoma in young (younger than 40 years) Chinese patients: Clinicopathology, family history, and postresection survival. *Medicine* **2016**, *95*, e2873. [CrossRef] [PubMed]

45. Anderson, W.F.; Camargo, M.C.; Fraumeni, J.F.; Correa, P.; Rosenberg, P.S.; Rabkin, C.S. Age-specific trends in incidence of non cardi- gastric cáncer in the US adults. *JAMA* **2010**, *303*, 1723–1728. [CrossRef] [PubMed]

46. Anderson, W.F.; Rabkin, C.S.; Turner, N.; Fraumeni, J.F.; Rosenberg, P.S.; Camargo, M.C. The changing face of noncardia gastric cancer incidence among US non-Hispanic Whites. *J. Natl. Cancer Inst.* **2018**. [CrossRef] [PubMed]

47. Ji, T.; Zhou, F.; Wang, J.; Zi, L. Risk factors for lymphonode metastasis of early gastric cancer in patients younger than 40. *Medicine* **2017**, *96*, 37. [CrossRef] [PubMed]

48. Braga-Neto, M.B.; Gomes carneiro, J.; de Castro Barbosa, A.M.; Silva, I.S.; Maia, D.C.; Maciel, F.S.; Alves de Alcantara, R.J.; Vasconcelos, P.R.L.; Braga, L.L.B.C. Clinical characteristics of distal gastric cáncer in Young adults from Northeastern Brazil. *BMC Cancer* **2018**, *18*, 131. [CrossRef] [PubMed]

49. Balakrish, M.; George, R.; Sharma, A.; Graham, D.Y.; Malaty, H.M. An investigation into recent increase in gastric cancer in the USA. *Dig. Dis. Sci.* **2018**. [CrossRef] [PubMed]

50. Carmel, R.; Johnson, C.S. Racial patterns in pernicious anemia. Early age of onset and increased frequency of intrinsic factor antibody in black women. *N. Engl. J. Med.* **1978**, *298*, 647–650. [CrossRef] [PubMed]

51. Neumann, W.L.; Coss, E.; Rugge, M.; Genta, R.M. Autoimmune atrophic gastritis-pathogenesis, pathology and management. *Nat. Rev. Gastroenterol. Hepatol.* **2013**, *10*, 529–541. [CrossRef] [PubMed]

52. Maeda, M.; Yamashita, S.; Shimazu, T.; Lida, N.; Takeshima, H.; Nakajima, T.; Oda, I.; Nanjo, S.; Kusano, C.; Mori, A.; et al. Novel epigenetic markers for gastric cáncer risk stratification in individuals after *Helicobacter pylori* eradication. *Gastric Cancer* **2018**. [CrossRef] [PubMed]

53. Leung, W.K.; Wong, I.O.L.; Cheung, K.S.; Yeung, K.F.; Chan, E.W.; Wong, A.Y.S.; Chen, L.; Wong, I.C.K.; Graham, D.Y. Effect of *Helicobacter pylori* treatment on incidence of gastric cancer in older individuals. *Gastroenterology* **2018**. [CrossRef] [PubMed]

54. Doorakkers, E.; Lagergren, J.; Engstrand, L.; Brusselaers, N. *Helicobacter pylori* eradication treatment and the risk of gastric adenocarcinoma in a western population. *Gut* **2018**. [CrossRef] [PubMed]

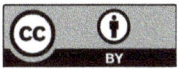

International Journal of
Molecular Sciences

MDPI

Review

Molecular Mechanisms of *H. pylori*-Induced DNA Double-Strand Breaks

Dawit Kidane

Division of Pharmacology and Toxicology, College of Pharmacy, The University of Texas at Austin, Dell Pediatric Research Institute, 1400 Barbara Jordan Blvd. R1800, Austin, TX 78723, USA; dawit.kidane@austin.utexas.edu; Tel.: +1-512-495-4720; Fax: +1-512-495-4945

Received: 16 August 2018; Accepted: 21 September 2018; Published: 23 September 2018

Abstract: Infections contribute to carcinogenesis through inflammation-related mechanisms. *H. pylori* infection is a significant risk factor for gastric carcinogenesis. However, the molecular mechanism by which *H. pylori* infection contributes to carcinogenesis has not been fully elucidated. *H. pylori*-associated chronic inflammation is linked to genomic instability via reactive oxygen and nitrogen species (RONS). In this article, we summarize the current knowledge of *H. pylori*-induced double strand breaks (DSBs). Furthermore, we provide mechanistic insight into how processing of oxidative DNA damage via base excision repair (BER) leads to DSBs. We review recent studies on how *H. pylori* infection triggers NF-κB/inducible NO synthase (iNOS) versus NF-κB/nucleotide excision repair (NER) axis-mediated DSBs to drive genomic instability. This review discusses current research findings that are related to mechanisms of DSBs and repair during *H. pylori* infection.

Keywords: *H. pylori*; RONS; BER; DSBs; NF-κB; NER

1. Introduction

Infection contributes to 20% of cancer worldwide [1]. *H. pylori* infection is one of the most common risk factors for gastric carcinogenesis [2]. More than 50% of the human population is infected with *H. pylori*, but few develop gastric cancer [3]. Several studies have shown that *H. pylori* infection causes chronic inflammation with different degrees of pathological severity, including chronic gastritis, peptic ulcers that eventually cause gastric adenocarcinoma, and gastric mucosa-associated lymphoid tissue (MALT) lymphoma [4–6]. Chronic gastritis that is associated with *H. pylori* infection is the first and early stage of inflammation. When accompanied by gastric epithelial cell injury, it may contribute to gastric cancer development [7–9]. *H. pylori* virulence factors that contribute to host-pathogen interaction have been characterized, which increase the risk of gastric cancer pathogenesis [4,10]. These virulence factors enhance the severity of the mucosal inflammatory response, which may largely be responsible for the virulence factor-associated increased risk of gastric cancer [10].

H. pylori causes chronic gastritis and contributes to genotoxic activity [11,12]. However, the molecular mechanisms by which *H. pylori* promotes genotoxic activity and the host response to genotoxic factors to drive gastric carcinogenesis require more study. Based on the current knowledge, *H. pylori* infection induces a genotoxic effect via two potential mechanisms. First, *H. pylori* infection enhances the infiltration of immune cells, including neutrophils and macrophages, to produce reactive oxygen species and nitrogen species (RONS) [13]. RONS can cause DNA base damage that leads to single strand breaks (SSBs) and the enhanced expression of oncogenes [14–16]. Alternatively, RONS activate the oxidant-sensitive transcription factor NF-κB, which induces the expression of oncogenes and cell-cycle regulators [17,18]. Activated NF-κB is translocated to the nucleus and it forms a protein complex with NER proteins (XPG and XPF) to cleave the promoter regions of the genes and cause double strand breaks (DSBs) that impact gene expression [11].

2. *H. pylori* Induces Inflammation-Dependent DNA Damage

Chronic inflammation is estimated to contribute to approximately 25% of human cancers [19]. Gastric inflammation in *H. pylori* infection may be induced via two different mechanisms. The first mechanism is initiated via physical contact between the pathogen and the host epithelial cells, producing direct cell damage or enhancing the ability of epithelial cells to release pro-inflammatory mediators (Figure 1). The second mechanism is likely promoted by *H. pylori* virulence factors (e.g., *CagA*, *VacA*) that may target the potential cell signaling pathways to stimulate immune responses. Interestingly, the *H. pylori CagA* positive strain enhances chemokine activation, such as IL-8, a potent neutrophil-activating chemotactic cytokine or chemokine [20,21]. Furthermore, chemokines that are released from infected gastric epithelial cells can stimulate neutrophil infiltration and T lymphocytes to enhance RONS-mediated gastritis [22,23]. Overall, *H. pylori*-mediated gastric inflammation is associated with humoral and cell-mediated immune cells.

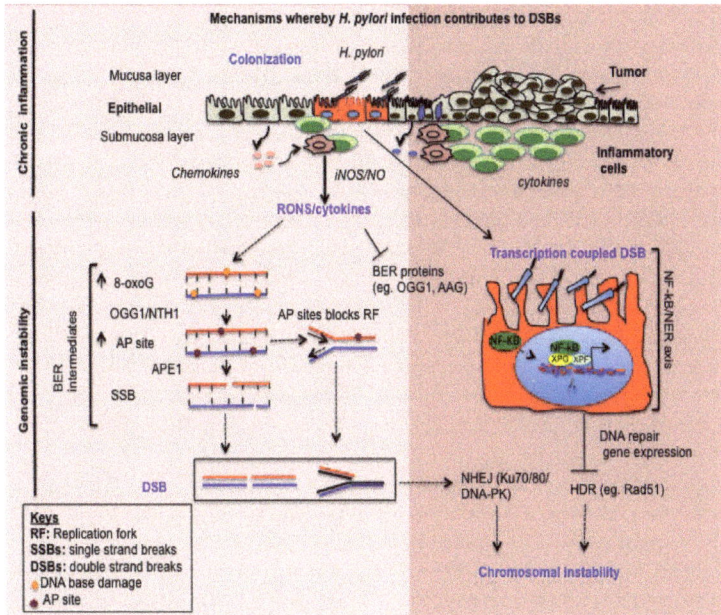

Figure 1. Molecular mechanisms of *H. pylori*-induced double strand breaks (DSBs). Schematic representation of how *H. pylori* induces DSBs. *H. pylori* infection causes DNA damage in gastric epithelial cells [24]. *H. pylori*-host cell interaction is a prerequisite for DSBs [25] (top panel). Persistence of the host-bacterium interaction leads to chronic inflammation and the release of inflammatory cytokines and chemokines, which contribute to oxidative DNA damage that is processed via base excision repair (BER) pathways (bottom panel). Processing oxidative DNA damage by DNA glycosylase (e.g., OGG1, NEIL1, etc.) contributes to accumulation of apurinic/apyrimidinic (AP) sites that are eventually converted to DSBs [26]. In addition, some cytokines (e.g., TNF-α) inhibit BER proteins to exacerbate genomic instability. The second pathway associated with *H. pylori*-mediated NF-κB activation leads to formation of a protein complex with nucleotide excision repair proteins (XPF and XPG), cleaves the promoter regions, and alters gene expression [11] including HR DNA repair proteins (Rad51). Alternatively, NF-κB/iNOS-mediated NO production leads to DNA damage and/or inhibits DNA repair proteins (AAG) that likely impact BER and cause DSBs. Note that solid arrow and dot arrow shows activation and alternative avenue for the down stream events respectively; T bar shows inhibition or suppression of protein activity or gene expression.

3. *H. pylori* Induces Base Excision Repair (BER) Intermediate-Dependent Double Strand Breaks (DSBs)

Chronic inflammatory conditions induce immune and epithelial cells to release RONS, which are capable of causing DNA damage and persistent cellular proliferation [27]. In addition, RONS accumulation may result in proto-oncogene activation, chromosomal aberrations, and DNA mutations [28,29]. There is considerable evidence that *H. pylori* itself induces genomic instability and epigenetic alteration in the host genome. However, there is little experimental evidence to provide mechanistic insight into how oxidative DNA damage leads to DSBs and how oxidative-damaged DNA processed via BER (Figure 1), which is thought to be the primary repair pathway against oxidative DNA damage [30]. The mechanism of *H. pylori*-induced host genomic instability remains poorly understood.

BER is crucial for maintaining genomic stability to prevent carcinogenesis [31–34]. BER is a major DNA repair pathway that removes the majority of oxidative and alkylating DNA damage without affecting the double helix DNA structure [30,35,36]. BER is the primary repair pathway of RONS-induced DNA damage during inflammation that occurs during *H. pylori* infection [37] (Table 1). Tight coordination of the different steps in BER is necessary to avoid genomic instability [38]. BER is initiated by the recognition and excision of the damaged base by specific DNA glycosylases. For example, the best characterized 8oxoG DNA lesions paired with cytosine are recognized and excised by bifunctional OGG1 glycosylase [39–42]. Subsequently, OGG1 remains bound to its abasic site (AP) and its turnover is stimulated by apurinic/apyrimidinic endonuclease1 (APE1) [43,44]. After AP site processing and end-remodeling, the single-nucleotide gap is filled by Pol β, and the nick is sealed by DNA ligase I to complete repair [45,46]. *H. pylori* can alter DNA repair gene expression and/or interfere with DNA repair activity [26,47,48]. Ding et al. reported live *H. pylori* upregulated APE1 expression in cultured gastric adenocarcinoma cell lines (AGS) and gastric epithelial cells that were isolated from uninfected human subjects [49]. Overexpressed APE1 likely interacts with other redox proteins to suppress ROS production [50]. In addition, Taller et al. show that coculture of *H. pylori* with gastric cancer cell lines induces DSBs in a contact-dependent manner [12]. DSBs in those cell lines lead to the activation of the ATM-dependent DNA damage response. *H. pylori*-induced DSBs likely cause chromosomal aberrations, such as deletions, insertions, and translocations, which are a major cause of the loss of heterozygosity.

Repair of oxidative DNA damage is critical for suppression of inflammation-associated carcinogenesis. However, host BER insufficiency caused by genetic polymorphism or loss of repair capacity likely exacerbates RONS-mediated DNA damage and cancer development [51–53] (Table 1). In addition, altered function of BER proteins causes aberrant function, including the processing of *H. pylori*-induced oxidative DNA damage that leads to SSBs [54] and mutation [47,48]. In vivo studies have shown that *H. pylori* infection in an OGG1 knockout mouse model enhances accumulation of 8oxoG DNA lesions and promotes resistance to inflammation [55–57]. In addition, loss of DNA glycosylase, such as *MYH* and alkyladenine DNA glycosylase (AAG), causes the accumulation of oxidative DNA damage lesions and promotes inflammation-associated tumor development [37,58,59]. *H. pylori* infection activates other BER proteins, such as PARP1 and enhances the inflammatory response, suggesting that the bacterium modulates the host PARP1 status to drive inflammation-associated gastric cancer [60]. However, cell culture experiments have shown that OGG1 downregulation in gastric epithelial cells decreases the formation of AP sites and suppress DSBs formation [26]. However, silencing of APE1 as part of the BER machinery failed to cause a significant level of *H. pylori*-induced DSBs [11].

Table 1. Interplay between *H. pylori* and relevant DNA repair gene products.

Gene	Role of Gene Products	Interplay between *H. pylori* & Gene	References
BER			
OGG1	removes 8oxoG and FapyG DNA lesions	absence causes increased mutation frequency, fewer DSBs and decreased inflammation	[26,55,61]
NEIL1	removes 8oxoG and Tg lesions	decreases mRNA in tumor; unknown role during infection	[34]
APE1	acts as a negative regulator of ROS and enhances chemokine release	enhances the expression of mRNA and protein	[49,62,63]
POLB	removes 5′-dRP group and adds a single nucleotide base	infection does not affect gene expression and protein level	[26]
XRCC1	scaffold protein enhance ligation	downregulated via promoter hypermethylation	[64,65]
NER			
XPG	cuts the 3′ of the DNA damage site; forms complex with NF-κB and promotes target gene expression	moderates change in gene expression	[11,66,67]
XPF	forms complex with NF-κB & promotes targeted gene expression	moderates change in gene expression	[11,66]
XPA	recognition bulk DNA adduct	increases IL-8 cytokine expression	[11,66]
NHEJ			
DNA-PK	increases cellular proliferation & facilitates NHEJ (nonhomologous DNA end-joining) repair	enhances activity and expression	[68]
Ku70/80	protects DNA DSB ends and prevents cell death	decreases protein level	[69]
DNA ligase IV	completes NHEJ repair by sealing DNA DSB regions	knock-down enhances DSBs	[11]
XRCC4	scaffold to hold DNA DSBs ends to enhance ligation	knock-down promotes DNA DSBs	[11]
HR			
NBS1	DNA DSB end processing/DDR	decreases expression and may impair DNA end processing and DDR	[66]
Rad51	strand exchange and enhances DSB repair	decreases gene expression; however, infection does not increase DSBs	[25]
RPA1	ssDNA binding and DDR	downregulates mRNA	[66]
Mre11	DSB end processing and DDR	decreases expression and impairs end processing and DDR	[66]

DSBs are the principle cytotoxic lesions generated by *H. pylori* infection. DSBs can be caused by the accumulation of unrepaired BER intermediates in DNA replication independently and/or arise when DNA replication forks encounter BER intermediates including DNA SSBs [70,71]. Few studies have shown that accumulation of AP sites in *H. pylori*-infected human gastric epithelial cells leads to DSBs [26]. Toller et al. [12] reported that a direct bacterium-host interaction is a prerequisite to DSBs, rather than the release of DNA-damaging components. Overall, these results suggest that DSB formation is mediated by BER intermediates that are generated from a direct response of the host-bacterium interaction (Figure 1).

4. NF-κB-iNOS Axis-Dependent DSB Formation

H. pylori infection induces DNA damage in gastric epithelial cells [24]. Contact-dependent interactions between *H. pylori* bacteria and gastric epithelial cells activate intracellular signaling events that have further downstream effects via activation of the transcription factor NF-κB [72]. NF-κB activation is effected through a series of phosphorylation and transactivation events, triggering a downstream signaling pathway that contributes to gastric inflammation in *H. pylori*-infected individuals [73,74]. *H. pylori*-mediated NF-κB activation leads to the upregulated expression of a variety of inflammatory mediators, including IL-8 [75], and regulates genes that govern the innate and adaptive immune response [76,77]. However, aberrant NF-κB activation has been reported to function as a tumor promoter in inflammation-associated cancer [78,79].

Moreover, the host response to *H. pylori* infection enhances NF-κB activation in immune and epithelial cells, resulting in inducible nitric oxide synthase (iNOS) [80–84]. iNOS is an inflammatory mediator that causes the production of nitric oxide (NO) by immune cells, such as macrophages, linking chronic inflammation and tumorigenesis [85–87]. iNOS is expressed in response to bacterial endotoxins and cytokines and leads to NO production that enhances carcinogenesis [88]. iNOS-mediated NO induces oxidized DNA and leads to mutations associated with the infection [89,90] and DSBs [91]. Furthermore, NO has a biphasic effect on NF-κB to exert both pro- and anti-inflammatory actions. Although the ability of NO to directly damage DNA has been studied to a limited degree [92], its role in promoting potentially mutagenic changes in DNA has received far less attention. NO prevents NF-κB transactivation via the stabilization of IκBα [93] and nitrosate, a specific cysteine residue on the p50 subunit of NF-κB that reduces its DNA-binding capacity [94,95]. Few studies have shown that NF-κB plays a significant role in inhibition of pathogen-induced apoptosis in immune cells [96], suggesting that NF-κB may play a pro-inflammatory role to induce persistent macrophage activation. Other studies have shown that DNA repair proteins that are involved in BER and SSBs (PARP1) interact with NF-κB to facilitate the interactions with DNA to promote the expression of pro-inflammatory cytokines and enhance the activity of iNOS [97–99].

iNOS-mediated NO enhances inactivation of DNA repair enzymes that eventually contribute to genomic instability, leading to cancer development [86]. NO can nitrosylate thiol and tyrosine residues of the DNA repair proteins, causing loss of their function [100,101]. Thus, determining the effect of iNOS-generated NO on DNA repair proteins is scientifically important to uncover the impact of *H. pylori*-triggered iNOS-mediated DNA repair defects (Figure 1). Few studies have shown that DNA repair proteins are vulnerable to oxidative damage from NO because of their active sites, such as sulphydryl, tyrosine, and phenol side chains [102]. DNA repair enzymes, such as MGMT, FpyG, and PARP may be inactivated by NO-mediated nitrosylation of the cysteine-rich residues of the active site [103,104]. The integrity of the genome may be challenged during exposure to high concentrations of NO by direct oxidative damage to DNA and by inhibiting the DNA repair capacity of the enzyme (Table 1).

5. NF-κB-Nucleotide Excision Repair (NER) Axis-Dependent DSB Formation

H. pylori infection increases NF-κB activation to promote the inflammatory immune response [105]. NF-κB modulates many DNA repair genes to facilitate repair and generate DNA DSBs [106,107]. Endonucleases XPF and XPG are critical components of NER that are responsible for excising the damaged DNA strand to remove the DNA lesion. The endonuclease XPG cuts the DNA strand approximately 5–6 nucleotides downstream of 3′ of the DNA damage site. In addition, the ERCC1-XPF protein complex performs an incision of the DNA strand 20–22 nucleotides upstream of the 5′ end of the DNA [108,109]. Although these two endonucleases are recruited and form complexes with NF-κB to make preincision complexes, proper assembly of all the factors seems to be required for dual incision at the promoter region of a given gene. XPF/XPG-mediated DSBs amplify NF-κB target inflammatory gene expression and promote host cell survival [11]. The NF-κB complex in XPG and XPF in the formation of the active DSBs at the chromatin region of the genome likely promotes a hub that controls gene expression (Figure 1). Furthermore, the expression level of XPG is significantly associated with an *H. pylori*-positive sample [110] (Table 1). However, silencing XPG strongly reduced the DSBs upon *H. pylori* infection, suggesting that NER-dependent DSBs contribute to genomic instability during infection. *H. pylori* infection modulates NER and enhances the interaction with NF-κB, likely providing a molecular basis for insights into how *H. pylori* infection induces transcription-associated DSBs (Figure 1).

6. *H. pylori* Impairs DSBs Repair

DSBs can be repaired via two major repair pathways [111,112]. Homologous recombination (HR) requires sequence homology of extensive DNA regions from an undamaged sister chromatid or homologous chromosomes. In contrast, nonhomologous DNA end-joining (NHEJ) occurs throughout the cell cycles and is processed without any sequence homology or few end homology sequences. *H. pylori*-induced DSBs are likely recognized by the MRE11-RAD50-NBS1 (MRN) complex [113,114], which is recognized and processed the DNA ends, resulting in the activation of ataxia telangiectasia mutated kinase (ATM) [115,116]. ATM is a major DNA damage response sensor of DSBs. It directly binds to the damaged DNA and phosphorylates target proteins, including H2AX protein at serine 139 of the histone (γH2AX) to mark DSBs sites [116–119]. Alternatively, ATM is involved in mediating the NF-κB response to DSBs [120].

In the NHEJ pathway, DNA-dependent protein kinase (DNA-PK) and Ku proteins play key roles in mediation of incompatible DNA ends. DNA-PK may function as a DNA damage sensor or scaffolding to assemble repair proteins including Ku proteins to bind the two ends of the break together. Then, ligase IV/XRCC4/XLF carries out the ligation reaction [121] to complete NHEJ repair. However, *H. pylori* causes an increase in Ku70/80, which may indicate that NHEJ-mediated repair contributes to genomic instability [69]. Recent evidence has shown that altered DNA-PK and Ku70/80 are associated with pathological processes in different types of cancer [122]. Moreover, Ku70 and DNA-PK are expressed in *H. pylori*-associated gastritis, intestinal metaplasia and gastric adenoma tissues [68]. Furthermore, Lim et al. [123] showed that activated NF-κB-Cox2 axis plays a significant role in enhancing the expression of KU70/80. In contrast, the loss of Ku proteins leads to an accumulation of DNA damage that eventually causes cell death in gastric epithelial cells [124].

Our previous study shows that DSBs significantly increase in the G1 stage of the cell cycle after *H. pylori* infection [26], suggesting that NHEJ repair might be involved in promotion of error-prone repair. When DSBs are generated during the S phase at DNA replication forks or after replication in the G2 phase of the cell cycle, HR may contribute to genome integrity (Figure 1). Few studies have shown that NF-κB interacts with HR proteins (e.g., CtIP-BRCA1 complexes) to stabilize BRCA1 and stimulate HR-mediated repair [125] Activation of multiple molecular targets by NF-κB enhances rapid activation of HR and may permit the accelerated proliferation of cells. However, *H. pylori* infection-mediated activation of the NF-κB/NER axis causes defects in HR that reduce the ability of DSB repair [11]. *H. pylori* infection modulates DSB repair efficiency to exacerbate genomic instability and facilitate gastric carcinogenesis.

7. Summary

H. pylori infection is a contributing factor for gastric cancer. This review highlights how *H. pylori*-associated DNA base damage in infected host cells is likely processed via BER to generate DSBs. In addition, this review provides a comprehensive overview of how *H. pylori*-associated DSBs are induced via the NF-κB/NER axis and NF-κB/iNOS axis, influencing DNA repair gene expression and enhancing genomic instability and carcinogenesis (Figure 1). Several studies have shown that *H. pylori* induces DSB and promotes gastric carcinogenesis. Host BER, NER, and NHEJ genetic variants could modify the process of carcinogenesis in *H. pylori* infected hosts. Alteration of the activity of enzymes that function in DNA repair as a result of genetic mutation could significantly impact gastric cancer risk. Other studies are needed to uncover the associations of the BER, NER and NHEJ genetic variants with increased susceptibility to gastric cancer in *H. pylori*-infected hosts. In addition, many questions remain regarding the mechanism of DSB formation and how breaks are processed via the NHEJ or HR pathways. Does *H. pylori* infection decrease tumor latency for carriers of BER variant genotypes? Future studies will likely explore how *H. pylori* manipulates host DNA repair genetics and how NHEJ processes DSBs. Therefore, the relevant DNA repair of the host genetics and *H. pylori* infection status of the host should be considered in studies of gastric cancer susceptibility in the future.

Funding: D.K. was supported by the United States National Institutes of Health (NIH/National Cancer Institute (NCI)) K01 CA154854 and start-up funds from The University of Texas at Austin, College of Pharmacy.

Acknowledgments: We would like to thank Stephanie D. Scott for editing the manuscript.

Conflicts of Interest: The author declares no conflict of interest.

References

1. Kuper, H.; Adami, H.O.; Trichopoulos, D. Infections as a major preventable cause of human cancer. *J. Int. Med.* **2000**, *248*, 171–183. [CrossRef]
2. De Martel, C.; Forman, D.; Plummer, M. Gastric cancer: Epidemiology and risk factors. *Gastroenterol. Clin.* **2013**, *42*, 219–240. [CrossRef] [PubMed]
3. Peek, R.M., Jr.; Blaser, M.J. *Helicobacter pylori* and gastrointestinal tract adenocarcinomas. *Nat. Rev. Cancer* **2002**, *2*, 28–37. [CrossRef] [PubMed]
4. Covacci, A.; Telford, J.L.; Del Giudice, G.; Parsonnet, J.; Rappuoli, R. Helicobacter pylori virulence and genetic geography. *Science* **1999**, *284*, 1328–1333. [CrossRef] [PubMed]
5. Montecucco, C.; Rappuoli, R. Living dangerously: How *Helicobacter pylori* survives in the human stomach. *Nat. Rev. Mol. Cell Biol.* **2001**, *2*, 457–466. [CrossRef] [PubMed]
6. Monack, D.M.; Mueller, A.; Falkow, S. Persistent bacterial infections: The interface of the pathogen and the host immune system. *Nat. Rev. Microbiol.* **2004**, *2*, 747–765. [CrossRef] [PubMed]
7. Correa, P. Human gastric carcinogenesis: A multistep and multifactorial process—First american cancer society award lecture on cancer epidemiology and prevention. *Cancer Res.* **1992**, *52*, 6735–6740. [PubMed]
8. Ohnishi, N.; Yuasa, H.; Tanaka, S.; Sawa, H.; Miura, M.; Matsui, A.; Higashi, H.; Musashi, M.; Iwabuchi, K.; Suzuki, M.; et al. Transgenic expression of *Helicobacter pylori* CagA induces gastrointestinal and hematopoietic neoplasms in mouse. *Proc. Natl. Acad. Sci. USA* **2008**, *105*, 1003–1008. [CrossRef] [PubMed]
9. Smoot, D.T.; Wynn, Z.; Elliott, T.B.; Allen, C.R.; Mekasha, G.; Naab, T.; Ashktorab, H. Effects of *Helicobacter pylori* on proliferation of gastric epithelial cells in vitro. *Am. J. Gastroenterol.* **1999**, *94*, 1508–1511. [CrossRef] [PubMed]
10. Dubreuil, J.D.; Giudice, G.D.; Rappuoli, R. *Helicobacter pylori* interactions with host serum and extracellular matrix proteins: Potential role in the infectious process. *Microbiol. Mol. Biol. Rev.* **2002**, *66*, 617–629. [CrossRef] [PubMed]
11. Hartung, M.L.; Gruber, D.C.; Koch, K.N.; Gruter, L.; Rehrauer, H.; Tegtmeyer, N.; Backert, S.; Muller, A. *H. Pylori*-induced DNA strand breaks are introduced by nucleotide excision repair endonucleases and promote NF-κB target gene expression. *Cell Rep.* **2015**, *13*, 70–79. [CrossRef] [PubMed]
12. Toller, I.M.; Neelsen, K.J.; Steger, M.; Hartung, M.L.; Hottiger, M.O.; Stucki, M.; Kalali, B.; Gerhard, M.; Sartori, A.A.; Lopes, M.; et al. Carcinogenic bacterial pathogen *Helicobacter pylori* triggers DNA double-strand breaks and a DNA damage response in its host cells. *Proc. Natl. Acad. Sci. USA* **2011**, *108*, 14944–14949. [CrossRef] [PubMed]
13. Suzuki, M.; Miura, S.; Mori, M.; Kai, A.; Suzuki, H.; Fukumura, D.; Suematsu, M.; Tsuchiya, M. Rebamipide, a novel antiulcer agent, attenuates *Helicobacter pylori* induced gastric mucosal cell injury associated with neutrophil derived oxidants. *Gut* **1994**, *35*, 1375–1378. [CrossRef] [PubMed]
14. Cerutti, P.A. Oxy-radicals and cancer. *Lancet* **1994**, *344*, 862–863. [CrossRef]
15. Feig, D.I.; Reid, T.M.; Loeb, L.A. Reactive oxygen species in tumorigenesis. *Cancer Res.* **1994**, *54*, 1890s–1894s. [PubMed]

16. Schreck, R.R. Tumor suppressor gene (*Rb* and *p53*) mutations in osteosarcoma. *Ped. Hematol. Oncol.* **1992**, *9*, ix–x. [CrossRef]

17. D'Angio, C.T.; Finkelstein, J.N. Oxygen regulation of gene expression: A study in opposites. *Mol. Genet. MeTable* **2000**, *71*, 371–380. [CrossRef] [PubMed]

18. Adler, V.; Yin, Z.; Tew, K.D.; Ronai, Z. Role of redox potential and reactive oxygen species in stress signaling. *Oncogene* **1999**, *18*, 6104–6111. [CrossRef] [PubMed]

19. Kawanishi, S.; Ohnishi, S.; Ma, N.; Hiraku, Y.; Murata, M. Crosstalk between DNA damage and inflammation in the multiple steps of carcinogenesis. *Int. J. Mol. Sci.* **2017**, *18*, 1808. [CrossRef] [PubMed]

20. Eck, M.; Schmausser, B.; Scheller, K.; Toksoy, A.; Kraus, M.; Menzel, T.; Muller-Hermelink, H.K.; Gillitzer, R. CXC chemokines Groα/IL-8 and IP-10/MIG in *Helicobacter pylori* gastritis. *Clin. Exp. Immunol.* **2000**, *122*, 192–199. [CrossRef] [PubMed]

21. Watanabe, N.; Shimada, T.; Ohtsuka, Y.; Hiraishi, H.; Terano, A. Proinflammatory cytokines and *Helicobacter pylori* stimulate CC-chemokine expression in gastric epithelial cells. *J. Physiol. Pharmacol.* **1997**, *48*, 405–413. [PubMed]

22. Nozawa, Y.; Nishihara, K.; Peek, R.M.; Nakano, M.; Uji, T.; Ajioka, H.; Matsuura, N.; Miyake, H. Identification of a signaling cascade for interleukin-8 production by *Helicobacter pylori* in human gastric epithelial cells. *Biochem. Pharmacol.* **2002**, *64*, 21–30. [CrossRef]

23. Naito, Y.; Yoshikawa, T. Molecular and cellular mechanisms involved in *Helicobacter pylori*-induced inflammation and oxidative stress. *Free Radic. Biol. Med.* **2002**, *33*, 323–336. [CrossRef]

24. Obst, B.; Wagner, S.; Sewing, K.F.; Beil, W. *Helicobacter pylori* causes DNA damage in gastric epithelial cells. *Carcinogenesis* **2000**, *21*, 1111–1115. [CrossRef] [PubMed]

25. Hanada, K.; Uchida, T.; Tsukamoto, Y.; Watada, M.; Yamaguchi, N.; Yamamoto, K.; Shiota, S.; Moriyama, M.; Graham, D.Y.; Yamaoka, Y. *Helicobacter pylori* infection introduces DNA double-strand breaks in host cells. *Infect. Immun.* **2014**, *82*, 4182–4189. [CrossRef] [PubMed]

26. Kidane, D.; Murphy, D.L.; Sweasy, J.B. Accumulation of abasic sites induces genomic instability in normal human gastric epithelial cells during *Helicobacter pylori* infection. *Oncogenesis* **2014**, *3*, e128. [CrossRef] [PubMed]

27. Perryman, S.V.; Sylvester, K.G. Repair and regeneration: Opportunities for carcinogenesis from tissue stem cells. *J. Cell Mol. Med.* **2006**, *10*, 292–308. [CrossRef] [PubMed]

28. Floyd, R.A. Role of oxygen free radicals in carcinogenesis and brain ischemia. *FASEB J.* **1990**, *4*, 2587–2597. [CrossRef] [PubMed]

29. Du, M.Q.; Carmichael, P.L.; Phillips, D.H. Induction of activating mutations in the human c-Ha-*ras*-1 proto-oncogene by oxygen free radicals. *Mol Carcinog* **1994**, *11*, 170–175. [CrossRef] [PubMed]

30. Dianov, G.L.; Hubscher, U. Mammalian base excision repair: The forgotten archangel. *Nucleic Acids Res.* **2013**, *41*, 3483–3490. [CrossRef] [PubMed]

31. Al-Tassan, N.; Chmiel, N.H.; Maynard, J.; Fleming, N.; Livingston, A.L.; Williams, G.T.; Hodges, A.K.; Davies, D.R.; David, S.S.; Sampson, J.R.; et al. Inherited variants of *MYH* associated with somatic g:C → t:A mutations in colorectal tumors. *Nat. Genet.* **2002**, *30*, 227–232. [CrossRef] [PubMed]

32. Farrington, S.M.; Tenesa, A.; Barnetson, R.; Wiltshire, A.; Prendergast, J.; Porteous, M.; Campbell, H.; Dunlop, M.G. Germline susceptibility to colorectal cancer due to base-excision repair gene defects. *Am. J. Hum. Genet.* **2005**, *77*, 112–119. [CrossRef] [PubMed]

33. Mahjabeen, I.; Masood, N.; Baig, R.M.; Sabir, M.; Inayat, U.; Malik, F.A.; Kayani, M.A. Novel mutations of OGG1 base excision repair pathway gene in laryngeal cancer patients. *Fam. Cancer* **2012**, *11*, 587–593. [CrossRef] [PubMed]

34. Shinmura, K.; Tao, H.; Goto, M.; Igarashi, H.; Taniguchi, T.; Maekawa, M.; Takezaki, T.; Sugimura, H. Inactivating mutations of the human base excision repair gene *NEIL1* in gastric cancer. *Carcinogenesis* **2004**, *25*, 2311–2317. [CrossRef] [PubMed]

35. Kim, Y.J.; Wilson, D.M., 3rd. Overview of base excision repair biochemistry. *Curr. Mol. Pharmacol.* **2012**, *5*, 3–13. [CrossRef] [PubMed]

36. Wallace, S.S.; Murphy, D.L.; Sweasy, J.B. Base excision repair and cancer. *Cancer Lett.* **2012**, *327*, 73–89. [CrossRef] [PubMed]

37. Meira, L.B.; Bugni, J.M.; Green, S.L.; Lee, C.W.; Pang, B.; Borenshtein, D.; Rickman, B.H.; Rogers, A.B.; Moroski-Erkul, C.A.; McFaline, J.L.; et al. DNA damage induced by chronic inflammation contributes to colon carcinogenesis in mice. *J. Clin. Investig.* **2008**, *118*, 2516–2525. [CrossRef] [PubMed]

38. Allinson, S.L.; Sleeth, K.M.; Matthewman, G.E.; Dianov, G.L. Orchestration of base excision repair by controlling the rates of enzymatic activities. *DNA Repair* **2004**, *3*, 23–31. [CrossRef] [PubMed]

39. Radicella, J.P.; Dherin, C.; Desmaze, C.; Fox, M.S.; Boiteux, S. Cloning and characterization of *hOGG1*, a human homolog of the *OGG1* gene of *Saccharomyces cerevisiae*. *Proc. Natl. Acad. Sci. USA* **1997**, *94*, 8010–8015. [CrossRef] [PubMed]

40. Aburatani, H.; Hippo, Y.; Ishida, T.; Takashima, R.; Matsuba, C.; Kodama, T.; Takao, M.; Yasui, A.; Yamamoto, K.; Asano, M. Cloning and characterization of mammalian 8-hydroxyguanine-specific DNA glycosylase/apurinic, apyrimidinic lyase, a functional mutm homologue. *Cancer Res.* **1997**, *57*, 2151–2156. [PubMed]

41. Fortini, P.; Parlanti, E.; Sidorkina, O.M.; Laval, J.; Dogliotti, E. The type of DNA glycosylase determines the base excision repair pathway in mammalian cells. *J. Biol. Chem.* **1999**, *274*, 15230–15236. [CrossRef] [PubMed]

42. Nishimura, S. Involvement of mammalian OGG1 (MMH) in excision of the 8-hydroxyguanine residue in DNA. *Free Radic. Biol. Med.* **2002**, *32*, 813–821. [CrossRef]

43. Mokkapati, S.K.; Wiederhold, L.; Hazra, T.K.; Mitra, S. Stimulation of DNA glycosylase activity of OGG1 by NEIL1: Functional collaboration between two human DNA glycosylases. *Biochemistry* **2004**, *43*, 11596–11604. [CrossRef] [PubMed]

44. Sidorenko, V.S.; Nevinsky, G.A.; Zharkov, D.O. Mechanism of interaction between human 8-oxoguanine-DNA glycosylase and ap endonuclease. *DNA Repair* **2007**, *6*, 317–328. [CrossRef] [PubMed]

45. Fortini, P.; Pascucci, B.; Parlanti, E.; D'Errico, M.; Simonelli, V.; Dogliotti, E. The base excision repair: Mechanisms and its relevance for cancer susceptibility. *Biochimie* **2003**, *85*, 1053–1071. [CrossRef] [PubMed]

46. Robertson, A.B.; Klungland, A.; Rognes, T.; Leiros, I. DNA repair in mammalian cells: Base excision repair: The long and short of it. *Cell. Mol. Life Sci.* **2009**, *66*, 981–993. [CrossRef] [PubMed]

47. Park, D.I.; Park, S.H.; Kim, S.H.; Kim, J.W.; Cho, Y.K.; Kim, H.J.; Sohn, C.I.; Jeon, W.K.; Kim, B.I.; Cho, E.Y.; et al. Effect of *Helicobacter pylori* infection on the expression of DNA mismatch repair protein. *Helicobacter* **2005**, *10*, 179–184. [CrossRef] [PubMed]

48. Kim, J.J.; Tao, H.; Carloni, E.; Leung, W.K.; Graham, D.Y.; Sepulveda, A.R. *Helicobacter pylori* impairs DNA mismatch repair in gastric epithelial cells. *Gastroenterology* **2002**, *123*, 542–553. [CrossRef] [PubMed]

49. Ding, S.Z.; O'Hara, A.M.; Denning, T.L.; Dirden-Kramer, B.; Mifflin, R.C.; Reyes, V.E.; Ryan, K.A.; Elliott, S.N.; Izumi, T.; Boldogh, I.; et al. Helicobacter pylori and h2o2 increase ap endonuclease-1/redox factor-1 expression in human gastric epithelial cells. *Gastroenterology* **2004**, *127*, 845–858. [CrossRef] [PubMed]

50. Den Hartog, G.; Chattopadhyay, R.; Ablack, A.; Hall, E.H.; Butcher, L.D.; Bhattacharyya, A.; Eckmann, L.; Harris, P.R.; Das, S.; Ernst, P.B.; et al. Regulation of Rac1 and reactive oxygen species production in response to infection of gastrointestinal epithelia. *PLoS Pathog.* **2016**, *12*, e1005382. [CrossRef] [PubMed]

51. Teoule, R.; Bert, C.; Bonicel, A. Thymine fragment damage retained in the DNA polynucleotide chain after gamma irradiation in aerated solutions. II. *Radiat. Res.* **1977**, *72*, 190–200. [CrossRef] [PubMed]

52. Altieri, F.; Grillo, C.; Maceroni, M.; Chichiarelli, S. DNA damage and repair: From molecular mechanisms to health implications. *Antioxid. Redox Signal.* **2008**, *10*, 891–937. [CrossRef] [PubMed]

53. Grollman, A.P.; Moriya, M. Mutagenesis by 8-oxoguanine: An enemy within. *Trends Genet.* **1993**, *9*, 246–249. [CrossRef]

54. Cooke, M.S.; Evans, M.D.; Dizdaroglu, M.; Lunec, J. Oxidative DNA damage: Mechanisms, mutation, and disease. *FASEB J.* **2003**, *17*, 1195–1214. [CrossRef] [PubMed]

55. Klungland, A.; Rosewell, I.; Hollenbach, S.; Larsen, E.; Daly, G.; Epe, B.; Seeberg, E.; Lindahl, T.; Barnes, D.E. Accumulation of premutagenic DNA lesions in mice defective in removal of oxidative base damage. *Proc. Natl. Acad. Sci. USA* **1999**, *96*, 13300–13305. [CrossRef] [PubMed]

56. Minowa, O.; Arai, T.; Hirano, M.; Monden, Y.; Nakai, S.; Fukuda, M.; Itoh, M.; Takano, H.; Hippou, Y.; Aburatani, H.; et al. *Mmh/Ogg1* gene inactivation results in accumulation of 8-hydroxyguanine in mice. *Proc. Natl. Acad. Sci. USA* **2000**, *97*, 4156–4161. [CrossRef] [PubMed]

57. Touati, E.; Michel, V.; Thiberge, J.M.; Ave, P.; Huerre, M.; Bourgade, F.; Klungland, A.; Labigne, A. Deficiency in OGG1 protects against inflammation and mutagenic effects associated with *H. pylori* infection in mouse. *Helicobacter* **2006**, *11*, 494–505. [CrossRef] [PubMed]

58. Cheadle, J.P.; Dolwani, S.; Sampson, J.R. Inherited defects in the DNA glycosylase MYH cause multiple colorectal adenoma and carcinoma. *Carcinogenesis* **2003**, *24*, 1281–1282; author reply 1283. [CrossRef] [PubMed]

59. Sakamoto, K.; Tominaga, Y.; Yamauchi, K.; Nakatsu, Y.; Sakumi, K.; Yoshiyama, K.; Egashira, A.; Kura, S.; Yao, T.; Tsuneyoshi, M.; et al. Mutyh-null mice are susceptible to spontaneous and oxidative stress induced intestinal tumorigenesis. *Cancer Res.* **2007**, *67*, 6599–6604. [CrossRef] [PubMed]

60. Nossa, C.W.; Blanke, S.R. Helicobacter pylori activation of PARP-1: Usurping a versatile regulator of host cellular health. *Gut Microbes* **2010**, *1*, 373–378. [CrossRef] [PubMed]

61. Mabley, J.G.; Pacher, P.; Deb, A.; Wallace, R.; Elder, R.H.; Szabo, C. Potential role for 8-oxoguanine DNA glycosylase in regulating inflammation. *FASEB J.* **2005**, *19*, 290–292. [CrossRef] [PubMed]

62. Bhattacharyya, A.; Chattopadhyay, R.; Burnette, B.R.; Cross, J.V.; Mitra, S.; Ernst, P.B.; Bhakat, K.K.; Crowe, S.E. Acetylation of apurinic/apyrimidinic endonuclease-1 regulates *Helicobacter pylori*-mediated gastric epithelial cell apoptosis. *Gastroenterology* **2009**, *136*, 2258–2269. [CrossRef] [PubMed]

63. O'Hara, A.M.; Bhattacharyya, A.; Mifflin, R.C.; Smith, M.F.; Ryan, K.A.; Scott, K.G.; Naganuma, M.; Casola, A.; Izumi, T.; Mitra, S.; et al. Interleukin-8 induction by helicobacter pylori in gastric epithelial cells is dependent on apurinic/apyrimidinic endonuclease-1/redox factor-1. *J. Immunol.* **2006**, *177*, 7990–7999. [CrossRef] [PubMed]

64. Wang, P.; Tang, J.T.; Peng, Y.S.; Chen, X.Y.; Zhang, Y.J.; Fang, J.Y. Xrcc1 downregulated through promoter hypermethylation is involved in human gastric carcinogenesis. *J. Dig. Dis.* **2010**, *11*, 343–351. [CrossRef] [PubMed]

65. Cannan, W.J.; Rashid, I.; Tomkinson, A.E.; Wallace, S.S.; Pederson, D.S. The human ligase iiialpha-xrcc1 protein complex performs DNA nick repair after transient unwrapping of nucleosomal DNA. *J. Biol. Chem.* **2017**, *292*, 5227–5238. [CrossRef] [PubMed]

66. Koeppel, M.; Garcia-Alcalde, F.; Glowinski, F.; Schlaermann, P.; Meyer, T.F. *Helicobacter pylori* infection causes characteristic DNA damage patterns in human cells. *Cell Rep.* **2015**, *11*, 1703–1713. [CrossRef] [PubMed]

67. Klungland, A.; Hoss, M.; Gunz, D.; Constantinou, A.; Clarkson, S.G.; Doetsch, P.W.; Bolton, P.H.; Wood, R.D.; Lindahl, T. Base excision repair of oxidative DNA damage activated by XPG protein. *Mol. Cell* **1999**, *3*, 33–42. [CrossRef]

68. Lee, H.S.; Choe, G.; Park, K.U.; Park, D.J.; Yang, H.K.; Lee, B.L.; Kim, W.H. Altered expression of DNA-dependent protein kinase catalytic subunit (DNA-PKcs) during gastric carcinogenesis and its clinical implications on gastric cancer. *Int. J. Oncol.* **2007**, *31*, 859–866. [CrossRef] [PubMed]

69. Bae, M.; Lim, J.W.; Kim, H. Oxidative DNA damage response in *Helicobacter pylori*-infected mongolian gerbils. *J. Cancer Prev.* **2013**, *18*, 271–275. [CrossRef] [PubMed]

70. Khanna, K.K.; Jackson, S.P. DNA double-strand breaks: Signaling, repair and the cancer connection. *Nat. Genet.* **2001**, *27*, 247–254. [CrossRef] [PubMed]

71. Mills, K.D.; Ferguson, D.O.; Alt, F.W. The role of DNA breaks in genomic instability and tumorigenesis. *Immunol. Rev.* **2003**, *194*, 77–95. [CrossRef] [PubMed]

72. Maeda, S.; Yoshida, H.; Ogura, K.; Mitsuno, Y.; Hirata, Y.; Yamaji, Y.; Akanuma, M.; Shiratori, Y.; Omata, M. H. Pylori activates NF-κB through a signaling pathway involving IκB kinases, NF-κB -inducing kinase, TRAF2, and TRAF6 in gastric cancer cells. *Gastroenterology* **2000**, *119*, 97–108. [CrossRef] [PubMed]

73. Bhattacharyya, A.; Pathak, S.; Kundu, M.; Basu, J. Mitogen-activated protein kinases regulate mycobacterium avium-induced tumor necrosis factor-α release from macrophages. *FEMS Immunol. Med. Microbiol.* **2002**, *34*, 73–80. [CrossRef]

74. Hayden, M.S.; Ghosh, S. Shared principles in NF-κB signaling. *Cell* **2008**, *132*, 344–362. [CrossRef] [PubMed]

75. De Luca, A.; Iaquinto, G. *Helicobacter pylori* and gastric diseases: A dangerous association. *Cancer Lett.* **2004**, *213*, 1–10. [CrossRef] [PubMed]

76. Lamb, A.; Chen, L.F. The many roads traveled by *Helicobacter pylori* to NF-κB activation. *Gut Microbes* **2010**, *1*, 109–113. [CrossRef] [PubMed]

77. Orlowski, R.Z.; Baldwin, A.S., Jr. NF-κB as a therapeutic target in cancer. *Trends Mol. Med.* **2002**, *8*, 385–389. [CrossRef]

78. Pikarsky, E.; Porat, R.M.; Stein, I.; Abramovitch, R.; Amit, S.; Kasem, S.; Gutkovich-Pyest, E.; Urieli-Shoval, S.; Galun, E.; Ben-Neriah, Y. NF-κB functions as a tumour promoter in inflammation-associated cancer. *Nature* **2004**, *431*, 461–466. [CrossRef] [PubMed]

79. Oussaief, L.; Ramirez, V.; Hippocrate, A.; Arbach, H.; Cochet, C.; Proust, A.; Raphael, M.; Khelifa, R.; Joab, I. NF-κB-mediated modulation of inducible nitric oxide synthase activity controls induction of the epstein-barr virus productive cycle by transforming growth factor β1. *J. Virol.* **2011**, *85*, 6502–6512. [CrossRef] [PubMed]

80. Viala, J.; Chaput, C.; Boneca, I.G.; Cardona, A.; Girardin, S.E.; Moran, A.P.; Athman, R.; Memet, S.; Huerre, M.R.; Coyle, A.J.; et al. Nod1 responds to peptidoglycan delivered by the *Helicobacter pylori* cag pathogenicity island. *Nat. Immunol.* **2004**, *5*, 1166–1174. [CrossRef] [PubMed]

81. Brandt, S.; Kwok, T.; Hartig, R.; Konig, W.; Backert, S. NF-κB activation and potentiation of proinflammatory responses by the *Helicobacter pylori* caga protein. *Proc. Natl. Acad. Sci. USA* **2005**, *102*, 9300–9305. [CrossRef] [PubMed]

82. Geem, D.; Medina-Contreras, O.; Kim, W.; Huang, C.S.; Denning, T.L. Isolation and characterization of dendritic cells and macrophages from the mouse intestine. *J. Vis. Exp.* **2012**. [CrossRef] [PubMed]

83. Geller, D.A.; Di Silvio, M.; Nussler, A.K.; Wang, S.C.; Shapiro, R.A.; Simmons, R.L.; Billiar, T.R. Nitric oxide synthase expression is induced in hepatocytes in vivo during hepatic inflammation. *J. Surg. Res.* **1993**, *55*, 427–432. [CrossRef] [PubMed]

84. Nussler, A.K.; Geller, D.A.; Sweetland, M.A.; Di Silvio, M.; Billiar, T.R.; Madariaga, J.B.; Simmons, R.L.; Lancaster, J.R., Jr. Induction of nitric oxide synthesis and its reactions in cultured human and rat hepatocytes stimulated with cytokines plus LPS. *Biochem. Biophys. Res. Commun.* **1993**, *194*, 826–835. [CrossRef] [PubMed]

85. Lowenstein, C.J.; Padalko, E. iNOS (NOS2) at a glance. *J. Cell Sci.* **2004**, *117*, 2865–2867. [CrossRef] [PubMed]

86. Choudhari, S.K.; Chaudhary, M.; Bagde, S.; Gadbail, A.R.; Joshi, V. Nitric oxide and cancer: A review. *World J. Surg. Oncol.* **2013**, *11*, 118. [CrossRef] [PubMed]

87. Thomsen, L.L.; Lawton, F.G.; Knowles, R.G.; Beesley, J.E.; Riveros-Moreno, V.; Moncada, S. Nitric oxide synthase activity in human gynecological cancer. *Cancer Res.* **1994**, *54*, 1352–1354. [PubMed]

88. Rieder, G.; Hofmann, J.A.; Hatz, R.A.; Stolte, M.; Enders, G.A. Up-regulation of inducible nitric oxide synthase in *Helicobacter pylori*-associated gastritis may represent an increased risk factor to develop gastric carcinoma of the intestinal type. *Int. J. Med. Microbiol.* **2003**, *293*, 403–412. [CrossRef] [PubMed]

89. Touati, E.; Michel, V.; Thiberge, J.M.; Wuscher, N.; Huerre, M.; Labigne, A. Chronic *Helicobacter pylori* infections induce gastric mutations in mice. *Gastroenterology* **2003**, *124*, 1408–1419. [CrossRef]

90. Wink, D.A.; Kasprzak, K.S.; Maragos, C.M.; Elespuru, R.K.; Misra, M.; Dunams, T.M.; Cebula, T.A.; Koch, W.H.; Andrews, A.W.; Allen, J.S.; et al. DNA deaminating ability and genotoxicity of nitric oxide and its progenitors. *Science* **1991**, *254*, 1001–1003. [CrossRef] [PubMed]

91. Baydoun, H.H.; Cherian, M.A.; Green, P.; Ratner, L. Inducible nitric oxide synthase mediates DNA double strand breaks in human T-cell leukemia virus type 1-induced leukemia/lymphoma. *Retrovirology* **2015**, *12*, 71. [CrossRef] [PubMed]

92. Nguyen, T.; Brunson, D.; Crespi, C.L.; Penman, B.W.; Wishnok, J.S.; Tannenbaum, S.R. DNA damage and mutation in human cells exposed to nitric oxide in vitro. *Proc. Natl. Acad. Sci. USA* **1992**, *89*, 3030–3034. [CrossRef] [PubMed]

93. Peng, H.B.; Libby, P.; Liao, J.K. Induction and stabilization of IκBα by nitric oxide mediates inhibition of NF-κB. *J. Biol. Chem.* **1995**, *270*, 14214–14219. [CrossRef] [PubMed]

94. Matthews, J.R.; Botting, C.H.; Panico, M.; Morris, H.R.; Hay, R.T. Inhibition of NF-κB DNA binding by nitric oxide. *Nucleic Acids Res.* **1996**, *24*, 2236–2242. [CrossRef] [PubMed]

95. Schroeder, R.A.; Punzalan, C.; Kuo, P.C. Endotoxin-mediated S-nitrosylation of p50 alters NF-κB -dependent gene transcription in ANA-1 murine macrophages. *J. Immunol.* **1999**, *162*, 4101–4108.

96. Park, J.M.; Greten, F.R.; Wong, A.; Westrick, R.J.; Arthur, J.S.; Otsu, K.; Hoffmann, A.; Montminy, M.; Karin, M. Signaling pathways and genes that inhibit pathogen-induced macrophage apoptosis—CREB and NF-κB as key regulators. *Immunity* **2005**, *23*, 319–329. [CrossRef] [PubMed]

97. Hassa, P.O.; Covic, M.; Hasan, S.; Imhof, R.; Hottiger, M.O. The enzymatic and DNA binding activity of PARP-1 are not required for NF-κB coactivator function. *J. Biol. Chem.* **2001**, *276*, 45588–45597. [CrossRef] [PubMed]

98. Ullrich, O.; Diestel, A.; Eyupoglu, I.Y.; Nitsch, R. Regulation of microglial expression of integrins by poly (ADP-ribose) polymerase-1. *Nat. Cell Biol.* **2001**, *3*, 1035–1042. [CrossRef] [PubMed]

99. Wang, J.; Hao, L.; Wang, Y.; Qin, W.; Wang, X.; Zhao, T.; Liu, Y.; Sheng, L.; Du, Y.; Zhang, M.; et al. Inhibition of poly (ADP-ribose) polymerase and inducible nitric oxide synthase protects against ischemic myocardial damage by reduction of apoptosis. *Mol. Med. Rep.* **2015**, *11*, 1768–1776. [CrossRef] [PubMed]

100. Ischiropoulos, H.; Zhu, L.; Beckman, J.S. Peroxynitrite formation from macrophage-derived nitric oxide. *Arch. Biochem. Biophys.* **1992**, *298*, 446–451. [CrossRef]

101. Kong, S.K.; Yim, M.B.; Stadtman, E.R.; Chock, P.B. Peroxynitrite disables the tyrosine phosphorylation regulatory mechanism: Lymphocyte-specific tyrosine kinase fails to phosphorylate nitrated cdc2(6-20)NH2 peptide. *Proc. Natl. Acad. Sci. USA* **1996**, *93*, 3377–3382. [CrossRef] [PubMed]

102. Starke, D.W.; Chen, Y.; Bapna, C.P.; Lesnefsky, E.J.; Mieyal, J.J. Sensitivity of protein sulfhydryl repair enzymes to oxidative stress. *Free Radic. Biol. Med.* **1997**, *23*, 373–384. [CrossRef]

103. Wink, D.A.; Laval, J. The Fpg protein, a DNA repair enzyme, is inhibited by the biomediator nitric oxide in vitro and in vivo. *Carcinogenesis* **1994**, *15*, 2125–2129. [CrossRef] [PubMed]

104. O'Connor, T.R.; Graves, R.J.; de Murcia, G.; Castaing, B.; Laval, J. Fpg protein of escherichia coli is a zinc finger protein whose cysteine residues have a structural and/or functional role. *J. Biol. Chem.* **1993**, *268*, 9063–9070. [PubMed]

105. Telford, J.L.; Covacci, A.; Rappuoli, R.; Chiara, P. Immunobiology of helicobacter pylori infection. *Curr. Opin. Immunol.* **1997**, *9*, 498–503. [CrossRef]

106. Le May, N.; Fradin, D.; Iltis, I.; Bougneres, P.; Egly, J.M. XPG and XPF endonucleases trigger chromatin looping and DNA demethylation for accurate expression of activated genes. *Mol. Cell* **2012**, *47*, 622–632. [CrossRef] [PubMed]

107. Le May, N.; Mota-Fernandes, D.; Velez-Cruz, R.; Iltis, I.; Biard, D.; Egly, J.M. NER factors are recruited to active promoters and facilitate chromatin modification for transcription in the absence of exogenous genotoxic attack. *Mol. Cell* **2010**, *38*, 54–66. [CrossRef] [PubMed]

108. Leibeling, D.; Laspe, P.; Emmert, S. Nucleotide excision repair and cancer. *J. Mol. Histol.* **2006**, *37*, 225–238. [CrossRef] [PubMed]

109. Friedberg, E.C. How nucleotide excision repair protects against cancer. *Nat. Rev. Cancer* **2001**, *1*, 22–33. [CrossRef] [PubMed]

110. Deng, N.; Liu, J.W.; Sun, L.P.; Xu, Q.; Duan, Z.P.; Dong, N.N.; Yuan, Y. Expression of XPG protein in the development, progression and prognosis of gastric cancer. *PLoS ONE* **2014**, *9*, e108704. [CrossRef] [PubMed]

111. Ivanov, E.L.; Haber, J.E. DNA repair: Rad alert. *Curr. Biol.* **1997**, *7*, R492–R495. [CrossRef]

112. Kanaar, R.; Hoeijmakers, J.H. Recombination and joining: Different means to the same ends. *Genes Funct.* **1997**, *1*, 165–174. [CrossRef] [PubMed]

113. Matsuura, S.; Tauchi, H.; Nakamura, A.; Kondo, N.; Sakamoto, S.; Endo, S.; Smeets, D.; Solder, B.; Belohradsky, B.H.; Der Kaloustian, V.M.; et al. Positional cloning of the gene for Nijmegen breakage syndrome. *Nat. Genet.* **1998**, *19*, 179–181. [CrossRef] [PubMed]

114. Carney, J.P.; Maser, R.S.; Olivares, H.; Davis, E.M.; Le Beau, M.; Yates, J.R., 3rd; Hays, L.; Morgan, W.F.; Petrini, J.H. The hmre11/hrad50 protein complex and nijmegen breakage syndrome: Linkage of double-strand break repair to the cellular DNA damage response. *Cell* **1998**, *93*, 477–486. [CrossRef]

115. Stracker, T.H.; Petrini, J.H. The mre11 complex: Starting from the ends. *Nat. Rev. Mol. Cell Biol.* **2011**, *12*, 90–103. [CrossRef] [PubMed]

116. Shiloh, Y.; Lehmann, A.R. Maintaining integrity. *Nat. Cell Biol.* **2004**, *6*, 923–928. [CrossRef] [PubMed]

117. Bakkenist, C.J.; Kastan, M.B. Phosphatases join kinases in DNA-damage response pathways. *Trends Cell Biol.* **2004**, *14*, 339–341. [CrossRef] [PubMed]

118. Dupre, A.; Boyer-Chatenet, L.; Gautier, J. Two-step activation of ATM by DNA and the Mre11–Rad50–Nbs1 complex. *Nat. Struct. Mol. Biol.* **2006**, *13*, 451–457. [CrossRef] [PubMed]

119. Burma, S.; Chen, B.P.; Murphy, M.; Kurimasa, A.; Chen, D.J. ATM phosphorylates histone H2AX in response to DNA double-strand breaks. *J. Biol. Chem.* **2001**, *276*, 42462–42467. [CrossRef] [PubMed]

120. Li, N.; Banin, S.; Ouyang, H.; Li, G.C.; Courtois, G.; Shiloh, Y.; Karin, M.; Rotman, G. ATM is required for IκB kinase (IKKk) activation in response to DNA double strand breaks. *J. Biol. Chem.* **2001**, *276*, 8898–8903. [CrossRef] [PubMed]

121. Ahnesorg, P.; Smith, P.; Jackson, S.P. XLF interacts with the XRCC4-DNA ligase IV complex to promote DNA nonhomologous end-joining. *Cell* **2006**, *124*, 301–313. [CrossRef] [PubMed]

122. Abe, T.; Ishiai, M.; Hosono, Y.; Yoshimura, A.; Tada, S.; Adachi, N.; Koyama, H.; Takata, M.; Takeda, S.; Enomoto, T.; et al. Ku70/80, DNA-PKcs, and artemis are essential for the rapid induction of apoptosis after massive DSB formation. *Cell. Signal.* **2008**, *20*, 1978–1985. [CrossRef] [PubMed]

123. Lim, J.W.; Kim, H.; Kim, K.H. Expression of Ku70 and Ku80 mediated by NF-κB and cyclooxygenase-2 is related to proliferation of human gastric cancer cells. *J. Biol. Chem.* **2002**, *277*, 46093–46100. [CrossRef] [PubMed]

124. Song, J.Y.; Lim, J.W.; Kim, H.; Morio, T.; Kim, K.H. Oxidative stress induces nuclear loss of DNA repair proteins Ku70 and Ku80 and apoptosis in pancreatic acinar AR42J cells. *J. Biol. Chem.* **2003**, *278*, 36676–36687. [CrossRef] [PubMed]

125. Volcic, M.; Karl, S.; Baumann, B.; Salles, D.; Daniel, P.; Fulda, S.; Wiesmuller, L. NF-κB regulates DNA double-strand break repair in conjunction with BRCA1–CtIP complexes. *Nucleic Acids Res.* **2012**, *40*, 181–195. [CrossRef] [PubMed]

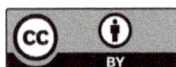

International Journal of
Molecular Sciences

MDPI

Review

The Reprimo Gene Family: A Novel Gene Lineage in Gastric Cancer with Tumor Suppressive Properties

Julio D. Amigo [1], Juan C. Opazo [2], Roddy Jorquera [5], Ignacio A. Wichmann [3,4,5],
Benjamin A. Garcia-Bloj [3], Maria Alejandra Alarcon [3,4], Gareth I. Owen [1,3,6]
and Alejandro H. Corvalán [3,4,5,*]

[1] Departamento de Fisiología, Facultad de Ciencias Biológicas, Pontificia Universidad Católica de Chile,
    8330025 Santiago, Chile; jamigo@bio.puc.cl (J.D.A.); gowen@bio.puc.cl (G.I.O.)
[2] Instituto de Ciencias Ambientales y Evolutivas, Facultad de Ciencias, Universidad Austral de Chile,
    5090000 Valdivia, Chile; jopazo@gmail.com
[3] Laboratory of Oncology, Facultad de Medicina, Pontificia Universidad Católica de Chile,
    8330034 Santiago, Chile; ignacio.wichmann@gmail.com (I.A.W.); garciabloj@gmail.com (B.A.G.-B.);
    mralarco@uc.cl (M.A.A.)
[4] Departamento de Oncología y Hematología, Facultad de Medicina, Pontificia Universidad Católica de Chile,
    8330034 Santiago, Chile
[5] CORE Biodata, Advanced Center for Chronic Diseases (ACCDiS), Pontificia Universidad Católica de Chile,
    8330024 Santiago, Chile; roddy.jorquera@gmail.com
[6] Millennium Institute on Immunology and Immunotherapy, Pontificia Universidad Católica de Chile,
    8331150 Santiago, Chile
*   Correspondence: corvalan@med.puc.cl; Tel.: +56-(2)-23548289

Received: 22 March 2018; Accepted: 21 April 2018; Published: 25 June 2018

Abstract: The reprimo (*RPRM*) gene family is a group of single exon genes present exclusively within
the vertebrate lineage. Two out of three members of this family are present in humans: *RPRM*
and *RPRM-Like* (*RPRML*). *RPRM* induces cell cycle arrest at G2/M in response to p53 expression.
Loss-of-expression of *RPRM* is related to increased cell proliferation and growth in gastric cancer.
This evidence suggests that *RPRM* has tumor suppressive properties. However, the molecular
mechanisms and signaling partners by which *RPRM* exerts its functions remain unknown. Moreover,
scarce studies have attempted to characterize *RPRML*, and its functionality is unclear. Herein,
we highlight the role of the *RPRM* gene family in gastric carcinogenesis, as well as its potential
applications in clinical settings. In addition, we summarize the current knowledge on the phylogeny
and expression patterns of this family of genes in embryonic zebrafish and adult humans. Strikingly,
in both species, *RPRM* is expressed primarily in the digestive tract, blood vessels and central nervous
system, supporting the use of zebrafish for further functional characterization of *RPRM*. Finally,
drawing on embryonic and adult expression patterns, we address the potential relevance of *RPRM* and
RPRML in cancer. Active investigation or analytical research in the coming years should contribute
to novel translational applications of this poorly understood gene family as potential biomarkers and
development of novel cancer therapies.

Keywords: gastric cancer; reprimo; tumor suppressive gene properties; development; evolution; biomarker

1. Introduction

The reprimo (*RPRM*) gene family is a novel and poorly understood single-exon intronless gene
family. *RPRM* genes are expressed across many species and are associated with developmental
patterning of the gastrointestinal tract, brain and blood vessels [1,2]. In humans, who have only *RPRM*
and *RPRM-Like* (*RPRML*), the *RPRM* gene appears to be involved in tumor suppression in tumors of
the gastrointestinal tract as well as in multiple other organs. Expression of *RPRM* is mainly induced

by p53 after DNA damage, though expression of this gene has also been associated to expression of p73, another member of the *p53* gene family [3]. Upregulation of RPRM results in cell cycle arrest at the G2/M checkpoint [4]. Epigenetic silencing of *RPRM*, mainly by DNA methylation of its promoter region, occurs at early stages of human cancer. Assessment of this biochemical DNA modification in body fluids has opened an interesting opportunity for translational applications of this family of genes, as cancer biomarkers.

Here, we describe and discuss the structure, genomic location and homologies of these poorly characterized genes. In addition, we explore the role in development as well as functional diversification of the *RPRM* family. In gastric cancer as well as in other human neoplasms, this family of single exon and intronless genes had led to the discovery of novel clinical applications such as non-invasive biomarkers for early diagnosis and disease monitoring and the development of new drugs for cancer therapies.

2. Structure and Genomic Location of the *RPRM* Gene Family

The *RPRM* gene family is composed of three members: *RPRM*, *RPRML* and *RPRM3*. While *RPRM* and *RPRML* are expressed in most of the vertebrate lineages, *RPRM3* is only found in cartilaginous fish (e.g., sharks and rays), bony fish (e.g., zebrafish) and coelacanths [1]. In humans, *RPRM* and *RPRML* are both single exon and intronless genes, which is an uncommon type of gene representing roughly 3% of the human genome [5]. *RPRM* and *RPRML* are located on the minus strand of chromosomes 2q23.3 and 17q21.32, respectively. *RPRM* spans 1.47 kb of genomic DNA and encodes a 109-amino acid protein with an estimated molecular weight of 11,774 Da. Similarly, *RPRML* spans 1.09 kb of genomic DNA encoding a 120-amino acid protein with an estimated molecular weight of 12,312 Da. *RPRM3* is also a single exon gene and intronless gene, that is located on the minus strand of chromosome 23q32.2 in zebrafish, *RPRM3* spans 1.794 kb of genomic DNA and encodes a 103-amino acid protein with an estimated molecular weight of 11,323 Da.

RPRM is a highly glycosylated protein which has two N-glycosylation sites at amino acids 7 and 18, a potential serine-phosphorylation site at residue 98, a predicted sumoylation site at position 82 and a potential transmembrane domain covering amino acids 56 to 76 (Figure 1) [6]. Furthermore, *RPRML* has predicted N-glycosylation sites at amino acids 2 and 27, a predicted sumoylation site at position 93 and a transmembrane site covering amino acids 67 to 87 (Figure 1). As other intronless gene families, such as *JUN* and *FOX*, the *RPRM* gene family is often implicated in cancer through their overrepresentation in cell growth and proliferation [7]. Functional analyses have suggested that *RPRM* is a transcriptional target for p53 and as a cell cycle arrest protein at the G2/M checkpoint, operating through inhibition of the nuclear translocation of the Cdc2/cyclin B1 complex [4].

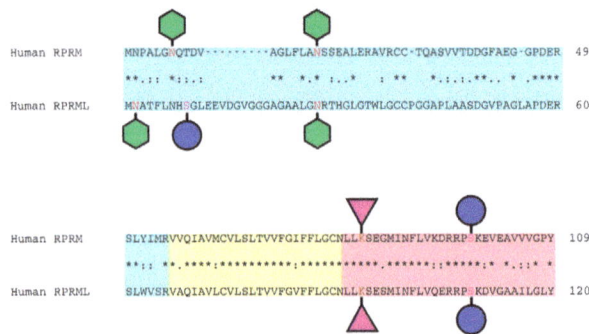

Figure 1. *Cont.*

⬡ Potential N-Glycosilation sites*

⬤ Potential Serine-Phosphorylation sites**

▽ Potential Sumoylation sites***

▪ N-terminal domain

▪ C-terminal domain

▪ Transmembrane domain

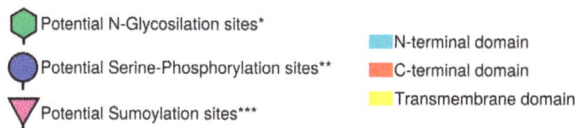

Figure 1. Domain structure and potential post-translational modification sites of human RPRM and RPRML proteins. Schematic representation shows the RPRM and RPRML putative *N*-glycosylation (green hexagons), serine-phosphorylation (blue circle) and sumoylation (purple triangle) sites. The N-terminal, transmembrane and C-terminal domains are represented by colored boxes (turquoise, yellow, and red, respectively). An * (asterisk) indicates positions which have a single, fully conserved residue. A: (colon) indicates conservation between groups of strongly similar properties—scoring >0.5 in the Gonnet PAM 250 matrix. A. (period) indicates conservation between groups of weakly similar properties—scoring 0.5 in the Gonnet PAM 250 matrix. Post-translational modification sites were predicted using *NetNGlyc (http://www.cbs.dtu.dk/services/NetNGlyc/), **NetPhos (http://www.cbs.dtu.dk/services/NetPhos/) and ***SumoPlot (http://www.abgent.com/sumoplot).

3. Evolution of the *RPRM* Gene Family

Based on current sequenced genome data, the evolutionary history of the *RPRM* gene family traces back to the last common ancestor of vertebrates, which lived between 676 and 615 million of years ago [1]. At that time the ancestor of vertebrates presumably had only a single *RPRM* gene in its genome, which likely performed many of the physiological functions that the current gene family performs today. Through time, this ancestral gene diversified as a consequence of the two rounds of whole genome duplications (WGDs), which occurred early in the evolutionary history of vertebrates [8,9]. Thus, the single copy gene present in the genome of the vertebrate ancestor gave rise to four *RPRM* genes [1], three of which were retained in actual vertebrates (Figure 2A). The presence of co-duplicated genes that are found on the chromosomes where the *RPRM* genes are located in actual species, and the fact that the genomic regions in which the *RPRM* genes are located derived from a single linkage group in the chordate ancestor support this hypothesis [10].

During the diversification of vertebrates the *RPRM* gene family was differentially retained, as not all *RPRM* genes are present in all main vertebrate groups (Figure 2A). Although it was previously claimed that the *RPRM* gene was not retained in birds [1], searches in the most recent version of bird genomes revealed the presence of the *RPRM* gene in this subgroup of amniotes. Thus, all groups of jawed vertebrates (gnathostomes) have retained this gene (Figure 2A). The *RPRML* gene has also been identified in all main groups of gnathostomes, whereas *RPRM3* was only retained in four distantly related vertebrate groups: cartilaginous fish (e.g., sharks, skates, and rays), holostean fish (e.g., bowfish, gars), teleost fish (e.g., zebrafish) and coelacanths (Figure 2A). In cyclostomes, the group that includes lampreys and hagfish, two *RPRM* genes has been identified (Figure 2A). However, phylogenetic reconstructions have failed in defining orthology. *RPRM* sequences of this group are recovered sister to each other, which might be due to features of their genomes (e.g., GC bias) that differ substantially from all other vertebrate genomes [11–13], making it difficult to recover the true evolutionary history using phylogenetic approaches.

More recently in vertebrate history, the *RPRM* gene family further expanded as a consequence of the teleost-specific genome duplication (TSGD) that occurred in the ancestor of this group between 325 and 275 million of years ago [14,15] (Figure 2A). Although the TSGD potentially doubled the number of all *RPRM* genes in the common ancestor of teleosts, only the *rprm* gene retained duplicated copies, termed *rprma* and *rprmb* (Figure 2A).

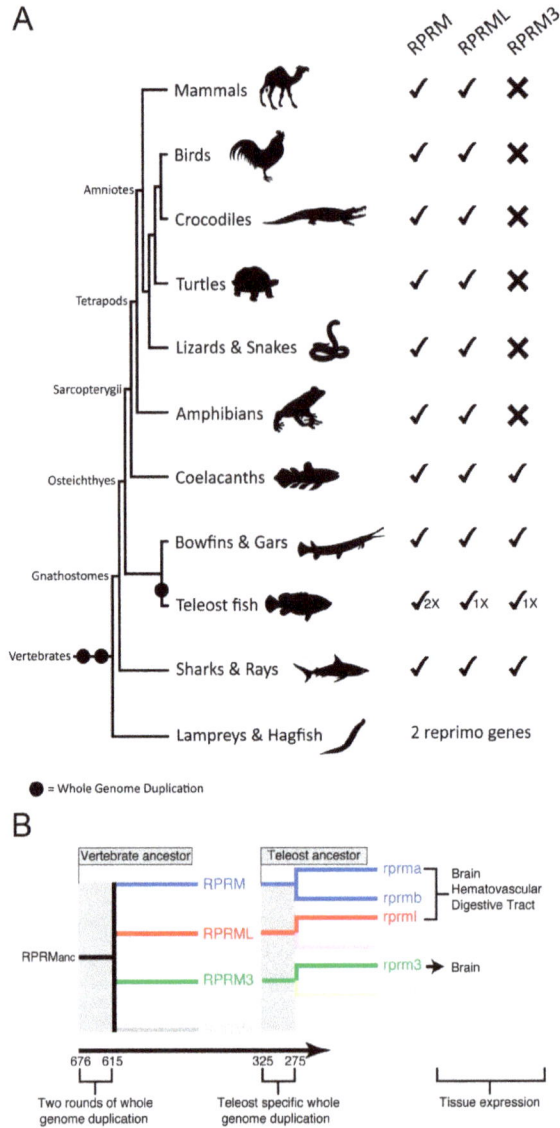

Figure 2. Evolution and diversification of *RPRM* genes in vertebrates. (**A**) During the diversification of vertebrates *RPRM* genes were differentially retained, as not all *RPRM* genes are present in all main groups of vertebrates. Thus, *RPRM* and *RPRML* genes were retained in all main groups of jawed vertebrates (gnathostomes), whereas *RPRM3* was only retained in four distantly related groups: cartilaginous fish (e.g., sharks, skates, and rays), holostean fish (e.g., bowfish and gars), teleost fish (e.g., zebrafish) and coelacanths. In the group that includes lampreys and hagfish, two *RPRM* genes have been identified, however, phylogenetic and synteny analyses have failed in defining orthology. (**B**) Schematic representation of the evolution of the *RPRM* gene family in teleost fish. On the left, the *RPRM* gene family diversified as a product of the two rounds of whole-genome duplication occurred in the vertebrate ancestor, as well as, a teleost-specific whole genome duplication. On the left, the expression territories of the three *RPRM* gene lineages present in teleost fish.

4. Developmental Expression Patterns of *RPRM* Gene Family

The use of animal models is the primary step to understand the process of human carcinogenesis and the development of new drugs for cancer therapies [16]. In this scenario, Zebrafish combines the complexity of a whole vertebrate animal with the easy-to-use and high-throughput characteristics of in vitro models [17,18]. Despite differences with teleosts, most of the genetic pathways that regulate development are similar between zebrafish and human [19]. In zebrafish embryos—both duplicated copies of *rprm* (*rprma* and *rprmb*) are expressed in a tissue-specific manner in the gastrointestinal tract, brain and blood vessels. Strikingly, expression of RPRM protein in adult human was also detected in the same organs [2]. Expression of *rprm3*, a gene that is lost in all tetrapods, is restricted to the central nervous system (CNS) in zebrafish embryos and larvae [2].

Our recent observations also indicate that the three *rprm* genes (*rprma*, *rprmb* and *rprml*) genes are expressed in the developing digestive tract in embryonic fish [2]. Importantly, in humans, *RPRM* is a gene which expression is lost in many human gastrointestinal malignancies and serves as a potential biomarker for non-invasive detection of gastric cancer (reviewed in the following section). The RPRM protein is located in epithelial cells lining the intestinal crypts and gastric glands and smooth muscle cells (SMCs) from the *Muscularis propria* [2], As in humans, the digestive tube of the zebrafish is organized in concentric layers of SMCs [20]. However, the role of *RPRM* genes during the differentiation process of gastrointestinal epithelial cells, which occurs during the migration of these cells from the base of gastric glands and intestinal crypts, remains to be determined. In this scenario, the zebrafish model organism offers an interesting alternative to dissect this role in developmental physiology.

Figueroa et al. [2] also show that, in zebrafish and humans, the *RPRM* and *RPRML* genes are expressed in vascular tissues. In humans, RPRM is expressed in endothelial and vascular smooth muscle cells (VSMCs). The expression of RPRM and RPRML in blood vessels suggests a potential involvement of *RPRM* during angiogenesis or vasculogenesis. Future studies require molecular manipulation of the *RPRM* gene family to unveil the role of *RPRM* genes in the formation and dynamics of the blood vessels.

As we recently reported, in embryonic zebrafish larvae, *rprma*, *rprmb* and *rprml* are expressed distinctly in the developing brain [21]. Some of the structures that express these genes include the forebrain, telencephalon and the olfactory epithelium (OE), among other sensory organs. For example, the expression of *rprma* is largely restricted to the peripheral nervous system at the OE, while *rprmb* transcripts are located in most posterior neuronal territories such as the optic tectum and trigeminal ganglia. In contrast to *rprma* and *rprmb*, expression of *rprml* is not detectable in the retina. In adult zebrafish and humans, the RPRM messenger and protein are both located in brain tissues. The human RPRM is expressed in grey and white matter neurons and glial cells from the brain cortex, a tissue that displays low mitotic rates during adulthood [2,21,22]. These findings suggest that the *RPRM* genes may play a key role in the regulation of cell proliferation in brain development and/or regeneration during adulthood [21]. Models that compare brain-specific gene expression profiles between wild-type animals and those with loss-of-function of *rprm* and *rprml* will help to define the expression and function of the *RPRM* gene family in the processes that contribute to brain development.

5. Functional Diversification of the *RPRM* Gene Family

Due to the three WGDs, the diversification of the *RPRM* gene family opens new opportunities for physiological innovation within this lineage. In the literature it has been difficult to probe the causal link between the WGDs and biological innovation [23], although for some well-studied gene families, this causal association has been demonstrated [24–26]. As mentioned above, expression profile analyses of the *RPRM* genes demonstrate that they exhibit unique—although partially overlapping—expression patterns during embryonic and larval vascular development [2]. On one hand, *rprma*, *rprmb* and *rprml* are all expressed in the digestive tube, blood vessels and brain; whereas *rprm3* possesses a unique expression profile restricted only to the brain. Importantly, the expression patterns of *rprma* and *rprmb* transcripts in the zebrafish resembled expression profiles of the RPRM protein in humans. This evidence suggests that the developmental expression pattern for the *RPRM* gene family is the same in fish and mammals [1]. Furthermore, the compartmentalization in humans of *RPRM* genes in partially overlapping territories seems to agree with the pattern described for teleost fish (Figure 2B) [27]. Future studies should elucidate the functional role of the *RPRM* gene family during the physiological processes such as gut, vascular and neuronal development across the vertebrate subphylum.

6. Role of the *RPRM* Gene Family in Human Carcinogenesis

In order to uncover the *RPRM* and *RPRML* tissue expression patterns in human samples, we have assessed in silico RNAseq data from the Genotype Tissue Expression (GTEx) database [28]. As shown in Figure 3A, *RPRM* has a variable expression across different tissues, whereas *RPRML* is expressed at very low levels in most tissues, except for brain compartments where expression levels are the highest. However, low transcript levels are expected for intronless genes, which generally express at lower levels than intron-containing genes despite having important biological roles [29]. Transcriptome studies in several vertebrate species reveal that *RPRM* genes are mainly expressed in the central nervous system. In accordance with this observation, our previous studies have shown that the transcript and protein for *RPRM* are expressed in the zebrafish and human brain [2]. In the case of cancer tissues, as shown in Figure 3B, both genes display down regulated expression in tumor tissues in comparison with non-tumor adjacent mucosa, including gastric cancer [30].

At experimental and clinical levels, only the *RPRM* gene has been examined in terms of biological functions and significance in human cancer. In gastric cancer cells, restoring the expression of *RPRM* by transfecting exogenous cDNA results in reduced colony formation and anchorage-independent growth [3,31]. Correspondingly, mouse xenografts models of gastric cancer cells deficient in *RPRM* expression have demonstrated enhanced tumor formation and volume [31,32]. In other tumors, such as breast cancer, pituitary tumors and renal cell carcinoma cell lines, overexpression of RPRM suppresses cell proliferation, cell migration, clonogenic capacity and invasiveness [33–35]. Furthermore, the role of RPRM in cell-cycle has also been explored. Ohki et al. [4] overexpressed RPRM through adenoviral infection in cells with wild-type (HeLa, Lovo, MCF7) and mutated (DLD1 and Saos2) p53, observing cell-cycle arrest in G2/M phase, independently of p53 mutational status. However, conflicting results have been reported in gastric cancer and pituitary cell lines where RPRM overexpression results in a significant increase in the sub-G1 population with minimal changes in S and G2/M populations [31,34]. Ectopic expression of RPRM cDNA in gastric cancer cell lines after exposure to DNA-damaging agents, such as 5-fluorouracil or cisplatin, results in an apoptotic phenotype 24 h after treatment [31]. In other types of tumors, with both wild-type and mutated *p53* gene, overexpression of RPRM induces an apoptotic phenotype after 4 days of adenoviral infection, suggesting that RPRM may also repress cell growth by induction of apoptosis [4]. Taken together, these results suggest that *RPRM* has tumor suppressive properties not only in gastric cancer but also in other tumors.

Clinical studies have shown that the loss of *RPRM* expression is as common event in gastric cancer [3,31,32,36] as in other tumors of the gastrointestinal tract including Barrett's-associated esophageal adenocarcinoma, pancreatic and colorectal carcinoma [37–41]. Loss of expression of *RPRM* has been also reported in non-digestive tumors including breast, renal cell carcinoma, adrenocortical and pituitary tumors [33–35,42,43]. Conversely, enhanced *RPRM* expression has been described in metastatic brain tumors [44].

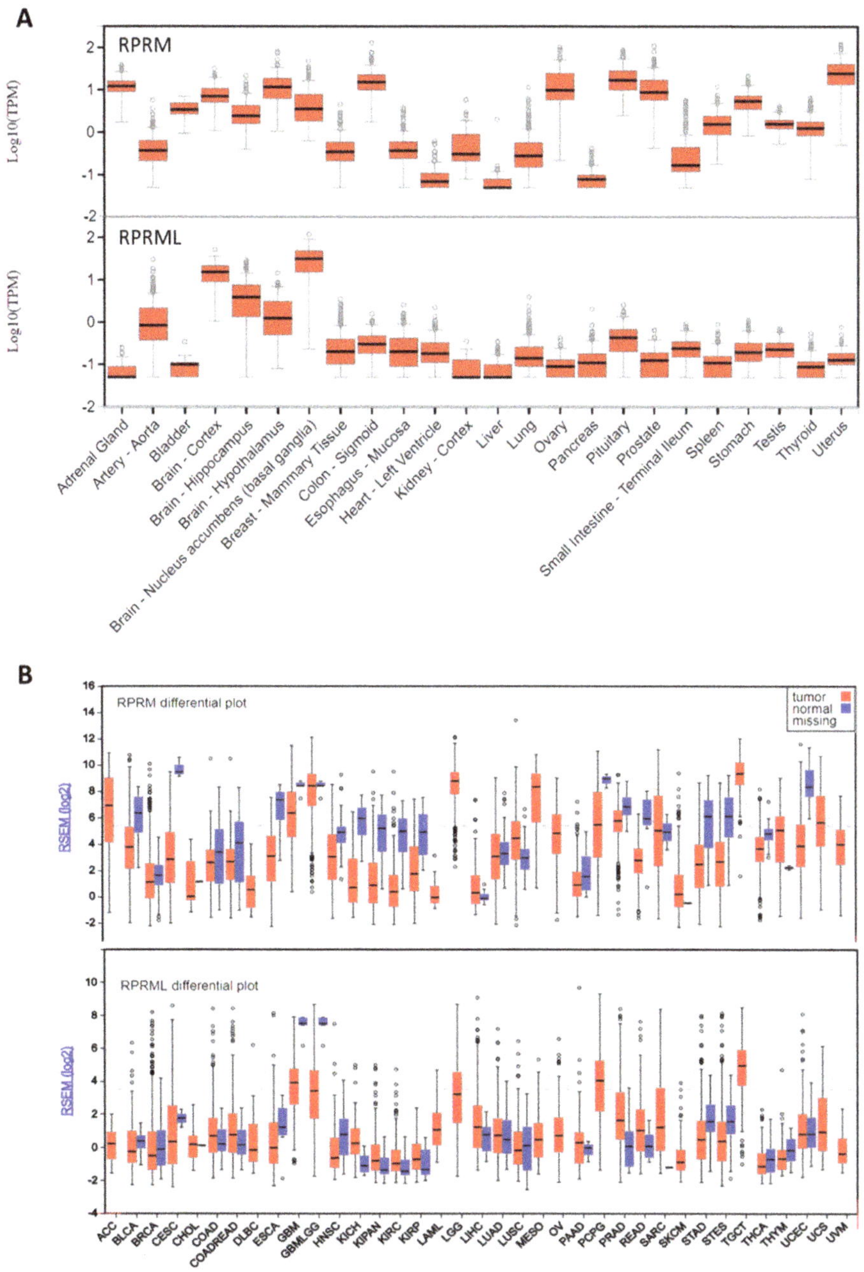

Figure 3. RNA expression of *RPRM* and *RPRML* across different tissues. (**A**) Tissue-specific expression profile from 570 human donors available in the Genotype-Tissue Expression (GTEx) database [28]. Data is expressed as log10 of Transcripts Per Kilobase Million (TPM). (**B**) Expression levels of human tumor and matched normal tissue samples from Broad Institute TCGA Genome Data Analysis Center [30]. Data is expressed as log2 of RSEM (RNA-Seq by Expectation Maximization).

RPRM is located within a CpG-enriched region of the genome. In these regions, a significant proportion of cytosines contain a methyl group in the fifth carbon when they are immediately preceded by a guanine (CpG sites). Although unevenly distributed across the genome, CpG sites generally cluster near gene promoters (CpG islands), thus controlling local chromatin structure and transcription factor binding [45]. In normal cells, a few ʿCpG islands are usually methylated (DNA methylation), maintaining genomic stability and controlling expression of tissue-specific, imprinted and housekeeping genes [46]. In contrast, an aberrant pattern of DNA methylation has been observed in some cancers characterized by a genome wide low methylation state that promotes transcriptional activation of oncogenes, genomic instability, and loss of imprinting, while some CpG islands, particularly those located in the promoter regions of tumor suppressor genes, show a local hypermethylated state that may result in gene silencing [47]. This is one of the most common epigenetic alterations found in human cancers. In the case of *RPRM*, bisulfite sequence experiments to evaluate the density of methylated CpG sites of the promoter region have correlated positively with the levels of the transcriptional expression of the gene [3]. Consequently, restoring the expression of *RPRM* by the use of demethylating agents, such as 5-aza-cytidine has confirmed that the expression of *RPRM* gene is regulated by DNA methylation in gastric cancer cells [3,32,48]. In other neoplasm similar results have been obtain confirming the role of DNA methylation as the main mechanisms of regulation of *RPRM* gene expression [35,49]. In addition, DNA methylation of *RPRM* has been associated with a compact chromatin structure and further increasing transcriptional silencing of the gene [49]. Interestingly, an in agreement with the enhanced *RPRM* expression in metastatic brain tumors [44], bisulfite sequence studies in pituitary tumors have shown that loss of *RPRM* is not due to hypermethylation of the promoter region [34]. This observation raises the possibility that other mechanisms, genetic and/or epigenetic (i.e., microRNAs), might contribute to *RPRM* gene regulation.

As previously mentioned, *RPRM* has been proposed as a transcriptional target for p53. In gastric cancer cells expressing wild-type p53, a significant down-regulation of RPRM has been described. Conversely, RPRM-induced changes were not seen in p53-deficient NCI-N87 cells. [50]. Analogous findings have been described by in silico analysis of the TCGA data, where a negative correlation between Survivin and RPRM expression was identified exclusively in patients with wild-type p53 protein status [50].

Based on a positive co-expression between RPRM and p73 proteins in a large cohort of tumor samples, the possibility that other members of the *p53* gene family participate in the regulation of *RPRM* has been raised [3]. Since cytoplasmic overexpression of RPRM inhibit nuclear translocation of the Cdc2-Cyclin/B1 complex inducing cell cycle arrest at the G2/M stage [4] further binding and or co-immunoprecipation experiments should contribute to clarify the role of p73 in the regulation of the expression of RPRM (Figure 4).

The clinical significance of the loss of RPRM expression in gastric cancer was first explored by Luo et al. [36]. This study analyzed RPRM protein expression along with tumor suppressor S100A2 (S100 calcium binding protein A2) in a cohort of 100 consecutive gastric cancer cases identifying loss of RPRM expression in up to 65% of cases. Interestingly, Luo et al. [36] found that there exists a positive relationship between the expressions of both genes. Furthermore, loss of RPRM expression was significantly associated with depth of tumor invasion, lymphatic vascular invasion and lymph node metastasis. These clinical findings have been confirmed by Saavedra et al. [3] showing also that loss of RPRM expression is particularly associated with the progression from stage I to stages III-IV (Japanese classification of gastric carcinoma) [51] in a cohort of Hispanic/Amerindian cases from Latin America, one of the highest regions in gastric cancer incidence worldwide [52]. Although none of the earlier studies were able to show that loss of expression of RPRM could influence overall survival in gastric cancer, our group has recently found that loss of RPRM expression does confer a worse prognosis only when accompanied with overexpression of Survivin, a well establish oncogene in gastric cancer [50,53]. Taken together, data suggest that *RPRM* requires a genetic background including other cancer-related genes, such as S100A2 and/or Survivin to drive the gastric carcinogenesis process.

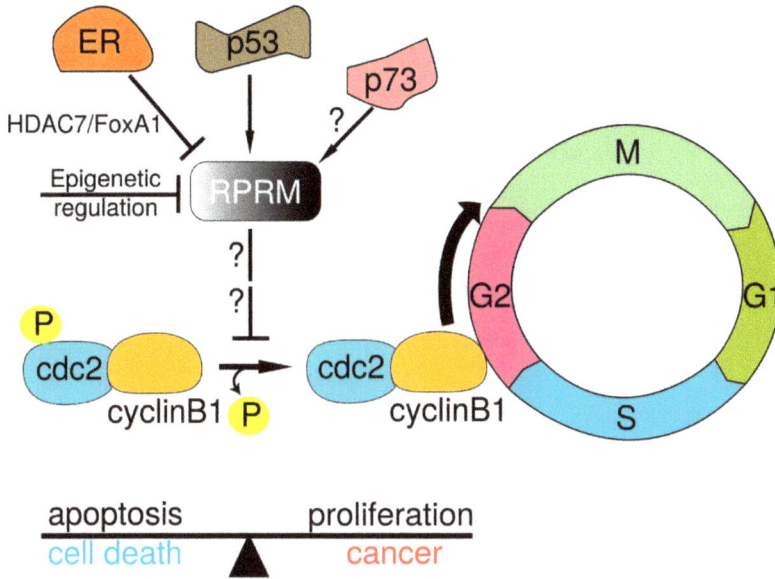

Figure 4. Schematic model of RPRM-mediated cell cycle and G2 arrest mechanisms. *RPRM* has been identified as a transcriptional target for: (1) p53 [4]; (2) histone deacetylase 7/FoxA1 (HDAC7/FoxA1) in an estrogen mediated mechanism [49]; and (3) for epigenetic silencing by hypermethylation of its promoter region [54]. A potential regulation by p73 it has also been proposed [3]. RPRM expression results in inhibited dephosphorylation of Cdc2, suppressing the activation of the Cdc2-Cyclin B1 complex. Thus, inducing cell cycle arrest at G2 suggesting a potential role for *RPRM* as a tumor suppressor gene [4]. The balance towards cell cycle arrest or proliferation can be shifted by multiple antagonistic effectors, amongst them *RPRM*. Straight lines with arrowheads indicate activation. Lines with no arrowhead indicate inhibition. Curved arrow on the bottom left indicates dephosphorylation of Cdc2/Cyclin B1 complex. Curved thick arrow on the bottom right indicates nuclear translocation of dephosphorylated Cdc2/Cyclin B1 at the G2/M checkpoint.

Interestingly, it has recently been shown that upregulation of endogenous RPRM expression by the use of CRISPR/dCas9 (Clustered Regularly Interspaced Short Palindromic Repeats and associated dead Cas9) system, a platform that utilizes a catalytically deactivated Cas9 (dCas9) linked to effector domains for gene expression regulation (i.e., Synergistic Activation Mediator (SAM) complex) reduced cell proliferation and increased apoptosis in gastric cancer cells [55]. This finding has been expanded to other genes with tumor suppressor properties embedded in a CpG-enriched region of the genome such as Maspin or METTL3 [55,56]. The use of this new tool will be useful not only for the understanding of the epigenetic modifications in an endogenous biological context but also for the potential cancer therapies based on these findings.

Studies have shown that across the gastric precancerous cascade, *RPRM* becomes increasingly hypermethylated, in association with loss of protein expression. These findings are particularly related with the transition from intestinal metaplasia to dysplasia and/or gastric cancer [57]. Consequently, no differences in methylation levels have been found between paired tumor and non-tumor adjacent cells [3]. Taken together, loss of expression and/or methylation of *RPRM* could be proposed as a late event in the gastric precancerous cascade. Methylation of the *RPRM* promoter region is associated with the infection of *Helicobacter pylori* particularly to cytotoxin-associated gene A (CagA) strains [58]. Accordingly, methylation of *RPRM* promoter region has been proposed as a tissue biomarker for the evaluation of *H. pylori* eradication [59].

Accordingly, with this line of evidence, follow-up studies examining DNA methylation levels of *RPRM* on the longitudinal progression of the gastric precancerous lesions after *H. pylori* eradication, have revealed an increasing level of the DNA methylation six-years prior the progression of gastric lesions [60]. Interestingly, these changes were independent of the effect of the duration of *H. pylori* infection and other clinical parameters [60].

Since *RPRML* is also located within a CpG-enriched region of the genome, as has been well documented in the case of *RPRM* [3,35,48,49] and also correlates with transcriptional silencing [3,32], the evaluation of *RPRML* methylation may yield similar findings to that of *RPRM*. To assess this issue, an exploratory in silico analysis of RNAseq expression data from paired gastric adenocarcinomas and non-tumor adjacent mucosa from The Cancer Genome Atlas (TCGA) database [0] is in progress. In addition, in vitro gain/loss of function experiments focused on evaluation of tumorigenic or tumor suppressive effects may provide insights on the role of *RPRML* in cancer.

7. Methylated *RPRM* Cell-Free DNA as a Potential Non-Invasive Biomarker in Gastric Cancer

The discovery of methylated cell-free DNA in body fluids has expanded the translational applications of DNA methylation of cancer-related genes [61,62]. Due to its relatively stable nature and availability, DNA methylation can be easily detected in serum, plasma and a variety of body fluids. Thus, the assessment of DNA methylation through cell-free DNA or liquid biopsy approaches has been proposed as a candidate for the diagnosis and management of cancer [63].

Our group was the first to propose the assessment of methylated cell-free DNA of the *RPRM* promoter gene region for non-invasive detection of gastric cancer with a sensitivity of 95.35% [95% CI: 84.19–99.43%] and specificity of 90.32% [95% CI: 74.25–97.96%] [48]. These values achieved the highest OR (OR = 191.33 [95% CI = 30.01, 1220.01]) in a comprehensive meta-analyses undertaken by Sapari el al. [64] after consolidation of 132 case-controls studies for potential biomarkers based on methylated DNA in gastric cancer. This approach has subsequently been extended to the detection of precancerous lesions [32,57,65]. Therefore, clinical trials addressing the role of *RPRM* as a non-invasive biomarker in gastric cancer should be performed.

8. Unanswered Questions and the *RPRM* Gene Family

There are many biological questions still to be answered regarding *RPRM* gene family. Protein structure and the biological relevance of post-translational modifications such as glycosylation, phosphorylation and sumoylation should be assessed (Figure 1). Furthermore, the regulation of expression and the translational applications of the *RPRM* gene family in cancer medicine need to be further elucidated, along with a potential role in other pathologies [4]. Originally described as a p53-dependent cell cycle arrest mediator (Figure 4), yet the functions and mechanisms by which RPRM acts still remain unknown. Evolutionary studies, developmental genetics and molecular biology approaches will prove useful tools in determining the origin and function of this single exon and intronless *RPRM* gene family [7,66]. The evaluation of different and complementary lines of evidence such as (1) selective pressures; (2) phenotypical variations as a consequence of loss- or gain-of-function; and (3) pre- and post-transcriptional and translational variations may deliver a better understanding of this gene family. From an evolutionary perspective, comparative genomics and phylogenetic analyses may provide evidence of co-evolution and potential relationships between *RPRM* and other gene families, and thus uncover new signaling partners. Questions regarding a "de novo" origin or retrotranscription of mRNA followed by insertion of the resulting DNA copy into the genome should be addressed to clarify the origin and evolution of the *RPRM* single exon gene family. Using molecular and genetic approaches, which rely on DNA sequence or RNA/protein expression alterations, it may be possible to establish the pathophysiological role of the *RPRM* genes in the regulation of cellular functions. Mutation of *RPRM* family genes will be useful to identify phenotypic defects generated by *RPRM* loss-of-function as well as to dissect the role of *RPRM* in developmental processes.

The function and role of the *RPRM* genes in gastric carcinogenesis should be expanded to incorporate *RPRML* (Figure 5); as to date, only the human *RPRM* gene has been examined. Importantly, the unique expression pattern of *rprml* suggests that this is a functional gene and will hopefully initiate studies into its presence and function in human gastric physiology and cancer tissues.

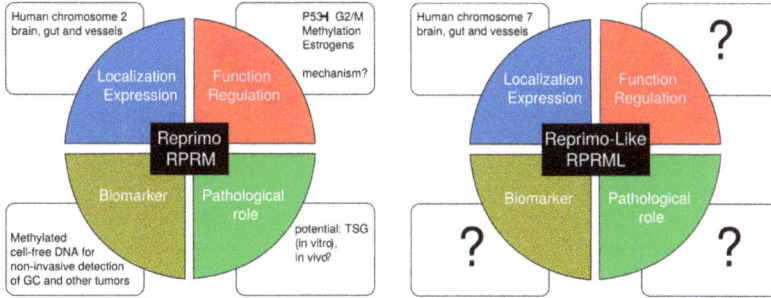

Figure 5. Unanswered questions in *RPRM* gene family. RPRM is as a p53-induced protein which induces cell cycle arrest at the G2/M checkpoint [4], through an unknown mechanism. Recently, *RPRM* genes have been shown to be expressed during brain, gut and blood vessel development [2]. Additional functions for *RPRM* include its role as a potential tumor suppressor gene (TSG), and a biomarker—through the assessment of the methylation status of its promoter region—for non-invasive detection of gastric cancer and other tumors [48,62]. Much like *RPRM*, *RPRML* is also expressed during embryonic development [2], but its role in physiological processes has never been investigated.

Although the ectopic expression of *RPRM* induces cell cycle arrest and apoptosis in vitro [4,34,55], unanswered questions still remain as to how transcriptional silencing of *RPRM* predisposes tissues to gastric cancer development. In multiple tumors, DNA methylation is the most common epigenetic mechanism of loss-of-expression of *RPRM* [62]. In fact, loss-of-expression by DNA methylation of the *RPRM* promoter region it is an indicator of cancer progression and the continuous use of demethylating agents such 5-aza -cytidine can restore *RPRM* gene function and dampen indicators of tumor progression [3]. In this scenario, more specific approaches to re-activate *RPRM* expression, for example through CRISPR/dCas9-based artificial transcription factors, may open the door to new translational opportunities in cancer therapeutics.

9. Concluding Remarks

The role of the *RPRM* gene family in vertebrate physiology and disease is still a bourgeoning field. A comprehensive characterization of the genetic interactions, signaling pathways, protein modifications and regulatory mechanisms of the *RPRM* gene family may shed light on its role in both physiological and oncological processes. *RPRM* is known to play a role in tumors of the stomach and has translational applications in the monitoring and treatment of disease. Whether other members of this gene family also have tumor suppressor properties or play relevant roles in other pathologies, remains a key question in need of further research. In this scenario, this family of single exon genes could lead to the discovery of novel biomarkers and therapeutic targets, together with the development of new drugs and clinical applications. The coming years should bring forth active investigation to help understand, define and utilize the *RPRM* gene family.

Acknowledgments: BMBF-CONICYT 20140027, CRP-ICGEB CH15-01 and CONICYT-ANILLO ACT1402 (JDA), IMII P09/016-F (GIO), Fondecyt grants 1160627 (JCO), 1180241 (GIO), 1151411 (AHC) and CONICYT-FONDAP 15130011 (AHC and GIO).

Conflicts of Interest: The authors declare no conflict of interest.

References

1. Wichmann, I.A.; Zavala, K.; Hoffmann, F.G.; Vandewege, M.W.; Corvalan, A.H.; Amigo, J.D.; Owen, G.I.; Opazo, J.C. Evolutionary history of the reprimo tumor suppressor gene family in vertebrates with a description of a new reprimo gene lineage. *Gene* **2016**, *591*, 245–254. [CrossRef] [PubMed]

2. Figueroa, R.J.; Carrasco-Avino, G.; Wichmann, I.A.; Lange, M.; Owen, G.I.; Siekmann, A.F.; Corvalan, A.H.; Opazo, J.C.; Amigo, J.D. Reprimo tissue-specific expression pattern is conserved between zebrafish and human. *PLoS ONE* **2017**, *12*, e0178274. [CrossRef] [PubMed]

3. Saavedra, K.; Valbuena, J.; Olivares, W.; Marchant, M.J.; Rodriguez, A.; Torres-Estay, V.; Carrasco-Avino, G.; Guzman, L.; Aguayo, F.; Roa, J.C.; et al. Loss of expression of reprimo, a p53-induced cell cycle arrest gene, correlates with invasive stage of tumor progression and p73 expression in gastric cancer. *PLoS ONE* **2015**, *10*, e0125834. [CrossRef] [PubMed]

4. Ohki, R.; Nemoto, J.; Murasawa, H.; Oda, E.; Inazawa, J.; Tanaka, N.; Taniguchi, T. Reprimo, a new candidate mediator of the p53-mediated cell cycle arrest at the G2 phase. *J. Biol. Chem.* **2000**, *275*, 22627–22630. [CrossRef] [PubMed]

5. Louhichi, A.; Fourati, A.; Rebai, A. Igd: A resource for intronless genes in the human genome. *Gene* **2011**, *488*, 35–40. [CrossRef] [PubMed]

6. Huret, J.L.; Ahmad, M.; Arsaban, M.; Bernheim, A.; Cigna, J.; Desangles, F.; Guignard, J.C.; Jacquemot-Perbal, M.C.; Labarussias, M.; Leberre, V.; et al. Atlas of genetics and cytogenetics in oncology and haematology in 2013. *Nucleic Acids Res.* **2013**, *41*, D920–D924. [CrossRef] [PubMed]

7. Grzybowska, E.A. Human intronless genes: Functional groups, associated diseases, evolution, and mRNA processing in absence of splicing. *Biochem. Biophys. Res. Commun.* **2012**, *424*, 1–6. [CrossRef] [PubMed]

8. Holland, P.W.; Garcia-Fernandez, J.; Williams, N.A.; Sidow, A. Gene duplications and the origins of vertebrate development. *Development* **1994**, *1994*, 125–133.

9. Dehal, P.; Boore, J.L. Two rounds of whole genome duplication in the ancestral vertebrate. *PLoS Boil.* **2005**, *3*, e314. [CrossRef] [PubMed]

10. Putnam, N.H.; Butts, T.; Ferrier, D.E.; Furlong, R.F.; Hellsten, U.; Kawashima, T.; Robinson-Rechavi, M.; Shoguchi, E.; Terry, A.; Yu, J.K.; et al. The amphioxus genome and the evolution of the chordate karyotype. *Nature* **2008**, *453*, 1064–1071. [CrossRef] [PubMed]

11. Qiu, H.; Hildebrand, F.; Kuraku, S.; Meyer, A. Unresolved orthology and peculiar coding sequence properties of lamprey genes: The KCNA gene family as test case. *BMC Genom.* **2011**, *12*, 325. [CrossRef] [PubMed]

12. Kuraku, S. Impact of asymmetric gene repertoire between cyclostomes and gnathostomes. *Semin. Cell Dev. Boil.* **2013**, *24*, 119–127. [CrossRef] [PubMed]

13. Smith, J.J.; Kuraku, S.; Holt, C.; Sauka-Spengler, T.; Jiang, N.; Campbell, M.S.; Yandell, M.D.; Manousaki, T.; Meyer, A.; Bloom, O.E.; et al. Sequencing of the sea lamprey (*Petromyzon marinus*) genome provides insights into vertebrate evolution. *Nat. Genet.* **2013**, *45*, 415–421. [CrossRef] [PubMed]

14. Meyer, A.; Van de Peer, Y. From 2R to 3R: Evidence for a fish-specific genome duplication (FSGD). *BioEssays* **2005**, *27*, 937–945. [CrossRef] [PubMed]

15. Kasahara, M. The 2R hypothesis: An update. *Curr. Opin. Immunol.* **2007**, *19*, 547–552. [CrossRef] [PubMed]

16. Gutierrez-Lovera, C.; Vazquez-Rios, A.J.; Guerra-Varela, J.; Sánchez, L.; de la Fuente, M. The potential of zebrafish as a model organism for improving the translation of genetic anticancer nanomedicines. *Gene* **2017**, *8*, 349. [CrossRef] [PubMed]

17. Vogel, G. Genomics: Sanger will sequence zebrafish genome. *Science* **2000**, *290*, 1671. [CrossRef] [PubMed]

18. Staton, C.A.; Reed, M.W.; Brown, N.J. A critical analysis of current in vitro and in vivo angiogenesis assays. *Int. J. Exp. Pathol.* **2009**, *90*, 195–221. [CrossRef] [PubMed]

19. MacRae, C.A.; Peterson, R.T. Zebrafish as tools for drug discovery. *Nat. Rev. Drug Discov.* **2015**, *14*, 721–731. [CrossRef] [PubMed]

20. Wallace, K.N.; Akhter, S.; Smith, E.M.; Lorent, K.; Pack, M. Intestinal growth and differentiation in zebrafish. *Mech. Dev.* **2005**, *122*, 157–173. [CrossRef] [PubMed]

21. Stanic, K.; Quiroz, A.; Wichmann, I.; Corvalan, A.H.; Owen, G.I.; Opazo, J.C.; Lemus, C.; Concha, M.; Amigo, J.D. Expression of *RPRM/rprm* in the olfactory system of embryonic zebrafish (*Danio rerio*). *Front. Neuroanat.* **2018**. [CrossRef] [PubMed]

22. Ming, G.L.; Song, H. Adult neurogenesis in the mammalian brain: Significant answers and significant questions. *Neuron* **2011**, *70*, 687–702. [CrossRef] [PubMed]

23. Van de Peer, Y.; Maere, S.; Meyer, A. The evolutionary significance of ancient genome duplications. *Nat. Rev. Genet.* **2009**, *10*, 725–732. [CrossRef] [PubMed]

24. Hoffmann, F.G.; Opazo, J.C.; Storz, J.F. Whole-genome duplications spurred the functional diversification of the globin gene superfamily in vertebrates. *Mol. Biol. Evol.* **2012**, *29*, 303–312. [CrossRef] [PubMed]

25. Hoffmann, F.G.; Opazo, J.C.; Storz, J.F. Differential loss and retention of cytoglobin, myoglobin, and globin-e during the radiation of vertebrates. *Genome Biol. Evol.* **2011**, *3*, 588–600. [CrossRef] [PubMed]

26. Storz, J.F.; Opazo, J.C.; Hoffmann, F.G. Gene duplication, genome duplication, and the functional diversification of vertebrate globins. *Mol. Phylogenet. Evol.* **2013**, *66*, 469–478. [CrossRef] [PubMed]

27. Braasch, I.; Gehrke, A.R.; Smith, J.J. The spotted gar genome illuminates vertebrate evolution and facilitates human-teleost comparisons. *Nat. Genet.* **2016**, *48*, 427–437. [CrossRef] [PubMed]

28. GTEx Consortium, T. The genotype-tissue expression (GTEx) project. *Nat. Genet.* **2013**, *45*, 580–585.

29. Shabalina, S.A.; Ogurtsov, A.Y.; Spiridonov, A.N.; Novichkov, P.S.; Spiridonov, N.A.; Koonin, E.V. Distinct patterns of expression and evolution of intronless and intron-containing mammalian genes. *Mol. Biol. Evol.* **2010**, *27*, 1745–1749. [CrossRef] [PubMed]

30. Broad Institute TCGA Genome Data Analysis Center. *Analysis-Ready Standardized TCGA Data from Broad GDAC Firehose 2016_01_28 Run*; Broad Institute of MIT and Harvard: Cambridge, MA, USA, 2016.

31. Ooki, A.; Yamashita, K.; Yamaguchi, K.; Mondal, A.; Nishimiya, H.; Watanabe, M. DNA damage-inducible gene, reprimo functions as a tumor-suppressor and is suppressed by promoter methylation in gastric cancer. *Mol. Cancer Res.* **2013**, *11*, 1362–1374. [CrossRef] [PubMed]

32. Lai, J.; Wang, H.; Luo, Q.; Huang, S.; Lin, S.; Zheng, Y.; Chen, Q. The relationship between DNA methylation and reprimo gene expression in gastric cancer cells. *Oncotarget* **2017**, *8*, 108610–108623. [CrossRef] [PubMed]

33. Morris, M.R.; Ricketts, C.; Gentle, D.; Abdulrahman, M.; Clarke, N.; Brown, M.; Kishida, T.; Yao, M.; Latif, F.; Maher, E.R. Identification of candidate tumour suppressor genes frequently methylated in renal cell carcinoma. *Oncogene* **2010**, *29*, 2104–2117. [PubMed]

34. Xu, M.; Knox, A.J.; Michaelis, K.A.; Kiseljak-Vassiliades, K.; Kleinschmidt-DeMasters, B.K.; Lillehei, K.O.; Wierman, M.E. Reprimo (RPRM) is a novel tumor suppressor in pituitary tumors and regulates survival, proliferation, and tumorigenicity. *Endocrinology* **2012**, *153*, 2963–2973. [CrossRef] [PubMed]

35. Buchegger, K.; Ili, C.; Riquelme, I.; Letelier, P.; Corvalan, A.H.; Brebi, P.; Huang, T.H.; Roa, J.C. Reprimo as a modulator of cell migration and invasion in the mda-mb-231 breast cancer cell line. *Biol. Res.* **2016**, *49*, 5. [CrossRef] [PubMed]

36. Luo, J.; Zhu, Y.; Yang, G.; Gong, L.; Wang, B.; Liu, H. Loss of reprimo and s100a2 expression in human gastric adenocarcinoma. *Diagn. Cytopathol.* **2011**, *39*, 752–757. [CrossRef] [PubMed]

37. Hamilton, J.P.; Sato, F.; Jin, Z.; Greenwald, B.D.; Ito, T.; Mori, Y.; Paun, B.C.; Kan, T.; Cheng, Y.; Wang, S.; et al. Reprimo methylation is a potential biomarker of barrett's-associated esophageal neoplastic progression. *Clin. Cancer Res.* **2006**, *12*, 6637–6642. [PubMed]

38. Nakazato, T.; Suzuki, Y.; Tanaka, R.; Abe, N.; Masaki, T.; Mori, T.; Ohkura, Y.; Sugiyama, M. Effect of reprimo down-regulation on malignant transformation of intraductal papillary mucinous neoplasm. *Pancreas* **2018**, *47*, 291–295. [CrossRef] [PubMed]

39. Sato, N.; Fukushima, N.; Hruban, R.H.; Goggins, M. CPG island methylation profile of pancreatic intraepithelial neoplasia. *Mod. Pathol.* **2008**, *21*, 238–244. [PubMed]

40. Chang, W.L.; Jackson, C.; Riel, S.; Cooper, H.S.; Devarajan, K.; Hensley, H.H.; Zhou, Y.; Vanderveer, L.A.; Nguyen, M.T.; Clapper, M.L. Differential preventive activity of sulindac and atorvastatin in Apc$^{+/Min-FCCC}$ mice with or without colorectal adenomas. *Gut* **2017**. [CrossRef] [PubMed]

41. Beasley, W.D.; Beynon, J.; Jenkins, G.J.; Parry, J.M. Reprimo 824 G>C and p53R2 4696 C>G single nucleotide polymorphisms and colorectal cancer: A case-control disease association study. *Int. J. Colorectal Dis.* **2008**, *23*, 375–381. [CrossRef] [PubMed]

42. Buchegger, K.; Riquelme, I.; Viscarra, T.; Ili, C.; Brebi, P.; Huang, T.H.; Roa, J.C. Reprimo, a potential p53-dependent tumor suppressor gene, is frequently hypermethylated in estrogen receptor alpha-positive breast cancer. *Int. J. Mol. Sci.* **2017**, *18*, 1525. [CrossRef] [PubMed]

43. Soon, P.S.; Gill, A.J.; Benn, D.E.; Clarkson, A.; Robinson, B.G.; McDonald, K.L.; Sidhu, S.B. Microarray gene expression and immunohistochemistry analyses of adrenocortical tumors identify IGF2 and Ki-67 as useful in differentiating carcinomas from adenomas. *Endocr. Relat. Cancer* **2009**, *16*, 573–583. [CrossRef] [PubMed]

44. Zohrabian, V.M.; Nandu, H.; Gulati, N.; Khitrov, G.; Zhao, C.; Mohan, A.; Demattia, J.; Braun, A.; Das, K.; Murali, R.; et al. Gene expression profiling of metastatic brain cancer. *Oncol. Rep.* **2007**, *18*, 321–328. [CrossRef] [PubMed]

45. Bernstein, B.E.; Meissner, A.; Lander, E.S. The mammalian epigenome. *Cell* **2007**, *128*, 669–681. [CrossRef] [PubMed]

46. Berdasco, M.; Esteller, M. Aberrant epigenetic landscape in cancer: How cellular identity goes awry. *Dev. Cell* **2010**, *19*, 698–711. [CrossRef] [PubMed]

47. Esteller, M.; Hamilton, S.R.; Burger, P.C.; Baylin, S.B.; Herman, J.G. Inactivation of the DNA repair gene o6-methylguanine-DNA methyltransferase by promoter hypermethylation is a common event in primary human neoplasia. *Cancer Res.* **1999**, *59*, 793–797. [PubMed]

48. Bernal, C.; Aguayo, F.R.; Villarroel, C.; Vargas, M.; Diaz, I.; Ossandón, F.J.; Santibáñez, E.; Palma, M.; Aravena, E.; Barrientos, C.; et al. Reprimo as a potential biomarker for early detection in gastric cancer. *Clin. Cancer Res.* **2008**, *14*, 6264–6269. [CrossRef] [PubMed]

49. Malik, S.; Jiang, S.; Garee, J.P.; Verdin, E.; Lee, A.V.; O'Malley, B.W.; Zhang, M.; Belaguli, N.S.; Oesterreich, S. Histone deacetylase 7 and foxa1 in estrogen-mediated repression of rprm. *Mol. Cell. Biol.* **2010**, *30*, 399–412. [CrossRef] [PubMed]

50. Cerda-Opazo, P.; Valenzuela-Valderrama, M.; Wichmann, I.; Rodriguez, A.; Contreras-Reyes, D.; Fernandez, E.; Carrasco-Aviño, G.; Corvalan, A.H.; Quest, A. Inverse expression of survivin and reprimo correlates with poor patient prognosis in gastric cancer. *Oncotarget* **2018**, *9*, 12853–12867. [CrossRef] [PubMed]

51. The Japanese Research Society for Gastric Cancer. Japanese classification of gastric carcinoma: 3rd English edition. *Gastric Cancer* **2011**, *14*, 101–112.

52. Torre, L.A.; Bray, F.; Siegel, R.L.; Ferlay, J.; Lortet-Tieulent, J.; Jemal, A. Global cancer statistics, 2012. *CA Cancer J. Clin.* **2015**, *65*, 87–108. [CrossRef] [PubMed]

53. Liu, J.L.; Gao, W.; Kang, Q.M.; Zhang, X.J.; Yang, S.G. Prognostic value of survivin in patients with gastric cancer: A systematic review with meta-analysis. *PLoS ONE* **2013**, *8*, e71930. [CrossRef] [PubMed]

54. Perri, F.; Longo, F.; Giuliano, M.; Sabbatino, F.; Favia, G.; Ionna, F.; Addeo, R.; Della Vittoria Scarpati, G.; Di Lorenzo, G.; Pisconti, S. Epigenetic control of gene expression: Potential implications for cancer treatment. *Crit. Rev. Oncol. Hematol.* **2017**, *111*, 166–172. [CrossRef] [PubMed]

55. Garcia-Bloj, B.; Moses, C.; Sgro, A.; Plani-Lam, J.; Arooj, M.; Duffy, C.; Thiruvengadam, S.; Sorolla, A.; Rashwan, R.; Mancera, R.L.; et al. Waking up dormant tumor suppressor genes with zinc fingers, tales and the crispr/dcas9 system. *Oncotarget* **2016**, *7*, 60535–60554. [CrossRef] [PubMed]

56. Chen, M.; Wei, L.; Law, C.T.; Tsang, F.H.; Shen, J.; Cheng, C.L.; Tsang, L.H.; Ho, D.W.; Chiu, D.K.; Lee, J.M.; et al. RNA N6-methyladenosine methyltransferase-like 3 promotes liver cancer progression through YTHDF2 dependent post-transcriptional silencing of SOCS2. *Hepatology* **2017**. [CrossRef]

57. Liu, L.; Yang, X. Implication of reprimo and *hMLH1* gene methylation in early diagnosis of gastric carcinoma. *Int. J. Clin. Exp. Pathol.* **2015**, *8*, 14977–14982. [PubMed]

58. Schneider, B.G.; Peng, D.F.; Camargo, M.C.; Piazuelo, M.B.; Sicinschi, L.A.; Mera, R.; Romero-Gallo, J.; Delgado, A.G.; Bravo, L.E.; Wilson, K.T.; et al. Promoter DNA hypermethylation in gastric biopsies from subjects at high and low risk for gastric cancer. *Int. J. Cancer* **2010**, *127*, 2588–2597. [CrossRef] [PubMed]

59. Maeda, M.; Yamashita, S.; Shimazu, T.; Iida, N.; Takeshima, H.; Nakajima, T.; Oda, I.; Nanjo, S.; Kusano, C.; Mori, A.; et al. Novel epigenetic markers for gastric cancer risk stratification in individuals after helicobacter pylori eradication. *Gastric Cancer* **2018**. [CrossRef] [PubMed]

60. Schneider, B.G.; Mera, R.; Piazuelo, M.B.; Bravo, J.C.; Zabaleta, J.; Delgado, A.G.; Bravo, L.E.; Wilson, K.T.; El-Rifai, W.; Peek, R.M., Jr.; et al. DNA methylation predicts progression of human gastric lesions. *Cancer Epidemiol. Biomark. Prev.* **2015**, *24*, 1607–1613. [CrossRef] [PubMed]

61. Duffy, M.J.; Napieralski, R.; Martens, J.W.; Span, P.N.; Spyratos, F.; Sweep, F.C.; Brunner, N.; Foekens, J.A.; Schmitt, M. Methylated genes as new cancer biomarkers. *Eur. J. Cancer* **2009**, *45*, 335–346. [CrossRef] [PubMed]

62. Padmanabhan, N.; Ushijima, T.; Tan, P. How to stomach an epigenetic insult: The gastric cancer epigenome. Nature reviews. *Gastroenterol. Hepatol.* **2017**, *14*, 467–478.

63. Leygo, C.; Williams, M.; Jin, H.C.; Chan, M.W.Y.; Chu, W.K.; Grusch, M.; Cheng, Y.Y. DNA methylation as a noninvasive epigenetic biomarker for the detection of cancer. *Dis. Markers* **2017**, *2017*, 3726595. [CrossRef] [PubMed]
64. Sapari, N.S.; Loh, M.; Vaithilingam, A.; Soong, R. Clinical potential of DNA methylation in gastric cancer: A meta-analysis. *PLoS ONE* **2012**, *7*, e36275. [CrossRef] [PubMed]
65. Wen, J.; Zheng, T.; Hu, K.; Zhu, C.; Guo, L.; Ye, G. Promoter methylation of tumor-related genes as a potential biomarker using blood samples for gastric cancer detection. *Oncotarget* **2017**, *8*, 77783–77793. [CrossRef] [PubMed]
66. Jorquera, R.; Ortiz, R.; Ossandon, F.; Cardenas, J.P.; Sepulveda, R.; Gonzalez, C.; Holmes, D.S. SinEx DB: A database for single exon coding sequences in mammalian genomes. *Database* **2016**. [CrossRef] [PubMed]

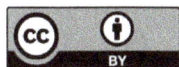

International Journal of
Molecular Sciences

MDPI

Review

Diffuse Gastric Cancer: A Summary of Analogous Contributing Factors for Its Molecular Pathogenicity

Shamshul Ansari [1], **Boldbaatar Gantuya** [1,2], **Vo Phuoc Tuan** [1,3] **and Yoshio Yamaoka** [1,4,*]

1   Department of Environmental and Preventive Medicine, Oita University Faculty of Medicine, Yufu-City, Oita 879-5593, Japan; shamshulansari483@yahoo.com (S.A.); medication_bg@yahoo.com (B.G.); vophuoctuandr@gmail.com (V.P.T.)
2   Department of Internal Medicine, Gastroenterology unit, Mongolian National University of Medical Sciences, Ulaanbaatar-14210, Mongolia
3   Department of Endoscopy, Cho Ray Hospital, Ho Chi Minh, Vietnam
4   Department of Medicine, Gastroenterology and Hepatology Section, Baylor College of Medicine, Houston, TX 77030, USA
*   Correspondence: yyamaoka@oita-u.ac.jp; Tel.: +81-97-586-5740; Fax: +81-97-586-5749

Received: 4 July 2018; Accepted: 14 August 2018; Published: 16 August 2018

Abstract: Gastric cancer is the third leading cause of cancer-related deaths and ranks as the fifth most common cancer worldwide. Incidence and mortality differ depending on the geographical region and gastric cancer ranks first in East Asian countries. Although genetic factors, gastric environment, and *Helicobacter pylori* infection have been associated with the pathogenicity and development of intestinal-type gastric cancer that follows the Correa's cascade, the pathogenicity of diffuse-type gastric cancer remains mostly unknown and undefined. However, genetic abnormalities in the cell adherence factors, such as E-cadherin and cellular activities that cause impaired cell integrity and physiology, have been documented as contributing factors. In recent years, *H. pylori* infection has been also associated with the development of diffuse-type gastric cancer. Therefore, in this report, we discuss the host factors as well as the bacterial factors that have been reported as associated factors contributing to the development of diffuse-type gastric cancer.

Keywords: gastric cancer; diffuse gastric cancer; hereditary diffuse gastric cancer; contributing factors

1. Introduction

Gastric cancer (GC) was the most common cancer as of 1975 [1] and because of the lack of sophisticated advancements, most of the GC cases were diagnosed at the advanced stages with poor prognosis [2]. However, relying on the development of advanced endoscopic techniques and national policy on *Helicobacter pylori* eradication, currently GC can be detected at earlier stages and better interventions can be provided to prevent its advance in some countries, such as Japan and Korea [3,4]. In fact, the declining trend in the global incidence and mortality of GC has been observed over past decades; however, it still ranks as the fifth most common cancer and the third leading cause of cancer-related mortality worldwide with an estimated number of 841,000 deaths, including 530,000 deaths and 11.7 million disability-adjusted life years (DALYs) for men in 2013 [5]. Hence, GC is still a significant public health issue and is still an area of focus for many international organizations in terms of both the prevention and control of the disease. The incidence and mortality of GC varies according to geographical region and it remains the highest in East Asian countries in comparison with other parts of the world [1].

GC is a multifactorial, morphologically heterogeneous disease where adenocarcinoma accounts for almost 90% of cases and lymphoma up to 5% [6,7]. Histologically, the adenocarcinomas originate from the glandular epithelium of gastric mucosa, whereas almost 90% of the primary gastrointestinal lymphomas are of B cell lineage with few T-cell or Hodgkin lymphomas [6,8]. In general, most GCs are sporadic (90%) and a positive family history exists in approximately 10% of cases, of which 1–3% are hereditary [9,10]. Based on differences in morphology, epidemiology, pathology, and genetic profiles, adenocarcinoma is classified as the well-differentiated or intestinal type gastric cancer (IGC) accounting for 60% of cases that typically show cohesive groups of tumor cells with a well-defined glandular architecture leading to expanding growth pattern. Poorly-differentiated or diffuse type gastric cancer (DGC) accounts for 30% cases; DGC lacks the intercellular adhesion, often observed with scattered signet-ring cell morphology predisposed to the diffuse invasion growth pattern throughout the stroma [11,12]. IGC is found in older patients and is associated more with environmental factors, such as high salty diet, smoking, obesity, and alcohol consumption [13–15], as well as *H. pylori* infection [16]. DGC is more commonly observed in younger patients [17,18]. IGC is the more common variant and its carcinogenic pathway is mainly caused by *H. pylori* infection, which predisposes a person to chronic gastritis, followed by atrophic gastritis, intestinal metaplasia, dysplasia, and finally carcinoma through the Correa's cascade [19]. The latter three lesions—atrophic gastritis, intestinal metaplasia, and dysplasia—are considered precancerous lesions. IGC accounts for the vast majority of GC. Although the pathogenicity of IGC has been well-characterized and studied, that of DGC mostly remains undefined and is considered to be primarily genetically determined and less associated with environmental factors and the inflammatory cascade. Even though DGC accounts for a lower proportion, an increasing incidence of DGC has been reported [20]. Moreover, a minor proportion of DGC (1–3%) has been inherently linked and associated with germline alterations in cellular physiology, which is known as hereditary-DGC (HDGC) [21–23]. Along with the worse prognosis characterized by early age of onset, rapid disease progression, being highly metastatic, inherited possibility within family in comparison associated with IGC, DGC has become a challenge for researchers and physicians. In practice, due to the clinical importance, several guidelines about diagnosis criteria, treatment, and monitoring of hereditary DGC (HDGC) were established and updated by a multidisciplinary group including clinical geneticists, gastroenterologists, surgeons, oncologists, pathologists, molecular biologists, and dieticians [24–26]. Nonetheless, the underlying molecular pathways of the disease have not yet been well-studied and understood. Notably, a report summarizing the molecular pathogenicity of GC in general has been published previously [27]. However, in this report, we summarized the current understanding of published knowledge to create a possible outline of the contributing factors involved in the molecular pathogenicity of DGC in order to gain deeper awareness about its mechanism (Table 1).

Table 1. Contributing factors for pathogenicity of diffuse type gastric cancer (DGC).

Factor	Mechanism	Effects	References
Host Factor			
E-cadherin (*CDH1*)	Mutational alterations	Deregulation of E-cadherin	[28,29]
	Over expression of transcription repressor	Down regulation of E-cadherin	[30–32]
	Post-translational modification	Glycosylation modification of E-cadherin	[33]
	Promoter hyper-methylation	E-cadherin inactivation	[34]
	Promoter polymorphism	Alterations in E-cadherin	[35]
Ras homolog gene family A (RHOA)	Mutational alterations	Loss of E-cadherin activity	[36]
Sphingosine-1-phosphate (S1P)	Synthesis	Development of DGC and lymphatic invasion	[37,38]
Adenomatous polyposis coli (APC)	Mutations leading to altered expression of APC protein	Accumulation of β-catenin leading to the activation of Wnt-signaling pathway	[39,40]

Table 1. *Cont.*

Factor	Mechanism	Effects	References
Host Factor			
Fibroblast growth factor receptor (FGFR2)	Overexpression	Inhibition in the cellular activities	[41,42]
Tumor protein 53 (TP53)	Mutational alteration	Loss of cell regulating mechanism	[43–46]
Helicobacter pylori			
Non-phosphorylated CagA	Binds with E-cadherin	Dissociation of E-cadherin-β-catenin complex	[47]
	Causes mutational alterations in TP53	Impairment of E-cadherin synthesis	[48,49]
	Causes hyper-methylation of CDH1	Reduced E-cadherin expression	[50,51]
High temperature requirement A (HtrA)	Causes cleavage of extracellular domain of E-cadherin	Disruption of normal cell junctions	[52–56]

2. Factors Associated with Molecular Pathogenicity of DGC

2.1. Role of E-Cadherin

For the normal maintenance of tissue morphogenesis and homeostasis, cell–cell adhesion is a critical phenomenon, also important for other cellular processes such as cell differentiation, cell survival, and cell migration, which are controlled by gene expression and signaling pathway activation [57]. E-cadherin (calcium-dependent classical cadherin), a trans-membrane glycoprotein consisting of three domains—extracellular, trans-membrane, and cytoplasmic—is involved in the cell–cell adhesion and tight adherent junctions that define cell differentiation and proliferation specificity of epithelial cells and invasion suppression [30,58–60]. The cytoplasmic domain of E-cadherin forms a protein complex with β- or γ-, p120-, and α-catenins linking the domain with the actin-myosin network that co-ordinates the specificity of cell shape, polarity, and function of the epithelial cells [61,62]. The extra-cellular domain of E-cadherin from the adjacent cells is involved in the cell adherence, providing a tight junction between the cells (Figure 1).

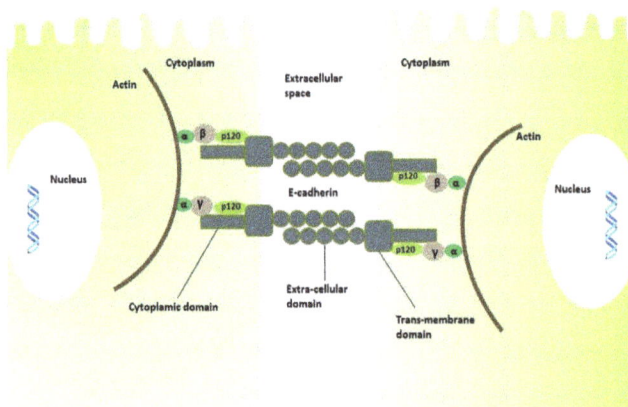

Figure 1. Cell–cell adhesion through E-cadherin. The extracellular domain of E-cadherin from adjacent cells is involved in cell adhesion and tight junction. The cytoplasmic domain forming a protein complex with catenins (α-, β-, and p120-) regulates the cytoskeleton protein and actin, which is an important protein for normal cell integrity.

The glycoprotein E-cadherin is encoded by the cadherin (*CDH1*) gene, which is located in chromosome 16q22.1 and contains 16 exons with a 4.5-kb mRNA [63]. E-cadherin is one of the major tumor suppressors in GC and the structural modifications in its encoding gene *CDH1* or alterations in its expression have been found as the common events that suppress the broad-ranging functions of E-cadherin during cancer progression and contribute to the morphogenetic effects in cancer [10,28,61]. The common mutations in *CDH1* are the well-known mechanism for its deregulation [29,64]. According to the human gene mutation database (HGMD), 121 variants have been reported for *CDH1* alterations to date [65,66]. In addition to the mutations, down regulation of E-cadherin expression can also occur via other mechanisms, such as overexpression of transcription repressor, alterations of microRNAs (miRNAs), protein trafficking deregulation, and post-translational modification of the protein [30–32]. Recently, glycosylation of E-cadherin has been suggested as another post-translational modification mechanism for its deregulation in many pathophysiological steps of tumor development and progression [33]. The alterations mediated by promoter hyper-methylation and epigenetic inactivation of *CDH1* has been found most commonly in DGC, playing a vital role as a second-hit mechanism in deregulation of the wild-type of *CDH1* in HDGC patients [34,67]. In a recent study, the substitution in *CDH1* encoding for the extracellular domain, such as NM_004360.3: c.2076T > C rs:1801552 in exon 13 together with c.348G > A as a new variant, were found to impair its cell adhesion function and contributed to the development of DGC [64]. On the other hand, substitution NM_004360.3: c.2253C > T rs:33964119 located in exon 14, encoding for the cytoplasmic domain of E-cadherin, was also found in DGC [64]. The cytoplasmic domain of E-cadherin binding with β-catenin plays a critical role in the inhibition of nuclear signaling pathways and tumor-suppression function [68]. In prior studies, the frequency of promoter polymorphism at the −160 position (C > A) of *CDH1* was found to be significantly greater in DGC than in the control groups. The three-marker haplotype (−160C > A, 48 + 6T > C, 2076C > T) was found to significantly contribute to DGC, whereas ATC and ACC haplotypes contributed to higher risk of the development of DGC [35,69,70]. Humar et al. also confirmed that the three-marker haplotype (−160C > A, 48 + 6T > C, 2076C > T) was associated with DGC [35]. In a recent study, impairment of E-cadherin expression was reported with a decreased membranous expression in early lesions of DGC [71].

Park et al. performed a study of gastro-duodenal epithelium-specific knockout of one allele of *CDH1* and both alleles of tumor protein 53 (TP53) and SMAD4 (a homologous gene product to the Caenorhabditis elegans gene (*SMA*) and the Drosophila gene 'mothers against decapetaplegic' (*MAD*)), which are the most vulnerable to being inactivated in human GCs. The loss of E-cadherin function together with SMAD4 was found, which underwent epithelium-mesenchymal transition (EMT) and co-operated to promote the development of metastatic progression of TP53-null DGC [72]. This result closely mimicked the human DGC and evaluated the possible role of E-cadherin and SMAD4 in the development of DGC. In addition to its role in cell–cell adhesion, E-cadherin and the cadherin-catenin complex have been demonstrated to modulate various signaling pathways in epithelial cells, such as Wnt signaling, Rho GTPases (a Ras homolog that hydrolyzes the guanosine triphosphate), and nuclear factor kappa-B (NF-κB) pathways [73]. Therefore, impairment of E-cadherin promotes dysfunctions of these signaling pathways, thereby influencing cell polarity, cell survival, invasion and metastasis of gastric cancer, and mainly promotes DGC through the EMT mechanism [74]. Therefore, the cellular events and deregulation in E-cadherin results in the disruption of normal cellular functions (Figure 2).

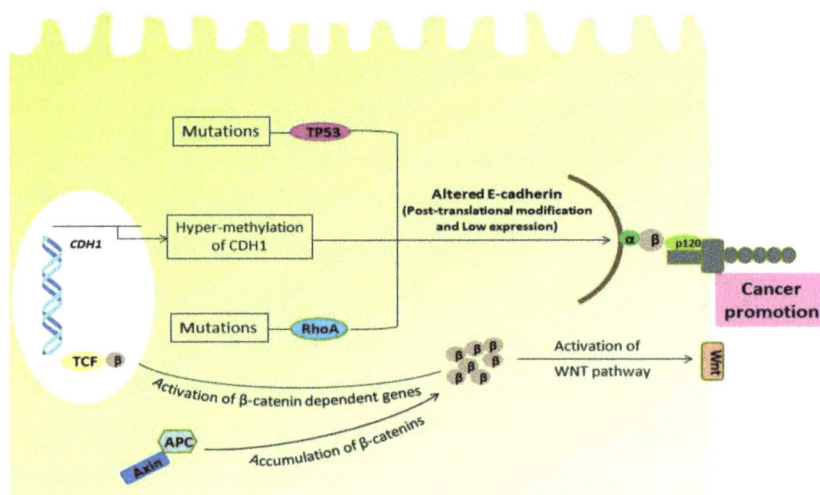

Figure 2. Pathogenicity and factors associated with the disruption of the normal cellular activity. Hyper-methylation of the *CDH1* gene and mutational alteration in TP53 protein causes the impaired synthesis of E-cadherin. The truncated APC causes accumulation of β-catenin, which activates the β-catenin-dependent genes and Wnt pathway, altering normal cellular functions. The Wnt pathway after its activation causes the accumulation of β-catenins in cytoplasm and its translocation into the nucleus where it transcriptionally activates the transcription factors belonging to the TCF family. The recurrent mutation in RhoA is able to alter the RhoA pathway, which has a deleterious effect on E-cadherin.

2.2. Alterations in Ras Homolog Gene Family A (RhoA)

Wang et al. conducted a study in 2014 utilizing primary mouse intestinal organoids and determined that the recurrent mutations in RHOA (Y42C and L57V) inhibit the cell death induced when anchorage-dependent cells detach from the surrounding extracellular matrix. This phenomenon is known as anoikis and it plays a key role in the development of DGC [75]. It is well known that the loss of E-cadherin leads to impairment of cellular adhesion, resulting in acute cell death via anoikis. In other words, the alterations or impairment in RHOA function somehow impairs E-cadherin function. Consequently, another study evaluated the role of RHOA mutations associated with DGC [36]. These RHOA mutations in hotspot sites were Y42C, G17E, R5Q/W, and L57V with Y42C being the most common mutation in the effector-binding region of RhoA. In 2014, The Cancer Genome Atlas (TCGA) identified a rate of RHOA mutations in DGC [76]. The TCGA network also found additional fusions in GTPase-activating proteins (GAPs), which are crucial in regulating RhoA activity. More importantly, these mutations were generally found in DGC and not in IGC. Consequently, Ushiku et al. also reported the RHOA mutations causing DGC in 2016 [77]. The impairment of RhoA results in the loss of its expression and activity that may play a role in the development of DGC [78]. RhoA, a member of the Rho family, is a small GTPase protein that plays a fundamental role in regulating diverse cellular processes, such as cell growth, cell survival, polarity, adhesion, cell migration, and differentiation [79–82]. The studies have shown that genetic alterations in the RhoA pathway, including recurrent RHOA mutations and RhoGAP fusion along with the *CDH1* mutations, are quite common in DGC but not in other variants of gastric cancer [36,76]. These results suggest a possible role of wild-type RhoA in the suppression of DGC development, whereas mutational alterations in RhoA lead to its development, inhibiting the tumor suppression activity (Figure 2).

2.3. Role of Sphingosine-1-Phosphate

Sphingosine-1-phosphate (S1P), a bioactive lipid mediator generated by sphingosine kinsase-1 (SphK1) inside the cancer cells, is a key regulatory molecule in cancer via cell proliferation, migration, invasion, and angiogenesis [83–88]. S1P, after being generated by cancer cells, is exported to the tumor microenvironment where binding to and signaling through specific G protein-coupled receptors, known as S1PR1-5, regulates many functions [85–91]. The experimental models conducted by Nagahashi et al. showed that S1P produced by SphK1 in cancer cells promotes lymph node metastasis in tumor microenvironments and promotes lymphangiogenesis [37]. In a recent study, Hanyu et al. reported the role of phosphorylated-SphK1 in the development of DGC and its lymphatic invasion [38].

2.4. Role of Adenomatous Polyposis Coli

The gene associated with human adenomatous polyposis coli (APC) is located on the long arm of chromosome 5, which encodes a protein of 312 kDa with 2843 amino acids that acts as a tumor-suppressive protein [92]. A Germline mutation of the APC gene and its inactivation has been found responsible for familial adenomatous polyposis (FAP) [93,94]. Mutations in the APC gene leading to the inactivation of this protein are involved in initiating the carcinogenesis events [92]. The wild-type APC gene product has been found to interact with and degrade β-catenin, whereas truncated APC promotes β-catenin accumulation, activating the members of Wnt signaling pathway that stimulates cell division within intestinal crypts [95]. Therefore, maintenance of low levels of cytosolic β-catenin by functioning APC proteins is essential to prevent excessive cell proliferation [39]. In a recent study by Ghatak et al., the role of somatic mutations in APC (g.127576C > A, g.127583C > T) in exon 14 altering the APC protein expression and cell cycle regulation was shown to contribute to the development of DGC [40].

2.5. Role of Fibroblast Growth Factor Receptor (FGFR)

The overexpression of receptor tyrosine kinases (RTKs) has been correlated with the progression and poor survival of GC, whereas the immuno-histochemical overexpression of RTKs variant (i.e., human epidermal growth factor receptor 2—HER2) was found to be associated more frequently in the development of IGC rather than DGC [96–98]. The role of genomic alterations in RTKs between IDC and DGC has been revealed in comprehensive genomic analysis performed in TGCA [76]. The fibroblast growth factor receptor (FGFR) family comprises another type of RTKs that interacts with fibroblast growth factors (FGFs) and regulates the essential developmental pathways participating in several biological functions, such as angiogenesis and wound repair [41]. FGFRs also regulate essential cell activities including cell proliferation, survival, migration and differentiation [41]. FGFR2 gene amplification and protein overexpression was found in the GC cell line originating from DGC and it has been recently reported in the development of GCs [99,100]. In a study, the significantly high expression of the FGFR2 protein was commonly reported in DGC rather than IGC [42]. A similar study also showed the significant association of FGFR2 protein overexpression with poor survival and peritoneal dissemination of GC [97]. Moreover, a significant correlation of overexpression of FGFR1 and FGFR2 with tumor progression and survival was found only in DGC, which was also associated with peritoneal dissemination [101]. Therefore, the findings of these studies suggest the possible role of FGFR1 and FGFR2 in DGC development and their association with peritoneal dissemination.

2.6. Role of Growth/Differentiation Factor 15 (GDF15)

The results of another study reported the association of growth/differentiating factor 15 (GDF15) with DGC; it was suggested that GDF15 may be the molecules involved in the progression of DGC [102]. Patients with DGC also showed significantly higher serum levels of GDF15, as analyzed by the ELISA method [102]. The secreted growth factors, such as transforming growth factor-β (TGF-β), platelet-derived growth factor (PDGF), and fibroblast growth factor-2 (FGF-2) released by cancer cells, play a key role in the activation of fibroblasts in DGC, and particularly in scirrhous GC [103]. The activated fibroblasts produce various growth factors that help in the progression of scirrhous GC and the secreted proteins play a major role in the molecular pathology of DGC progression [103].

2.7. Li-Fraumeni Syndrome with Germline Mutations in Tumor Protein 53 (TP53)

Li-Fraumeni syndrome is genetically inherited in an autosomal dominant manner that is characterized by an accumulation of brain tumors, sarcomas, and breast cancer. Li-Fraumeni syndrome is caused by an alteration in *TP53* (tumor protein 53 or p53), which is a tumor suppressive gene [104]. Upon activation under the cellular stress, the p53 protein performs several functions such as induction of cell cycle arrest and apoptosis, inhibition of cell growth, and interaction with DNA repair proteins [43]. The mutational alteration in *TP53* is considered one of the most prevalent genetic alterations in GC. However, the association of *TP53* mutation with histological-type CG is conflicting [105]. The truncating germline *TP53* mutation was reported in a family characterized by having both HDGC and Li-Fraumeni syndrome [106]. Several other studies highlighted a significant association of the TP53 mutations with the development of DGC rather than IGC [44,45]. The frequent mutations at *TP53*, CKLF-like MARVEL transmembrane domain-containing protein-2 (*CMTM2*), *CDH1*, and *RHOA* were reported in DGC [46].

2.8. Role of Alteration in Other Genes

In addition to the alterations in the E-cadherin gene (*CDH1*), the mutations in the catenin alpha-1 (*CTNNA1*), breast cancer gene (*BRCA2*), serine/threonine kinase-11 (*STK11*), succinate dehydrogenase subunit-B (*SDHB*), serine protease-1 (*PRSS1*), ataxia-telangiectasia mutated gene (*ATM*), macrophage scavenger receptor-1 (*MSR1*), and partner and localizer of BRCA2 (*PALB2*) genes have been reported in the development of DGC [107]. In a recent study, the high frequency mutations for DGC were also reported in lysine methyl-transferase-2D gene (*KMT2D*), AT-rich interactive domain-containing protein 1A (*ARID1A*), *APC*, and phosphatidylinositol 3-kinase catalytic subunit (*PIK3CA*), in addition to high frequency mutations in *TP53*, *CDH1*, and *RHOA* [108]. Alterations in new candidates such as insulin receptor gene (*INSR*), F-box only protein 24 (*FBXO24*), and dot1-like histone lysine methyltransferase (*DOT1L*) have also been reported for DGC susceptibility [109]. Choi et al. found a novel mutation at *CMTM2* in addition to the previously known mutations and they suggested that it may play a crucial role in development of DGC [46]. CMTM2 is a chemokine-like factor that regulates vesicular transport or membrane apposition events belonging to the CMTM family (e.g., CMTM3, CMTM4, CMTM7, and CMTM8), which play a role in the tumor suppression [110–113].

3. *Helicobacter pylori* Infection and DGC

H. pylori colonizes the gastric epithelium and persists for several decades. Chronic infections have been found to cause chronic gastritis and atrophic gastritis, a precancerous lesion of gastric cancer. Based on the strong linking evidence of this bacterium with the development of peptic ulcers and gastric cancer, the International Agency for Research on Cancer (IARC) categorized this bacterium as a group I carcinogen (strong carcinogen) in 1994 [114,115]. *H. pylori* infection was initially believed to be associated with the development of IGC, which arises from chronic gastritis, atrophic gastritis, intestinal metaplasia, and dysplasia, whereas the sequence of events for DGC is poorly understood, though it is thought that at least a subset of DGC is due to genetic abnormalities [19,116]. However, unlike HDGC, *H. pylori* and/or Epstein-Barr virus (EBV) infections have been reported to play an essential role in the development of sporadic DGC [117–119]. Several other studies have also reported the association of *H. pylori* infection with the development of DGC [120–122]. A recent study reported that patients with current infections were prone to developing DGC compared to patients with past infections [123,124]. Similarly, the association of *H. pylori* was found in 85.36% of DGC [125]. There appears to be little difference in the sero-prevalence of *H. pylori* between the two types of cancers, even after adjusting for age. Serological studies confirmed that *H. pylori* infection is associated with both histological types of GC. The studies suggested that patients with a low *H. pylori*-IgG titer are more prone to developing IGC, whereas those with high *H. pylori*-IgG titer are at high risk for developing DGC [18,122,126]. The progression of gastric mucosal atrophy associated with a decrease in *H. pylori* titer may be attributable to the association between past infection or low *H. pylori*-IgG titer and IGC [123]. Gong et al. also reported the association of high *H. pylori*-IgG titer with the development of DGC [124].

H. pylori infection has been reported to inhibit several factors responsible for cell–cell adhesion and DGC pathogenicity. Yang et al. demonstrated the cleavage of E-cadherin by *H. pylori* strains SS1 and 26695, producing cytoplasmic fragments to induce apoptosis. Strain SS1 was found to cleave E-cadherin more efficiently at 12 hour and 24 hour [127]. After translocation into the gastric epithelium, the non-phosphorylated CagA binding with E-cadherin results in the separation of E-cadherin and β-catenin complex, which causes accumulation of β-catenin in the cytoplasm and nucleus, which ultimately trans-activates the β-catenin-dependent gene involved in cancer progression [47]. The aberrant activation of β-catenin disrupts the normal apical-junctional complexes, which lead to the loss of cellular polarity [128]. The binding of CagA with E-cadherin results in its down-regulation, together with decreased expression of p120 and aberrant localization from membrane to cytoplasm, which interacts with Rho GTPases and promotes motility and metastasis [129]. Moreover, the unusual localization of p120 to the nucleus, preventing transcriptional repression of the matrix metalloproteinase-7 (*mmp7*) gene, is involved in gastric carcinogenesis [130]. In a recent study, *H. pylori* infection was found to degrade the membrane-bound β-catenin [131]. *H. pylori* infection has been also shown to cause TP53 mutation and a decreased p27 protein expression [48,49]. Non-phosphorylated CagA, in addition to E-cadherin, have been shown to target the phospholipase C-γ, the adaptor protein Grb2, the hepatocyte growth factor receptor c-Met, and other components, leading to the proinflammatory and mitogenic responses that disrupts cell–cell adhesion, cell polarity, and other cellular physiology [132].

Impairment of myelocytomatosis oncogene (*MYC*) expression occurs in a broad range of human cancers, indicating a crucial role in tumor progression [133,134]. The *MYC* gene, located on chromosome 8q24, encoding a transcriptional factor, plays a key role in the regulation of cell cycle progression, growth, proliferation and apoptosis [135,136]. The results of a study indicated that the MYC protein plays a key role in association with *H. pylori* for diffuse type gastric carcinogenesis, whereas it was concluded that the MYC protein is not associated with the tumorigenic pathway of IGC [137].

Aberrant DNA hypermethylation and inactivation of the *CDH1* gene have been found in DGC [34,67]. *H. pylori* infection can induce aberrant hypermethylation of multiple genes, including *CDH1*, leading to the reduction in E-cadherin expression in gastric mucosa, which increases the risk for DGC [50,51]. *H. pylori* serine protease high temperature requirement A (HtrA) is a highly active protein under extreme conditions and degrades the miss-folded protein in bacterial periplasm that enhances the bacterial survival in adverse conditions [138]. In an in vitro infection experiment, the HtrA protein was shown to cleave the extracellular domain of E-cadherin, which led to the opening of the cell junctions in polarized cell monolayers [52]. The results of several other studies identified the *H. pylori* HtrA protein as an E-cadherin targeting protease that directly cleaves-off the extracellular domain of E-cadherin disrupting cell–cell adhesion, leading to cancer development [53–56]. Moreover, a study conducted by Abdi et al. reported the *H. pylori* vacA d1 type as a potent bacterial virulence factor significantly associated with the development of DGC [139]. Therefore, *H. pylori* proteins, such as CagA, VacA, and HtrA, have regulatory effects on many cellular pathways, and in addition to their role in IGC, they also contribute to the development and prognosis of DGC (Figure 3).

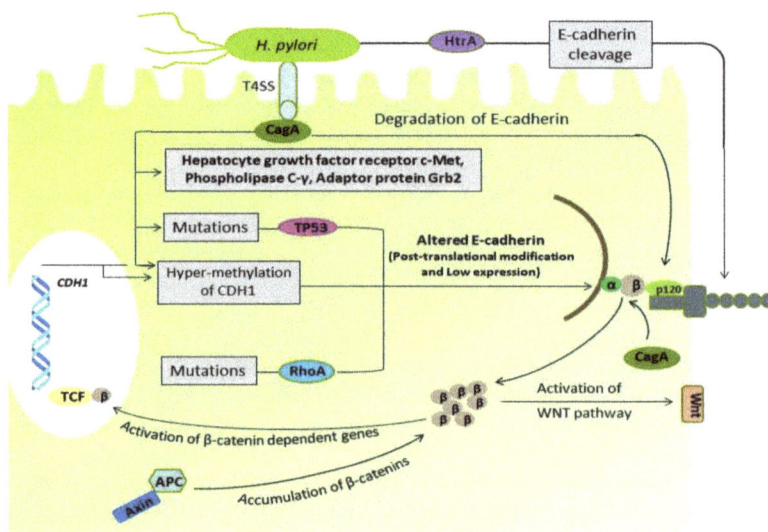

Figure 3. *H. pylori* CagA has an inducible effect on the CDH1 methylation and TP53 mutational alteration. CagA can directly degrade the β-catenin from the E-cadherin-catenins complex. CagA can also degrade the E-cadherin directly. Bacterial HtrA protein can cleave the extracellular domain of E-cadherin.

4. Hereditary Diffuse Gastric Cancer (HDGC) and Germline Mutations

Although the majority of the DGC cases are sporadic, approximately 1–3% of cases are characterized by inherited syndrome, known as hereditary DGC (HDGC)—an autosomal-dominant cancer susceptibility syndrome characterized by signet ring cell (diffuse) gastric cancer [21,22]. In DGC, the somatic mutations of E-cadherin are described in up to 40–70% of cases, whereas the germline mutations of E-cadherin (*CDH1*), causing loss of its function, are the only proven cause of HDGC, found in approximately 40% of cases [23,140,141]. In 1994, Becker et al. first reported evidence of an inherited form of DGC associated with E-cadherin mutations in specimens from sporadic DGC [113]. In 1998, Guilford et al. found multiple cases of early-onset DGC in Maori ethnic peoples of New Zealand that were carriers of a three germline truncating mutation in the E-cadherin (*CDH1*) gene [23]. Several other publications emerged confirming the association of autosomal-dominant pattern of inheritance with germline mutations of the *CDH1* gene in the following years [26,71,90,107,140–145]. Sporadic DGC has shown germline mutations for *CDH1* in a hot spot region between exons 7 and 9, whereas genetic alterations scattered over the entire gene length have been observed for HDGC [146]. Individuals with germline *CDH1* mutations have a single functional *CDH1* allele, whereas the germline *CDH1* alterations in the entire coding region of the other allele may contain small frameshifts, splice-site, nonsense, and missense mutations, as well as large rearrangements. The mutations causing the truncating or pre-matured types are pathogenic, whereas several missense mutations cause impairment of E-cadherin function [147]. Moreover, germline *CDH1* mutations resulting in the complete loss of E-cadherin expression is observed in about 80% of the cases due to the occurrence of premature stop codons causing truncating or non-functional E-cadherin [148,149]. Also, missense-type mutations substituting a single amino acid resulted in full-length E-cadherin in the remaining 20% of HDGC cases [147,148,150,151].

The second hit molecular mechanism causing the inactivation of the remaining functional allele by promoter hyper-methylation was demonstrated to be the most frequent cause of a second hit that leads to the inactivation of both alleles of the E-cadherin (*CDH1*) gene, which is the trigger event for the development of DGC [31,152–154]. The second mutation or deletion is an apparently less frequent cause of second hit molecular inactivation of E-cadherin [31,153].

The International Gastric Cancer Linkage Consortium has defined the well-characterized criteria for ruling out HDGC: two GC cases in a family with one individual with confirmed DGC at any age; or three confirmed cases in a family with GC in first- or second-degree relatives regardless of age; or a single case of GC before 40 years of age; or a family history of GC and lobular breast cancer, one diagnosed before 50 years of age [26]. In families meeting the consortium criteria for HDGC carrying the germline mutations are predisposed to an extreme risk of developing DGC from a relatively young age. Based on the familial trace-out of HDGC cases from around the world, the estimated cumulative risk of developing DGC by the age of 80 years has been documented to be 70% for men (95% confidence interval 59–80%) and 56% for women (95% confidence interval 44–69%) [155]. In addition to the risk for DGC, women carrying *CDH1* mutations also possess a cumulative risk of 42% for developing breast cancer, typically the lobular type [155]. However, mutations in *CDH1* are not always associated with the development of GC. In another study, a *CDH1* pathogenic mutation was recorded in a patient but no history of DGC was found in three generations of that family [156]. Similarly, in another study, there was *CDH1* germline missense mutation without any reported history of DGC [157]. Moreover, approximately 60 to 70% of families that fulfill the current testing criteria for HDGC do not possess the germline *CDH1* mutations [152,155]. There has been a few, rare, and highly penetrant familial GC genes; several other familial cancer syndromes also exist for which the GC has a low penetrance feature [158]. Moreover, only about 40% of the probands meeting the 2010 consortium criteria carry germline *CDH1* alterations [159,160]; of the remaining 60%, a small percentage is due to *CDH1* deletions not detected by conventional DNA sequencing and others have shown mutations in other genes such as *CTNNA1* [161], *MAP3K6* [162], *INSR*, *FBXO24*, and *DOT1L* [109]. Hansford et al. showed results from targeted sequencing of 55 cancer-associated genes in 144 families with HDGC who did not possess the detectable germline *CDH1* mutations [155]. They identified two families with germline mutations in *CTNNA1* as well as germline mutations causing truncated type of BRCA2, PRSS1, ATM, PALB2, SDHB, STK11, and MSR1 [155].

CTNNA1 encodes α-catenin, forming a complex with β-catenin to bind the cytoplasmic domain of E-cadherin to the cytoskeleton, is involved in cell–cell adhesion [152]. In a recent study, the comparison of caudal type homeobox-2 protein (CDX2) association with sporadic or HDGC showed that all HDGC cases were negative for CDX2, whereas 19 out of 20 sporadic DGC cases showed CDX2 expression, indicating that sporadic and HDGC may arise via different molecular carcinogenic pathways [163]. Other germline mutations described for familial DGC are in mitogene-activated protein kinase kinase kinase 6 (MAP3K6) and myeloid differentiation primary response protein 88 (MYD88), but their significance in causing DGC is not yet known [162,164]. In summary, germline *CDH1* mutation—however not limited—is frequently associated with the development of HDGC, whereas the mutations in *TP53* and *RHOA*, in addition to the *CDH1* mutations, are documented in sporadic-type DGC. However, the detailed molecular mechanisms underlying the development of DGC have not yet been clarified in detail [36,46,76].

5. Conclusions

Although the detailed pathogenicity of DGC is not well described, the combined information presented in this report indicates that development of DGC involves multiple factors of cell signaling pathways, cell–cell adhesion, and *H. pylori* infection. The E-cadherin and cell-signaling pathways play a vital role in the maintenance of cell integrity and normal cell function. Deregulation and alterations in these molecules disrupt the normal cellular functions that contribute to the initiation and progression of gastric cancer. The alterations in E-cadherin have been known as a factor strongly associated factor with DGC, with other less frequently associated and newly identified factors. Despite its role in IDC, *H. pylori* has been found to influence the development of DGC. However, more details and further investigations are needed.

Author Contributions: Conceptualization, Y.Y.; Literature Review, S.A., B.G. and V.P.T.; Manuscript Writing, S.A.; Figure Preparation, S.A.; Final Manuscript Preparation, S.A., B.G. and V.P.T.; Manuscript Supervision, Y.Y.; Funding Acquisition, Y.Y.

Funding: This work was funded by grants-in-aid for Scientific Research from the Ministry of Education, Culture, Sports, Science, and Technology (MEXT) of Japan (221S0002, 16H06279, 15H02657 and 16H05191), by the Japan Society for the Promotion of Science (Core-to-Core Program), and by National Institutes of Health (DK62813). Shamshul Ansari, Boldbaatar Gantuya and Vo Phuoc Tuan are PhD students supported by the Japanese Government (MEXT) Scholarship Program for 2015 (S.A. and V.P.T.) and 2014 (B.G.).

Conflicts of Interest: The authors declare no conflict of interest.

References

1. Ferlay, J.; Soerjomataram, I.; Dikshit, R.; Eser, S.; Mathers, C.; Rebelo, M.; Parkin, D.M.; Forman, D.; Bray, F. Cancer incidence and mortality worldwide: Sources, methods and major patterns in GLOBOCAN 2012. *Int. J. Cancer* **2015**, *136*, 359–386. [CrossRef] [PubMed]

2. Hartgrink, H.H.; Jansen, E.P.; van Grieken, N.C.; van de Velde, C.J. Gastric cancer. *Lancet* **2009**, *374*, 477–490. [CrossRef]

3. Hamashima, C.; Shibuya, D.; Yamazaki, H.; Inoue, K.; Fukao, A.; Saito, H.; Sobue, T. The Japanese guidelines for gastric cancer screening. *Jpn. J. Clin. Oncol.* **2008**, *38*, 259–267. [CrossRef] [PubMed]

4. Choi, I.J. Endoscopic gastric cancer screening and surveillance in high-risk groups. *Clin. Endosc.* **2014**, *47*, 497–503. [CrossRef] [PubMed]

5. Fitzmaurice, C.; Dicker, D.; Pain, A.; Hamavid, H.; Moradi-Lakeh, M.; MacIntyre, M.F.; Allen, C.; Hansen, G.; Woodbrook, R.; Wolfe, C.; et al. The global burden of cancer 2013. *JAMA Oncol.* **2015**, *1*, 505–527. [CrossRef] [PubMed]

6. Ajani, J.A.; Lee, J.; Sano, T.; Janjigian, Y.Y.; Fan, D.; Song, S. Gastric adenocarcinoma. *Nat. Rev. Dis. Primer* **2017**, *3*, 17036. [CrossRef] [PubMed]

7. Ferrucci, P.F.; Zucca, E. Primary gastric lymphoma pathogenesis and treatment: What has changed over the past 10 years? *Br. J. Haematol.* **2007**, *136*, 521–538. [CrossRef] [PubMed]

8. Ghimire, P.; Wu, G.Y.; Zhu, L. Primary gastrointestinal lymphoma. *World J. Gastroenterol.* **2011**, *17*, 697–707. [CrossRef] [PubMed]

9. Henson, D.E.; Dittus, C.; Younes, M.; Nguyen, H.; Albores-Saavedra, J. Differential trends in the intestinal and diffuse types of gastric carcinoma in the United States, 1973–2000: Increase in the signet ring cell type. *Arch. Pathol. Lab. Med.* **2004**, *128*, 765–770. [PubMed]

10. Paredes, J.; Figueiredo, J.; Albergaria, A.; Oliveira, P.; Carvalho, J.; Ribeiro, A.S.; Caldeira, J.; Costa, A.M.; Simoes-Correia, J.; Oliveira, M.J.; et al. Epithelial E- and P-cadherins: Role and clinical significance in cancer. *Biochim. Biophys. Acta* **2012**, *1826*, 297–311. [CrossRef] [PubMed]

11. Flejou, J. WHO Classification of digestive tumors: The fourth edition. *Ann. Pathol.* **2011**, *31*, 27–31.

12. Lauren, P. The two histological main types of gastric carcinoma: Diffuse and so-called intestinal-type carcinoma. An attempt at a histo-clinical classification. *Acta. Pathol. Microbiol. Scand.* **1965**, *64*, 31–49. [CrossRef] [PubMed]

13. Lee, S.; Lee, J.; Choi, I.J.; Kim, Y.W.; Ryu, K.W.; Kim, Y.I.; Oh, J.K.; Tran, B.T.; Kim, J. Dietary inflammatory index and the risk of gastric cancer in a Korean population. *Oncotarget* **2017**, *8*, 85452–85462. [CrossRef] [PubMed]

14. Peleteiro, B.; Lopes, C.; Figueiredo, C.; Lunet, N. Salt intake and gastric cancer risk according to *Helicobacter pylori* infection, smoking, tumour site and histological type. *Br. J. Cancer* **2011**, *104*, 198–207. [CrossRef] [PubMed]

15. Rota, M.; Pelucchi, C.; Bertuccio, P.; Matsuo, K.; Zhang, Z.F.; Ito, H.; Hu, J.; Johnson, K.C.; Palli, D.; Ferraroni, M.; et al. Alcohol consumption and gastric cancer risk-A pooled analysis within the StoP project consortium. *Int. J. Cancer* **2017**, *141*, 1950–1962. [CrossRef] [PubMed]

16. Binh, T.T.; Tuan, V.P.; Dung, H.D.Q.; Tung, P.H.; Tri, T.D.; Thuan, N.P.M.; Khien, V.V.; Hoan, P.Q.; Suzuki, R.; Uchida, T.; et al. Advanced non-cardia gastric cancer and *Helicobacter pylori* infection in Vietnam. *Gut Pathog.* **2017**, *9*, 46. [CrossRef] [PubMed]

17. Ellison-Loschmann, L.; Sporle, A.; Corbin, M.; Cheng, S.; Harawira, P.; Gray, M.; Whaanga, T.; Guillford, P.; Koea, J.; Pearce, N. Risk of stomach cancer in Aotearoa/New Zealand: A Māori population based case-control study. *PLoS ONE* **2017**, *12*, E0181581. [CrossRef] [PubMed]

18. Lee, J.Y.; Gong, E.J.; Chung, E.J.; Park, H.W.; Bae, S.E.; Kim, E.H.; Kim, J.; Do, Y.S.; Kim, T.H.; Chang, H.S.; et al. The characteristics and prognosis of diffuse-type early gastric cancer diagnosed during health check-ups. *Gut Liver* **2017**, *11*, 807–812. [CrossRef] [PubMed]

19. Correa, P. Human gastric carcinogenesis: A multistep and multifactorial process-first American Cancer Society award lecture on cancer epidemiology and prevention. *Cancer Res.* **1992**, *52*, 6735–6740. [PubMed]

20. Crew, K.D.; Neugut, A.I. Epidemiology of gastric cancer. *World J. Gastroenterol.* **2006**, *12*, 354–362. [CrossRef] [PubMed]

21. Petrovchich, I.; Ford, J.M. Genetic predisposition to gastric cancer. *Semin. Oncol.* **2016**, *43*, 554–559. [CrossRef] [PubMed]

22. Carneiro, F.; Charlton, A.; Huntsman, D.G. Hereditary diffuse gastric cancer. In *WHO Classification of Tumours of the Digestive System*, 4th ed.; Bosman, D.T., Carneiro, F., Hruban, R.H., Theise, N.D., Eds.; International Agency for Research on Cancer: Lyon, France, 2010; Volume 3, pp. 59–63.

23. Guilford, P.; Hopkins, J.; Harraway, J.; McLeod, M.; McLeod, N.; Harawira, P.; Taite, H.; Scoular, R.; Miller, A.; Reeve, A.E. E-cadherin germline mutations in familial gastric cancer. *Nature* **1998**, *392*, 402–405. [CrossRef] [PubMed]

24. Kluijt, I.; Sijmons, R.H.; Hoogerbrugge, N.; Plukker, J.T.; de Jong, D.; van Krieken, J.H.; van Hillegersberg, R.; Ligtenberg, M.; Bleiker, E.; Cats, A.; et al. Familial gastric cancer: Guidelines for diagnosis, treatment and periodic surveillance. *Fam. Cancer* **2012**, *11*, 363–369. [CrossRef] [PubMed]

25. Fitzgerald, R.C.; Hardwick, R.; Huntsman, D.; Carneiro, F.; Guilford, P.; Blair, V.; Chung, D.C.; Norton, J.; Ragunath, K.; Van Krieken, J.H.; et al. Hereditary diffuse gastric cancer: Updated consensus guidelines for clinical management and directions for future research. *J. Med. Genet.* **2010**, *47*, 436–444. [CrossRef] [PubMed]

26. Van der Post, R.S.; Vogelaar, I.P.; Carneiro, F.; Guilford, P.; Huntsman, D.; Hoogerbrugge, N.; Caldas, C.; Schreiber, K.E.; Hardwick, R.H.; Ausems, M.G.; et al. Hereditary diffuse gastric cancer: Updated clinical guidelines with an emphasis on germline CDH1 mutation carriers. *J. Med. Genet.* **2015**, *52*, 361–374. [CrossRef] [PubMed]

27. Tan, P.; Yeoh, K.G. Genetics and Molecular Pathogenesis of Gastric Adenocarcinoma. *Gastroenterology* **2015**, *149*, 1153–1162. [CrossRef] [PubMed]

28. Jeanes, A.; Gottardi, C.J.; Yap, A.S. Cadherins and cancer: How does cadherin dysfunction promote tumor progression? *Oncogene* **2008**, *27*, 6920–6929. [CrossRef] [PubMed]

29. Cho, S.Y.; Park, J.W.; Liu, Y.; Park, Y.S.; Kim, J.H.; Yang, H.; Um, H.; Ko, W.R.; Lee, B.I.; Kwon, S.Y.; et al. Sporadic early-onset diffuse gastric cancers have high frequency of somatic CDH1 alterations, but low frequency of somatic RHOA mutations compared with late-onset cancers. *Gastroenterology* **2017**, *153*, 536–549. [CrossRef] [PubMed]

30. Van Roy, F.; Berx, G. The cell–cell adhesion molecule E-cadherin. *Cell Mol. Life Sci.* **2008**, *65*, 3756–3788. [CrossRef] [PubMed]

31. Grady, W.M.; Willis, J.; Guilford, P.J.; Dunbier, A.K.; Toro, T.T.; Lynch, H.; Wiesner, G.; Ferguson, K.; Eng, C.; Park, J.G.; et al. Methylation of the CDH1 promoter as the second genetic hit in hereditary diffuse gastric cancer. *Nat. Genet.* **2000**, *26*, 16–17. [CrossRef] [PubMed]

32. Carvalho, S.; Catarino, T.A.; Dias, A.M.; Kato, M.; Almeida, A.; Hessling, B.; Figueiredo, J.; Gartner, F.; Sanches, J.M.; Ruppert, T.; et al. Preventing E-cadherin aberrant *N*-glycosylation at Asn-554 improves its critical function in gastric cancer. *Oncogene* **2016**, *35*, 1619–1631. [CrossRef] [PubMed]

33. Pinho, S.S.; Seruca, R.; Gartner, F.; Yamaguchi, Y.; Gu, J.; Taniguchi, N.; Reis, C.A. Modulation of E-cadherin function and dysfunction by *N*-glycosylation. *Cell Mol. Life Sci.* **2011**, *68*, 1011–1020. [CrossRef] [PubMed]

34. Liu, Y.C.; Shen, C.Y.; Wu, H.S.; Hsieh, T.Y.; Chan, D.C.; Chen, C.J.; Yu, J.C.; Yu, C.P.; Ham, H.J.; Chen, P.J.; et al. Mechanisms inactivating the gene for E-cadherin in sporadic gastric carcinomas. *World J. Gastroenterol.* **2006**, *12*, 2168–2173. [CrossRef] [PubMed]

35. Humar, B.; Graziano, F.; Cascinu, S.; Catalano, V.; Ruzzo, A.M.; Magnani, M.; Toro, T.; Burchill, T.; Futschik, M.E.; Merriman, T.; et al. Association of CDH1 haplotypes with susceptibility to sporadic diffuse gastric cancer. *Oncogene* **2002**, *21*, 8192–8195. [CrossRef] [PubMed]

36. Kakiuchi, M.; Nishizawa, T.; Ueda, H.; Gotoh, K.; Tanaka, A.; Hayashi, A.; Yamamoto, S.; Tatsuno, K.; Katoh, H.; Watanabe, Y.; et al. Recurrent gain-of-function mutations of RHOA in diffuse-type gastric carcinoma. *Nat. Genet.* **2014**, *46*, 583–587. [CrossRef] [PubMed]

37. Nagahashi, M.; Ramachandran, S.; Kim, E.Y.; Allegood, J.C.; Rashid, O.M.; Yamada, A.; Zhao, R.; Milstien, S.; Zhou, H.; Spiegel, S.; et al. Sphingosine-1-phosphate produced by sphingosine kinase 1 promotes breast cancer progression by stimulating angiogenesis and lymphangiogenesis. *Cancer Res.* **2012**, *72*, 726–735. [CrossRef] [PubMed]

38. Hanyu, T.; Nagahashi, M.; Ichikawa, H.; Ishikawa, T.; Kobayashi, T.; Wakai, T. Expression of phosphorylated sphingosine kinase 1 is associated with diffuse type and lymphatic invasion in human gastric cancer. *Surgery* **2017**. [CrossRef] [PubMed]

39. Dumas, Y.R.; He, X. Wnt signaling: What the X@# is WTX? *EMBO J.* **2011**, *30*, 1415–1417.

40. Ghatak, S.; Chakraborty, P.; Sarkar, S.R.; Chowdhury, B.; Bhaumik, A.; Kumar, N.S. Novel APC gene mutations associated with protein alteration in diffuse type gastric cancer. *BMC Med. Genet.* **2017**, *18*, 61. [CrossRef] [PubMed]

41. Turner, N.; Grose, R. Fibroblast growth factor signalling: From development to cancer. *Nat. Rev. Cancer* **2010**, *10*, 116–129. [CrossRef] [PubMed]

42. Hattori, Y.; Itoh, H.; Uchino, S.; Hosokawa, K.; Ochiai, A.; Ino, Y.; Ishii, H.; Sakamoto, H.; Yamaguchi, N.; Yanagihara, K.; et al. Immunohistochemical detection of K-sam protein in stomach cancer. *Clin. Cancer Res.* **1996**, *2*, 1373–1381. [PubMed]

43. Levine, A. The p53 tumor-suppressor gene. *N. Engl. J. Med.* **1992**, *326*, 1350–1352. [CrossRef] [PubMed]

44. Kohno, Y.; Yamamoto, H.; Hirahashi, M.; Kumagae, Y.; Nakamura, M.; Oki, E.; Oda, Y. Reduced MUTYH, MTH1, and OGG1 expression and TP53 mutation in diffuse-type adenocarcinoma of gastric cardia. *Hum. Pathol.* **2016**, *52*, 145–152. [CrossRef] [PubMed]

45. Ge, S.; Li, B.; Li, Y.; Li, Z.; Liu, Z.; Chen, Z.; Wu, J.; Gao, J.; Shen, L. Genomic alterations in advanced gastric cancer endoscopic biopsy samples using targeted next-generation sequencing. *Am. J. Cancer Res.* **2017**, *7*, 1540–1553. [PubMed]

46. Choi, J.H.; Kim, Y.B.; Ahn, J.M.; Kim, M.J.; Bae, W.J.; Han, S.U.; Woo, H.G.; Lee, D. Identification of genomic aberrations associated with lymph node metastasis in diffuse-type gastric cancer. *Experimen. Mol. Med.* **2018**, *50*, 6. [CrossRef] [PubMed]

47. Oliveira, M.J.; Costa, A.M.; Costa, A.C.; Ferreira, R.M.; Sampaio, P.; Machado, J.C.; Seruca, R.; Mareel, M.; Figueiredo, C. CagA associates with c-Met, E-cadherin, and p120-catenin in a multiproteic complex that suppresses *Helicobacter pylori*-induced cell-invasive phenotype. *J. Infect. Dis.* **2009**, *200*, 745–755. [CrossRef] [PubMed]

48. Kim, S.; Meitner, P.; Konkin, T.; Cho, Y.; Resnick, M.; Moss, S. Altered expression of Skp2, c-Myc and p27 proteins but not mRNA after *Helicobacter pylori* eradication in chronic gastritis. *Mod. Pathol.* **2006**, *19*, 49–58. [CrossRef] [PubMed]

49. Andre, A.; Ferreira, M.; Mota, R.; Ferrasi, A.; Pardini, M.; Rabenhorst, S. Gastric adenocarcinoma and *Helicobacter pylori*: Correlation with p53 mutation and p27 immunoexpression. *Cancer Epidemiol.* **2010**, *34*, 618–625. [CrossRef] [PubMed]

50. Yamamoto, E.; Suzuki, H.; Takamaru, H.; Yamamoto, H.; Toyota, M.; Shinomura, Y. Role of DNA methylation in the development of diffuse-type gastric cancer. *Digestion* **2011**, *83*, 241–249. [CrossRef] [PubMed]

51. Perri, F.; Cotugno, R.; Piepoli, A.; Merla, A.; Quitadamo, M.; Gentile, A.; Pilotto, A.; Annese, V.; Andriulli, A. Aberrant DNA methylation in non-neoplastic gastric mucosa of *Helicobacter pylori* infected patients and effect of eradication. *Am. J. Gastroenterol.* **2007**, *102*, 1361–1371. [CrossRef] [PubMed]

52. Hoy, B.; Lower, M.; Weydig, C.; Carra, G.; Tegtmeyer, N.; Geppert, T.; Schroder, P.; Sewald, N.; Backert, S.; Schneider, G.; et al. *Helicobacter pylori* HtrA is a new secreted virulence factor that cleaves E-cadherin to disrupt intercellular adhesion. *EMBO Rep.* **2010**, *11*, 798–804. [CrossRef] [PubMed]

53. Tegtmeyer, N.; Moodley, Y.; Yamaoka, Y.; Pernitzsch, S.R.; Schmidt, V.; Traverso, F.R.; Schmidt, T.P.; Rad, R.; Yeoh, K.G.; Bow, H.; et al. Characterization of worldwide *Helicobacter pylori* strains reveals genetic conservation and essentiality of serine protease HtrA. *Mol. Microbiol.* **2016**, *99*, 925–944. [CrossRef] [PubMed]

54. Schmidt, T.P.; Goetz, C.; Huemer, M.; Schneider, G.; Wessler, S. Calcium binding protects E-cadherin from cleavage by *Helicobacter pylori* HtrA. *Gut Pathog.* **2016**, *8*, 29. [CrossRef] [PubMed]

55. Schmidt, T.P.; Pema, A.M.; Fugmann, T.; Bohm, M.; Jan, H.; Haller, S.; Gotz, C.; Tegtmeyer, N.; Hoy, B.; Rau, T.T.; et al. Identification of E-cadherin signature motifs functioning as cleavage sites for *Helicobacter pylori* HtrA. *Sci. Rep.* **2016**, *6*, 23264. [CrossRef] [PubMed]

56. Hoy, B.; Geppert, T.; Boehm, M.; Reisen, F.; Plattner, P.; Gadermaier, G.; Sewald, N.; Ferreira, F.; Briza, P.; Schneider, G.; et al. Distinct roles of secreted HtrA proteases from gram-negative pathogens in cleaving the junctional protein and tumor suppressor E-cadherin. *J. Biol. Chem.* **2012**, *287*, 10115–10120. [CrossRef] [PubMed]

57. Green, K.J.; Getsios, S.; Troyanovsky, S.; Godsel, L.M. Intercellular junction assembly, dynamics, and homeostasis. *Cold Spring Harb. Perspect. Biol.* **2010**, *2*. [CrossRef] [PubMed]

58. Gumbiner, B.; Stevenson, B.; Grimaldi, A. The role of the cell adhesion molecule uvomorulin in the formation and maintenance of the epithelial junctional complex. *J. Cell Biol.* **1988**, *107*, 1575–1587. [CrossRef] [PubMed]

59. Berx, G.; Nollet, F.; van Roy, F. Dysregulation of the E-cadherin/catenin complex by irreversible mutations in human carcinomas. *Cell Adhes. Commun.* **1998**, *6*, 171–184. [CrossRef] [PubMed]

60. Stemmler, M.P. Cadherins in development and cancer. *Mol. Bio. Syst.* **2008**, *4*, 835–850. [CrossRef] [PubMed]

61. Berx, G.; van Roy, F. Involvement of members of the cadherin superfamily in cancer. *Cold Spring Harb. Perspect. Biol.* **2009**, *1*. [CrossRef] [PubMed]

62. Wheelock, M.J.; Johnson, K.R. Cadherins as modulators of cellular phenotype. *Ann. Rev. Cell. Dev. Biol.* **2003**, *19*, 207–325. [CrossRef] [PubMed]

63. Liu, X.; Chu, K.-M. E-cadherin and gastric cancer: Cause, consequence, and applications. *Biomed. Res. Int.* **2014**, *2014*. [CrossRef] [PubMed]

64. Moridnia, A.; Tabatabaiefar, M.A.; Zeinalian, M.; Minakari, M.; Kheirollahi, M.; Moghaddam, N.A. Novel variants and copy number variation in CDH1 gene in Iranian patients with sporadic diffuse gastric cancer. *J. Gastrointest. Cancer* **2018**. (ahead of print). [CrossRef] [PubMed]

65. Moran, C.J.J.M.; McAnena, O.J. CDH1 associated gastric cancer: A report of a family and review of the literature. *Eur. J. Surg. Oncol.* **2005**, *31*, 259–264. [CrossRef] [PubMed]

66. Pinheiro, H.B.-C.R.; Seixas, S.; Carvalho, J.; Senz, J.; Oliveira, P.; Inácio, P.; Gusmao, L.; Rocha, J.; Huntsman, D.; Seruca, R.; et al. Allele-specific CDH1 down-regulation and hereditary diffuse gastric cancer. *Hum. Mol. Genet.* **2010**, *19*, 943–952. [CrossRef] [PubMed]

67. Tamura, G. Alterations of tumor suppressor and tumor-related genes in the development and progression of gastric cancer. *World J. Gastroenterol.* **2006**, *12*, 192–198. [CrossRef] [PubMed]

68. Ghaffari, S.; Rafati, M.; Sabokbar, T.; Dastan, J. A novel truncating mutation in the E-cadherin gene in the first Iranian family with hereditary diffuse gastric cancer. *Eur. J. Surg. Oncol.* **2010**, *36*, 559–562. [CrossRef] [PubMed]

69. Chu, C.M.; Chen, C.J.; Chan, D.C.; Wu, H.S.; Liu, Y.C.; Shen, C.Y.; Chang, T.M.; Yu, J.C.; Harn, H.J.; Yu, C.P.; et al. CDH1 polymorphisms and haplotypes in sporadic diffuse and intestinal gastric cancer: A case–control study based on direct sequencing analysis. *World J. Surg. Oncol.* **2014**, *12*, 80. [CrossRef] [PubMed]

70. Medina-Franco, H.; Ramos-De la Medina, A.; Vizcaino, G.; Medina-Franco, J.L. Single nucleotide polymorphisms in the promoter region of the E-cadherin gene in gastric cancer: Case–control study in a young Mexican population. *Ann. Surg. Oncol.* **2007**, *14*, 2246–2249. [CrossRef] [PubMed]

71. Gullo, I.; Devezas, V.; Baptista, M.; Garrido, L.; Castedo, S.; Morais, R.; Wen, X.; Rios, E.; Pinheiro, J.; Pinto-Ribeiro, I.; et al. The phenotypic heterogeneity of hereditary diffuse gastric cancer: The report of one family with early-onset disease. *Gastroint. Endos.* **2018**. [CrossRef] [PubMed]

72. Park, J.W.; Jang, S.H.; Park, D.M.; Lim, N.J.; Deng, C.; Kim, D.Y.; Green, J.E.; Kim, H.K. Cooperativity of E-cadherin and Smad4 Loss to promote diffuse-type gastric adenocarcinoma and metastasis. *Mol. Cancer Res.* **2014**, *12*, 1088–1099. [CrossRef] [PubMed]

73. Gall, T.M.H.; Frampton, A.E. Gene of the month: Ecadherin (CDH1). *J. Clin. Pathol.* **2013**, *66*, 928–932. [CrossRef] [PubMed]

74. Park, J.W.; Kim, M.S.; Voon, D.C.; Kim, S.J.; Bae, J.; Mun, D.G.; Ko, S.I.; Kim, H.K.; Lee, S.W.; Kim, D.Y. Multi-omics analysis identifies pathways and genes involved in diffuse-type gastric carcinogenesis induced by E-cadherin, p53, and Smad4 loss in mice. *Mol. Carcinog.* **2018**. [CrossRef] [PubMed]

75. Wang, K.; Yuen, S.T.; Xu, J.; Lee, S.P.; Yan, H.H.; Shi, S.T.; Siu, H.C.; Deng, S.; Chu, K.M.; Law, S.; et al. Whole-genome sequencing and comprehensive molecular profiling identify new driver mutations in gastric cancer. *Nat. Genet.* **2014**, *46*, 573–582. [CrossRef] [PubMed]

76. Cancer Genome Atlas Research Network. Comprehensive molecular characterization of gastric adenocarcinoma. *Nature* **2014**, *513*, 202–209. [CrossRef] [PubMed]

77. Ushiku, T.; Ishikawa, S.; Kakiuchi, M.; Tanaka, A.; Katoh, H.; Aburatani, H.; Lauwers, G.Y.; Fukayama, M. RHOA mutation in diffuse-type gastric cancer: A comparative clinicopathology analysis of 87 cases. *Gastric Cancer* **2016**, *19*, 403–411. [CrossRef] [PubMed]

78. Miyamoto, S.; Nagamura, Y.; Nakabo, A.; Okabe, A.; Yanagihara, K.; Fukami, K.; Sakai, R.; Yamaguchi, H. Aberrant alternative splicing of RHOA is associated with loss of its expression and activity in diffuse-type gastric carcinoma cells. *Biochem. Biophys. Res. Commun.* **2018**, *495*, 1942–1947. [CrossRef] [PubMed]

79. Etienne-Manneville, S.; Hall, A. Rho GTPases in cell biology. *Nature* **2002**, *420*, 629–635. [CrossRef] [PubMed]

80. Heasman, S.J.; Ridley, A.J. Mammalian Rho GTPases: New insights into their functions from in vivo studies. *Nat. Rev. Mol. Cell Biol.* **2008**, *9*, 690–701. [CrossRef] [PubMed]

81. Guan, R.; Xu, X.; Chen, M.; Hu, H.; Ge, H.; Wen, S.; Zhou, S.; Pi, R. Advances in the studies of roles of Rho/Rho-kinase in diseases and the development of its inhibitors. *Eur. J. Medicinal Chem.* **2013**, *70*, 613–622. [CrossRef] [PubMed]

82. Thumkeo, D.; Watanabe, S.; Narumiya, S. Physiological roles of Rho and Rho effectors in mammals. *Eur. J. Cell Biol.* **2013**, *92*, 303–315. [CrossRef] [PubMed]

83. Pyne, N.J.; Pyne, S. Sphingosine 1-phosphate and cancer. *Nat. Rev. Cancer* **2010**, *10*, 489–503. [CrossRef] [PubMed]

84. Liang, J.; Nagahashi, M.; Kim, E.Y.; Harikumar, K.B.; Yamada, A.; Huang, W.C.; Hait, N.C.; Allegood, J.C.; Price, M.M.; Avni, D.; et al. Sphingosine-1-phosphate links persistent STAT3 activation, chronic intestinal inflammation, and development of colitisassociated cancer. *Cancer Cell.* **2013**, *23*, 107–120. [CrossRef] [PubMed]

85. Anelli, V.; Gault, C.R.; Snider, A.J.; Obeid, L.M. Role of sphingosine kinase-1 in paracrine/transcellular angiogenesis and lymphangiogenesis in vitro. *FASEB J.* **2010**, *24*, 2727. [CrossRef] [PubMed]

86. Nagahashi, M.; Matsuda, Y.; Moro, K.; Tsuchida, J.; Soma, D.; Hirose, Y.; Kobayashi, T.; Kosugi, S.; Takabe, K.; Komatsu, M.; et al. DNA damage response and sphingolipid signaling in liver diseases. *Surg. Today* **2016**, *46*, 995–1005. [CrossRef] [PubMed]

87. Takabe, K.; Spiegel, S. Export of sphingosine-1-phosphate and cancer progression. *J. Lipid Res.* **2014**, *55*, 1839. [CrossRef] [PubMed]

88. Nagahashi, M.; Takabe, K.; Terracina, K.P.; Soma, D.; Hirose, Y.; Kobayashi, T.; Matsuda, Y.; Wakai, T. Sphingosine-1-phosphate transporters as targets for cancer therapy. *Biomed. Res. Int.* **2014**, *2014*, 651727. [CrossRef] [PubMed]

89. Spiegel, S.; Milstien, S. The outs and the ins of sphingosine-1-phosphate in immunity. *Nat. Rev. Immunol.* **2011**, *11*, 403–415. [CrossRef] [PubMed]

90. Takabe, K.; Kim, R.H.; Allegood, J.C.; Mitra, P.; Ramchandran, S.; Nagahashi, M.; Harikumar, K.B.; Hait, N.C.; Milstien, S.; Spiegel, S. Estradiol induces export of sphingosine 1-phosphate from breast cancer cells via ABCC1 and ABCG2. *J. Biol. Chem.* **2010**, *285*, 10477–10486. [CrossRef] [PubMed]

91. Takabe, K.; Paugh, S.W.; Milstien, S.; Spiegel, S. "Inside-out" signaling of sphingosine- 1-phosphate: Therapeutic targets. *Pharmacol. Rev.* **2008**, *60*, 181. [CrossRef] [PubMed]

92. Powell, S.M.; Zilz, N.; Beazer-Barclay, Y.; Bryan, T.M.; Hamilton, S.R.; Thibodeau, S.N.; Vogelstein, B.; Kinzler, K.W. APC mutations occur early during colorectal tumorigenesis. *Nature* **1992**, *359*, 235–237. [CrossRef] [PubMed]

93. Nishisho, I.; Nakamura, Y.; Mivoshi, Y.; Miki, Y.; Ando, H.; Horii, A. Mutations of chromosomes 5q21 genes in FAP and cokorctal cancer patients. *Science* **1991**, *253*, 665–669. [CrossRef] [PubMed]

94. Groden, J.; Thliveris, A.; Samovitz, W.S.; Carlson, M.I.; Gilbert, L.; Albertsen, H.; Joslyn, G.; Stevens, J.; Spirio, L.; Robertson, M.; et al. Identification and characterization of the familial adenomatous polyposis coli gene. *Cell* **1991**, *66*, 589–600. [CrossRef]

95. Behrens, J.; Von-Kries, J.P.; Kuhl, M.; Bruhn, L.; Wedlich, D.; Grosschedl, R.; Birchmeier, W. Functional interaction of β-catenin with the transcription factor LEF-1. *Nature* **1996**, *382*, 638–642. [CrossRef] [PubMed]

96. Deng, N.; Goh, L.K.; Wang, H.; Das, K.; Tao, J.; Tan, I.B.; Zhang, S.; Lee, M.; Wu, J.; Lim, K.H.; et al. A comprehensive survey of genomic alterations in gastric cancer reveals systematic patterns of molecular exclusivity and co-occurrence among distinct therapeutic targets. *Gut* 2012, *61*, 673–684. [CrossRef] [PubMed]

97. Nagatsuma, A.K.; Aizawa, M.; Kuwata, T.; Doi, T.; Ohtsu, A.; Fujii, H.; Ochiai, A. Expression profiles of HER2, EGFR, MET and FGFR2 in a large cohort of patients with gastric adenocarcinoma. *Gastric Cancer* 2015, *18*, 227–238. [CrossRef] [PubMed]

98. Chua, T.C.; Merrett, N.D. Clinicopathologic factors associated with HER2-positive gastric cancer and its impact on survival outcomes-a systematic review. *Int. J. Cancer* 2012, *130*, 2845–2856. [CrossRef] [PubMed]

99. Hattori, Y.; Odagiri, H.; Nakatani, H.; Miyagawa, K.; Naito, K.; Sakamoto, H.; Katoh, O.; Yoshida, T.; Sugimura, T.; Terada, M. K-sam, an amplified gene in stomach cancer, is a member of the heparin binding growth factor receptor genes. *Proc. Natl. Acad. Sci. USA* 1990, *87*, 5983–5987. [CrossRef] [PubMed]

100. Inokuchi, M.; Otsuki, S.; Fujimori, Y.; Sato, Y.; Nakagawa, M.; Kojima, K. Therapeutic targeting of fibroblast growth factor receptors in gastric cancer. *Gastroenterol. Res. Pract.* 2015, *2015*, 796380. [CrossRef] [PubMed]

101. Inokuchi, M.; Murase, H.; Otsuki, S.; Kawano, T.; Kojima, K. Different clinical significance of FGFR1–4 expression between diffuse-type and intestinal-type gastric cancer. *World J. Surg. Oncol.* 2017, *15*, 2. [CrossRef] [PubMed]

102. Ishige, T.; Nishimura, M.; Satoh, M.; Fujimoto, M.; Fukuyo, M.; Semba, T.; Kado, S.; Tsuchida, S.; Sawai, S.; Matsushita, K.; et al. Combined secretomics and transcriptomics revealed cancer-derived GDF15 is involved in diffuse-type gastric cancer progression and fibroblast activation. *Sci. Rep.* 2016, *6*, 21681. [CrossRef] [PubMed]

103. Yashiro, M.; Hirakawa, K. Cancer-stromal interactions in scirrhous gastric carcinoma. *Cancer Microenviron.* 2010, *3*, 127–135. [CrossRef] [PubMed]

104. Hata, K.; Yamamoto, Y.; Kiyomatsu, T.; Tanaka, T.; Kazama, S.; Nozawa, H.; Kawai, K.; Tanaka, J.; Nishikawa, T.; Otani, K.; et al. Hereditary gastrointestinal cancer. *Surg. Today* 2016, *46*, 1115–1122. [CrossRef] [PubMed]

105. Bellini, M.F.; Cadamuro, A.C.T.; Succi, M.; Proenc, M.A.; Silva, A.E. Alterations of the TP53 gene in gastric and esophageal carcinogenesis. *J. Biomed. Biotechnol.* 2012, *2012*, 891961. [CrossRef] [PubMed]

106. Kim, I.J.; Kang, H.C.; Park, H.W.; Jang, S.G.; Han, S.Y.; Lim, S.K.; Lee, M.R.; Chang, H.J.; Ku, J.L.; Yang, H.K.; et al. A TP53 -truncating germline mutation (E287X) in a family with characteristics of both hereditary diffuse gastric cancer and Li-Fraumeni syndrome. *J. Hum. Genet.* 2004, *49*, 591–595. [CrossRef] [PubMed]

107. Kaurah, P.; MacMillan, A.; Boyd, N.; Senz, J.; De Luca, A.; Chun, N.; Suriano, G.; Zaor, S.; Van Manen, L.; Gilpin, C.; et al. Founder and recurrent CDH1 mutations in families with hereditary diffuse gastric cancer. *JAMA* 2007, *297*, 2360–2372. [CrossRef] [PubMed]

108. Ge, S.; Xia, X.; Ding, C.; Zhen, B.; Zhou, Q.; Feng, J.; Yuan, J.; Chen, R.; Li, Y.; Ge, Z.; et al. A proteomic landscape of diffuse-type gastric cancer. *Nat. Commun.* 2018, *9*, 1012. [CrossRef] [PubMed]

109. Donner, I.; Kiviluoto, T.; Ristimaki, A.; Aaltonen, L.A.; Vahteristo, P. Exome sequencing reveals three novel candidate predisposition genes for diffuse gastric cancer. *Fam. Cancer* 2015, *14*, 241–246. [CrossRef] [PubMed]

110. Liu, G.; Xin, Z.C.; Chen, L.; Tian, L.; Yuan, Y.M.; Song, W.D.; Jiang, X.J.; Guo, Y.L. Expression and localization of CKLFSF2 in human spermatogenesis. *Asian J. Androl.* 2007, *9*, 189–198. [CrossRef] [PubMed]

111. Plate, M.; Li, T.; Wang, Y.; Mo, X.; Zhang, Y.; Ma, D.; Han, W. Identification and characterization of CMTM4, a novel gene with inhibitory effects on HeLa cell growth through Inducing G2/M phase accumulation. *Mol. Cells* 2010, *29*, 355–361. [CrossRef] [PubMed]

112. Zhang, W.; Mendoza, M.C.; Pei, X.; Ilter, D.; Mahoney, S.J.; Zhang, Y.; Ma, D.; Blenis, J.; Wang, Y. Down-regulation of CMTM8 induces epithelial to mesenchymal transition-like changes via c-MET/extracellular signal-regulated kinase (ERK) signaling. *J. Biol. Chem.* 2012, *287*, 11850–11858. [CrossRef] [PubMed]

113. Li, H.; Li, J.; Su, Y.; Fan, Y.; Guo, X.; Li, L.; Su, X.; Rong, R.; Ying, J.; Mo, X.; et al. A novel 3p22.3 gene CMTM7 represses oncogenic EGFR signaling and inhibits cancer cell growth. *Oncogene* 2014, *33*, 3109–3118. [CrossRef] [PubMed]

114. Schistosomes, liver flukes and *Helicobacter pylori*. IARC working group on the evaluation of carcinogenic risks to humans. Lyon, 7–14 June 1994. *IARC Monogr. Eval. Carcinog. Risks Hum.* 1994, *61*, 1–241.

115. IARC *Helicobacter pylori* Working Group. Helicobacter pylori Eradication as a Strategy for Preventing Gastric Cancer. Lyon, France 2014: International Agency for Research on Cancer (IARC Working Group Reports,

No. 8). Available online: http://www.iarc.fr/en/publications/pdfsonline/wrk/wrk8/index.php. (accessed on 6 December 2013).

116. Becker, K.F.; Atkinson, M.J.; Reich, U.; Becker, I.; Nekarda, H.; Siewert, J.R.; Hofler, H. E-cadherin gene mutations provide clues to diffuse type gastric carcinomas. *Cancer Res.* **1994**, *54*, 3845–3852. [PubMed]

117. Uemura, N.; Okamoto, S.; Yamamoto, S.; Matsumura, N.; Yamaguchi, S.; Yamakido, M.; Taniyama, K.; Sasaki, N.; Schlemper, R.J. *Helicobacter pylori* infection and the development of gastric cancer. *N. Engl. J. Med.* **2001**, *345*, 784–789. [CrossRef] [PubMed]

118. Komoto, K.; Haruma, K.; Kamada, T.; Tanaka, S.; Yoshihara, M.; Sumii, K.; Kajiyama, G.; Talley, N.J. *Helicobacter pylori* infection and gastric neoplasia: Correlations with histological gastritis and tumor histology. *Am. J. Gastroenterol.* **1998**, *93*, 1271–1276. [CrossRef] [PubMed]

119. Nishibayashi, H.; Kanayama, S.; Kiyohara, T.; Yamamoto, K.; Miyazaki, Y.; Yasunaga, Y.; Shinomura, Y.; Takeshita, T.; Takeuchi, T.; Morimoto, K.; et al. *Helicobacter pylori*-induced enlarged-fold gastritis is associated with increased mutagenicity of gastric juice, increased oxidative DNA damage, and an increased risk of gastric carcinoma. *J. Gastroenterol. Hepatol.* **2003**, *18*, 1384–1391. [CrossRef] [PubMed]

120. Misra, V.; Misra, S.P.; Singh, M.K.; Singh, P.A.; Dwivedi, M. Prevalence of *Helicobacter pylori* in patients with gastric cancer. *Indian J. Pathol. Microbiol.* **2007**, *50*, 702–707. [PubMed]

121. Awad, H.A.; Hajeer, M.H.; Abulihya, M.W.; Al-Chalabi, M.A.; Al-Khader, A.A. Epidemiologic characteristics of gastric malignancies among Jordan University Hospital patients. *Saudi Med. J.* **2017**, *38*, 965–967. [CrossRef] [PubMed]

122. Watanabe, M.; Kato, J.; Inoue, I.; Yoshimura, N.; Yoshida, T.; Mukoubayashi, C.; Deguchi, H.; Enomoto, S.; Ueda, K.; Maekita, T.; et al. Development of gastric cancer in nonatrophic stomach with highly active inflammation identified by serum levels of pepsinogen and *Helicobacter pylori* antibody together with endoscopic rugal hyperplastic gastritis. *Int. J. Cancer* **2012**, *131*, 2632–2642. [CrossRef] [PubMed]

123. Kwak, H.W.; Choi, I.J.; Cho, S.J.; Lee, J.Y.; Kim, C.G.; Kook, M.C.; Ryu, K.W.; Kim, Y.W. Characteristics of gastric cancer according to *Helicobacter pylori* infection status. *J. Gastroenterol. Hepatol.* **2014**, *29*, 1671–1677. [CrossRef] [PubMed]

124. Gong, E.J.; Lee, J.Y.; Bae, S.E.; Park, Y.S.; Choi, K.D.; Song, H.J.; Lee, G.H.; Jung, H.Y.; Jeong, W.J.; Cheon, G.J.; et al. Characteristics of non-cardia gastric cancer with a high serum anti-*Helicobacter pylori* IgG titer and its association with diffuse-type histology. *PLoS ONE* **2018**, *13*, e0195264. [CrossRef] [PubMed]

125. Jindal, Y.; Singh, A.; Kumar, R.; Varma, K.; Misra, V.; Misra, S.P.; Dwivedi, M. Expression of alpha methylacyl CoA racemase (AMACR) in gastric adenocarcinoma and its correlation with *Helicobacter pylori* infection. *J. Clin. Diag. Res.* **2016**, *10*, 10–12. [CrossRef] [PubMed]

126. Tatemichi, M.; Sasazuki, S.; Inoue, M.; Tsugane, S. Clinical significance of IgG antibody titer against *Helicobacter pylori*. *Helicobacter* **2009**, *14*, 231–236. [CrossRef] [PubMed]

127. Yang, Y.; Du, J.; Liu, F.; Wang, X.; Li, X.; Li, Y. Role of caspase-3/E-cadherin in *Helicobacter pylori*-induced apoptosis of gastric epithelial cells. *Oncotarget* **2017**, *8*, 59204–59216. [CrossRef] [PubMed]

128. Bagnoli, F.; Buti, L.; Tompkins, L.; Covacci, A.; Amieva, M.R. *Helicobacter pylori* CagA induces a transition from polarized to invasive phenotypes in MDCK cells. *Proc. Natl. Acad. Sci. USA* **2005**, *102*, 16339–16344. [CrossRef] [PubMed]

129. Zhang, X.Y.; Zhang, P.Y.; Aboul-Soud, M.A. From inflammation to gastric cancer: Role of *Helicobacter pylori*. *Oncol. Lett.* **2017**, *13*, 543–548. [CrossRef] [PubMed]

130. Ogden, S.R.; Wroblewski, L.E.; Weydig, C.; Romero-Gallo, J.; O'Brien, D.P.; Israel, D.A.; Krishna, U.S.; Fingleton, B.; Reynolds, A.B.; Wessler, S.; et al. p120 and Kaiso regulate *Helicobacter pylori*-induced expression of matrix metalloproteinase-7. *Mol. Biol. Cell* **2008**, *19*, 4110–4121. [CrossRef] [PubMed]

131. Das, L.; Kokate, S.B.; Dixit, P.; Rath, S.; Rout, N.; Singh, S.P.; Crowe, S.E.; Bhattacharyya, A. Membrane-bound β-catenin degradation is enhanced by ETS2-mediated Siah1 induction in *Helicobacter pylori*-infected gastric cancer cells. *Oncogenesis* **2017**, *6*, e327. [CrossRef] [PubMed]

132. Murata-Kamiya, N.; Kurashima, Y.; Teishikata, Y.; Yamahashi, Y.; Saito, Y.; Higashi, H.; Aburatani, H.; Akiyama, T.; Peek, R.M. Jr.; Azuma, T.; et al. *Helicobacter pylori* CagA interacts with E-cadherin and deregulates the beta-catenin signal that promotes intestinal transdifferentiation in gastric epithelial cells. *Oncogene* **2007**, *26*, 4617–4626. [CrossRef] [PubMed]

133. Pelengaris, S.; Khan, M. The many faces of c-MYC. *Arch. Biochem. Biophys.* **2003**, *416*, 129–136. [CrossRef]

134. Faria, M.; Patrocínio, R.; Moraes-Filho, M.; Rabenhorst, S. Expressão das proteínas BCL-2 e BAX em tumores astrocíticos humanos. *JPBML* **2006**, *4*, 271–278. [CrossRef]

135. Pelengaris, S.; Khan, M.; Evan, G. c-MYC: More than just a matter of life and death. *Nat. Rev. Cancer* **2002**, *2*, 764–776. [CrossRef] [PubMed]

136. Calcagno, D.; Leal, M.; Seabra, A.; Khayat, A.; Chen, E.; Demachki, S.; Assumpção, P.; Faria, M.; Rabenhorst, S.; Ferreira, M.; et al. Interrelationship between chromosome 8 aneuploidy, C-MYC amplification and increased espression in individuals from northern Brazil with gastric adenocarcinoma. *World J. Gastroenterol.* **2006**, *12*, 6207–6211. [CrossRef] [PubMed]

137. De Lima Silva-Fernandes, I.J.; Alves, M.K.S.; Lima, V.P.; Pereira de Lima, M.A.; Barros, M.A.P.; Ferreira, M.V.P.; Rabenhorst, S.H.B. Differential expression of MYC in *Helicobacter pylori*-related intestinal and diffuse gastric tumors. *Virchows Arch.* **2011**, *458*, 725–731. [CrossRef] [PubMed]

138. Hoy, B.; Brandstetter, H.; Wessler, S. The stability and activity of recombinant *Helicobacter pylori* HtrA under stress conditions. *J. Basic Microbiol.* **2013**, *53*, 402–409. [CrossRef] [PubMed]

139. Abdi, E.; Latifi-Navid, S.; Zahri, S.; Yazdanbod, A.; Safaralizadeh, R. *Helicobacter pylori* genotypes determine risk of non-cardia gastric cancer and intestinal- or diffuse-type GC in Ardabil: A very high-risk area in Northwestern Iran. *Microb. Pathog.* **2017**, *107*, 287–292. [CrossRef] [PubMed]

140. Guilford, P.J.; Hopkins, J.B.; Grady, W.M.; Markowitz, S.D.; Willis, J.; Lynch, H.; Rajput, A.; Wiesner, G.L.; Lindor, N.M.; Burgart, L.J.; et al. E-cadherin germline mutations define an inherited cancer syndrome dominated by diffuse gastric cancer. *Hum. Mutat.* **1999**, *14*, 249–255. [CrossRef]

141. Brooks-Wilson, A.R.; Kaurah, P.; Suriano, G.; Leach, S.; Senz, J.; Grehan, N.; Butterfield, Y.S.; Jeyes, J.; Schinas, J.; Bacani, J.; et al. Germline E-cadherin mutations in hereditary diffuse gastric cancer: Assessment of 42 new families and review of genetic screening criteria. *J. Med. Genet.* **2004**, *41*, 508–517. [CrossRef] [PubMed]

142. More, H.; Humar, B.; Weber, W.; Ward, R.; Christian, A.; Lintott, C.; Graziano, F.; Ruzzo, A.M.; Acosta, E.; Boman, B.; et al. Identification of seven novel germline mutations in the human E-cadherin (CDH1) gene. *Hum. Mutat.* **2007**, *28*, 203. [CrossRef] [PubMed]

143. Feroce, I.; Serrano, D.; Biffi, R.; Andreoni, B.; Galimberti, V.; Sonzogni, A.; Bottiglieri, L.; Botteri, E.; Trovato, C.; Marabelli, M.; et al. Hereditary diffuse gastric cancer in two families: A case report. *Oncol. Lett.* **2017**, *14*, 1671–1674. [CrossRef] [PubMed]

144. Zylberberg, H.M.; Sultan, K.; Rubin, S. Hereditary diffuse gastric cancer: One family's story. *World J. Clin. Cases* **2018**, *6*, 1–5. [CrossRef] [PubMed]

145. Hakkaart, C.; Ellison-Loschmann, L.; Day, R.; Sporle, A.; Koea, J.; Harawira, P.; Cheng, S.; Gray, M.; Whaanga, T.; Pearce, N.; et al. Germline CDH1 mutations are a significant contributor to the high frequency of early-onset diffuse gastric cancer cases in New Zealand Māori. *Fam. Cancer* **2018**. [CrossRef] [PubMed]

146. Corso, G.; Marrelli, D.; Pascale, V.; Vindigni, C.; Roviello, F. Frequency of CDH1 germline mutations in gastric carcinoma coming from high- and low-risk areas: Metanalysis and systematic review of the literature. *BMC Cancer* **2012**, *12*, 8. [CrossRef] [PubMed]

147. Oliveira, C.; Pinheiro, H.; Figueiredo, J.; Seruca, R.; Carneiro, F. Familial gastric cancer: Genetic susceptibility, pathology, and implications for management. *Lancet Oncol.* **2015**, *16*, 60–70. [CrossRef]

148. Oliveira, C.; Pinheiro, H.; Figueiredo, J.; Seruca, R.; Carneiro, F. E-cadherin alterations in hereditary disorders with emphasis on hereditary diffuse gastric cancer. *Prog. Mol. Biol. Transl. Sci.* **2013**, *116*, 337–359. [PubMed]

149. Guilford, P.; Humar, B.; Blair, V. Hereditary diffuse gastric cancer: Translation of CDH1 germline mutations into clinical practice. *Gastric Cancer* **2010**, *13*, 1–10. [CrossRef] [PubMed]

150. Suriano, G.; Oliveira, C.; Ferreira, P.; Machado, J.C.; Bordin, M.C.; De Wever, O.; Bruyneel, E.A.; Moguilevsky, N.; Grehan, N.; Porter, T.R.; et al. Identification of CDH1 germline missense mutations associated with functional inactivation of the E-cadherin protein in young gastric cancer probands. *Hum. Mol. Genet.* **2003**, *12*, 575–582. [CrossRef] [PubMed]

151. Figueiredo, J.; Seruca, J. Germline missense mutants in hereditary diffuse gastric cancer. *Spotlight Fam. Hered. Gastric Cancer* **2013**, *7*, 77–86.

152. Van der Post, R.S.; Carneiro, F. Emerging concepts in gastric neoplasia heritable gastric cancers and polyposis disorders. *Surg. Pathol.* **2017**, *10*, 931–945. [CrossRef] [PubMed]

153. Kluijt, I.; Siemerink, E.J.; Ausems, M.G.; van Os, T.A.; de Jong, D.; Simoes-Correia, J.; van Krieken, J.H.; Ligtenberg, M.J.; Figueiredo, J.; van Riel, E.; et al. CDH1-related hereditary diffuse gastric cancer syndrome: Clinical variations and implications for counseling. *Int. J. Cancer* **2012**, *131*, 367–376. [CrossRef] [PubMed]

154. Barber, M.E.; Save, V.; Carneiro, F.; Dwerryhouse, S.; Lao-Sirieix, P.; Hardwick, R.H.; Caldas, C.; Fitzgerald, R.C. Histopathological and molecular analysis of gastrectomy specimens from hereditary diffuse gastric cancer patients has implications for endoscopic surveillance of individuals at risk. *J. Pathol.* **2008**, *216*, 286–294. [CrossRef] [PubMed]

155. Hansford, S.; Kaurah, P.; Li-Chang, H.; Woo, M.; Senz, J.; Pinheiro, H.; Schrader, K.A.; Schaeffer, D.F.; Shumansky, K.; Zogopoulos, G. Hereditary diffuse gastric cancer syndrome: CDH1 mutations and beyond. *JAMA Oncol.* **2015**, *1*, 23–32. [CrossRef] [PubMed]

156. Huynh, J.M.; Laukaitis, C.M. Panel testing reveals nonsense and missense CDH1 mutations in families without hereditary diffuse gastric cancer. *Mol. Genet. Genom. Med.* **2016**, *4*, 232–236. [CrossRef] [PubMed]

157. Lajus, T.B.P.; Sales, R.M.D. CDH1 germ-line missense mutation identified by multigene sequencing in a family with no history of diffuse gastric cancer. *Gene* **2015**, *568*, 215–219. [CrossRef] [PubMed]

158. Boland, C.R.; Yurgelun, M.B. Historical Perspective on Familial Gastric Cancer. *Cell. Mol. Gastroenterol. Hepatol.* **2017**, *3*, 192–200. [CrossRef] [PubMed]

159. Pinheiro, H.; Oliveira, C.; Seruca, R.; Carneiro, F. Hereditary diffuse gastric cancer-pathophysiology and clinical management. *Best Pract. Res. Clin. Gastroenterol.* **2014**, *28*, 1055–1068. [CrossRef] [PubMed]

160. Oliveira, C.; Senz, J.; Kaurah, P.; Pinheiro, H.; Sanges, R.; Haegert, A.; Corso, G.; Schouten, J.; Fitzgerald, R.; Vogelsang, H.; et al. Germline CDH1 deletions in hereditary diffuse gastric cancer families. *Hum. Mol. Genet.* **2009**, *18*, 1545–1555. [CrossRef] [PubMed]

161. Majewski, I.J.; Kluijt, I.; Cats, A.; Scerri, T.S.; de Jong, D.; Kluin, R.J.; Hansford, S.; Hogervorst, F.B.; Bosma, A.J.; Hofland, I.; et al. An α-E-catenin (CTNNA1) mutation in hereditary diffuse gastric cancer. *J. Pathol.* **2013**, *229*, 621–629. [CrossRef] [PubMed]

162. Gaston, D.; Hansford, S.; Oliveira, C.; Nightingale, M.; Pinheiro, H.; Macgillivray, C.; Kaurah, P.; Rideout, A.L.; Steele, P.; Soares, G.; et al. Germline mutations in MAP3K6 are associated with familial gastric cancer. *PLoS Genet.* **2014**, *10*, e1004669. [CrossRef] [PubMed]

163. Lee, H.E.; Smyrk, T.C.; Zhang, L. Histologic and immunohistochemical differences between hereditary and sporadic diffuse gastric carcinoma. *Human Pathol.* **2018**, *74*, 64–72. [CrossRef] [PubMed]

164. Vogelaar, I.P.; Ligtenberg, M.J.; van der Post, R.S.; de Voer, R.M.; Kets, C.M.; Jansen, T.J.; Jacobs, L.; Schreibelt, G.; de Vries, I.J.; Netea, M.G.; et al. Recurrent candidiasis and early-onset gastric cancer in a patient with a genetically defined partial MYD88 defect. *Fam. Cancer* **2016**, *15*, 289–296. [CrossRef] [PubMed]

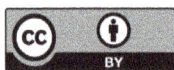

International Journal of
Molecular Sciences

MDPI

Review

Predicting the Functional Impact of *CDH1* Missense Mutations in Hereditary Diffuse Gastric Cancer

Soraia Melo [1,2,3], Joana Figueiredo [1,2], Maria Sofia Fernandes [1,2,4], Margarida Gonçalves [1,5], Eurico Morais-de-Sá [1,5], João Miguel Sanches [4] and Raquel Seruca [1,2,3,*]

1   Instituto de Investigação e Inovação em Saúde (i3S), University of Porto, 4200-135 Porto, Portugal; soraiam@ipatimup.pt (S.M.); jfigueiredo@ipatimup.pt (J.F.); sfernandes@ipatimup.pt (M.S.F.); m.goncalves@i3s.up.pt (M.G.); eurico.sa@ibmc.up.pt (E.M.-d.-S.)
2   Institute of Molecular Pathology and Immunology, University of Porto (IPATIMUP), 4200-135 Porto, Portugal
3   Medical Faculty, University of Porto, 4200-135 Porto, Portugal
4   Institute for Systems and Robotics (ISR), Instituto Superior Técnico (IST), 1049-001 Lisboa, Portugal; jmrs@tecnico.ulisboa.pt
5   Instituto de Biologia Molecular e Celular (IBMC), Universidade do Porto, 4200-135 Porto, Portugal
*   Correspondence: rseruca@ipatimup.pt

Received: 10 October 2017; Accepted: 30 November 2017; Published: 12 December 2017

Abstract: The role of E-cadherin in Hereditary Diffuse Gastric Cancer (HDGC) is unequivocal. Germline alterations in its encoding gene (*CDH1*) are causative of HDGC and occur in about 40% of patients. Importantly, while in most cases *CDH1* alterations result in the complete loss of E-cadherin associated with a well-established clinical impact, in about 20% of cases the mutations are of the missense type. The latter are of particular concern in terms of genetic counselling and clinical management, as the effect of the sequence variants in E-cadherin function is not predictable. If a deleterious variant is identified, prophylactic surgery could be recommended. Therefore, over the last few years, intensive research has focused on evaluating the functional consequences of *CDH1* missense variants and in assessing E-cadherin pathogenicity. In that context, our group has contributed to better characterize *CDH1* germline missense variants and is now considered a worldwide reference centre. In this review, we highlight the state of the art methodologies to categorize *CDH1* variants, as neutral or deleterious. This information is subsequently integrated with clinical data for genetic counseling and management of *CDH1* variant carriers.

Keywords: Hereditary Diffuse Gastric Cancer; E-cadherin; *CDH1* missense variants; functional characterization; diagnostic tools

1. Introduction

In this review article, a special focus is given to a particular type of gastric cancer, the Hereditary Diffuse Gastric Cancer (HDGC). Herein, important aspects of HDGC are discussed, including the molecular mechanisms involved, how E-cadherin deregulation affects the development of the disease, and more importantly the translation of this knowledge into clinical practice.

An overview is given of the role of E-cadherin in normal epithelia and cancer, how distinct missense mutations in the E-cadherin encoding gene, *CDH1*, differently disturb E-cadherin expression and function, what are the recommendations and guidelines for the classification and management of *CDH1* mutation carriers, and what strategies are available, or being developed, to predict *CDH1* variants pathogenicity. The latter includes in silico tools, in vitro assays for the analysis of E-cadherin expression profiles, intracellular organization, cell-cell adhesion status and invasive and migratory properties, and finally an in vivo approach taking advantage of the fly *Drosophila melanogaster*.

We describe the technological developments and state of the art methodologies that have emerged, and how bench results are used to help clinicians and genetic counselors in the management of HDGC patients and families. In order to collect the available literature, related to germline E-cadherin missense mutations in the HDGC context, the PubMed database was accessed and publications searched from November 1982 to September 2017. Search terms included: *CDH1*, E-cadherin, E-cadherin in cancer, gastric cancer, familial and Hereditary Diffuse Gastric Cancer, E-cadherin dysfunction, E-cadherin germline mutation, *CDH1*/E-cadherin missense mutation, and in vitro and in vivo functional assays. Overall, this review brings together issues that are of interest to researchers, clinicians, and genetic counseling experts.

2. The Role of E-Cadherin in Normal Epithelia and Cancer

Cell-cell adhesion is critical for the maintenance of tissue morphogenesis and homeostasis, but is also crucial for a plethora of other cellular processes, including cell differentiation, survival, and migration through the control of gene expression and the activation of signaling pathways [1]. Particularly relevant in cell-cell adhesion are the classical cadherins, such as E-cadherin, that play a key role in calcium-dependent cell-cell interactions, in establishing tight adherent junctions, and in defining cell differentiation specificity [2]. In fact, the cytoplasmic tail of E-cadherin forms a protein complex with β-, p120- and α-catenins that links this adhesion molecule with the actin-myosin network, coordinating the shape, polarity, and function of the cells in an epithelium [3,4]. Given the broad-ranging functions of E-cadherin on tissue organization, it is not surprising that alterations in its expression or structural modifications in its encoding gene *CDH1* are common events during cancer progression and contribute to the aberrant morphogenetic effects in cancer [3,5,6]. Indeed, most human carcinomas partially or completely lose E-cadherin as they progress towards malignancy, supporting the role of E-cadherin and downstream targets in cancer development [3,7].

3. E-Cadherin Deregulation Mechanisms

Mutations in the *CDH1* gene are a well-known mechanism of E-cadherin deregulation, as thoroughly described in Section 4. In addition, downregulation of E-cadherin expression can occur via other mechanisms including overexpression of transcription repressors, alterations of microRNAs (miRNAs), deregulation of protein trafficking, and aberrant post-translational regulation of the protein [7–9]. The transcriptional activity of E-cadherin can be negatively regulated by a multitude of transcriptional repressors like SNAIL, with expression levels increased in ductal breast carcinomas [10], but also Slug, zinc finger E-box-binding homeobox 1 (ZEB1), and ZEB2 [11,12]. Inhibition of members of miR-200 family of miRNAs, which directly target the transcriptional repressors of E-cadherin (ZEB1 and ZEB2), was shown to induce the reduction of E-cadherin mRNA levels, and miR-9 and miR-101 have also been implicated in the complex network of E-cadherin regulation [13]. Further, deregulation of exocytic and endocytic pathways is known to control the delivery and internalization of E-cadherin, with consequences for protein turnover, recycling, sequestration, and degradation [14]. In particular, the disruption of the binding of type Iγ phosphatidylinositol phosphate kinase (PIPKIγ) to E-cadherin modulates the intracellular trafficking, inducing aberrant E-cadherin transport and blocking the gathering of the adherent junctions [15]. Another key molecule in the endocytic pathway is the ADP-ribosylation factor 6 (ARF6) [16,17], whose activation through epithelial growth factor receptor (EGFR) signaling induces E-cadherin internalization into early endosomes [18]. In fact, abnormal activation of proto-oncogenes such as EGFR, c-Met, and Src also results in increased phosphorylation of tyrosine residues in the E-cadherin-catenin complex [7], which leads to internalization and ubiquitination of the protein through the recruitment of E3-ubiquitin ligase Hakai [19]. More recently, post-translational glycosylation of E-cadherin has also been suggested as a mechanism of deregulation in many pathophysiological steps of tumour development and progression [20]. More specifically, E-cadherin extracellular domain has four potential *N*-glycosylation sites essential for its correct folding and transport to the cell membrane [20]. The abrogation of one of those specific residues (Asn633) was demonstrated to target E-cadherin for endoplasmic reticulum-associated degradation (ERAD) [21]. At the cytoplasmic region, E-cadherin undergoes *O*-glycosylation (*O*-GlcNAc) that blocks the transport of newly synthesised molecules to the cell surface and prevents the process of intercellular adhesion via p120-catenin [22].

4. The Hereditary Diffuse Gastric Cancer and Its Genetic Signature

The deregulation of E-cadherin is particularly well established in gastric cancer. More specifically, in the diffuse type of gastric cancer, E-cadherin somatic mutations were described in up to 40–70% of the cases. Moreover, germline loss-of-function mutations are the only proven cause of the cancer syndrome HDGC, occurring in approximately 40% of cases [23–25]. In fact, the first evidence of an inherited form of diffuse gastric cancer (DGC) associated with E-cadherin was observed in 1994, when Becker and colleagues identified somatic E-cadherin mutations in specimens of sporadic DGC [26]. Later on, Guilford P. et al. presented a large kindred from New Zealand with multiple cases of early onset DGC (EODGC) that were carriers of a causative germline mutation in the E-cadherin gene [23]. In the following years, several other publications emerged, confirming the autosomal-dominant pattern of inheritance associated with germline mutations of the *CDH1* gene [24,25,27–31]. Inactivation of the remaining functional allele, by a second hit molecular mechanism, leads to biallelic inactivation of the E-cadherin gene and is the trigger event for the development of diffuse type gastric cancer in germline mutation carriers [8,32,33]. Interestingly, hypermethylation was demonstrated to be the most frequent cause of a second-hit *CDH1* inactivation in HDGC tumours, whereas a second mutation or deletion is apparently less frequent [8,32]. In the sporadic forms of DGC, a hot spot region between exons 7 and 9 is observed for *CDH1* germline mutations, while in the hereditary forms of DGC, the *CDH1* genetic alterations are scattered over the entire gene length [34]. To date, 155 different mutations were identified in members of these families, and no correlation has been reported between the clinical phenotype and the location/type of the mutation presented [25,35]. Furthermore, in about 80% of the cases, *CDH1* germline mutations are of the truncating type, resulting in the complete loss of E-cadherin expression due to the occurrence of premature stop codons [36,37]. However, in about 20% of the HDGC patients, mutations are of the missense type, resulting in full-length E-cadherin molecules with a single amino acid substitution [27,35,36,38]. In the latter, the impact on protein function is not predictable and, for that reason, *CDH1* germline missense mutations represent a serious problem in terms of genetic counselling and clinical surveillance [27,35,36,38].

5. Management of *CDH1* Germline Missense Mutation Carriers

The clinical and functional relevance of *CDH1* missense mutations is still controversial, in part because normal protein length and an apparent regular level of expression are observed. Therefore, upon identification of a *CDH1* missense variant, it is mandatory that additional studies are performed to assess how this alteration could perturb the expression and function of E-cadherin, as well as related signaling and cellular mechanisms [25,35,39]. Altogether, those features will determine E-cadherin putative pathogenicity. In clinical terms, this information is extremely valuable, as once a germline missense mutation is detected and classified as deleterious, *CDH1* mutant carriers enter a surveillance programme similar to that offered to carriers of truncating mutations, possibly involving prophylactic surgery [25,35,39]. Thus, in the last decade, and due to the lack of comprehensive tools, Seruca's group established a multidisciplinary approach to evaluate the pathogenicity of germline *CDH1* missense variants and classify them as neutral or deleterious (pathogenic variants) (Figure 1) [27,38,40–42]. The pipeline is extensive and relies on familial data, in silico studies, expression analysis, and functional characterization of *CDH1* missense mutants in vitro and in vivo [27,40–42]. Based on the results of these analyses, and upon clinical recommendations, a subset of patients with deleterious germline missense mutations performed prophylactic gastrectomy and the histopathological examination of the stomach revealed the presence of cancer foci in all the specimens, supporting the reliability and the accuracy of this evaluation [33,43]. Regrettably, for about 17% of missense mutations, the current pipeline is not sufficient to ensure a confident result, and the functional relevance of the missense variants remains undetermined. Therefore, carriers of unclassified missense variants should be closely monitored and managed by clinicians, and an intensive endoscopic surveillance programme should be carried out.

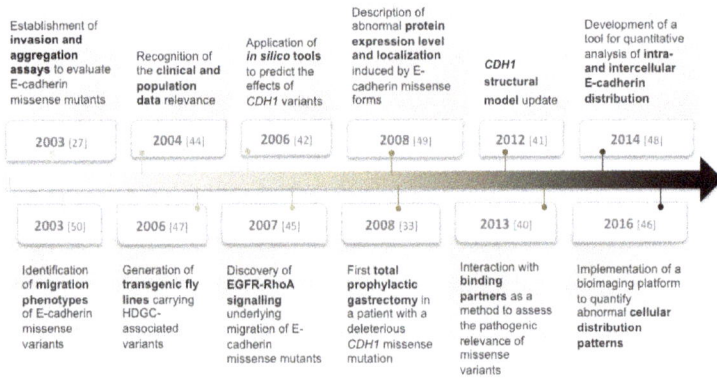

Figure 1. Timeline with the key findings and technological developments important to evaluate the pathogenicity of *CDH1* germline missense variants, in the context of Hereditary Diffuse Gastric Cancer (HDGC) [27,33,40–42,44–50].

6. Clinical and Familial Data Collection for Classification of *CDH1* Germline Missense Mutation Carriers

In the last meeting of the International Gastric Cancer Linkage Consortium (IGCLC), the clinical criteria and guidelines for HDGC family screening and surveillance were re-established [25]. In particular, the Consortium proposed that the analysis of genetic and familial data should be the first approach in the evaluation of a *CDH1* missense variant. Moreover, special attention should be given to the presence of gastric and lobular breast cancer (LBC) within the family, as well as the occurrence of cleft/lip congenital malformations [25]. The genealogy allows the analysis of co-segregation of the mutation with the disease within pedigrees and, thus, the identification of inheritance patterns in the family. Fitzgerald and Caldas [44] proposed that, in the case of *CDH1* germline missense variants, at least 4 affected family members need to be screened and present the same alteration. Unfortunately, for most of the families, it is not possible to perform these studies, since geneticists are frequently confronted with families of small size and/or with a low number of affected members within a family, which prevents segregation analysis [42,44]. It is interesting that, and still not yet well understood why, HDGC families with germline *CDH1* missense mutations often display a low disease penetrance [35,42]. Besides the segregation analyses, it is mandatory to evaluate other genetic parameters, such as mutation recurrence in unrelated HDGC families and mutation frequency in healthy controls [25,27,44]. Variant frequency in a control or a general population can be assessed by searching publicly available population databases such as 1000 Genomes Project (http://browser.1000genomes.org), Exome Variant Server (http://evs.gs.washington.edu/EVS), or dbSNP Database (http://www.ncbi.nlm.nih.gov/snp). However, one should be aware that these databases can have limitations as low-quality data and may lack details on the origin of the study or information regarding any possible associated phenotype [51].

7. In Silico Predictions of *CDH1* Missense Mutation Pathogenicity

In silico tools are continuously being developed to improve the knowledge and interpretation of DNA variants. Predictions can provide useful information regarding the effect of the variant on the primary and alternative gene transcripts, as well as the potential impact of the variant on protein structure and function [41,42]. Most of the existing algorithms take into account the degree of conservation of a particular nucleotide among species, the location and context within the protein sequence, the biochemical properties of the amino acid substitution, the putative impact of the variant in protein native-state, and the possible effect in splice sites [41,42]. The use of multiple software programs for sequence variant interpretation is also recommended, as these programs are based on distinct algorithms that result in different outputs [51]. To infer the impact of *CDH1* germline missense mutations using in silico analysis, SIFT and PolyPhen2 have become the standard tools [30,41,42,52–56]. SIFT-Sorting Intolerant From Tolerant (http://sift.jcvi.org/) predicts the impact of a particular amino acid replacement in protein function [57,58]. The method takes into consideration the evolutionary conservation of amino acids within species. Highly conserved residues are expected to be important for protein function, whereas those with a low degree of conservation are likely to tolerate a number of substitutions without affecting the molecule and its cellular function. SIFT workflow ends in a scaled probability, termed the SIFT score, that ranges from 0 to 1 [57]. A substitution is classified as damaging if the score value is below 0.05 [41,42]. It is noteworthy that the software does not use protein structural information, lacking possible compensatory effects of neighbouring positions [59]. In contrast, PolyPhen-2—Polymorphism Phenotyping v2 (http://genetics.bwh.harvard.edu/pph2/) [60,61] employs a machine-learning classification along with a multiple protein sequence alignment pipeline, which combines structural and comparative evolutionary considerations to evaluate effects on protein stability and function [61]. Given that an amino acid replacement in a protein sequence can change many of its chemical and physical properties, resulting in unfolding and decreased stability of polypeptides, structural modelling has become a major tool. Indeed, FoldX (http://foldxsuite.crg.eu/) [62] has been extensively explored to determine the structural impact of *CDH1* missense mutations. Specifically, this theoretical tool calculates how sequence variants, in comparison to the wild-type, affect the native-state stability of the structures ($\Delta\Delta G = \Delta GMut - \Delta GWT$), and if the stability change ($\Delta\Delta G$) is higher than >0.8 kcal/mol, the missense variant is considered destabilizing [62]. Such mutations are associated with high turnover of the protein in the cell, protein premature degradation and, consequently, loss of E-cadherin function [41]. This model covers most of E-cadherin, including the prodomain, the extracellular domain, and the β-catenin binding domain [41]. However, the juxtamembrane region remains to be structurally characterized.

An additional tool is the Netgene2 algorithm (http://www.cbs.dtu.dk/services/NetGene2/) that investigates the potential of *CDH1* variants to cause alternative splicing and processing of introns in nuclear pre-mRNA [63,64]. Nevertheless, the identification of cryptic splice sites in *CDH1* mutated gene is limited due to the lack of transcript data available. Overall, in silico predictions can be very useful for gathering information, but should be used with caution, as a complementary tool, and not as the sole source of evidence to classify a missense variant [41,42].

8. Characterization of *CDH1* Missense Mutations In Vitro

8.1. CDH1 Germline Missense Mutation Categorization According to Protein Expression

As previously mentioned, *CDH1* germline variants can result in a normal length protein with localization of the molecule at the membrane. However, missense mutations frequently lead to abnormal E-cadherin levels and expression patterns through mechanisms of trafficking deregulation and premature degradation of the molecule that are most often difficult to detect and interpret [17,49]. Therefore, our group developed a strategy to quantify and map E-cadherin expression for all *CDH1* germline variants by combining Western-blotting, immunocytochemistry, and bioimaging techniques (Figure 2). Briefly, our approach involves the use of an immortalized cell line in which *CDH1* variants are induced. Chinese Hamster Ovary (CHO) cells, which are negative for E-cadherin expression, are transfected with vectors encoding the wild-type E-cadherin or the diverse variants identified at the germline level [27,40–42,49,50,52–56,65–67]. Upon transfection, protein expression is assessed by Western blot (Figure 2A). Low E-cadherin levels strongly indicate structural destabilization and degradation of the protein by mechanisms of Protein Quality Control (PQC) [41,49]. Occasionally, a band mobility shift can also be detected, indicating that the mutation could affect glycosylation sites [9,68].

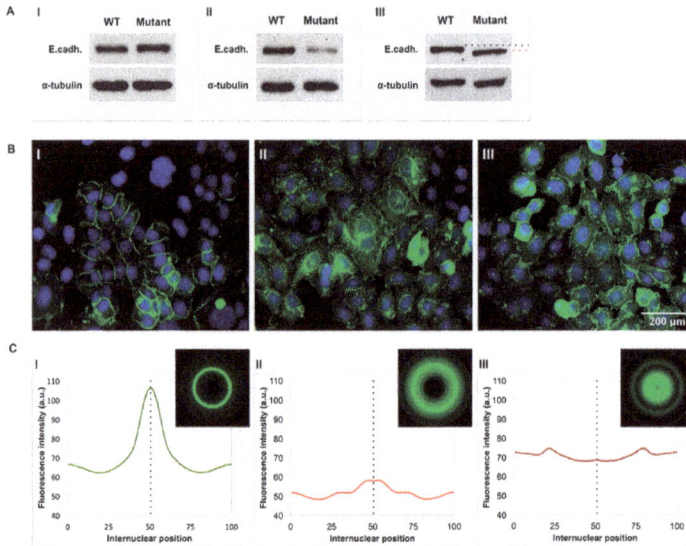

Figure 2. Representative E-cadherin expression profiles in cells with *CDH1* missense variants found in the context of HDGC. (**A**) Chinese Hamster Ovary (CHO) cells transfected with different *CDH1* missense variants were analysed for total E-cadherin expression levels by Western blot. Demonstrative images of normal expression level (**AI**), low expression (**AII**) and abnormal glycosylation (**AIII**) of the protein are shown. Small dots in (**AIII**) represent band mobility shift of total E-cadherin. Tubulin was used as a loading control. (**B**) Immunofluorescence (IF) images (400×) of E-cadherin with a membrane phenotype (**BI**), diffuse subcellular localization (**BII**), and cytoplasmic accumulation (**BIII**). E-cadherin is labelled in green and nuclei are counterstained with DAPI (blue). (**C**) Average intensity of E-cadherin internuclear profiles (IN) and the corresponding virtual illustration, obtained through IF images of cells expressing *CDH1* with distinct missense mutations. Examples for each type of protein accumulation are illustrated. Protein at the membrane, diffused throughout the cytoplasm and perinuclear accumulation of the protein are represented in (**CI**), (**CII**), and (**CIII**), respectively. (a.u.), arbitrary units. The data are in accordance to previously described methods [40,48,49] and emphasize the diversity of *CDH1* missense variants phenotypes.

Subsequently, immunostaining with monoclonal antibodies is used for E-cadherin analysis at the cellular and intercellular level (Figure 2B). The qualitative evaluation of E-cadherin expression and localization is performed by the classical approach, which involves visual inspection under a fluorescence microscope. Still, this process is strongly operator-dependent and based on subjective criteria. To overcome this limitation, we developed an objective and quantitative methodology that extracts detailed information on E-cadherin distribution intracellularly and at boundaries of contiguous cells (adherens junctions) [48,69]. This tool generates an inter- and intra-cellular expression profile for the wild-type and mutated forms of E-cadherin, and deviations from the reference are used to classify the level of E-cadherin dysfunction (Figure 2C) [48]. Typically, deleterious variants show aberrant peaks of E-cadherin cytoplasmic accumulation, or low and diffuse expression throughout the cell, as a result of trafficking anomalies [17,48,49,69]. For each E-cadherin variant, features such as

Int. J. Mol. Sci. **2017**, *18*, 2687

mean fluorescence intensity at the membrane, position of the maximum fluorescence intensity, and Maximum Mean Ratio (MMR) are computed and subject to analysis. The mean fluorescence intensity, measured at the middle axis between two juxtaposed cells, reflects the number of molecules present at the membrane and is significantly lower in dysfunctional mutants than in wild-type cells [48]. To quantify the variation of the fluorescence signals along the inter-nuclear space, the MMR parameter is used. High MMR values are associated with a strong and well-defined pattern of expression at the membrane, while a low MMR level indicates diffuse protein expression at the membrane and aberrant expression patterns throughout the cell. Accordingly, deleterious variants show a lower MMR when compared to the wild-type form [48].

In conclusion, quantification and characterization of E-cadherin expression patterns is crucial to detect deregulated post-translational mechanisms induced by *CDH1* pathogenic mutations.

8.2. CDH1 Germline Missense Mutation Classification According to Its Impact on Intercellular Organization and Cell-Cell Adhesion Status

Cell adhesion is an essential mechanism in the formation and maintenance of cell architecture in the epithelium [1]. Importantly, functional impairment of E-cadherin and eventual loss of the molecule is typically associated with decreased cell-cell interaction and tissue remodelling [3,5,6]. Recently, to characterize defects in the epithelial structure and morphology that can arise from E-cadherin mutants, we developed a platform that identifies and quantifies cellular distribution patterns using in situ microscopy images [46]. More specifically, we used DAPI-stained nuclei to create artificial cellular networks, from which we could extract quantitative data regarding cell distribution and organization (Figure 3A). The software creates digital meshes composed of triangles centred in triplets of neighbouring nuclei, and explores their topological features, such as area, edges length, and angles [46]. Pathogenic mutations with impact in cellular organization, present triangles with higher areas and edges when compared with the wild-type cell counterparts. At the individual cell level, the assessment of E-cadherin binding with its different cytoplasmic protein partners is important as part of the missense mutation studies [40]. Notably, the cytoplasmic domain of E-cadherin has a crucial role in its function, because it supports the assembly of a complex of cytosolic proteins, including α-, β-, p120-, and γ-catenins, which provides anchorage to the actin cytoskeleton to form stable cell-cell contact [2,3]. Nonetheless, this domain also has an essential role in protein trafficking and regulation at the membrane [14,70]. The association of β-catenin and PIPKIγ to E-cadherin cytoplasmic portion is necessary for newly synthesized E-cadherin molecules to be delivered to the basolateral membrane [15,71]. For maintenance and stability of the molecules at the membrane, p120-ctn binds to the juxtamembrane domain of E-cadherin and simultaneously blocks the interaction with the endocytic machinery, such as with clathrin adaptor proteins and Hakai [19,72,73]. Importantly, Hakai binds directly to E-cadherin and, being an E3 ubiquitin-ligase, it ubiquitinates and induces E-cadherin endocytosis [19]. To verify the interaction of E-cadherin with its various interactors, we use an indirect approach, the in situ Proximity ligation assay (PLA) [40]. This assay, which is a PCR-based system, relies on the affinity between two proteins requiring their proximal binding to get an amplification signal that can be detected at the cellular level [74,75]. Therefore, we have used in situ PLA to determine which *CDH1* missense variants, located at the cytoplasmic domain of the protein, affect the correct interplay with the corresponding binding partners [40]. Using this strategy, we have identified E-cadherin mutations that impair the association of E-cadherin/β-catenin, some located outside of the E-cadherin β-catenin binding domain [40]. Further, we have also demonstrated that E-cadherin mutations affecting the p120-binding domain are more available to be targeted by Hakai and to be degraded, and in this way to behave functionally as a truncated mutation [40]. Interestingly, the PLA results point out that each mutation behaviour is unique, as it interacts differently with its binding partners, produces its own phenotype, and possibly plays different roles in signal transduction. For these reasons, we believe that each E-cadherin missense mutation is likely to induce cell-specific biological behaviour.

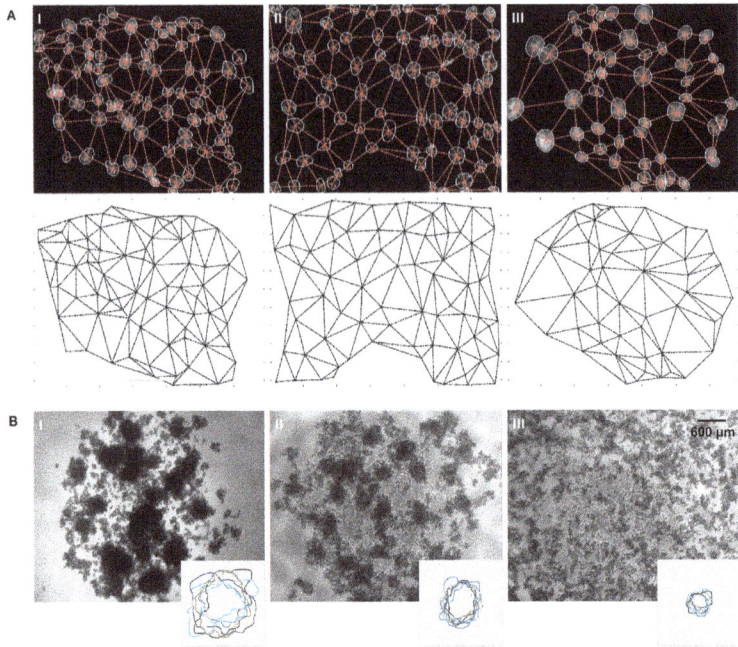

Figure 3. Intercellular organization and cell adhesive properties induced by *CDH1* germline missense variants. (**A**) Patterns of cellular distribution elicited by E-cadherin variants. In the upper panel, cell nuclei are overlapped with the corresponding network. In the lower panel, the final networks are presented. (**AI**) Illustrates a more regular and cohesive cellular topology, while (**AII**) depicts an intermediate cellular organization, and (**AIII**) represents a scatter and disorganized phenotype. (**B**) Adhesiveness of cells expressing E-cadherin variants evaluated by slow-aggregation assays and corresponding outlines of cellular aggregates. Variants preserving a functional adhesion complex display compact cellular aggregates (**BI**), while dysfunctional E-cadherin forms present small cellular aggregates (**BII**) or an isolated phenotype (**BIII**). The images illustrate different adhesiveness effects on E-cadherin missense variants cells as firstly described in [40,46].

Furthermore, due to the pivotal role of E-cadherin in cell-cell adhesion, understanding how E-cadherin impacts this cellular effect is of major relevance. Indeed, we have established a functional in vitro cell model to determine the impact of *CDH1* variants on cell compaction, a direct indicator of cell-cell adhesion competence [27,42,65]. In this assay, a single-cell suspension is seeded on soft-agar, and cells with a competent adhesion complex spontaneously aggregate (Figure 3B). Accordingly, cells transfected with the wild-type protein form compact cellular aggregates, while cells expressing dysfunctional E-cadherin form small cellular aggregates with different degrees of cohesion, or a completely isolated phenotype. The areas and density of the aggregates are subsequently quantified for a complete evaluation of cellular adhesiveness. Overall, using these different approaches, we established a system for a thorough characterization of *CDH1* variants with respect to their effect on cellular topology, stability of the cadherin-catenin complex, and strength of cell-cell interactions.

8.3. Invasive and Migratory Properties of Cells with CDH1 Germline Missense Mutations

Gastric cancer of the diffuse type is a highly invasive and lethal cancer, as cells that lose E-cadherin can evade apoptosis stimuli and acquire increased cell invasive potential, determining the fast and silent progression of the disease [34,36,76]. Therefore, assessing the ability of directed migration and spread throughout the extracellular matrix is of major importance in the study of E-cadherin missense variants [45,50,77–79].

A series of methodologies is used to evaluate the invasive and migratory properties of cells with *CDH1* germline missense mutations. Most frequently, the motile/migratory behaviour of the cells, transfected with the wild-type protein or the missense variants, is evaluated using wound reepithelialisation systems (Figure 4A). The method requires unilateral adhesion and transient attachment to a substrate, usually fibronectin, and provides information regarding migration velocity, persistence, and directionality during wound healing [80,81]. By exploiting this approach, we have identified a subset of germline E-cadherin missense variants that are associated with particular cellular phenotypes and biological behaviours [50]. Indeed, missense mutations clustering in the extracellular region of E-cadherin lead to cytoskeleton rearrangements and fibroblastic morphology, which provide cells with increased motility [50]. Cells expressing those variants migrate in an isolated and random way, and faster than the wild-type cells or the cells with variants affecting the intracellular portion of E-cadherin [50]. Further, we verified that E-cadherin-dependent migration is mediated by reduced E-cadherin/EGFR interaction and, consequently, by aberrant activation of EGFR and RhoA-GTP [45,79]. In contrast, intracellular mutants, such as V832M, display piled-up structures of round cells and migrate collectively and in a directed manner across the wound due to a reduced affinity between β-catenin and α-catenin [50]. Alternatively, the effects of the *CDH1* deleterious variants in cell motility can also be analysed independently of a wound stimulus by time-lapse scanning microscopy. This assay, although corroborating the wound healing data, is only used as a complementary tool [79]. To evaluate the invasive ability of E-cadherin mutant cells, matrigel invasion chambers are the in vitro preferred system [27,40–42,49,53–56,65,66]. The matrigel matrix contains structural proteins such as collagen, fibronectin, laminin, and proteoglycans, but also a panel of growth factors, which reconstitute the basement membrane composition and provide proper conditions for cell interaction with the surrounding microenvironment [82,83]. Upon seeding, invasive cells are able to degrade the matrix and reach the lower side of the filter through the pores (Figure 4B,C). The total number of invasive cells is then counted using a fluorescent microscope. In contrast, non-invasive cells do not migrate through the membrane and remain in an epithelium-like structure on top of the matrigel (Figure 4B). Remarkably, about 60% of the variants studied to date were shown to be invasive [27,40–42,49,53–56,65,66].

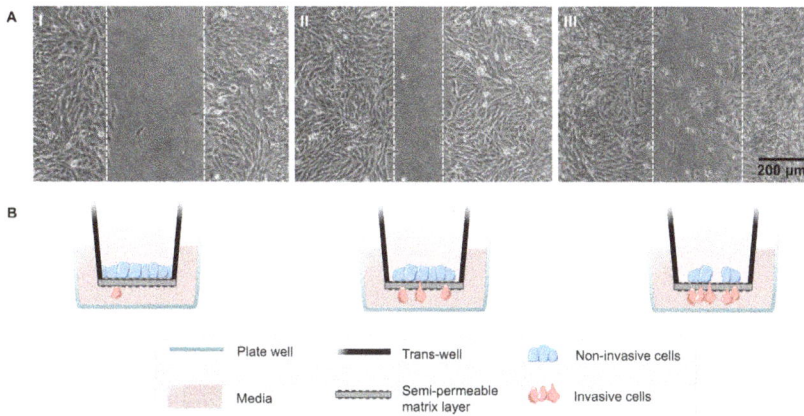

Figure 4. *Cont.*

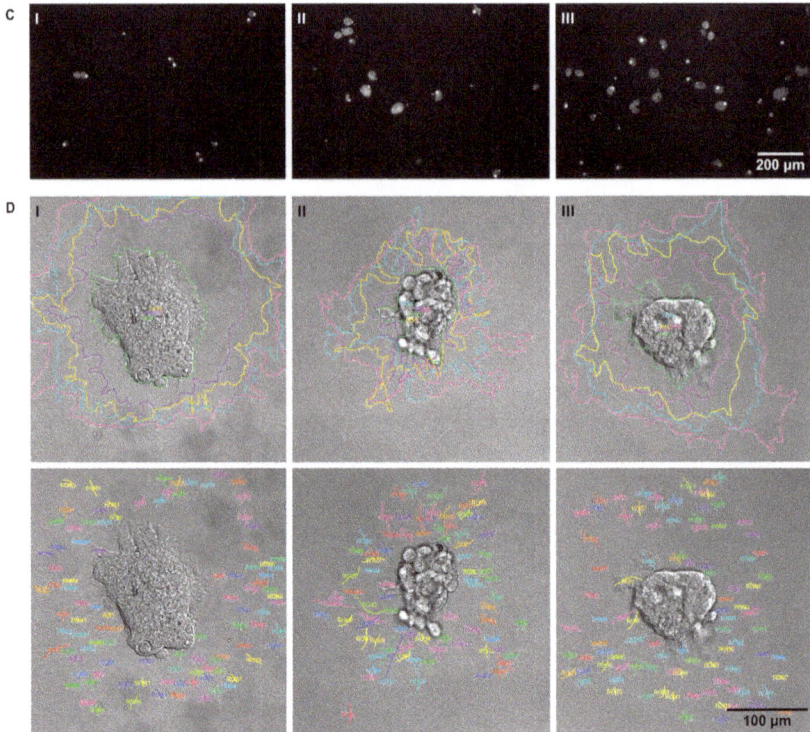

Figure 4. Effect of *CDH1* germline missense variants on the invasive and migratory properties of cells. (**A**) Migratory behaviour of Chinese Hamster Ovary (CHO) cells transfected with *CDH1* variants. Panel (**AI**) illustrates cells with decreased motility, (**AII**) exhibits a compact front of migration with unidirectional movement of cells, and (**AIII**) shows random colonization of the wound. Pictures were captured in phase contrast microscopy (200×), 8 h after wound incision. (**B**) Illustrative scheme of the non-invasive, invasive, and highly invasive phenotypes. (**C**) Invasive behaviour of cells expressing *CDH1* variants in matrigel-coated insert wells. The invasive cells on the lower part of the insert membranes were stained with DAPI. (**CI**) Represents cells with a non-invasive phenotype, (**CII**) represents cells with an invasive phenotype, and (**CIII**) shows cells with a high invasion rate. (**D**) Structural organization (upper panel) and protrusion formation (lower panel) of cellular spheroids embedded in collagen were monitored by time-lapse (400×). The area, as well as protrusion trajectories over time, are marked by colored traces. Cells forming compact aggregates and short protrusions are displayed in (**DI**). (**DII**) Shows a small multicellular structure with lower number of cells but more extended protrusions. In (**DIII**), cells form a more extensive and disorganized structure with large protrusions, indicating a highly invasive phenotype. The data in panels (**A–C**) are in accordance with previously described methods [27,50,79]. Novel strategies and phenotypes to better evaluate *CDH1* mutation variants are illustrated in panel (**D**).

As the process through which invasive cells leave the epithelium and cross the basement membrane involves proteolytic degradation by the matrix metalloproteinase (MMPs) [84], additional assays can be performed to evaluate whether cells harbouring deleterious variants of E-cadherin lead to increased protease secretion. Although informative, this assay is not routinely used. Very recently, and taking advantage of the morphological changes that cells undergo to escape the epithelium and invade adjacent tissues, we have established an innovative approach using 3D culture systems. In order to analyse structural organization, protrusion formation, and dissemination of cells with

E-cadherin variants, spheroids of wild-type and mutant cells are embedded in collagen and monitored by time-lapse. The aggregate area, the number of cells that disseminate, as well as the number and extension of protrusive structures can be easily evaluated (Figure 4D). In line with this, our next step is to track different cytoskeletal markers in these cells, and to develop new algorithms and software applications to analyse their patterns and dynamics. We envision that our combined strategy will be able to identify deleterious E-cadherin variants more efficiently and provide novel insights into the clinical surveillance of *CDH1* mutation carriers.

9. Assessment of *CDH1* Germline Missense Mutation Aggressiveness through an In Vivo Strategy

In addition to in vitro studies, the use of animal models is of major relevance to better understand the molecular mechanisms of cancer development. While mice models are frequently used in in vivo studies, there are many limitations associated with this model in the context of gastric cancer [85–87]. Therefore, the use of alternative organisms has been suggested to study specific features of cancer development. In particular, *Drosophila melanogaster* has received much attention as it is an inexpensive, genetically tractable organism that can recapitulate key events of human carcinogenesis, allowing investigation of cell morphology, invasion, and metastatic growth. Moreover, there is a high degree of conservation in terms of the basic mechanisms and signaling pathways in flies and man. Junctional complexes and overall epithelial organization are similar enough, in vertebrates and invertebrates, to assume that most cellular and molecular mechanisms involved in epithelial maintenance and reorganization are conserved [88]. Taking into account these similarities, the *Drosophila's* potential has been explored to unravel the cascade of events that follow E-cadherin loss of function due to missense mutations and to understand how they contribute to cancer progression in the tissue, in an in vivo context. Suriano G. and colleagues [47] generated transgenic fly lines carrying cDNAs of wild-type human E-cadherin (hEcad) and two missense mutant forms obtained from HDGC patients: hEcad-A634V, which affects the extracellular protein domain, and hEcad-V832M, affecting the intracellular portion. Using a GAL4/UAS system, the different hE-cadherin forms were expressed in the *Drosophila*-developing wing epithelium (the so-called wing imaginal disc) that forms a simple monolayer epithelium and allows the inspection of an altered pattern of E-cadherin sub-cellular localization [47]. Interestingly, it was observed that cells expressing the wild-type protein remain confined to normal epithelial fold as a result of proper cell-cell interaction [47]. In contrast, the mutant cells expressing A634V and V832M forms were found to infiltrate neighbouring regions of wing epithelium [47]. Remarkably, the mutants exhibited unlike behaviours regarding its invasive pattern, possibly due to distinctive abilities to support cell-cell adhesion. The A634V mutant still retains homophilic adhesion, invading as a group of cells, whereas the hE-cadherin V832M has a stronger effect on the adhesive capabilities and invades as smaller groups of cells or even individually [47]. Furthermore, it was shown that the fly β-catenin homolog, Armadillo (Arm), could mediate the distinct migratory and invasive behaviours of the different E-cadherin forms. In accordance, overexpression of hE-cadherin V832M in *Drosophila* imaginal disc exposed a weaker interaction with Arm at the plasma membrane and, thus, the availability of Arm for the canonical Wtn-Notch signaling activation [47]. Those results recapitulated the in vitro findings for both mutations [50], validating the applicability of the in vivo assays in the characterization of HDGC-associated germline missense mutations. More recently, we are using the *Drosophila* ovary as a model to evaluate novel HDGC-associated *CDH1* variants and their impact on epithelial organization and cell migration (data not shown). More specifically, we are able to easily analyse the influence of *CDH1* variants on the monolayered follicular epithelium (Figure 5) and also the effects of specific human cadherin transgenes on the collective migration of epithelial cysts formed by border cells. To date, all the mutants studied affected E-cadherin expression at the membrane and frequently disrupted epithelial organization, mimicking what is observed in biological samples from HDGC patients [35,36]. Additionally, to investigate migration dynamics of cells carrying E-cadherin variants in vivo, the fly dorsal closure model is also being tested. Particularly, using live imaging and fluorescently tagged transgenes, we are able to monitor closure rates, zippering velocity, and epithelial cohesion, as well as leading edge morphology and orientation in opposing migratory epidermis towards the dorsal midline of the embryos [89,90]. In conclusion, the use of the *Drosophila* model could have a huge impact in the current pipeline for the characterization of *CDH1* variants, as well as for research purposes in the context of targeting interactors and signaling pathways mediated by E-cadherin dysfunction.

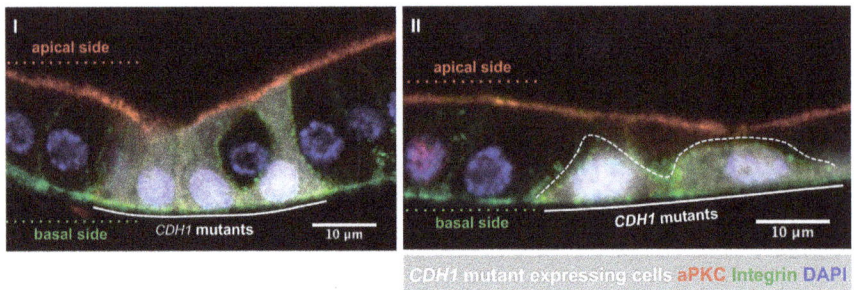

Figure 5. Expression of human *CDH1* mutants in the *Drosophila* follicular epithelium and their effects on tissue organization. (**I**) The expression of *CDH1* mutants promotes the disruption of epithelial organization, inducing epithelial invagination; (**II**) Cell extrusion from the monolayer occurs through loss of contact with the apical surface of the tissue. Staining is as follows: DAPI labels the nuclei, aPKC in red delineates the apical side, whereas integrins are labelled in green. Mosaic expression of *CDH1* (labelled in white) enables direct comparison between wild-type and genetically manipulated clones. The original data in *Drosophila* heighten the potential of novel strategies to evaluate *CDH1* missense variants in the context of HDGC.

10. Conclusions

Alterations in *CDH1*/E-cadherin are the proven cause for HDGC and LBC [34,36,76]. In these cancers, loss of E-cadherin function alters cell morphology and epithelial architecture, disrupts cell-cell adhesion, and increases cancer invasion, contributing to the high mortality rate of gastric cancer [3,4]. In case a germline pathogenic mutation is identified, the carrier is counselled to perform the ablation of the target organ, since the disease is silent and has a very poor prognosis. The clinical guidelines for truncating mutations are well established, but *CDH1* missense sequence variants still pose a clinical burden for geneticists and clinicians [27,35,36]. Therefore, and in the absence of appropriate clinical and familial data, the characterization of these *CDH1* variants and their classification, as neutral or deleterious, is mandatory.

As a reference centre of the IGCLC, our group has established a series of functional assays and developed novel approaches to assess the pathogenic role of all *CDH1* germline sequence variants detected worldwide (from New Zealand, Europe, and Asia to North and South America) and show their added value in genetic counselling [27,40,42,46,48]. In close collaboration with experimental biologists, bioinformaticians, and bioengineers, we show herein how these methods contribute to ameliorating the classification of E-cadherin germline mutations. Based on our multidisciplinary approach, curative prophylactic gastrectomy has already been performed in carriers of germline missense mutations and histopathological examination of the gastrectomies revealed the presence of invasive cancer in all the specimens, supporting the reliability of this working model [33,43]. We envisage that, in the near future, the development of novel and user-friendly tools will further improve the identification and management of deleterious variant carriers reported in genetic screening.

Acknowledgments: This work was supported by Fundo Europeu de Desenvolvimento Regional (FEDER) through the Operational Programme for Competitiveness Factors (COMPETE), Norte Portugal Regional Programme—NORTE 2020 (through the PORTUGAL 2020 Partnership Agreement), and National Funds through the Portuguese Foundation for Science and Technology (FCT), under the projects NORTE-01-0145-FEDER-000029, PTDC/BIM-ONC/0171/2012, PTDC/BIM-ONC/0281/2014, PTDC/BBB-IMG/0283/2014; doctoral grant SFRH/BD/108009/2015-SM and post-doctoral grant SFRH/BPD/87705/2012-JF. We acknowledge the American Association of Patients with Hereditary Gastric Cancer "No Stomach for Cancer" for funding the projects "Today's present, tomorrow's future on the study of germline E-cadherin missense mutations" and "Today's Present, Tomorrow's Future on the Study of Germline E-Cadherin Missense Mutations: A Step Forward on Providing Informed Genetic Counseling to Everyone".

Author Contributions: Raquel Seruca, Joana Figueiredo, and Maria Sofia Fernandes contributed to the conceptual design and supervision of the manuscript. The review was drafted by Soraia Melo, Raquel Seruca, Joana Figueiredo, Maria Sofia Fernandes, João Miguel Sanches, Eurico Morais-de-Sá, and Margarida Gonçalves. Soraia Melo compiled all relevant references and the existing data. All authors contributed to this review providing input to the respective subsections and approved the final version before submission.

Conflicts of Interest: The authors declare no conflict of interest.

Abbreviations

ARF6	ADP-ribosylation factor 6
Arm	Armadillo
CHO	Chinese Hamster Ovary
DGC	Diffuse Gastric Cancer
DAPI	4′,6-diamidino-2-phenylindole
EGFR	Epithelial growth factor receptor
EODGC	Early onset Diffuse Gastric Cancer
ERAD	Endoplasmic reticulum-associated degradation
HDGC	Hereditary Diffuse Gastric Cancer
hEcad	Human E-cadherin
IGCLC	International Gastric Cancer Linkage Consortium
LBC	Lobular Breast Cancer
miRNAs	MicroRNAs
MMPs	Matrix metalloproteinase
MMR	Maximum Mean Ratio
PIPKIγ	Type Iγ phosphatidylinositol phosphate Kinase
PLA	Proximity ligation assay
PolyPhen-2	Polymorphism Phenotyping v2
PQC	Protein Quality Control
SIFT	Sorting Intolerant From Tolerant
ZEB	Zinc finger E-box-binding homeobox

References

1. Green, K.J.; Getsios, S.; Troyanovsky, S.; Godsel, L.M. Intercellular junction assembly, dynamics, and homeostasis. *Cold Spring Harb. Perspect. Biol.* **2010**, *2*. [CrossRef] [PubMed]
2. Gumbiner, B.; Stevenson, B.; Grimaldi, A. The role of the cell adhesion molecule uvomorulin in the formation and maintenance of the epithelial junctional complex. *J. Cell Biol.* **1988**, *107*, 1575–1587. [CrossRef] [PubMed]
3. Berx, G.; van Roy, F. Involvement of members of the cadherin superfamily in cancer. *Cold Spring Harb. Perspect. Biol.* **2009**, *1*. [CrossRef] [PubMed]
4. Wheelock, M.J.; Johnson, K.R. Cadherins as modulators of cellular phenotype. *Ann. Rev. Cell Dev. Biol.* **2003**, *19*, 207–325. [CrossRef] [PubMed]
5. Jeanes, A.; Gottardi, C.J.; Yap, A.S. Cadherins and cancer: How does cadherin dysfunction promote tumor progression? *Oncogene* **2008**, *27*, 6920–6929. [CrossRef] [PubMed]
6. Paredes, J.; Figueiredo, J.; Albergaria, A.; Oliveira, P.; Carvalho, J.; Ribeiro, A.S.; Caldeira, J.; Costa, A.M.; Simoes-Correia, J.; Oliveira, M.J.; et al. Epithelial E- and P-cadherins: Role and clinical significance in cancer. *Biochim. Biophys. Acta* **2012**, *1826*, 297–311. [CrossRef] [PubMed]

7.   Van Roy, F.; Berx, G. The cell-cell adhesion molecule E-cadherin. *Cell. Mol. Life Sci.* **2008**, *65*, 3756–3788. [CrossRef] [PubMed]
8.   Grady, W.M.; Willis, J.; Guilford, P.J.; Dunbier, A.K.; Toro, T.T.; Lynch, H.; Wiesner, G.; Ferguson, K.; Eng, C.; Park, J.G.; et al. Methylation of the CDH1 promoter as the second genetic hit in hereditary diffuse gastric cancer. *Nat. Genet.* **2000**, *26*, 16–17. [CrossRef] [PubMed]
9.   Carvalho, S.; Catarino, T.A.; Dias, A.M.; Kato, M.; Almeida, A.; Hessling, B.; Figueiredo, J.; Gartner, F.; Sanches, J.M.; Ruppert, T.; et al. Preventing E-cadherin aberrant N-glycosylation at Asn-554 improves its critical function in gastric cancer. *Oncogene* **2016**, *35*, 1619–1631. [CrossRef] [PubMed]
10. Cheng, C.W.; Wu, P.E.; Yu, J.C.; Huang, C.S.; Yue, C.T.; Wu, C.W.; Shen, C.Y. Mechanisms of inactivation of E-cadherin in breast carcinoma: Modification of the two-hit hypothesis of tumor suppressor gene. *Oncogene* **2001**, *20*, 3814–3823. [CrossRef] [PubMed]
11. Hajra, K.M.; Chen, D.Y.; Fearon, E.R. The SLUG zinc-finger protein represses E-cadherin in breast cancer. *Cancer Res.* **2002**, *62*, 1613–1618. [PubMed]
12. Perez-Moreno, M.A.; Locascio, A.; Rodrigo, I.; Dhondt, G.; Portillo, F.; Nieto, M.A.; Cano, A. A new role for E12/E47 in the repression of E-cadherin expression and epithelial-mesenchymal transitions. *J. Biol. Chem.* **2001**, *276*, 27424–27431. [CrossRef] [PubMed]
13. Carvalho, J.; van Grieken, N.C.; Pereira, P.M.; Sousa, S.; Tijssen, M.; Buffart, T.E.; Diosdado, B.; Grabsch, H.; Santos, M.A.; Meijer, G.; et al. Lack of microRNA-101 causes E-cadherin functional deregulation through EZH2 up-regulation in intestinal gastric cancer. *J. Pathol.* **2012**, *228*, 31–44. [CrossRef] [PubMed]
14. Bryant, D.M.; Stow, J.L. The ins and outs of E-cadherin trafficking. *Trends Cell Biol.* **2004**, *14*, 427–434. [CrossRef] [PubMed]
15. Ling, K.; Bairstow, S.F.; Carbonara, C.; Turbin, D.A.; Huntsman, D.G.; Anderson, R.A. Type I gamma phosphatidylinositol phosphate kinase modulates adherens junction and E-cadherin trafficking via a direct interaction with mu 1B adaptin. *J. Cell Biol.* **2007**, *176*, 343–353. [CrossRef] [PubMed]
16. Palacios, F.; Price, L.; Schweitzer, J.; Collard, J.G.; D'Souza-Schorey, C. An essential role for ARF6-regulated membrane traffic in adherens junction turnover and epithelial cell migration. *EMBO J.* **2001**, *20*, 4973–4986. [CrossRef] [PubMed]
17. Figueiredo, J.; Simoes-Correia, J.; Soderberg, O.; Suriano, G.; Seruca, R. ADP-ribosylation factor 6 mediates E-cadherin recovery by chemical chaperones. *PLoS ONE* **2011**, *6*. [CrossRef] [PubMed]
18. Morishige, M.; Hashimoto, S.; Ogawa, E.; Toda, Y.; Kotani, H.; Hirose, M.; Wei, S.; Hashimoto, A.; Yamada, A.; Yano, H.; et al. GEP100 links epidermal growth factor receptor signalling to Arf6 activation to induce breast cancer invasion. *Nat. Cell Biol.* **2008**, *10*, 85–92. [CrossRef] [PubMed]
19. Fujita, Y.; Krause, G.; Scheffner, M.; Zechner, D.; Leddy, H.E.; Behrens, J.; Sommer, T.; Birchmeier, W. Hakai, a c-Cbl-like protein, ubiquitinates and induces endocytosis of the E-cadherin complex. *Nat. Cell Biol.* **2002**, *4*, 222–231. [CrossRef] [PubMed]
20. Pinho, S.S.; Seruca, R.; Gartner, F.; Yamaguchi, Y.; Gu, J.; Taniguchi, N.; Reis, C.A. Modulation of E-cadherin function and dysfunction by N-glycosylation. *Cell. Mol. Life Sci.* **2011**, *68*, 1011–1020. [CrossRef] [PubMed]
21. Zhou, F.; Su, J.; Fu, L.; Yang, Y.; Zhang, L.; Wang, L.; Zhao, H.; Zhang, D.; Li, Z.; Zha, X. Unglycosylation at Asn-633 made extracellular domain of E-cadherin folded incorrectly and arrested in endoplasmic reticulum, then sequentially degraded by ERAD. *Glycoconj. J.* **2008**, *25*, 727–740. [CrossRef] [PubMed]
22. Zhu, W.; Leber, B.; Andrews, D.W. Cytoplasmic O-glycosylation prevents cell surface transport of E-cadherin during apoptosis. *EMBO J.* **2001**, *20*, 5999–6007. [CrossRef] [PubMed]
23. Guilford, P.; Hopkins, J.; Harraway, J.; McLeod, M.; McLeod, N.; Harawira, P.; Taite, H.; Scoular, R.; Miller, A.; Reeve, A.E. E-cadherin germline mutations in familial gastric cancer. *Nature* **1998**, *392*, 402–405. [CrossRef] [PubMed]
24. Guilford, P.J.; Hopkins, J.B.; Grady, W.M.; Markowitz, S.D.; Willis, J.; Lynch, H.; Rajput, A.; Wiesner, G.L.; Lindor, N.M.; Burgart, L.J.; et al. E-cadherin germline mutations define an inherited cancer syndrome dominated by diffuse gastric cancer. *Hum. Mutat.* **1999**, *14*, 249–255. [CrossRef]
25. Van der Post, R.S.; Vogelaar, I.P.; Carneiro, F.; Guilford, P.; Huntsman, D.; Hoogerbrugge, N.; Caldas, C.; Schreiber, K.E.; Hardwick, R.H.; Ausems, M.G.; et al. Hereditary diffuse gastric cancer: Updated clinical guidelines with an emphasis on germline CDH1 mutation carriers. *J. Med. Genet.* **2015**, *52*, 361–374. [CrossRef] [PubMed]

26. Becker, K.F.; Atkinson, M.J.; Reich, U.; Becker, I.; Nekarda, H.; Siewert, J.R.; Hofler, H. E-cadherin gene mutations provide clues to diffuse type gastric carcinomas. *Cancer Res.* **1994**, *54*, 3845–3852. [PubMed]

27. Suriano, G.; Oliveira, C.; Ferreira, P.; Machado, J.C.; Bordin, M.C.; De Wever, O.; Bruyneel, E.A.; Moguilevsky, N.; Grehan, N.; Porter, T.R.; et al. Identification of CDH1 germline missense mutations associated with functional inactivation of the E-cadherin protein in young gastric cancer probands. *Hum. Mol. Genet.* **2003**, *12*, 575–582. [CrossRef] [PubMed]

28. Brooks-Wilson, A.R.; Kaurah, P.; Suriano, G.; Leach, S.; Senz, J.; Grehan, N.; Butterfield, Y.S.; Jeyes, J.; Schinas, J.; Bacani, J.; et al. Germline E-cadherin mutations in hereditary diffuse gastric cancer: Assessment of 42 new families and review of genetic screening criteria. *J. Med. Genet.* **2004**, *41*, 508–517. [CrossRef] [PubMed]

29. Kaurah, P.; MacMillan, A.; Boyd, N.; Senz, J.; De Luca, A.; Chun, N.; Suriano, G.; Zaor, S.; Van Manen, L.; Gilpin, C.; et al. Founder and recurrent CDH1 mutations in families with hereditary diffuse gastric cancer. *JAMA* **2007**, *297*, 2360–2372. [CrossRef] [PubMed]

30. More, H.; Humar, B.; Weber, W.; Ward, R.; Christian, A.; Lintott, C.; Graziano, F.; Ruzzo, A.M.; Acosta, E.; Boman, B.; et al. Identification of seven novel germline mutations in the human E-cadherin (CDH1) gene. *Hum. Mutat.* **2007**, *28*, 203. [CrossRef] [PubMed]

31. Kluijt, I.; Siemerink, E.J.; Ausems, M.G.; van Os, T.A.; de Jong, D.; Simoes-Correia, J.; van Krieken, J.H.; Ligtenberg, M.J.; Figueiredo, J.; van Riel, E.; et al. CDH1-related hereditary diffuse gastric cancer syndrome: Clinical variations and implications for counseling. *Int. J. Cancer* **2012**, *131*, 367–376. [CrossRef] [PubMed]

32. Oliveira, C.; de Bruin, J.; Nabais, S.; Ligtenberg, M.; Moutinho, C.; Nagengast, F.M.; Seruca, R.; van Krieken, H.; Carneiro, F. Intragenic deletion of CDH1 as the inactivating mechanism of the wild-type allele in an HDGC tumour. *Oncogene* **2004**, *23*, 2236–2240. [CrossRef] [PubMed]

33. Barber, M.E.; Save, V.; Carneiro, F.; Dwerryhouse, S.; Lao-Sirieix, P.; Hardwick, R.H.; Caldas, C.; Fitzgerald, R.C. Histopathological and molecular analysis of gastrectomy specimens from hereditary diffuse gastric cancer patients has implications for endoscopic surveillance of individuals at risk. *J. Pathol.* **2008**, *216*, 286–294. [CrossRef] [PubMed]

34. Corso, G.; Marrelli, D.; Pascale, V.; Vindigni, C.; Roviello, F. Frequency of CDH1 germline mutations in gastric carcinoma coming from high- and low-risk areas: Metanalysis and systematic review of the literature. *BMC Cancer* **2012**, *12*, 8. [CrossRef] [PubMed]

35. Oliveira, C.; Pinheiro, H.; Figueiredo, J.; Seruca, R.; Carneiro, F. Familial gastric cancer: Genetic susceptibility, pathology, and implications for management. *Lancet Oncol.* **2015**, *16*, e60–e70. [CrossRef]

36. Oliveira, C.; Pinheiro, H.; Figueiredo, J.; Seruca, R.; Carneiro, F. E-cadherin alterations in hereditary disorders with emphasis on hereditary diffuse gastric cancer. *Prog. Mol. Biol. Transl. Sci.* **2013**, *116*, 337–359. [CrossRef] [PubMed]

37. Guilford, P.; Humar, B.; Blair, V. Hereditary diffuse gastric cancer: Translation of CDH1 germline mutations into clinical practice. *Gastric Cancer* **2010**, *13*, 1–10. [CrossRef] [PubMed]

38. Figueiredo, J.; Seruca, J. Germline missense mutants in hereditary diffuse gastric cancer. *Spotlight Fam. Hered. Gastric Cancer* **2013**, *7*, 77–86. [CrossRef]

39. Corso, G.; Figueiredo, J.; Biffi, R.; Trentin, C.; Bonanni, B.; Feroce, I.; Serrano, D.; Cassano, E.; Annibale, B.; Melo, S.; et al. E-cadherin germline mutation carriers: Clinical management and genetic implications. *Cancer Metastasis Rev.* **2014**, *33*, 1081–1094. [CrossRef] [PubMed]

40. Figueiredo, J.; Soderberg, O.; Simoes-Correia, J.; Grannas, K.; Suriano, G.; Seruca, R. The importance of E-cadherin binding partners to evaluate the pathogenicity of E-cadherin missense mutations associated to HDGC. *Eur. J. Hum. Genet.* **2013**, *21*, 301–309. [CrossRef] [PubMed]

41. Simoes-Correia, J.; Figueiredo, J.; Lopes, R.; Stricher, F.; Oliveira, C.; Serrano, L.; Seruca, R. E-cadherin destabilization accounts for the pathogenicity of missense mutations in hereditary diffuse gastric cancer. *PLoS ONE* **2012**, *7*. [CrossRef] [PubMed]

42. Suriano, G.; Seixas, S.; Rocha, J.; Seruca, R. A model to infer the pathogenic significance of CDH1 germline missense variants. *J. Mol. Med.* **2006**, *84*, 1023–1031. [CrossRef] [PubMed]

43. Betes, M.; Alonso-Sierra, M.; Valenti, V.; Patino, A. A multidisciplinary approach allows identification of a new pathogenic CDH1 germline missense mutation in a hereditary diffuse gastric cancer family. *Dig. Liv. Dis.* **2017**, *49*, 825–826. [CrossRef] [PubMed]

44. Fitzgerald, R.C.; Caldas, C. Clinical implications of E-cadherin associated hereditary diffuse gastric cancer. *Gut* **2004**, *53*, 775–778. [CrossRef] [PubMed]

45. Mateus, A.R.; Seruca, R.; Machado, J.C.; Keller, G.; Oliveira, M.J.; Suriano, G.; Luber, B. EGFR regulates RhoA-GTP dependent cell motility in E-cadherin mutant cells. *Hum. Mol. Genet.* **2007**, *16*, 1639–1647. [CrossRef] [PubMed]

46. Mestre, T.; Figueiredo, J.; Ribeiro, A.S.; Paredes, J.; Seruca, R.; Sanches, J.M. Quantification of topological features in cell meshes to explore E-cadherin dysfunction. *Sci. Rep.* **2016**, *6*. [CrossRef] [PubMed]

47. Pereira, P.S.; Teixeira, A.; Pinho, S.; Ferreira, P.; Fernandes, J.; Oliveira, C.; Seruca, R.; Suriano, G.; Casares, F. E-cadherin missense mutations, associated with hereditary diffuse gastric cancer (HDGC) syndrome, display distinct invasive behaviors and genetic interactions with the Wnt and Notch pathways in Drosophila epithelia. *Hum. Mol. Genet.* **2006**, *15*, 1704–1712. [CrossRef] [PubMed]

48. Sanches, J.M.; Figueiredo, J.; Fonseca, M.; Duraes, C.; Melo, S.; Esmenio, S.; Seruca, R. Quantification of mutant E-cadherin using bioimaging analysis of in situ fluorescence microscopy. A new approach to CDH1 missense variants. *Eur. J. Hum. Genet.* **2014**. [CrossRef] [PubMed]

49. Simoes-Correia, J.; Figueiredo, J.; Oliveira, C.; van Hengel, J.; Seruca, R.; van Roy, F.; Suriano, G. Endoplasmic reticulum quality control: A new mechanism of E-cadherin regulation and its implication in cancer. *Hum. Mol. Genet.* **2008**, *17*, 3566–3576. [CrossRef] [PubMed]

50. Suriano, G.; Oliveira, M.J.; Huntsman, D.; Mateus, A.R.; Ferreira, P.; Casares, F.; Oliveira, C.; Carneiro, F.; Machado, J.C.; Mareel, M.; et al. E-cadherin germline missense mutations and cell phenotype: Evidence for the independence of cell invasion on the motile capabilities of the cells. *Hum. Mol. Genet.* **2003**, *12*, 3007–3016. [CrossRef] [PubMed]

51. Richards, S.; Aziz, N.; Bale, S.; Bick, D.; Das, S.; Gastier-Foster, J.; Grody, W.W.; Hegde, M.; Lyon, E.; Spector, E.; et al. Standards and guidelines for the interpretation of sequence variants: A joint consensus recommendation of the American College of Medical Genetics and Genomics and the Association for Molecular Pathology. *Genet. Med.* **2015**, *17*, 405–424. [CrossRef] [PubMed]

52. Garziera, M.; De Re, V.; Geremia, S.; Seruca, R.; Figueiredo, J.; Melo, S.; Simoes-Correia, J.; Caggiari, L.; De Zorzi, M.; Canzonieri, V.; et al. A novel CDH1 germline missense mutation in a sporadic gastric cancer patient in north-east of Italy. *Clin. Exp. Med.* **2013**, *13*, 149–157. [CrossRef] [PubMed]

53. Vogelaar, I.P.; Figueiredo, J.; van Rooij, I.A.; Simoes-Correia, J.; van der Post, R.S.; Melo, S.; Seruca, R.; Carels, C.E.; Ligtenberg, M.J.; Hoogerbrugge, N.; et al. Identification of germline mutations in the cancer predisposing gene CDH1 in patients with orofacial clefts. *Hum. Mol. Genet.* **2013**, *22*, 919–926. [CrossRef] [PubMed]

54. Brito, L.A.; Yamamoto, G.L.; Melo, S.; Malcher, C.; Ferreira, S.G.; Figueiredo, J.; Alvizi, L.; Kobayashi, G.S.; Naslavsky, M.S.; Alonso, N.; et al. Rare Variants in the Epithelial Cadherin Gene Underlying the Genetic Etiology of Nonsyndromic Cleft Lip with or without Cleft Palate. *Hum. Mutat.* **2015**, *36*, 1029–1033. [CrossRef] [PubMed]

55. Corso, G.; Roviello, F.; Paredes, J.; Pedrazzani, C.; Novais, M.; Correia, J.; Marrelli, D.; Cirnes, L.; Seruca, R.; Oliveira, C.; et al. Characterization of the P373L E-cadherin germline missense mutation and implication for clinical management. *Eur. J. Surg. Oncol.* **2007**, *33*, 1061–1067. [CrossRef] [PubMed]

56. Zhang, L.; Xiao, A.; Ruggeri, J.; Bacares, R.; Somar, J.; Melo, S.; Figueiredo, J.; Simoes-Correia, J.; Seruca, R.; Shah, M.A. The germline CDH1 c.48 G>C substitution contributes to cancer predisposition through generation of a pro-invasive mutation. *Mutat. Res.* **2014**, *770*, 106–111. [CrossRef] [PubMed]

57. Kumar, P.; Henikoff, S.; Ng, P.C. Predicting the effects of coding non-synonymous variants on protein function using the SIFT algorithm. *Nat. Protoc.* **2009**, *4*, 1073–1081. [CrossRef] [PubMed]

58. Sim, N.L.; Kumar, P.; Hu, J.; Henikoff, S.; Schneider, G.; Ng, P.C. SIFT web server: Predicting effects of amino acid substitutions on proteins. *Nucleic Acids Res.* **2012**, *40*, W452–W457. [CrossRef] [PubMed]

59. Saunders, C.T.; Baker, D. Evaluation of structural and evolutionary contributions to deleterious mutation prediction. *J. Mol. Biol.* **2002**, *322*, 891–901. [CrossRef]

60. Ramensky, V.; Bork, P.; Sunyaev, S. Human non-synonymous SNPs: Server and survey. *Nucleic Acids Res.* **2002**, *30*, 3894–3900. [CrossRef] [PubMed]

61. Adzhubei, I.A.; Schmidt, S.; Peshkin, L.; Ramensky, V.E.; Gerasimova, A.; Bork, P.; Kondrashov, A.S.; Sunyaev, S.R. A method and server for predicting damaging missense mutations. *Nat. Methods* **2010**, *7*, 248–249. [CrossRef] [PubMed]

62. Schymkowitz, J.; Borg, J.; Stricher, F.; Nys, R.; Rousseau, F.; Serrano, L. The FoldX web server: An online force field. *Nucleic Acids Res.* **2005**, *33*, W382–W388. [CrossRef] [PubMed]
63. Brunak, S.; Engelbrecht, J.; Knudsen, S. Prediction of human mRNA donor and acceptor sites from the DNA sequence. *J. Mol. Biol.* **1991**, *220*, 49–65. [CrossRef]
64. Hebsgaard, S.M.; Korning, P.G.; Tolstrup, N.; Engelbrecht, J.; Rouze, P.; Brunak, S. Splice site prediction in Arabidopsis thaliana pre-mRNA by combining local and global sequence information. *Nucleic Acids Res.* **1996**, *24*, 3439–3452. [CrossRef] [PubMed]
65. Suriano, G.; Mulholland, D.; de Wever, O.; Ferreira, P.; Mateus, A.R.; Bruyneel, E.; Nelson, C.C.; Mareel, M.M.; Yokota, J.; Huntsman, D.; et al. The intracellular E-cadherin germline mutation V832 M lacks the ability to mediate cell-cell adhesion and to suppress invasion. *Oncogene* **2003**, *22*, 5716–5719. [CrossRef] [PubMed]
66. Suriano, G.; Yew, S.; Ferreira, P.; Senz, J.; Kaurah, P.; Ford, J.M.; Longacre, T.A.; Norton, J.A.; Chun, N.; Young, S.; et al. Characterization of a recurrent germ line mutation of the E-cadherin gene: Implications for genetic testing and clinical management. *Clin. Cancer Res.* **2005**, *11*, 5401–5409. [CrossRef] [PubMed]
67. Simoes-Correia, J.; Silva, D.I.; Melo, S.; Figueiredo, J.; Caldeira, J.; Pinto, M.T.; Girao, H.; Pereira, P.; Seruca, R. DNAJB4 molecular chaperone distinguishes WT from mutant E-cadherin, determining their fate in vitro and in vivo. *Hum. Mol. Genet.* **2014**, *23*, 2094–2105. [CrossRef] [PubMed]
68. Carvalho, S.; Oliveira, T.; Bartels, M.F.; Miyoshi, E.; Pierce, M.; Taniguchi, N.; Carneiro, F.; Seruca, R.; Reis, C.A.; Strahl, S.; et al. O-mannosylation and N-glycosylation: Two coordinated mechanisms regulating the tumour suppressor functions of E-cadherin in cancer. *Oncotarget* **2016**, *7*, 65231–65246. [CrossRef] [PubMed]
69. Figueiredo, J.; Ribeiro, A.S.; Mestre, T.; Esménio, S.; Fonseca, M.; Paredes, J.; Seruca, R.; Sanches, J.M. Capturing quantitative features of protein expression from in situ fluorescence microscopic images of cancer cell populations. In *Fluorescence Imaging and Biological Quantification*; CRC Press: Roca Raton, FL, USA, 2017; Volume 15, pp. 279–297.
70. D'Souza-Schorey, C. Disassembling adherens junctions: Breaking up is hard to do. *Trends Cell Biol.* **2005**, *15*, 19–26. [CrossRef] [PubMed]
71. Chen, Y.T.; Stewart, D.B.; Nelson, W.J. Coupling assembly of the E-cadherin/beta-catenin complex to efficient endoplasmic reticulum exit and basal-lateral membrane targeting of E-cadherin in polarized MDCK cells. *J. Cell Biol.* **1999**, *144*, 687–699. [CrossRef] [PubMed]
72. Davis, M.A.; Ireton, R.C.; Reynolds, A.B. A core function for p120-catenin in cadherin turnover. *J. Cell Biol.* **2003**, *163*, 525–534. [CrossRef] [PubMed]
73. Xiao, K.; Garner, J.; Buckley, K.M.; Vincent, P.A.; Chiasson, C.M.; Dejana, E.; Faundez, V.; Kowalczyk, A.P. p120-Catenin regulates clathrin-dependent endocytosis of VE-cadherin. *Mol. Biol. Cell* **2005**, *16*, 5141–5151. [CrossRef] [PubMed]
74. Soderberg, O.; Gullberg, M.; Jarvius, M.; Ridderstrale, K.; Leuchowius, K.J.; Jarvius, J.; Wester, K.; Hydbring, P.; Bahram, F.; Larsson, L.G.; et al. Direct observation of individual endogenous protein complexes in situ by proximity ligation. *Nat. Methods* **2006**, *3*, 995–1000. [CrossRef] [PubMed]
75. Weibrecht, I.; Leuchowius, K.J.; Clausson, C.M.; Conze, T.; Jarvius, M.; Howell, W.M.; Kamali-Moghaddam, M.; Soderberg, O. Proximity ligation assays: A recent addition to the proteomics toolbox. *Expert Rev. Proteom.* **2010**, *7*, 401–409. [CrossRef] [PubMed]
76. Hansford, S.; Kaurah, P.; Li-Chang, H.; Woo, M.; Senz, J.; Pinheiro, H.; Schrader, K.A.; Schaeffer, D.F.; Shumansky, K.; Zogopoulos, G.; et al. Hereditary Diffuse Gastric Cancer Syndrome: CDH1 Mutations and Beyond. *JAMA Oncol.* **2015**, *1*, 23–32. [CrossRef] [PubMed]
77. Ferreira, A.C.; Suriano, G.; Mendes, N.; Gomes, B.; Wen, X.; Carneiro, F.; Seruca, R.; Machado, J.C. E-cadherin impairment increases cell survival through Notch-dependent upregulation of Bcl-2. *Hum. Mol. Genet.* **2012**, *21*, 334–343. [CrossRef] [PubMed]
78. Ferreira, P.; Oliveira, M.J.; Beraldi, E.; Mateus, A.R.; Nakajima, T.; Gleave, M.; Yokota, J.; Carneiro, F.; Huntsman, D.; Seruca, R.; et al. Loss of functional E-cadherin renders cells more resistant to the apoptotic agent taxol in vitro. *Exp. Cell Res.* **2005**, *310*, 99–104. [CrossRef] [PubMed]
79. Mateus, A.R.; Simoes-Correia, J.; Figueiredo, J.; Heindl, S.; Alves, C.C.; Suriano, G.; Luber, B.; Seruca, R. E-cadherin mutations and cell motility: A genotype-phenotype correlation. *Exp. Cell Res.* **2009**, *315*, 1393–1402. [CrossRef] [PubMed]

80. Keren, K.; Pincus, Z.; Allen, G.M.; Barnhart, E.L.; Marriott, G.; Mogilner, A.; Theriot, J.A. Mechanism of shape determination in motile cells. *Nature* **2008**, *453*, 475–480. [CrossRef] [PubMed]
81. Vitorino, P.; Meyer, T. Modular control of endothelial sheet migration. *Genes Dev.* **2008**, *22*, 3268–3281. [CrossRef] [PubMed]
82. Kleinman, H.K.; Martin, G.R. Matrigel: Basement membrane matrix with biological activity. *Semin. Cancer Biol.* **2005**, *15*, 378–386. [CrossRef] [PubMed]
83. Kleinman, H.K.; McGarvey, M.L.; Liotta, L.A.; Robey, P.G.; Tryggvason, K.; Martin, G.R. Isolation and characterization of type IV procollagen, laminin, and heparan sulfate proteoglycan from the EHS sarcoma. *Biochemistry* **1982**, *21*, 6188–6193. [CrossRef] [PubMed]
84. Jodele, S.; Blavier, L.; Yoon, J.M.; DeClerck, Y.A. Modifying the soil to affect the seed: Role of stromal-derived matrix metalloproteinases in cancer progression. *Cancer Metastasis Rev.* **2006**, *25*, 35–43. [CrossRef] [PubMed]
85. Humar, B.; Blair, V.; Charlton, A.; More, H.; Martin, I.; Guilford, P. E-cadherin deficiency initiates gastric signet-ring cell carcinoma in mice and man. *Cancer Res.* **2009**, *69*, 2050–2056. [CrossRef] [PubMed]
86. Mimata, A.; Fukamachi, H.; Eishi, Y.; Yuasa, Y. Loss of E-cadherin in mouse gastric epithelial cells induces signet ring-like cells, a possible precursor lesion of diffuse gastric cancer. *Cancer Sci.* **2011**, *102*, 942–950. [CrossRef] [PubMed]
87. Shimada, S.; Mimata, A.; Sekine, M.; Mogushi, K.; Akiyama, Y.; Fukamachi, H.; Jonkers, J.; Tanaka, H.; Eishi, Y.; Yuasa, Y. Synergistic tumour suppressor activity of E-cadherin and p53 in a conditional mouse model for metastatic diffuse-type gastric cancer. *Gut* **2012**, *61*, 344–353. [CrossRef] [PubMed]
88. Locascio, A.; Nieto, M.A. Cell movements during vertebrate development: Integrated tissue behaviour versus individual cell migration. *Curr. Opin. Genet. Dev.* **2001**, *11*, 464–469. [CrossRef]
89. Goodwin, K.; Ellis, S.J.; Lostchuck, E.; Zulueta-Coarasa, T.; Fernandez-Gonzalez, R.; Tanentzapf, G. Basal Cell-Extracellular Matrix Adhesion Regulates Force Transmission during Tissue Morphogenesis. *Dev. Cell* **2016**, *39*, 611–625. [CrossRef] [PubMed]
90. Gorfinkiel, N.; Blanchard, G.B.; Adams, R.J.; Martinez Arias, A. Mechanical control of global cell behaviour during dorsal closure in Drosophila. *Development* **2009**, *136*, 1889–9188. [CrossRef] [PubMed]

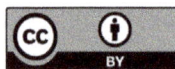

International Journal of
Molecular Sciences

MDPI

Review

Autoimmunity and Gastric Cancer

Nicola Bizzaro [1], Antonio Antico [2] and Danilo Villalta [3,*]

[1]   Laboratorio di Patologia Clinica, Azienda Sanitaria Universitaria Integrata, 33100 Udine, Italy;
      nic.bizzaro@gmail.com
[2]   Laboratorio Analisi ULSS 4, 36014 Santorso, Italy; antonio.antico@aulss7.veneto.it
[3]   Immunologia e Allergologia, Presidio Ospedaliero S. Maria degli Angeli, 33170 Pordenone, Italy
*   Correspondence: danilo.villalta@aas5.sanita.fvg.it; Tel.: +30-0434-399647

Received: 19 December 2017; Accepted: 24 January 2018; Published: 26 January 2018

Abstract: Alterations in the immune response of patients with autoimmune diseases may predispose to malignancies, and a link between chronic autoimmune gastritis and gastric cancer has been reported in many studies. Intestinal metaplasia with dysplasia of the gastric corpus-fundus mucosa and hyperplasia of chromaffin cells, which are typical features of late-stage autoimmune gastritis, are considered precursor lesions. Autoimmune gastritis has been associated with the development of two types of gastric neoplasms: intestinal type and type I gastric carcinoid. Here, we review the association of autoimmune gastritis with gastric cancer and other autoimmune features present in gastric neoplasms.

Keywords: autoimmune diseases; autoimmune gastritis; gastric cancer; *Helicobacter pylori* infection; intrinsic factor antibodies; parietal cell antibodies

1. Introduction

Immune dysregulation is believed to play a pathogenic role in the development of both autoimmunity and neoplasia, and autoimmune conditions have been described in patients with neoplastic diseases. Antinuclear antibodies, the hallmark of many autoimmune rheumatic diseases, have been reported in the sera of patients with malignant tumors [1–3]; anti-La antibodies which are characteristically detected in sera of patients with Sjögren's syndrome, and anti-CENP-B antibodies, a marker of systemic sclerosis, were detected in patients with breast cancer [4,5]. Similarly, anti-dsDNA antibodies which are of both diagnostic and prognostic value in systemic lupus erythematosus (SLE), were also reported to be present in the sera of patients with various types of cancer [6,7]; the presence of rheumatoid factor was found to correlate with poor prognosis in different types of neoplastic diseases including gastrointestinal cancer [8]. Also, organ-specific antibodies were reported in malignancies; among these are anti-smooth muscle antibodies, anti-parietal cell antibodies and anti-thyroid antibodies [9,10].

Conversely, an increased incidence of malignancies has been observed among patients with autoimmune diseases [11]. According to the Bradford Hill postulates [12] that evaluate the degree in which an autoimmune disease is conditioning a higher probability to develop a malignant neoplasm, a link has been found for rheumatoid arthritis, SLE, Sjögren's syndrome and celiac disease in association with lymphoproliferative diseases [13,14]; idiopathic inflammatory myositis with solid tumors [15]; and systemic sclerosis in association with breast and gastrointestinal cancer [16]. In addition, recent research has shown that neoplastic transformation of autoimmune gastritis is as high as 10% and that autoimmune gastritis should be considered a pre-neoplastic disorder with an annual incidence of gastric cancer of 0.3% [17].

Here, we review the association of autoimmune gastritis with gastric cancer and other autoimmune features present in gastric neoplasms.

1.1. Autoimmune Gastritis

Autoimmune gastritis (AIG) is an organ-specific disease characterized by a chronic inflammation of the mucosa of the stomach that evolves in atrophic gastritis causing malabsorption of essential elements and eventually microcytic iron-deficient anemia [18] or pernicious anemia due to vitamin B_{12} deficiency [19]. As the lesion progresses, the parietal and principal cells of the mucosa may be replaced by cells containing mucus, similar to the intestinal ones. Two types of metaplasia are considered to be associated with gastric carcinogenesis in humans: intestinal metaplasia, and spasmolytic polypeptide-expressing metaplasia (SPEM). Goblet cells in intestinal metaplasia express appropriate intestinal markers, including Muc2 and Trefoil factor 3 (TFF3), while the mucous metaplastic lineages in SPEM display morphological characteristics more typical of deep antral gland cells or Brunner's glands, with expression of Muc6 and Trefoil factor 2 (TFF2). Importantly, recent investigations support the origin of SPEM through transdifferentiation from mature principal cells following parietal cell loss [20]. Both intestinal metaplasia and SPEM have been associated with the progression to intestinal-type gastric cancer [21].

Similar to other autoimmune conditions, AIG is more common in females than in males (3:1 ratio). AIG is generally asymptomatic up to an advanced stage of atrophy and/or dysplasia of the mucosa [22]. For this reason, AIG is a frequently underdiagnosed disease, with an estimated prevalence of nearly 2% in the third decade to 12% in the eighth decade [17,23,24]. The prevalence is even higher in patients affected by other autoimmune diseases, especially autoimmune thyroid diseases (AITD) and type 1 diabetes (T1DM) [25,26]. These associations define the multiple autoimmune diseases (MAS) type 3B and 4 [27].

Chronic autoimmune gastritis (type A) is etiologically and histologically distinct from type B gastritis associated with *Helicobacter pylori* (*H. pylori*) infection [28]. Different from *H. pylori* gastritis which is mainly localized in the antrum, AIG is restricted to the gastric body and fundus because inflammatory aggression affects the cells of the oxytocin glands [29]. However, there is a peculiar form of AIG that may develop in genetically predisposed subjects during *H. pylori* infection [30]. The finding of anti-parietal cell antibodies in 20–30% of patients with *H. pylori* infection and of anti-*H. pylori* antibodies in patients with AIG, suggests that there is a link between *H. pylori* and gastric autoimmunity [31–33].

H. pylori infection could induce AIG through mechanisms of molecular mimicry and/or epitope spreading; a high homology has been demonstrated between the β subunit of Hp urease and the subunit β of gastric ATPase [34]. The activation of gastric Th1 cells reactive to different peptides of *H. pylori* wall that cross-react with gastric H^+K^+-ATPase, results in an inflammatory process in which T-cell-derived IFN-γ enables parietal cells to act as APCs and to become targets of cross-reactive epitope recognition resulting in killing or apoptotic suicide. Apoptotic parietal cells would thus allow cross-priming of T cells that are specific to private gastric ATPase epitopes [35,36].

Although histological healing of the mucosa of the body has been reported in patients in whom *H. pylori* had been eradicated [37,38], a direct correlation between *H. pylori* infection and AIG remains controversial [39–41]. To this end, it has to be noted that while the bacterium is present in the initial stages of gastritis, in the atrophic stage the bacterium is no longer recognizable because hypocloridry and mucosal destruction result in environmental conditions unsuitable for *H. pylori* survival.

1.2. Cell-Mediated Autoimmunity

In AIG, cell-mediated autoimmunity plays a primary role sustained by $CD4^+CD25^-$ Th1 resting lymphocyte effectors [42]. Most of these self-reactive cells produce IFN-γ and TNF-α and possess cytolytic capacities, with perforin and Fas/Fas ligand-mediated mechanisms, which they express in well-defined gene restriction conditions dictated by the MHC system [43]. They induce gastric parietal cell death by apoptosis and perforin/granzyme B pathway, in particular through IFN-γ, which increases the expression of Fas and MHC class II molecules on gastric parietal cells.

The evidence that in the guinea pigs a single injection of an IFN-γ neutralizing antibody prevents the development of gastritis makes it clear that this cytokine is active in the genesis of the disease [44].

Moreover, the role of CD4$^+$CD25$^-$ Th1 lymphocytes in the pathogenesis of AIG has been demonstrated by their isolation in the paragastric lymph nodes in experimental murine models and the development of atrophic gastritis with appearance of parietal cell antibodies in association with a decrease in CD4$^+$CD25$^+$ T-cell tolerance [45].

The main target of immunological injury is the gastric H$^+$/K$^+$-adenosine-triphosphate enzyme (ATPase), a protein of the membrane that coats the secretory canaliculi of the parietal cells and is responsible for the secretion of hydrogen ions in exchange for potassium ions (proton pump) [46,47]. The gastric H$^+$/K$^+$-ATPase is formed by a catalytic 100 kDa α subunit and a 60–90 kDa β subunit; CD4$^+$ T cells react to H$^+$/K$^+$-ATPase α chain and marginally to the β chain. Induced by a triggering factor not yet entirely identified, the CD4$^+$CD25$^-$ T-cells, together with macrophages and B lymphocytes, infiltrate the submucosa, the lamina propria and the gastric glands causing the loss of parietal, principal and P/D1 ghrelin-producing cells [48,49], the principal and P/D1 cells being destroyed as bystanders of the parietal cells.

1.3. Humoral Autoimmunity

Patients with AIG have been shown to have two types of antibodies, one to parietal cells (PCAs) and the other to intrinsic factor (IFA) or its binding site in the small bowel.

PCAs are present at a high frequency in AIG (80–90%), especially in early stages of the disease [50,51] and bind to both α and β subunits of gastric H$^+$/K$^+$-ATPase. Antibody reactivity to the α catalytic subunit includes epitopes on the cytosolic side of the secretory membrane. Antibody reactivity to the β subunit requires that the antigen is linked in a disulfide-bond and glycosylated, thus, suggesting that autoepitopes are located in the luminal domain of the glycoprotein [47,52].

In the later stages of the disease, the incidence of PCA decreases due to the progression of atrophy and the loss of gastric parietal cells and, thus, the decrease in antigenic rate [53,54]. It is currently unknown if these autoantibodies play a pathogenic role in AIG but their finding in serum in the subclinical stage, especially in patients with autoimmune endocrine disease, is predictive of the presence of AIG [55].

Human intrinsic factor (IF) is a 60-kDa glycoprotein secreted by gastric parietal cells. Its action is high affinity binding and transport of vitamin B$_{12}$. The complex IF-vitamin B$_{12}$ reaches terminal ileum where it is absorbed after binding to specific receptors in the membranes of cells of ileal lumen [56]. IFAs are considered specific markers for AIG and are present both in blood serum and in the gastric juice of 30–50% of AIG patients [57]. In serum, two specific types of IFA, both of the IgG class, have been described: type 1 (blocking antibodies) that react with the binding site for vitamin B$_{12}$ and are found in 70% of IFA-positive patients, and type 2 (binding or precipitating antibody) that recognizes a site away from B$_{12}$ binding sites and impedes binding of IF-vitamin B$_{12}$ to the receptors in the ileal mucosa. Type 2 IFAs are found in about 30% of AIG patients, and are rarely present in the absence of type I autoantibodies [58].

2. Autoimmune Gastritis and Gastric Cancer

The incidence of gastric neoplasms is higher in patients with AIG compared to the general population [59,60]. Prospective studies have shown that 4–9% of patients with AIG, or its more severe form pernicious anemia, have gastric carcinoid tumors, whose frequency is 13-times higher than that of control subjects [44]. In addition, AIG progression to atrophic gastritis, associated with intestinal metaplasia, may predispose to gastric adenocarcinoma in more than 10% of patients [44].

Two recent studies, one with over 4.5 million adult male veterans admitted to US Veterans Affairs hospitals in the United States [61] and the other including nine million individuals from Sweden [62], reported that individuals with AIG/pernicious anemia had a three-fold increased risk of developing not only stomach carcinoid and adenocarcinomas, but also small intestinal adenocarcinomas and esophageal squamous cell carcinomas.

Nguyen and coworkers [63], using a transgenic mouse model of AIG, investigated the potential link between AIG and gastric cancer using CD4$^+$ T cells expressing a T-cell receptor specific for a peptide from the gastric H$^+$/K$^+$ ATPase proton pump. By 2–4 months of age, all mice developed chronic gastritis that resulted from large numbers of CD4$^+$ T cells that infiltrated the gastric mucosa and produced large amounts of IFNγ and smaller amounts of IL-17. At this stage of the disease, mice also developed several molecular features similar to those that precede gastric cancer in humans, including SPEM.

For these reasons, autoimmune gastritis should be considered a precancerous lesion, and the European MAPS (Management of Precancerous Conditions and Lesions in the Stomach) guidelines [64] recommend a three-yearly endoscopic and bioptic follow-up for all patients with extensive atrophy (stage III and IV of the OLGA classification [65]) (Table 1 and Figure 1).

Table 1. Clinical presentation, serology, pathology and neoplastic risk of autoimmune gastritis.

Clinical Presentation	No symptoms or dyspepsia	
	Anemia (iron deficiency, vitamin B12 deficiency)	
	Coexisting autoimmune diseases:	Autoimmune thyroid diseases (Hashimoto and Graves) Type 1 diabetes Addison disease Polyglandular autoimmune syndromes type III
Serology	Gastrin 17 Pepsinogen I Pepsinogen II Parietal cell autoantibodies Intrinsic factor autoantibodies	>10 pmol/L <30 µg/L normal (3–15 µg/L) pos 90–95% pos 30–50%
Pathology	Corpus/fundus restricted gastritis	
Neoplastic Risk	Gastric carcinoid: increased according to gastric (oxyntic) atrophy score to the corpus and fundus of the stomach	
	Gastric adenocarcinoma: increased according to pangastric atrophy score	

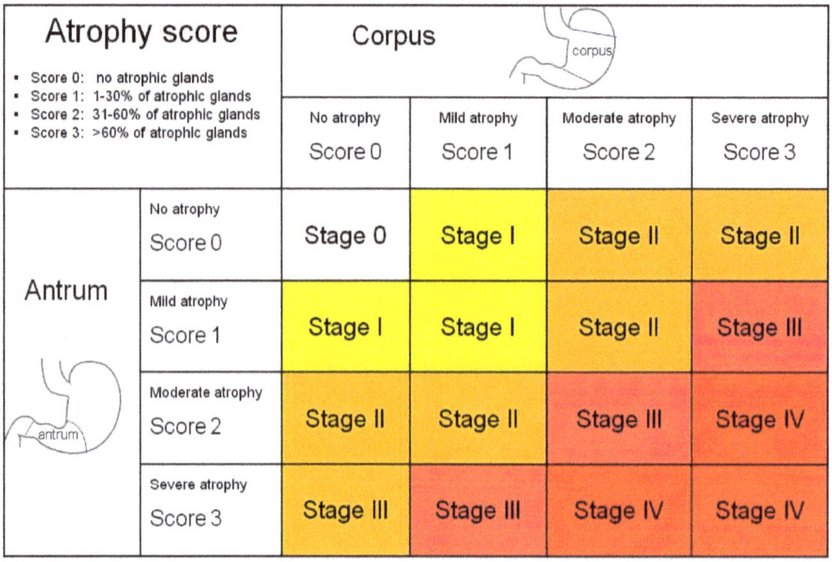

Figure 1. OLGA (operative link for gastritis assessment) staging system for gastritis. Modified from Rugge M. et al. [65].

Gastric atrophy is a key step towards gastric neoplasms, as studies of resected stomachs from patients with intestinal-type gastric cancer have shown gastric atrophy in every case [66]. Atrophy and metaplasia (including SPEM), occur in a setting of inflammation and a complex milieu of cytokines [67]. Studies in humans and mouse models of gastritis and gastric cancer identified important roles for cytokines in regulating oxyntic atrophy, hyperplasia, metaplasia, and progression to gastric cancer. Several reports showed that IL-17A promotes tumorigenesis. In particular: (a) level of IL-17 mRNA in gastric tumors was associated with the depth of tumor, lymph-vascular invasion and lymph node involvement [68]; (b) gastric cancer patients have higher levels of IL-17 in serum and in cancer tissues than the general population [69]; (c) genetic data show that IL-17A and IL-17F polymorphisms increase gastric cancer risk [70]; (d) there are increased Th17 cells infiltrating tumors on patients with advanced gastric cancer [71].

Kuai and coworkers have demonstrated that tumor cells produce IL-8, a cytokine of the CXC chemokine family, as an autocrine growth factor, which promotes tumor growth, tissue invasion, metastatic spread and chemoresistance of gastric cancer cells [72]. Genotypes of TNF, IL10, IL1B, and the interleukin-1 receptor antagonist (IL-1RA) are also reported to confer greater risk of gastric cancer [73]. IL-1β was able to directly induce DNA methylation, which may link inflammation-induced epigenetic changes and the development of gastric diseases [74]. Several additional cytokines (IL-22, IL-23, IL-32, IL-33) have been also implicated in gastric cancer progression [75–77]. Taken together, these findings show that diverse cytokines and different combinations of cytokines might promote gastric oncogenesis and/or metastasis. The risk may depend on the types of cytokines made by different subsets of differentiated CD4$^+$ helper T cells responding to *H. pylori* or self-antigens such as H$^+$/K$^+$ adenosine triphosphatase (ATPase) in the case of autoimmune gastritis [73].

However, more information on cytokines that influence gastric cancer development is needed, in particular in light of the development of new biological entities for targeting specific cytokines. In fact, a better understanding of the cytokine pathway promoting gastric cancer development and progression may be used to obtain additional therapeutic options for patients with chronic atrophic gastritis and gastric cancer.

Overall, AIG has been associated with the development of two types of gastric neoplasms: intestinal type and type I gastric carcinoid [78].

2.1. Intestinal-Type Gastric Cancer

As previously mentioned, the two known factors predisposing gastric cancer in patients with AIG are intestinal metaplasia and concurrent *H. pylori* infection, which is the most common cause of intestinal metaplasia of the gastric mucosa [79]. It should be noted that *H. pylori* eradication in patients with precancerous lesions (gastric atrophy, intestinal metaplasia or gastric dysplasia) does not significantly reduce the incidence of gastric cancer [80]. However, not all patients with *H. pylori* gastritis develop gastric cancer. Chances are higher when there are some virulence factors. For example, *H. pylori* cagA-positive strains have been shown to pose a significantly greater risk of developing peptic ulcers and gastric cancer than cagA-negative strains [81,82]. Another well-known virulence factor is the vacuolating cytotoxin A (vacA) protein [83].

The pathway of gastric cancer development, mainly of the intestinal histological type, was described by Correa [84]: chronic inflammation leads to tissue atrophy, which is further followed by intestinal metaplasia. Unknown genetic, metabolic or environmental triggers eventually lead to the development of adenocarcinoma. In a recent systematic review, an annual incidence of gastric adenocarcinoma of 0.27% per person-year was demonstrated, with an overall relative risk of 6.8 [60]. In another study, in which 877 Danish patients with gastric cancer were examined, 12 (1.3%) had a previous diagnosis of AIG [85]. According to the typical distribution of lesions in AIG, these tumors were localized to the body and to the fundus of the stomach, while they were mainly affecting the antral and pyloric region in patients without AIG (*H. pylori* infection was not investigated).

2.2. Type I Gastric Carcinoid

Hypergastrinemia resulting from the loss of HCl secretion by gastric parietal cells leads to the development of hyperplasia of the enterochromaffin cells with possible evolution into a carcinoid tumor. Carcinoid tumor in patients with AIG represents about 10% of all carcinoid tumors and about 1% of gastric neoplasms [86,87].

There are three types of gastric carcinoid characterized by different levels of gastrin: (a) type I associated with a very high gastrinemia resulting from AIG; (b) type II which is present in patients with multiple endocrine neoplasia (MEN) and show elevated levels of gastrin; (c) type III presenting as Zollinger–Ellison syndrome which is the most aggressive variant and showing a normal gastrin level [88]. In type I carcinoid, lesions are characterized by the secretion of gastrin in response to the loss of the negative feedback due to the loss of parietal cells, which produce hydrochloric acid. Hypergastrinemia, in turn, has trophic effects on enterochromaffin cells. Hyperplasia and subsequent dysplasia of enterochromaffin cells may progress toward the gastric carcinoid type I over time [89]. In addition, chronic achlorhydria increases the production of gastrin by the G cells in the antrum, which then stimulates enterochromaffin cells that lead to their hyperplasia. Patients with type I gastric carcinoid are generally asymptomatic, although dyspeptic symptoms may be present. For this reason, diagnosis is usually performed during endoscopic examination [90].

2.3. Cancer Stem Cells

Recently, a cancer stem/initiating cell concept was proposed to explain cancer development.

According to Visvader [91], either stem or progenitor cells can act as targets for tumor initiation. Several diverse cancers are hierarchically organized and sustained by a subpopulation of self-renewing cells that can generate the full repertoire of tumor cells (both tumorigenic and non-tumorigenic cells). Stem cells have been favored candidates for targets of transformation because of their inherent capacity for self-renewal and their longevity, which would allow the sequential accumulation of genetic or epigenetic mutations required for oncogenesis.

Indeed, it has been demonstrated that, as one of the possible mechanisms of gastric carcinogenesis, chronic inflammation induced by *Helicobacter pylori* infection can increase the number of tissue stem/progenitor cells, promote their proliferation, and alter the properties of stem cells toward intestinal metaplasia to cancer [92]. Thus, an intestinal phenotype in the stomach would be not just a differentiated metaplasia in the stomach, but a phenotype of stem cell abnormality with precancerous lesion susceptible to gastric carcinogenesis after chronic inflammation [92].

3. Autoantibodies as Markers of Gastric Cancer

Cancer cells can induce an immunological response resulting in the production of autoantibodies against tumor antigens which can be used as biomarkers to detect cancer at an early stage. Indeed, the immune system is capable of sensing at least some tumor-associated antigens before many standard clinical tests for cancer diagnosis [93], so that detection of tumor-associated autoantibodies could have both diagnostic and prognostic relevance [94,95]. Availability of early and specific markers would be an important advance in cancer management because currently a significant proportion of individuals are diagnosed late, presenting with advanced disease at which time the opportunities for successful treatment are drastically reduced and treatment costs significantly increased [95]. The use of autoantibodies as biomarkers in cancer immunodiagnosis is further justified by the fact that these antibodies are generally absent or present in very low concentration in normal individuals and in non-cancer conditions [96]. Importantly, although no evidence of correlation between antibody concentration and cancer stage emerged from most studies [94], usually a marked decrease in antibody levels is seen after surgical removal of solid tumors, indicating that they can be used in monitoring the efficacy of surgical treatment and in patient follow up.

Most tumor-associated autoantigens are cellular proteins and belong to three main classes: (a) antigens resulting from genetic mutations or rearrangements; (b) viral antigens; and (c) antigens that are ectopically expressed. Somatic mutations can increase immunogenicity by producing new antigenic epitopes via point mutations, frame shifts, or coding sequence extensions or truncations [95]. Several techniques are used for their detection, including serological analysis of tumor antigens by recombinant cDNA expression cloning (SEREX), phage display, serological proteome analysis (SERPA), multiple affinity protein profiling (MAPPing), and protein microarrays [97].

Currently, there are some candidate autoantibodies as clinically useful biomarkers for gastric cancer; namely, anti-p53, anti-carcinoembryonic antigen (CEA), anti-mucin, anti-survivin, and anti-livin autoantibodies.

p53 is a tumor suppressor gene that plays a critical role in oncology. Its protein participates in the regulation of the cell-cycle, acts as a transcriptional transactivator/repressor, helps in DNA repair, suppresses cell growth, induces apoptosis and has many other functions [98]. The production of anti-p53 autoantibodies is strongly related to p53 protein overexpression in the tumor tissue [99]. Autoantibodies against the p53 protein were detected for the first time in sera of patients with breast cancer [100] and then in many other solid tumors. In gastric cancer, 20% of all patients and 46% of patients with p53-positive tumors have high levels of anti-p53 antibodies [101]. Regardless of the moderate sensitivity, there is consensus on the very high specificity (around 96%) of p53 antibodies for malignancy [102,103]. Several studies have also demonstrated that anti-p53 antibodies are more prevalent in advanced gastric cancers with a prevalence of regional lymph node involvement [95,101, 104,105] recognizing the poor prognostic value of p53 autoantibody markers in gastric carcinoma.

Antibodies to CEA, an oncofetal glycoprotein commonly measured as a tumor marker, may be found in 46–56% of gastrointestinal tumors, especially in cancer at an early stage, even with undetectable circulating CEA [7,106]. However, they are also found in 10% of healthy individuals suggesting they could be part of the natural autoantibody repertoire. Anti-CEA antibodies are associated with the host immune response against the tumor and show a good prognostic value for survival [99,107]. Antibodies to mucin [108], surviving, and livin [109] have also been detected in patients with gastric cancer, with a prevalence of 75%, 40%, and 50%, respectively. They could represent new tumor markers not only for diagnosis but also for postoperative monitoring of gastric cancer patients, particularly in those lacking anti-p53 antibodies [95].

Autoantibodies to the extracellular protein kinase A (ECPKA), a cAMP-dependent intracellular enzyme, are markedly up-regulated in the sera of cancer patients, have been found in many malignant tumors, including gastric cancer. Although these antibodies measure malignant transformation in all cells and are not specific to one type of cancer, they have a sensitivity of 90% with a specificity of 87% and could be used as a universal screening method to detect serum tumor markers [110].

However, notwithstanding their high diagnostic specificity, in clinical practice, autoantibody response has been seen to be highly variable from patient to patient, probably due to diverse immune responses resulting from the highly heterogeneous nature of cancer and inherent genotypic (and epigenetic) variations within a population [95]. In addition, contrary to what occurs in autoimmune diseases, assays that measure a single tumor-associated autoantibody appear to have little diagnostic use for cancer due to their low frequency, rarely exceeding 30%. A possible strategy for overcoming this limitation due to individual variability and poor diagnostic sensitivity could be combining known autoantibody markers with other biomarkers for gastric cancer, such as tumor markers like carcinoembryonic antigen (CEA) [111], CA19-9 [112], and CA72-4 [113] markers related to chronic atrophic gastritis (e.g., parietal cell antibodies, *H. pylori* antibodies and serum pepsinogens I and II, gastrin [114]), microRNAs [115] or glycosylation signatures [116].

Another strategy to increase diagnostic sensitivity is to associate multiple antibody markers. To this end, Werner et al. studied 329 gastric cancer patients, 321 healthy controls and 124 participants with other diseases of the upper digestive tract by multiplex serology using a fluorescent bead-based glutathione S-transferase (GST) capture immunosorbent assay [117]. Among 64 candidate autoantibodies directed against gastric tumor-associated antigens, they identified five antibodies: MAGEA4, CTAG1, TP53, ERBB2_C, and SDCCAG8. At 98% specificity, sensitivity for gastric cancer detection for single antibodies was not higher than 12%, while a combination of the five antibodies enabled recognition of 32% of early-stage gastric cancer with a specificity of 87% [117].

Using an ELISA assay to detect autoantibodies towards an antigenic panel containing a seven-marker combination (p53, Koc, p62, c-myc, IMP1, survivin and p16), in a cohort of 383 patients (88 with gastric adenocarcinoma, 79 with gastric dysplasia, 76 with chronic atrophic gastritis, and 140 individuals with normal gastric mucosa), Zhou et al. reported a sensitivity of 64% for adenocarcinoma with a specificity of 87%. The area under the receiver operating characteristic (ROC) curve was 0.730. Sensitivity for gastric cancer did not increase with the addition of other autoantibodies to tumor-associated antigens [118].

In a similar study by Wang and coworkers, autoantibodies against eight tumor-associated recombinant antigens (IMP1, p62, Koc, p53, c-myc, cyclin B1, survivin and p16) determined by ELISA and Western blot, showed 56.1% sensitivity for gastric cancer detection, at 86.2% specificity. The highest frequency (27%) was found for cyclin B1 [119].

Thus, a substantial number of autoantibodies present in patients with gastric cancer have been identified. Although some of the autoantibodies are highly specific, their low diagnostic sensitivity has limited their application in clinical practice and assays that measure a single tumor-associated autoantibody appear to have little diagnostic utility for cancer detection. In the future, availability of new multiplex technology for the simultaneous detection of many autoantibodies might prove to be able to overcome these limitations by providing cancer-specific autoantibody profiles to be used for population screening for the early detection of gastric cancer.

4. Conclusions

There is evidence that the incidence of gastric neoplasms is higher in patients with autoimmune gastritis compared to the general population. Many studies in humans and in mouse models of gastritis indicate that chronic inflammation stimulates gastric cells to produce inflammatory cytokines which play a relevant role in regulating oxyntic atrophy, hyperplasia, metaplasia, and progression to gastric cancer by up-regulating expression of progenitor cells. Recent data on gastric cancer stem cell involvement may provide insights into the molecular pathway of carcinogenesis, eventually leading to development of new therapeutic approaches to target early-stage gastric cancer.

Conflicts of Interest: The authors declare no conflict of interest.

References

1. Burnham, T.K. Antinuclear antibodies in patients with malignancies. *Lancet* **1972**, *2*, 436–437. [CrossRef]
2. Zermosky, J.O.; Gormy, M.K.; Jarczewska, K. Malignancy associated with antinuclear antibodies. *Lancet* **1972**, *2*, 1035–1036. [CrossRef]
3. Solans-Laqué, R.; Pérez-Bocanegra, C.; Salud-Salvia, A.; Fonollosa-Plá, V.; Rodrigo, M.J.; Armadans, L.; Simeón-Aznar, C.P.; Vilardell-Tarres, M. Clinical significance of antinuclear antibodies in malignant diseases: Association with rheumatic and connective tissue paraneoplastic syndromes. *Lupus* **2004**, *13*, 159–164. [CrossRef] [PubMed]
4. Atalay, C.; Atalay, G.; Yilmaz, K.B.; Altinok, M. The role of anti-CENP-B and anti-SS-B antibodies in breast cancer. *Neoplasma* **2005**, *52*, 32–35. [PubMed]
5. Toubi, E.; Shoenfeld, Y. protective autoimmunity in cancer. *Oncol. Rep.* **2007**, *17*, 245–251. [PubMed]
6. Lv, S.; Zhang, J.; Wu, J.; Zheng, X.; Chu, Y.; Xiong, S. Origin and anti-tumor effects of anti-dsDNA autoantibodies in cancer patients and tumor-bearing mice. *Immunol. Lett.* **2005**, *99*, 217–227. [CrossRef] [PubMed]
7. Konstadoulakis, M.M.; Syrigos, K.N.; Albanopoulos, C.; Mayers, G.; Golematis, B. The presence of anti-carcinoembryonic antigen (CEA) antibodies in the sera of patients with gastrointestinal malignancies. *J. Clin. Immunol.* **1994**, *14*, 310–313. [CrossRef] [PubMed]

8. Schattner, A.; Shani, A.; Talpaz, M.; Bentwich, Z. Rheumatoid factors in the sera of patients with gastrointestinal carcinoma. *Cancer* **1983**, *52*, 2156–2161. [CrossRef]

9. Betterle, C.; Peserico, A.; Bersani, G.; Ninfo, V.; del Prete, G.F.; Stefani, R.; Nitti, D. Circulating antibodies in malignant melanoma patients. *Dermatologica* **1979**, *159*, 24–29. [CrossRef] [PubMed]

10. Molander, S.; Jønsson, V.; Andersen, L.P.; Bennetzen, M.; Christiansen, M.; Hou-Jensen, K.; Madsen, H.O.; Ryder, L.P.; Permin, H.; Wiik, A. Pseudolymphoma and ventricular maltoma in patients with chronic gastritis, ulcer and Helicobacter pylori infection. *Ugeskr. Laeger* **2000**, *162*, 791–795. [PubMed]

11. Tomer, Y.; Shoenfeld, Y. Autoantibodies, autoimmunity and cancer. In *Cancer and Autoimmunity*; Shoenfeld, Y., Gershwin, M.E., Eds.; Elsevier Science: Amsterdam, The Netherlands, 2000; pp. 141–150.

12. Bradford-Hill, A. The environment and disease: Association or causation? *Proc. R. Soc. Med.* **1965**, *58*, 295–300.

13. Mellemkjaer, L.; Andersen, V.; Linet, M.S.; Gridley, G.; Hoover, R.; Olsen, J.H. Non-Hodgkin's lymphoma and other cancers among a cohort of patients with systemic lupus erythematosus. *Arthritis Rheum.* **1997**, *40*, 761–768. [CrossRef] [PubMed]

14. Valesini, G.; Priori, R.; Bavoillot, D.; Osborn, J.; Danieli, M.G.; del Papa, N.; Gerli, R.; Pietrogrande, M.; Sabbadini, M.G.; Silvestris, F.; et al. Differential risk of non-Hodgkin's lymphoma in Italian patients with primary Sjögren's syndrome. *J. Rheumatol.* **1997**, *24*, 2376–2380. [PubMed]

15. Villa, A.R.; Kraus, A.; Alarcon-Segovia, D. Autoimmune rheumatic diseases and cancer: Evidence of causality? In *Cancer and Autoimmunity*; Shoenfeld, Y., Gershwin, M.E., Eds.; Elsevier Science: Amsterdam, The Netherlands, 2000; pp. 111–117.

16. Moinzadeh, P.; Fonseca, C.; Hellmich, M.; Shah, A.A.; Chighizola, C.; Denton, C.; Ong, V.H. Association of anti-RNA polymerase III autoantibodies and cancer in scleroderma. *Arthritis Res. Ther.* **2014**, *16*, R53. [CrossRef] [PubMed]

17. Toh, BH. Diagnosis and classification of autoimmune gastritis. *Autoimmun. Rev.* **2014**, *13*, 459–462. [CrossRef] [PubMed]

18. Marignani, M.; Delle Fave, G.; Mecarocci, S.; Bordi, C.; Angeletti, S.; D'Ambra, G.; Aprile, M.R.; Corleto, V.D.; Monarca, B.; Annibale, B. High prevalence of atrophic body gastritis in patients with unexplained microcytic and macrocytic anemia. *Am. J. Gastroenterol.* **1999**, *94*, 766–772. [PubMed]

19. Bizzaro, N.; Antico, A. Diagnosis and classification of pernicious anemia. *Autoimmun. Rev.* **2014**, *13*, 565–568. [CrossRef] [PubMed]

20. Weis, V.G.; Goldenring, J.R. Current understanding of SPEM and its standing in the preneoplastic process. *Gastric Cancer* **2009**, *12*, 189–197. [CrossRef] [PubMed]

21. Kokkola, A.; Sjoblom, S.M.; Haapiainen, R.; Sipponen, P.; Puolakkainen, P.; Jarvinen, H. The risk of gastric carcinoma and carcinoid tumours in patients with pernicious anemia: A prospective follow-up study. *Scand. J. Gastroenterol.* **1998**, *33*, 88–92. [PubMed]

22. Dixon, M.F.; Genta, R.M.; Yardley, J.H.; Correa, P. Classification and grading of gastritis. The updated Sydney System. International Workshop on the Histopathology of Gastritis, Houston 1994. *Am. J. Surg. Pathol.* **1996**, *20*, 1161–1181. [CrossRef] [PubMed]

23. Hawa, M.; Beyan, H.; Leslie, R.D. Principles of autoantibodies as disease-specific markers. *Autoimmunity* **2004**, *37*, 253–256. [CrossRef] [PubMed]

24. Weck, M.N.; Brenner, H. Prevalence of chronic atrophic gastritis in different parts of the world. *Cancer Epidemiol. Biomarkers Prev.* **2006**, *15*, 1083–1094. [CrossRef] [PubMed]

25. Weetman, A.P. Non-thyroid antibodies in autoimmune thyroid disease. *Best Pract. Res. Clin. Endocrinol. Metab.* **2005**, *19*, 17–32. [CrossRef] [PubMed]

26. Van den Driessche, A.; Eenkhoorn, V.; van Gaal, L.; de Block, C. Type 1 diabetes and autoimmune polyglandular syndrome: A clinical review. *Neth. J. Med.* **2009**, *67*, 376–387. [PubMed]

27. Betterle, C.; Presotto, F. Autoimmune polyendocrine syndromes (APS) or multiple autoimmune syndromes (MAS). In *Handbook of Systemic Autoimmune Diseases. Endocrine Manifestations of Systemic Autoimmune Diseases*; Walker, S.A., Jara, L.J., Eds.; Elsevier Science: Amsterdam, The Netherlands, 2008; pp. 135–148.

28. Strickland, R.G.; Mackay, I.R. The reappraisal of the nature and significance of chronic atrophic gastritis. *Am. J. Dig. Dis.* **1973**, *18*, 426–440. [CrossRef] [PubMed]

29. Toh, B.H.; Sentry, J.W.; Alderuccio, F. The causative H^+/K^+ ATPase antigen in the pathogenesis of autoimmune gastritis. *Immunol. Today* **2000**, *21*, 348–354. [CrossRef]

30. Weck, M.N.; Brenner, H. Association of Helicobacter pylori infection with chronic atrophic gastritis: Meta-analyses according to type of disease definition. *Int. J. Cancer* **2008**, *123*, 874–881. [CrossRef] [PubMed]

31. Ma, J.Y.; Borch, K.; Sjostrand, S.E.; Janzon, L.; Mardh, S. Positive correlation between H, K-adenosine triphosphatase autoantibodies and Helicobacter pylori antibodies in patients with pernicious anemia. *Scand. J. Gastroenterol.* **1994**, *29*, 961–965. [CrossRef] [PubMed]

32. Faller, G.; Kirchner, T. Immunological and morphogenic basis of gastric mucosa atrophy and metaplasia. *Virchows. Arch.* **2005**, *446*, 1–9. [CrossRef] [PubMed]

33. Claeys, D.; Faller, G.; Appelmelk, B.; Negrini, R.; Kirchner, T. The gastric H^+/K^+ ATPase is a major autoantigen in chronic Helicobacter pylori gastritis with body mucosa atrophy. *Gastroenterology* **1998**, *115*, 340–347. [CrossRef]

34. Amedei, A.; Bergman, M.P.; Appelmelk, B.; Azzurri, A.; Benagiano, M.; Tamburini, C.; van der Zee, R.; Telford, J.L.; Vandenbroucke-Grauls, C.M.J.E.; D'Elios, M.M.; et al. Molecular mimicry between Helicobacter pylori antigens and H^+K^+-adenotriphosphatase in human gastric autoimmunity. *J. Exp. Med.* **2003**, *198*, 1147–1156. [CrossRef] [PubMed]

35. D'Elios, M.M.; Appelmelk, B.J.; Amedei, A.; Bergman, M.P.; Del Prete, G.F. Gastric autoimmunity: The role of Helicobacter pylori and molecular mimicry. *Trends Mol. Med.* **2004**, *10*, 316–323. [CrossRef] [PubMed]

36. Plebani, M.; Basso, D. Le malattie autoimmuni del tratto gastro-enterico. In *Il Laboratorio Nelle Malattie Autoimmuni D'organo*; Tozzoli, R., Bizzaro, N., Villalta, D., Tonutti, E., Pinchera, A., Eds.; Esculapio: Bologna, Italy, 2009; pp. 313–332.

37. Faller, G.; Winter, M.; Steininger, H.; Lehn, N.; Meining, A.; Bayerdorffer, E.; Kirchner, T. Decrease of antigastric autoantibodies in Helicobacter pylori gastritis after cure of infection. *Pathol. Res. Pract.* **1999**, *195*, 243–246. [CrossRef]

38. Ohkusa, T.; Fujiki, K.; Takashimizu, I.; Kuma, G.A.J.; Tanizawa, T.; Eishi, Y.; Yokoyama, T.; Watanabe, M. Improvement in atrophic gastritis and intestinal metaplasia in patients in whom Helicobacter pylori was eradicated. *Ann. Intern. Med.* **2001**, *134*, 380–386. [CrossRef] [PubMed]

39. Oksanen, A.; Sipponen, P.; Karttunen, R.; Miettinen, A.; Veijola, L.; Sarna, S.; Rautelin, H. Atrophic gastritis and Helicobacter pylori infection in outpatients referred for gastroscopy. *Gut* **2000**, *46*, 460–463. [CrossRef] [PubMed]

40. De Block, C.E.; de Leeuw, I.H.; Bogers, J.J.; Pelckmans, P.A.; Ieven, M.; van Marck, E.A.; van Hoof, V.; Máday, E.; van Acker, K.L.; van Gaal, L.F. Helicobacter pylori, parietal cell antibodies and autoimmune gastropathy in type 1 diabetes mellitus. *Aliment. Pharmacol. Ther.* **2002**, *16*, 281–289. [CrossRef] [PubMed]

41. Annibale, B.; Aprile, M.R.; D'Ambra, G.; Caruana, P.; Bordi, C.; Delle Fave, G. Cure of Helicobacter pylori infection in atrophic body gastritis patients does not improve mucosal atrophy but reduces hypergastrinemia and its related effects on body ECL-cell hyperplasia. *Aliment. Pharmacol. Ther.* **2000**, *14*, 625–634. [CrossRef] [PubMed]

42. D'Elios, M.M.; Bergman, M.P.; Azzurri, A.; Amedei, A.; Benagiano, M.; de Pont, J.J.; Cianchi, F.; Vandenbroucke-Grauls, C.M.; Romagnani, S.; Appelmelk, B.J.; et al. $H(^+),K(^+)$- ATPase (proton pump) is the target autoantigen of Th1-type cytotoxic T cells in autoimmune gastritis. *Gastroenterology* **2001**, *120*, 377–386. [CrossRef] [PubMed]

43. Vergelli, M.; Hemmer, B.; Muraro, P.A.; Tranquill, L.; Biddison, W.E.; Sarin, A.; McFarland, H.F.; Martin, R. Human autoreactive CD4 T cell clones use perforin or Fas/Fas ligand-mediated pathways for target cell lysis. *J. Immunol.* **1997**, *158*, 2756–2761. [PubMed]

44. De Block, C.E.M.; de Leeuw, I.H.; van Gaal, L.F. Autoimmune gastritis in type 1 diabetes: A clinically oriented review. *J. Clin. Endocrinol. Metab.* **2008**, *93*, 363–371. [CrossRef] [PubMed]

45. Alderuccio, F.; Sentry, J.W.; Marshall, A.C.; Biondo, M.; Toh, B.H. Animal models of human disease: Experimental autoimmune gastritis and pernicious anemia. *Clin. Immunol.* **2002**, *102*, 48–58. [CrossRef] [PubMed]

46. Toh, B.H.; Van Driel, I.R.; Gleeson, P.A. Mechanisms of disease: Pernicious anemia. *N. Engl. J. Med.* **1997**, *337*, 1441–1448. [CrossRef] [PubMed]

47. Callaghan, J.M.; Khan, M.A.; Alderuccio, F.; van Driel, I.R.; Gleeson, P.A.; Toh, B.H. Alpha and beta subunits of the gastric H^+/K^+-ATPase are concordantly targeted by parietal cell autoantibodies associated with autoimmune gastritis. *Autoimmunity* **1993**, *16*, 289–295. [CrossRef] [PubMed]

Int. J. Mol. Sci. **2018**, *19*, 377

48. Asano, M.; Toda, M.; Sakaguchi, N.; Sakaguchi, S. Autoimmune disease as a consequence of developmental abnormality of a T cell subpopulation. *J. Exp. Med.* **1996**, *184*, 387–396. [CrossRef] [PubMed]
49. Taguchi, O.; Takahashi, T. Administration of anti-interleukin-2 receptor alfa antibody in vivo induces localized autoimmune disease. *Eur. J. Immunol.* **1996**, *26*, 1608–1612. [CrossRef] [PubMed]
50. Zittoun, J. Biermer's disease. *Rev. Prat.* **2001**, *51*, 1542–1546. (In French) [PubMed]
51. Toh, B.H.; Alderuccio, F. Pernicious anaemia. *Autoimmunity* **2004**, *37*, 357–361. [CrossRef] [PubMed]
52. Toh, B.H.; Chan, J.; Kyaw, T.; Alderuccio, F. Cutting edge issues in autoimmune gastritis. *Clin. Rev. Allergy Immunol.* **2012**, *42*, 269–278. [CrossRef] [PubMed]
53. Antico, A. L'autoimmunità gastrica. In *Il Laboratorio Nelle Malattie Autoimmuni D'organo*; Tozzoli, R., Bizzaro, N., Villalta, D., Tonutti, E., Pinchera, A., Eds.; Esculapio: Bologna, Italy, 2009; pp. 333–343.
54. Antico, A.; Tampoia, M.; Villalta, D.; Tonutti, E.; Tozzoli, R.; Bizzaro, N. Clinical usefulness of the serological gastric biopsy for the diagnosis of chronic autoimmune gastritis. *Clin. Dev. Immunol.* **2012**, *2012*, 520970. [CrossRef] [PubMed]
55. Tozzoli, R.; Kodermaz, G.; Perosa, A.R.; Tampoia, M.; Zucano, A.; Antico, A.; Bizzaro, N. Autoantibodies to parietal cells as predictors of atrophic body gastritis: A five-year prospective study in patients with autoimmune thyroid diseases. *Autoimmun. Rev.* **2010**, *10*, 80–83. [CrossRef] [PubMed]
56. Seetharam, B.; Alpers, D.H.; Allen, R.H. Isolation and characterization of the ileal receptor for intrinsic factor-cobalamin. *J. Biol. Chem.* **1981**, *256*, 3785–3790. [PubMed]
57. Carmel, R. Reassessment of the relative prevalence of antibodies to gastric parietal cell and to intrinsic factor in patients with pernicious anaemia: Influence of patient age and race. *Clin. Exp. Immunol.* **1992**, *89*, 74–77. [CrossRef] [PubMed]
58. Conn, D.A. Detection of type I and II antibodies to intrinsic factor. *Med. Lab. Sci.* **1986**, *43*, 148–151. [PubMed]
59. Vannella, L.; Sbrozzi-Vanni, A.; Lahner, E.; Bordi, C.; Pilozzi, E.; Corleto, V.D.; Osborn, J.F.; Delle, F.G.; Annibale, B. Development of type I gastric carcinoid in patients with chronic atrophic gastritis. *Aliment. Pharmacol. Ther.* **2011**, *33*, 1361–1369. [CrossRef] [PubMed]
60. Vannella, L.; Lahner, E.; Osborn, J.; Annibale, B. Systematic review: Gastric cancer incidence in pernicious anaemia. *Aliment Pharmacol. Ther.* **2013**, *37*, 375–382. [CrossRef] [PubMed]
61. Landgren, A.M.; Landgren, O.; Gridley, G.; Dores, G.M.; Linet, M.S.; Morton, L.M. Autoimmune disease and subsequent risk of developing alimentary tract cancers among 4.5 million US male veterans. *Cancer* **2011**, *117*, 1163–1171. [CrossRef] [PubMed]
62. Hemminki, K.; Liu, X.; Ji, J.; Sundquist, J.; Sundquist, K. Effect of autoimmune diseases on mortality and survival in subsequent digestive tract cancers. *Ann. Oncol.* **2012**, *23*, 2179–2184. [CrossRef] [PubMed]
63. Nguyen, T.L.; Khurana, S.S.; Bellone, C.J.; Capoccia, B.J.; Sagartz, J.E.; Kesman, R.A., Jr.; Mills, J.C.; DiPaolo, R.J. Autoimmune gastritis mediated by CD4+ T cells promotes the development of gastric cancer. *Cancer Res.* **2013**, *73*, 2117–2126. [CrossRef] [PubMed]
64. Dinis-Ribeiro, M.; Areia, M.; de Vries, A.C.; Marcos-Pinto, R.; Monteiro-Soare, M.; O'Connor, A.; Pereira, C.; Pimentel-Nunes, P.; Correia, R.; Ensari, A.; et al. Management of precancerous conditions and lesions in the stomach (MAPS): Guideline from European Society of Gastrointestinal Endoscopy (ESGE), European Helicobacter Study Group (EHSG), European Society of Pathology (ESP), and the Sociedade Portoguesa de Endoscopia Digestiva (SPED). *Virchows. Arch.* **2012**, *460*, 74–94.
65. Rugge, M.; Correa, P.; di Mario, F.; El-Omar, E.; Fiocca, R.; Geboes, K.; Genta, R.M.; Graham, D.Y.; Hattori, T.; Malfertheiner, P.; et al. OLGA staging for gastritis: A tutorial. *Dig. Liver. Dis.* **2008**, *40*, 650–658. [CrossRef] [PubMed]
66. El Zimaity, H.M.; Ota, H.; Graham, D.Y.; Akamatsu, T.; Katsuyama, T. Patterns of gastric atrophy in intestinal type gastric carcinoma. *Cancer* **2002**, *94*, 1428–1436. [CrossRef] [PubMed]
67. Epplein, M.; Xiang, Y.B.; Cai, Q.; Peek, R.M., Jr.; Lin, H.; Correa, P.; Gao, J.; Wu, J.; Michel, A.; Pawlita, M.; et al. Circulating cytokines and gastric cancer risk. *Cancer Causes Control.* **2013**, *24*, 2245–2250. [CrossRef] [PubMed]
68. Lida, T.; Iwahashi, M.; Katsuda, M.; Nakamori, M.; Nakamura, M.; Naka, T.; Ojima, T.; Ueda, K.; Hayata, K.; Nakamura, Y. Tumor-infiltrating CD4+ Th 17 cells produce IL-17 in tumor microenvironment and promote tumor progression in human gastric cancer. *Oncol. Rep.* **2011**, *25*, 1271–1277.
69. Meng, X.Y.; Zhou, C.H.; Ma, J.; Jiang, C.; Ji, P. Expression of interleukin-17 and its clinical significance in gastric cancer patients. *Med. Oncol.* **2012**, *29*, 3024–3028. [CrossRef] [PubMed]

70. Dai, Z.M.; Zhang, T.S.; Lin, S.; Zhang, W.G.; Liu, D.; Cao, X.M.; Li, H.B.; Wang, M.; Liu, X.H.; Liu, K.; et al. Role of IL-17A rs2275913 and IL-17F rs763780 polymorphisms in risk of cancer development: An update meta-analysis. *Sci. Rep.* **2016**, *6*, 20439. [CrossRef] [PubMed]

71. Muruyama, T.; Kono, K.; Mizukami, Y.; Kawaguchi, Y.; Mimura, K.; Watanabe, M.; Izawa, S.; Fujii, H. Distribution of Th17 cells and FoxP3(+) regulatory T cells in tumor-infiltrating lymphocytes, tumor-draining lymph nodes and peripheral blood lymphocytes in patients with gastric cancer. *Cancer Sci.* **2010**, *101*, 1947–1954. [CrossRef] [PubMed]

72. Kuai, W.X.; Wang, Q.; Yang, X.Z.; Zhao, Y.; Yu, R.; Tang, X.J. Interleukin-8 associates with adhesion, migration, invasion and chemosensitivity of human gastric cancer cells. *World J. Gastroenterol.* **2012**, *18*, 979–985. [CrossRef] [PubMed]

73. Bockerstett, K.A.; DiPaolo, R.J. Regulation of gastric carcinogenesis by inflammatory cytokines. *Cell Mol. Gastroenterol. Hepatol.* **2017**, *4*, 47–53. [CrossRef] [PubMed]

74. Huang, F.Y.; Chan, A.O.; Rashid, A.; Wong, D.K.; Seto, W.K.; Cho, C.H.; Lai, C.L.; Yuen, M.F. Interleukin 1β increases the risk of gastric cancer through induction of aberrant DNA methylation in a mouse model. *Oncol. Lett.* **2016**, *11*, 2919–2924. [CrossRef] [PubMed]

75. Al-Sammak, F.; Kalinski, T.; Winert, S.; Link, A.; Wex, T.; Malfertheiner, P. Gastric epithelial expression of IL-12 cytokine family in Helicobacter pylori infection in human: Is it head or tail of the coin? *PLoS ONE* **2013**, *8*, e75192. [CrossRef] [PubMed]

76. Tsai, C.Y.; Wang, C.S.; Tsai, M.M.; Chi, H.C.; Cheng, W.L.; Tseng, Y.H.; Chen, C.Y.; Lin, C.D.; Wu, J.I.; Wang, L.H.; et al. Interleukin-32 increase human gastric cancer cell invasion associated with tumor progression and metastasis. *Clin. Cancer Res.* **2014**, *20*, 2276–2288. [CrossRef] [PubMed]

77. Buzzelli, J.N.; Chalinor, H.V.; Pavlic, D.I.; Sutton, P.; Menheniott, T.R.; Giraud, A.S.; Judd, L.M. IL33 is a stomach alarmin that initiates a skewed Th2 response to injury and infection. *Cell. Mol. Gastroenterol. Hepatol.* **2015**, *1*, 203–221.e3. [CrossRef] [PubMed]

78. Lahner, E.; Esposito, G.; Galli, G.; Annibale, B. Atrophic gastritis and pre-malignant gastric lesions. *Transl. Gastrointest. Cancer* **2015**, *4*, 272–281.

79. Schneller, J.; Gupta, R.; Mustafa, J.; Villanueva, R.; Straus, E.W.; Raffaniello, R.D. Helicobacter pylori infection is associated with a high incidence of intestinal metaplasia in the gastric mucosa of patients at inner-city hospitals in New York. *Dig. Dis. Sci.* **2006**, *51*, 1801–1809. [CrossRef] [PubMed]

80. Wong, B.C.; Lam, S.K.; Wong, W.M.; Chen, J.S.; Zheng, T.T.; Feng, R.E.; Lai, K.C.; Cheng, W.H.; Yuen, S.T.; Leung, S.Y.; et al. Helicobacter pylori eradication to prevent gastric cancer in a high-risk region of China: A randomized controlled trial. *JAMA* **2004**, *291*, 187–194. [CrossRef] [PubMed]

81. Yamaoka, Y. Mechanisms of disease: Helicobacter pylori virulence factors. *Nat. Rev. Gastroenterol. Hepatol.* **2010**, *7*, 629–641. [CrossRef] [PubMed]

82. Yong, X.; Tang, B.; Li, B.-S.; Xie, R.; Hu, C.J.; Luo, G.; Qin, Y.; Dong, H.; Yang, S.M. Helicobacter pylori virulence factor CagA promotes tumorigenesis of gastric cancer via multiple signaling pathways. *Cell Commun. Signal.* **2015**, *13*, 1–13. [CrossRef] [PubMed]

83. Van Doorn, L.J.; Figueiredo, C.; Sanna, R.; Plaisier, A.; Schneeberger, P.; de Boer, W.; Quint, W. Clinical relevance of the cagA, vacA, and iceA status of Helicobacter pylori. *Gastroenterology* **1998**, *115*, 58–66. [CrossRef]

84. Correa, P.; Piazuelo, M.B. The gastric precancerous cascade. *J. Dig. Dis.* **2012**, *13*, 2–9. [CrossRef] [PubMed]

85. Elsborg, L.; Mosbech, J. Pernicious anaemia as a risk factor in gastric cancer. *Acta Med. Scand.* **1979**, *206*, 315–318. [CrossRef] [PubMed]

86. Nikou, G.C.; Angelopoulos, T.P. Current concepts on gastric carcinoid tumors. *Gastroenterol. Res. Pract.* **2012**, *2012*, 287825. [CrossRef] [PubMed]

87. Vanoli, A.; La Rosa, S.; Luinetti, O.; Klersy, C.; Manca, R.; Alvisi, C.; Rossi, S.; Trespi, E.; Zangrandi, A.; Sessa, F.; et al. Histologic changes in type A chronic atrophic gastritis indicating increased risk of neuroendocrine tumor development: The predictive role of dysplastic and severely hyperplastic enterochromaffin-like cell lesions. *Hum. Pathol.* **2013**, *44*, 1827–1837. [CrossRef] [PubMed]

88. Zhou, K.; Ho, W. Gastric carcinoids: Classification and Diagnosis. In *Management of Pancreatic Neuroendocrine Tumors*; Pisegna, R.J., Ed.; Springer: New York, NY, USA, 2015; pp. 83–93.

89. Burkitt, M.D.; Pritchard, D.M. Review article: Pathogenesis and management of gastric carcinoid tumours. *Aliment Pharmacol. Ther.* **2006**, *24*, 1305–1320. [CrossRef] [PubMed]

90. Minalyan, A.; Benhammou, N.J.; Artashesyan, A.; Lewis, S.M.; Pisegna, J.R. Autoimmune atrophic gastritis: Current perspectives. *Clin. Exp. Gastroenterol.* **2017**, *1*, 19–27. [CrossRef] [PubMed]

91. Visvader, J.E. Cells of origin in cancer. *Nature* **2011**, *469*, 314–322. [CrossRef] [PubMed]

92. Shibata, W.; Sue, S.; Tsumura, S.; Ishii, Y.; Sato, T.; Kameta, E.; Sugimori, M.; Yamada, H.; Kaneko, H.; Sasaki, T.; et al. Helicobacter-induced gastric inflammation alters the properties of gastric tissue stem/progenitor cells. *BMC Gastroenterol.* **2017**, *17*, 145. [CrossRef] [PubMed]

93. Tan, E.M. Autoantibodies as reporters identifying aberrant cellular mechanisms in tumorigenesis. *J. Clin. Investig.* **2001**, *108*, 1411–1415. [CrossRef] [PubMed]

94. Werner, S.; Chen, H.; Tao, S.; Brenner, H. Systematic review: Serum autoantibodies in the early detection of gastric cancer. *Int. J. Cancer* **2015**, *136*, 2243–2252. [CrossRef] [PubMed]

95. Macdonald, I.K.; Parsy-Kowalska, C.B.; Chapman, C.J. Autoantibodies: Opportunities for early cancer detection. *Trends Cancer* **2017**, *3*, 198–213. [CrossRef] [PubMed]

96. Liu, W.; Peng, B.; Lu, Y.; Xu, W.; Qian, W.; Zhang, J.Y. Autoantibodies to tumor-associated antigens as biomarkers in cancer immunodiagnosis. *Autoimmun. Rev.* **2011**, *10*, 331–335. [CrossRef] [PubMed]

97. Zaenker, P.; Ziman, M.R. Serologic autoantibodies as diagnostic cancer biomarkers—A review. *Cancer Epidemiol. Biomarkers Prev.* **2013**, *22*, 2161–2181. [CrossRef] [PubMed]

98. Flammann, H.T.; Kuhn, HM. P53 autoantibodies and cancer: Specificity, diagnosis and monitoring. In *Cancer and Autoimmunity*; Shoenfeld, Y., Gershwin, M.E., Eds.; Elsevier Science: Amsterdam, The Netherlands, 2000; pp. 181–188.

99. Saif, M.W.; Zalonis, A.; Syrigos, K. The clinical significance of autoantibodies in gastrointestinal malignancies: An overview. *Expert Opin. Biol. Ther.* **2007**, *7*, 493–507. [CrossRef] [PubMed]

100. Crawford, L.V.; Pim, D.C.; Bulbrook, R.D. Detection of antibodies against the cellular protein p53 in sera from patients with breast cancer. *Int. J. Cancer* **1982**, *30*, 403–408. [CrossRef] [PubMed]

101. Wurl, P.; Weigmann, F.; Meye, A.; Fittkau, M.; Rose, U.; Berger, D.; Rath, F.W.; Dralle, H.; Taubert, H. Detection of p53 autoantibodies in sera of gastric cancer patients and their prognostic relevance. *Scand. J. Gastroenterol.* **1997**, *32*, 1147–1151. [CrossRef] [PubMed]

102. Soussi, T. p53 Antibodies in the sera of patients with various types of cancer: A review. *Cancer Res.* **2000**, *60*, 1777–1788. [PubMed]

103. Shimada, H.; Ochiai, T.; Nomura, F. Japan p53 Antibody Research Group. Titration of serum p53 antibodies in 1085 patients with various types of malignant tumors: A multiinstitutional analysis by the Japan p53 Antibody Research Group. *Cancer* **2003**, *97*, 682–689. [CrossRef] [PubMed]

104. Shiota, G.; Ishida, M.; Noguchi, N.; Takano, Y.; Oyama, K.; Okubo, M.; Katayama, S.; Harada, K.; Hori, K.; Ashida, K.; et al. Clinical significance of serum P53 antibody in patients with gastric cancer. *Res. Commun. Mol. Pathol. Pharmacol.* **1998**, *99*, 41–51. [PubMed]

105. Maehara, Y.; Kakeji, Y.; Watanabe, A.; Baba, H.; Kusumoto, H.; Kohnoe, S.; Sugimachi, K. Clinical implications of serum anti-p53 antibodies for patients with gastric carcinoma. *Cancer* **1999**, *85*, 302–308. [CrossRef]

106. Ura, Y.; Ochi, Y.; Hamazu, M.; Ishida, M.; Nakajima, K.; Watanabe, T. Studies on circulating antibody against carcinoembryonic antigen (CEA) and CEA-like antigen in cancer patients. *Cancer Lett.* **1985**, *25*, 283–295. [CrossRef]

107. Albanopoulos, K.; Armakolas, A.; Konstadoulakis, M.M.; Leandros, E.; Tsiompanou, E.; Katsaragakis, S.; Alexiou, D.; Androulakis, G. Prognostic significance of circulating antibodies against carcinoembryonic antigen (anti-CEA) in patients with colon cancer. *Am. J. Gastroenterol.* **2000**, *95*, 1056–1061. [CrossRef] [PubMed]

108. Nakamura, H.; Hinoda, Y.; Nakagawa, N.; Makiguchi, Y.; Itoh, F.; Endo, T.; Imai, K. Detection of circulating anti-MUC1 mucin core protein antibodies in patients with colorectal cancer. *J. Gastroenterol.* **1998**, *33*, 354–361. [CrossRef] [PubMed]

109. Yagihashi, A.; Asanuma, K.; Nakamura, M.; Araya, J.; Mano, Y.; Torigoe, T.; Kobayashi, D.; Watanabe, N. Detection of anti-survivin antibody in gastrointestinal cancer patients. *Clin. Chem.* **2001**, *47*, 1729–1731. [PubMed]

110. Cho-Chung, Y.S. Autoantibody biomarkers in the detection of cancer. *Biochim. Biophys. Acta.* **2006**, *1762*, 587–591. [CrossRef] [PubMed]

111. Qiu, L.L.; Hua, P.Y.; Ye, L.L.; Wang, Y.C.; Qiu, T.; Bao, H.Z.; Wang, L. The detection of serum anti-p53 antibodies from patients with gastric carcinoma in China. *Cancer Detect Prev.* **2007**, *31*, 45–49. [CrossRef] [PubMed]

112. Shimizu, K.; Ueda, Y.; Yamagishi, H. Titration of serum p53 antibodies in patients with gastric cancer: A single-institute study of 40 patients. *Gastric Cancer* **2005**, *8*, 214–219. [CrossRef] [PubMed]

113. Shimada, H.; Noie, T.; Ohashi, M.; Oba, K.; Takahashi, Y. Clinical significance of serum tumor markers for gastric cancer: A systematic review of literature by the Task Force of the Japanese Gastric Cancer Association. *Gastric Cancer* **2014**, *17*, 26–33. [CrossRef] [PubMed]

114. Di Mario, F.; Cavallaro, L.G. Non-invasive tests in gastric diseases. *Dig. Liver Dis.* **2008**, *40*, 523–530. [CrossRef] [PubMed]

115. Majeed, W.; Iftikhar, A.; Khaliq, T.; Aslam, B.; Muzaffar, H.; Atta, K.; Mahmood, A.; Waris, S. Gastric carcinoma: Recent trends in diagnostic biomarkers and molecular targeted therapies. *Asian Pac. J. Cancer Prev.* **2016**, *17*, 3053–3060. [PubMed]

116. Zayakin, P.; Ancans, G.; Silina, K.; Meistere, I.; Kalnina, Z.; Andrejeva, D.; Endzelinš, E.; Ivanova, L.; Pismennaja, A.; Ruskule, A.; et al. Tumor-associated autoantibody signature for the early detection of gastric cancer. *Int. J. Cancer* **2013**, *132*, 137–147. [CrossRef] [PubMed]

117. Werner, S.; Chen, H.; Butt, J.; Michel, A.; Knebel, P.; Holleczek, B.; Zörnig, I.; Eichmüller, S.B.; Jäger, D.; Pawlita, M.; et al. Evaluation of the diagnostic value of 64 simultaneously measured autoantibodies for early detection of gastric cancer. *Sci. Rep.* **2016**, *6*, 25467. [CrossRef] [PubMed]

118. Zhou, S.L.; Ku, J.W.; Fan, Z.M.; Yue, W.B.; Du, F.; Zhou, Y.F. Detection of autoantibodies to a panel of tumor-associated antigens for the diagnosis values of gastric cardia adenocarcinoma. *Dis. Esophagus* **2015**, *28*, 371–379. [CrossRef] [PubMed]

119. Wang, P.; Song, C.; Xie, W.; Ye, H.; Wang, K.; Dai, L.; Zhang, Y.; Zhang, J. Evaluation of diagnostic value in using a panel of multiple tumor-associated antigens for immunodiagnosis of cancer. *J. Immunol. Res.* **2014**, *2014*, 512540. [CrossRef] [PubMed]

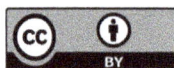

International Journal of
Molecular Sciences

MDPI

Review

Common Variable Immunodeficiency and Gastric Malignancies

Patrizia Leone, Angelo Vacca, Franco Dammacco and Vito Racanelli *

Department of Biomedical Sciences and Human Oncology, Unit of Internal Medicine, University of Bari
Medical School, 70124 Bari, Italy; patrizia.leone@uniba.it (P.L.); angelo.vacca@uniba.it (A.V.);
francesco.dammacco@uniba.it (F.D.)
* Correspondence: vito.racanelli1@uniba.it; Tel.: +39-080-5478-050; Fax: +39-080-5478-045

Received: 21 December 2017; Accepted: 31 January 2018; Published: 2 February 2018

Abstract: Common variable immunodeficiency (CVID) is an immunodeficiency disorder with a high
incidence of gastrointestinal manifestations and an increased risk of gastric carcinoma and lymphoma.
This review discusses the latest advancements into the immunological, clinical and diagnostic
aspects of gastric malignances in patients with CVID. The exact molecular pathways underlying
the relationships between CVID and gastric malignancies remain poorly understood. These include
genetics, immune dysregulation and chronic infections by *Helicobacter pylori*. Further studies are
needed to better stratify the risk for cancer in these patients, to elaborate surveillance programs aimed
at preventing these complications, and to develop new and more effective therapeutic approaches.

Keywords: common variable immunodeficiency; gastric cancer; human immunoglobulins;
lymphoproliferative disorders

1. Introduction

Common variable immunodeficiency (CVID) comprises a heterogeneous group of relatively
rare disorders characterized by remarkable decrease of two or three major immunoglobulin isotypes
(IgG, IgA, and IgM), often associated to defects in cell-mediated immunity [1]. Several immunological
studies of large cohorts of CVID patients have demonstrated phenotypic and functional abnormalities
of B cells [2,3], T cells [4–6], and antigen-presenting cells [7,8]. These abnormalities include mutations
that occur in genes essential for the co-operation between B and T cells in the germinal center, as well
as for intrinsic signaling pathways of such cells. A flow cytometry-based analysis of CVID patients
revealed a marked reduction of mature class-switched $CD27^+IgD^-IgM^-$ memory B cells and/or an
increased number of $CD19^+CD21^-$ immature B cells [3]. In addition, a decreased number of $CD4^+$
naïve T cells and regulatory T cells has been detected in the patients' peripheral blood, possibly
ascribable to defective generation of T cell precursors in the bone marrow [4]. Bone marrow biopsies
have in fact shown the absence or a significant decrease of plasma cells and, conversely, an increase of
diffuse and nodular T cell infiltrates [9].

The diagnosis of CVID obviously requires the exclusion of other causes of
hypogammaglobulinemia [10]. The mean age at diagnosis is 29 years for males and 33 years
for females, although the condition can be diagnosed at any age without gender predominance [11].
The prevalence varies widely worldwide, ranging from 1:100,000 to 1:10,000 of the general
population [12]. Although CVID is clinically highly variable and heterogeneous, severe, recurrent,
and chronic bacterial infections of the respiratory and gastrointestinal tracts are the major
characterizing features. In addition, approximately half of the patients suffer from non-infectious
complications, including autoimmune, lung and gastrointestinal disease, benign lymphoproliferation,
and malignancies [11]. In particular, the gastrointestinal tract [13] and the lymphoid tissue are among

the most affected systems [14–16], as shown by the fact that CVID patients have an almost 47-fold increased risk for gastric cancer and a 30-fold increased risk for lymphoma [17].

In this paper, we will provide an overview of the main clinical, diagnostic and immunological features of gastric malignancies in patients with CVID, with special emphasis for gastric carcinoma and lymphoproliferative disorders.

2. Genetic Abnormalities

CVID is a polygenic disease which is the result of numerous genetic immune defects, summarized in Table 1. The mode of inheritance is mostly autosomal dominant, and autosomal recessive in about 20% of the cases. The most frequently identified mutations have been discovered in the tumor necrosis factor (TNF) receptor superfamily member 13B (TNFRSF13B) gene encoding TACI (transmembrane activator and calcium-modulating cyclophilin ligand interactor), a B cell-specific TNF receptor superfamily member. Both homozygous and heterozygous coding variants have been identified in patients with CVID [18,19]. TACI is preferentially expressed on marginal zone B cells, CD27+ memory B cells, and plasma cells. Its ligands are the B cell-activating factor (BAFF) and the proliferation-inducing ligand (APRIL) involved in cell survival, apoptosis, and isotype switching [20].

Defects of TACI impair BAFF and APRIL signaling, and consequently plasma cell survival, maturation and class switch recombination, Ig production [21,22], and the removal of autoreactive B cells at the central B cell tolerance checkpoint, thus increasing the susceptibility of CVID patients to autoimmune diseases [23]. A181E and C104R are the two most frequent TNFRSF13B variants in these patients [18,19,24], although the mentioned mutations are neither necessary nor sufficient to cause CVID. While healthy individuals with a single pathogenic TNFRSF13B allele have a normal B cell phenotype, this is not the case for CVID patients with the same TNFRSF13B status, suggesting that the disease expression depends on the loss of compensating forces. Further studies are needed to elucidate the additional genetic and environmental factors that act in concert to generate the disease.

Homozygous and heterozygous mutations in the BAFF receptor (BAFF-R) gene, and single nucleotide polymorphisms resulting in BAFF-R missense mutations have been reported in CVID patients [25]. BAFF-R is required for B cell maturation and survival [26], and its mutations are associated to impairment in the proliferation, differentiation, and maturation of B lymphocytes [27]. Animal studies, carried out with both knockout and transgenic models, demonstrated that disruption of BAFF-R results in an immunological phenotype similar to that observed in CVID, suggesting that BAFF-R may be involved in the pathogenesis of CVID [28].

Biallelic deleterious mutations in members of the CD19 B-cell receptor complex (CD19, CD21, and CD81) and CD20 could also be involved in the onset of CVID [29–31]. Homozygous deletion in the inducible co-stimulator (ICOS) gene has been associated with adult-onset CVID [32]. ICOS belongs to the family of co-stimulatory T cell molecules and is expressed by antigen-activated T cells. Its unique ligand is ICOS-L expressed constitutively on B cells [33]. ICOS:ICOS-L interaction plays an important role in mediating T-B cell cooperation and promoting the terminal differentiation of B cells into memory cells and plasma cells. Patients with ICOS deletion displayed a reduced number of naïve, switched and memory B cells as well as low serum Ig levels [32]. This is further supported by the results achieved in ICOS and ICOS-L knockout mice, both showing a defect in germinal center formation and in humoral immune responses, due to the lack of T cell-mediated help to the B cells [34].

Table 1. Genetic immune defects in common variable immunodeficiency.

Gene	Defect	References
TNFRSF13B	Homozygous and heterozygous mutations	[18,19,24]
BAFF-R	Homozygous and heterozygous mutations	[25]
CD20	Homozygous mutations	[29]
CD19-B-cell receptor complex	Homozygous mutations	[30,31]
ICOS	Homozygous deletions	[32]
Genes implicated in DNA repair *(MSH5, MSH2, MLH1, RAD50 and NBS1)*	Heterozygous non-synonymous mutations	[35]
CARD11	Heterozygous single nucleotide polymorphisms	[36]
Bob1	Heterozygous single nucleotide polymorphisms	[36]
MHC region	Single nucleotide polymorphisms	[37]
ADAM	Single nucleotide polymorphisms	[37]
CTLA4	Heterozygous nonsense mutations Frameshift deletion Intronic mutations	[38]
PIK3CD	Heterozygous splice site mutations Gain-of-function mutations	[39]
NFκB2	Heterozygous frameshift mutation Heterozygous nonsense mutation	[40]
PLCG2	Deletions	[41]
LRBA	Homozygous mutations	[42]
CD27	Homozygous mutations	[43]

TNFRSF13B, tumor necrosis factor receptor superfamily member 13B; BAFF-R, B cell-activating factor receptor; ICOS, inducible costimulatory; CARD, caspase activation and recruitment domain; Bob1, B cell-specific transcriptional co-activator; ADAM, disintegrin and metalloproteinas genes; CTLA4, cytotoxic T lymphocyte antigen-4; PIK3CD, phosphatidylinositol-4,5-bisphosphate 3-kinase catalytic subunit delta; NFκB2, nuclear factor kappa B2; PLCG2, phospholipase C gamma 2; LRBA, lipopolysaccharide-responsive beige-like anchor.

The described mutations, however, account for less than 15% of CVID cases. The remaining 85% of the patients do not have a known genetic defect and it is likely that other genes besides those already identified may be involved in the pathogenesis of the CVID. For example, single nucleotide polymorphisms in genes implicated in deoxyribonucleic acid (DNA) repair (MSH5, MSH2, MLH1, RAD50, and NBS1) and in genes involved in B cell development, encoding the caspase activation and recruitment domain (CARD)11 and the B cell-specific transcriptional co-activator Bob1, could be associated with CVID [35,36]. Furthermore, a genome-wide association study, using single nucleotide polymorphism arrays and copy number variation, revealed a strong relationship between CVID and the MHC region as well as between CVID and a disintegrin and metalloproteinase genes (ADAM) [37].

In addition, a CVID-like syndrome, characterized by hypogammaglobulinemia, progressive loss of circulating B cells, immune dysregulation, and lymphocytic infiltration of target organs was demonstrated to be caused by heterozygous mutations in: (a) cytotoxic T lymphocyte antigen-4 (CTLA4) involved in T and B lymphocyte homeostasis [38]; (b) phosphatidylinositol-4,5-bisphosphate 3-kinase catalytic subunit delta (PIK3CD) gene, resulting in hyperactivation of the PI3K signaling pathway important for B and T cell development, differentiation, and function [39]; (c) nuclear factor kappa B2 (NFκB2) required for B cell development and antibody production [40]; (d) phospholipase C gamma 2 (PLCG2) causing gain of PLCγ(2) function, a signaling molecule expressed in B cells [41]; (e) lipopolysaccharide-responsive beige-like anchor (LRBA) causing severe defects in B cell development and activation [42]; and (f) CD27, a lymphocyte costimulatory molecule implicated in B cell and plasma cell function, survival, and differentiation [43].

3. Common Variable Immunodeficiency and Gastric Cancer

Many studies reported an increased risk of gastric cancer in CVID patients [15–17,44,45]. The first evidence was described in 1985 when a prospective study of 220 patients with CVID followed for 11 years showed a 47-fold increased risk of stomach cancer [17]. A multicenter study which examined 176 Danish and Swedish patients with CVID and their relatives reported a risk of stomach cancer 10-fold higher for CVID subjects, whereas no increased risk was found for this or any other type of cancer among 626 relatives of CVID patients. This suggests that the increased risk of gastric cancer is related to the immunodeficiency per se, rather than to specific genetic alterations shared with their relatives [45]. In an analysis of the Australasian Society of Clinical Immunology and Allergy primary immunodeficiency disease registry of 1132 subjects from 79 centers, it was shown that only subjects with CVID and ataxia telangiectasia had an increased risk of cancer. A high relative risk in relation to an age-matched general population was observed for non-Hodgkin's lymphoma (NHL), leukemia, and gastric cancer [16].

In a recent study, the incidence of cancer in patients with primary immunodeficiency diseases enrolled in the United States Immune Deficiency Network registry was assessed compared with age-adjusted cancer incidence in the Surveillance, Epidemiology and End Results Program database. An increased risk of NHL, gastric cancer, and skin cancer was observed in 1285 patients with CVID. Gastric cancer, in particular, was more common than expected ($n = 2$ in men and $n = 3$ in women vs. expected rates of $n = 0.4$ in men ($p = 0.011$) and $n = 0.7$ in women ($p = 0.005$)) [44].

The exact mechanisms underlying an enhanced frequency of gastric cancer in patients with CVID are unknown, but a possible sequence of events is schematized in Figure 1. The weakened immunity to potentially carcinogenic pathogens, such as *Helicobacter pylori* (HP), and the impaired tumor cell surveillance should obviously be considered predisposing factors to gastric cancer. Several studies have in fact ascribed the higher incidence of gastric cancer to HP infection (reviewed in [46]) and achlorhydria [17]. Eradication of HP in patients with non-atrophic gastritis has been demonstrated to prevent the subsequent development of gastric cancer [47]. Data from prospective studies revealed a two to nine fold increased risk of gastric cancer in the general population with HP infection [48,49]. More recently, however, gastric cancer appears rarer in CVID, possibly due to the more common use of antibiotics that would eradicate HP. Probably, the gastrointestinal defects associated with CVID, such as the decreased production of gastric IgA (with bactericidal activity against HP) and hydrochloric acid, may result in enhanced HP colonization and gastric inflammation, thus promoting carcinogenesis [50].

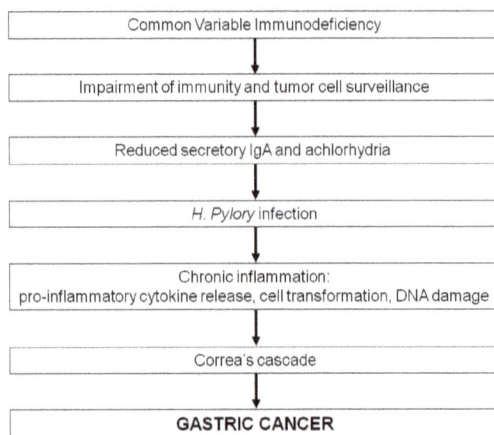

Figure 1. Hypothetical mechanisms of gastric cancer in patients with CVID.

HP causes chronic gastritis by stimulating the release of pro-inflammatory cytokines and favoring achlorhydria; in addition, certain strains produce virulence factors with oncogenic effects on the gastric epithelium. It induces upregulation of oncogenes and silencing of tumor suppressor genes, triggering a stepwise cascade of events ranging from intestinal metaplasia to dysplasia to neoplasia, the so called Correa's cascade (Figure 1) [51]. Moreover, an inflammatory response is generated, in that replicating cells are invaded by neutrophils and monocytes, which release reactive oxygen species (ROS) and reactive nitrogen species (RNS), thus inducing DNA breaks and point mutations in genes critical for cell replication and death [52]. It should also be emphasized that hypochlorhydria and achlorhydria may result in impaired defense against HP infection and enhanced bacterial overgrowth, including nitrate reducing strains, with consequent increased levels of N-nitroso compounds in the gastric juice. This endogenous nitrosation can promote the progression from gastric atrophy to intestinal metaplasia, dysplasia, and eventually carcinoma [46,53,54].

4. Features of CVID-Associated Gastric Cancer

CVID-associated gastric cancer typically displays peculiar features. First, it is diagnosed in patients younger than the overall gastric cancer population. Second, it is moderately to poorly differentiated intestinal-type adenocarcinoma, containing a high number of intra-tumoral lymphocytes. Third, it arises in a background of gastritis characterized by severe atrophy, pan-gastric distribution, intestinal metaplasia, plasma cell paucity, lymphoid nodular aggregates, and apoptotic activity [55]. This latter feature, which is reminiscent of gastritis from HP, may also underlie autoimmune gastritis given that autoimmunity is a well-known complication of CVID and pernicious anemia affects approximately 10% of patients [46]. Pernicious anemia is readily suspected by a low serum vitamin B12 and macrocytic red blood cells, although a precise diagnosis in CVID patients is more difficult because of the lack of typical anti-parietal cell and anti-intrinsic factor autoantibodies. Tissue damage in autoimmune gastritis is indeed mediated not only by autoantibodies targeting the parietal cell proton pump and intrinsic factor, but also by sensitized T cells. When fully developed, autoimmune gastritis displays dense and diffuse lymphoplasmacytic inflammation with the oxyntic epithelia replaced by atrophic (and metaplastic) mucosa, creating the phenotypic background in which gastric intestinal-type adenocarcinomas may arise [56,57]. Several studies have also addressed the role of HP infection in the pathogenesis of autoimmune gastritis, and there is evidence to support a mechanism of molecular mimicry between HP antigens and the proton pump [58]. Epidemiological studies suggest that a significant number of patients with autoimmune gastritis suffered from, or still have, HP infection and anti-proton pump autoantibodies have consistently been demonstrated in HP-infected patients.

An additional, potential abnormality that can be identified in patients with CVID-associated gastric cancer is granuloma resembling sarcoidosis [59]. Whether the granuloma reflects a primary T-cell defect, or an abnormal response to infectious agents is presently unknown. In any case, fungal and mycobacterial special stains are always appropriate when granulomas are identified, given that tuberculosis has been described in the setting of CVID [60].

5. Gastric Cancer Screening and Prevention in CVID Patients

Gastric cancer is the fourth most common cancer and the second leading cause of cancer death worldwide [61]. There is no ideal protocol for gastric cancer screening in high-risk CVID individuals, and prerequisites of screening programs differ from country to country because of the variable cancer incidence and mortality in each country, ethnic differences, and socio-economic conditions [62]. Consensus exists, however, over the usefulness of a risk assessment primarily based on the diagnosis of HP infection and/or pernicious anemia.

Rather than on HP antibody test, the diagnosis of HP infection is usually based on urea breath test (UBT), stool antigen immunoassay and/or endoscopic biopsy. UBT is largely preferred being widely available, accurate, and noninvasive, with a sensitivity and specificity of roughly 90% [63]. An additional noninvasive method is the stool test, characterized by sensitivity in the range of 69–92%

and specificity of approximately 75–89% [64]. HP infection is often asymptomatic, thus accounting for its uncommon detection and eradication at an early stage. Following its eradication, HP rarely recurs in the general population [65]. Whether this rare recurrence is also common to patients with CVID, given their lack of secretory IgA on the gastric mucosa, has not been established.

The diagnosis of pernicious anemia can be made by showing the presence of megaloblastic or macrocytic anemia, and measuring serum vitamin B_{12} and iron levels. Therefore, a screening protocol to target patients with CVID who are at the highest risk of gastric cancer should include three easy, non-invasive tests such as UBT, serum B_{12}, and serum iron [65].

Regardless of the presence of pernicious anemia or HP infection, patients with CVID should be considered at increased risk for gastric cancer [15–17,44,45]. We propose a step-by-step evaluation of all patients with CVID, with invasiveness increasing stepwise according to the risk (Figure 2). The initial screening should focus on noninvasive tests, such as UBT to detect HP infection and the measurement of serum vitamin B_{12} and iron to detect the presence of pernicious anemia. If patients are positive for HP infection, HP eradication should follow standard practice, repeating the UBT after one month to demonstrate that treatment was effective. Because HP infection is the major cause of gastric cancer, eradication of infection should be the most effective method to prevent its occurrence [47]. However, only few studies have reported the effects of screening and treating this pathogen at the population levels [66], given the lack of infrastructures for delivery of systematic screening services, the lack of standardization to ensure that each subject receives the correct diagnostic testing and antibiotic treatment, and limitation of resources.

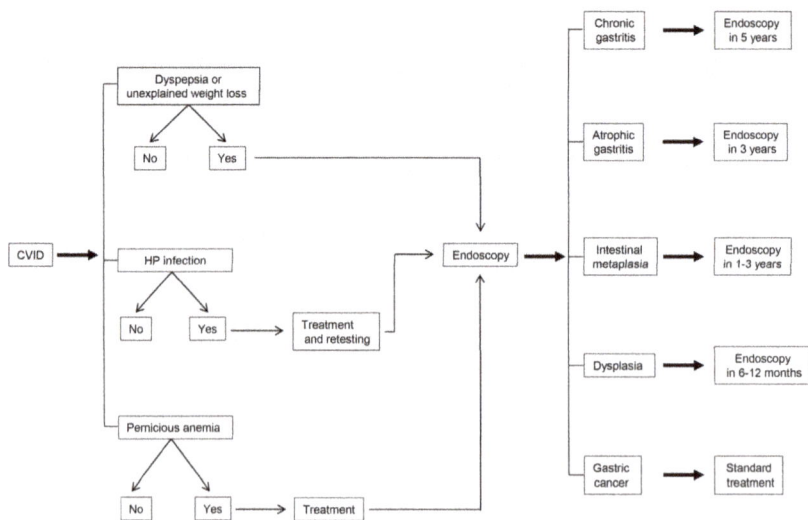

Figure 2. Protocol of screening and surveillance for gastric cancer in patients with CVID.

If patients have low serum vitamin B_{12} and iron concentrations, their replacement should obviously be effected. In addition, in patients negative for pernicious anemia it is advisable to repeat the screening tests yearly, in that pernicious anemia or gastritis may appear later on.

During regular follow-up for CVID, patients with low serum levels of vitamin B_{12}, patients with positive UBT and those with dyspeptic symptoms or unexplained weight loss should undergo upper gastrointestinal endoscopy, including biopsies of the antrum and fundus. Patients with premalignant lesions should receive endoscopic surveillance.

In the absence of established guidelines, it seems reasonable to adopt the following procedure: (a) no follow-up endoscopy in patients with normal histopathology and (b) repeat endoscopy after a time interval ranging from a few months to 5 years, depending on the histopathological diagnosis [67,68] (Figure 2). The time intervals for follow-up of gastric precancerous lesions are based upon data on estimated rates of progression to gastric cancer. Progression rates to cancer vary from: 0 to 1.8% per year for atrophic gastritis, 0 to 10% per year for intestinal metaplasia, and 0 to 73% per year for dysplasia [69]. Obviously, the time intervals of follow-up should be personalized in each individual patient depending on location, severity and extent of gastric pathology and the occurrence of other risk factors for gastric cancer.

6. CVID and Gastric Lymphoma

Lymphoproliferative disorders are common in CVID. Gastrointestinal lymphoid hyperplasia and/or splenomegaly are found in at least 20% of the patients with CVID [70]. Splenomegaly has in fact been reported in 26% of a cohort of 2212 European patients [15]. The cause of CVID-associated gastrointestinal lymphoproliferation is not known, but the potential role of bacterial, protozoal (mainly *Giardia lamblia*), and viral gastrointestinal infections should be kept in mind. Their eradication may be difficult for some patients.

Biopsies of lymph nodes usually show atypical or reactive lymphoid hyperplasia, but granulomatous inflammation may also be found. Typical features are the lack of plasma cells and the presence of ill-defined germinal centers in lymph nodes and other lymphoid tissues [71]. These same tissues should be examined for B- and T-cell clonality, using fluorescence markers, cytogenetics, and/or molecular analysis to rule out lymphoid malignancy. In lymph nodes with B-cell infiltrates, examination for EBV-encoded RNAs by in situ hybridization should be performed, often showing an expansion of transitional $CD19^+CD38^{++}IgM^{high}$ B cells or $CD19^+CD38^{low}CD21^{low}$ B cells [72]. Given that patients with CVID may have unusual lymphoid structures with loss of characteristic boundaries, it is important that the biopsies be examined by an experienced pathologist, in that the presence of clonal lymphocytes is not in itself diagnostic of lymphoma because these cells can be found in CVID lymphoid tissue showing reactive hyperplasia [70].

The risk for lymphoma in CVID is estimated to lie between 1.4% and 7% [16,44,45,73]. About 2–8% of subjects with CVID are diagnosed with NHL, in step with the longer survival of these patients [70]. In a study carried out on 248 consecutive CVID patients, who have been followed-up for 1–25 years, 23 patients were diagnosed with lymphoid malignancies. Specifically, 19 patients had NHL, three Hodgkin's disease, and one Waldenström's macroglobulinemia [74]. In this context, it is worth emphasizing that: (a) NHL occurs rarely in the pediatric population [75] and (b) in most cases it is usually B cell in type, extranodal, EBV-negative and more frequent in females than males [76]. A study of 98 CVID patients who have been followed-up for periods of 1–13 years showed an eight- to 13-fold increase in cancer in general and a 438-fold increase in lymphoma for females [76]. An earlier report based on a European cohort of 176 patients found three of the four NHL in women [45].

Extranodal marginal zone NHL arising in mucosal sites, named also mucosa-associated lymphoid tissue (MALT) lymphomas or "maltomas", can also affect CVID patients. In the earlier literature, 10 cases of extranodal marginal zone lymphoma complicating CVID have been reported [73], but probably many more cases are clinically hidden. Extranodal marginal zone lymphomas are low-grade B cell lymphomas that occur in organs with lymphoid infiltration, due to long-term infectious or autoimmune stimulation [14]. A causal relationship is likely to exist between HP infection and extranodal marginal zone lymphoma with gastric location, in that HP infection is present in more than 90% of the patients with this type of lymphoma [77].

Finally, a subset of CVID patients with T cell lymphoma should be mentioned. Gottesman et al. described the occurrence of a peripheral extranodal T cell lymphoma arising in the bone marrow, liver and central nervous system of a patient with CVID. Immunohistochemical phenotyping and gene rearrangement studies revealed a T cell origin of this lymphoma. It was not associated with EBV infection of the lymphoma cells [78]. Recently, Jesus et al. illustrated a case of CVID associated with hepato-splenic T-cell lymphoma mimicking juvenile systemic lupus erythematosus. The autopsy showed a diffuse involvement of bone marrow, spleen, liver, and lungs. The lymphoma cells were positive for CD3 and negative for CD20 and lysozyme expression [79]. CD8$^+$ granulomatous cutaneous T-cell lymphoma is a rarely encountered entity that appears to be associated with immunodeficiency, as reported by Gammon et al. in a retrospective review of four cases. Patients were characterized by an asymptomatic papulo-nodular eruption occurring in association with immunodeficiency [80].

Usually, patients with splenomegaly alone may not need treatment. Likewise, persistent hypertrophy of lymph nodes should suggest to review the diagnosis in order to exclude lymphoma but, again, this does not imply that treatment should be given. The administration of corticosteroids is commonly associated to regression of these phenomena, but they may recur when steroids are tapered. A rapid increase in adenopathy or splenomegaly should prompt evaluation for possible malignant transformation. Lymphoma may be difficult to distinguish from polyclonal lymphoid proliferation. Clonal analysis can be misleading because oligoclonal lymphocyte subpopulations have been found in biopsies, irrespective of histology [70]. Treatment follows the current protocols for immunocompetent patients.

7. Conclusions

CVID seems to be a predisposing factor to gastric malignancies. The reasons for this increased susceptibility are still unclear and additional animal models of CVID are needed to establish mechanisms of its relationship to cancer. The impaired immunity to potentially carcinogenic pathogens, the weakened tumor cell surveillance, and T and B cell defects are no doubt predisposing factors.

Due to the great heterogeneity of CVID patients, there are no set rules regarding their therapy and follow-up. Although treatment obviously requires the infusion of human immunoglobulins, an unsettled point is whether an adequate immunoglobulin replacement is sufficient to prevent the increased risk of malignancy. Bacterial and viral infections must be treated. Low-dose corticosteroids can be administered to ameliorate gastrointestinal lymphoproliferative disorders, but higher doses should be avoided to prevent the risk of opportunistic infections [12]. Treatment of gastric cancer and lymphoma must follow the current protocols for immunocompetent patients. Further studies are recommended to better identify patients at high risk of gastric neoplasias and to better treat them.

Acknowledgments: This work was supported by the Italian Association for Cancer Research (AIRC) and by Fondo di Sviluppo e Coesione 2007-2013—APQ Ricerca Regione Puglia "Programma regionale a sostegno della specializzazione intelligente e della sostenibilità sociale ed ambientale—FutureInResearch".

Author Contributions: Patrizia Leone and Vito Racanelli wrote the manuscript. Franco Dammacco and Angelo Vacca critically revised the manuscript for important intellectual content. All authors reviewed the report, approved the draft submission, and agreed to be accountable for all aspects of this study.

Conflicts of Interest: The authors declare no conflict of interest.

References

1. Abbott, J.K.; Gelfand, E.W. Common Variable Immunodeficiency: Diagnosis, Management, and Treatment. *Immunol. Allergy Clin. N. Am.* **2015**, *35*, 637–658. [CrossRef] [PubMed]
2. Anzilotti, C.; Kienzler, A.K.; Lopez-Granados, E.; Gooding, S.; Davies, B.; Pandit, H.; Lucas, M.; Price, A.; Littlewood, T.; van der Burg, M.; et al. Key stages of bone marrow B-cell maturation are defective in patients with common variable immunodeficiency disorders. *J. Allergy Clin. Immunol.* **2015**, *136*, 487–490. [CrossRef] [PubMed]
3. Warnatz, K.; Denz, A.; Drager, R.; Braun, M.; Groth, C.; Wolff-Vorbeck, G.; Eibl, H.; Schlesier, M.; Peter, H.H. Severe deficiency of switched memory B cells (CD27$^+$IgM$^-$IgD$^-$) in subgroups of patients with common variable immunodeficiency: A new approach to classify a heterogeneous disease. *Blood* **2002**, *99*, 1544–1551. [CrossRef] [PubMed]
4. Arandi, N.; Mirshafiey, A.; Jeddi-Tehrani, M.; Abolhassani, H.; Sadeghi, B.; Mirminachi, B.; Shaghaghi, M.; Aghamohammadi, A. Evaluation of CD4$^+$CD25$^+$FOXP3$^+$ regulatory T cells function in patients with common variable immunodeficiency. *Cell. Immunol.* **2013**, *281*, 129–133. [CrossRef] [PubMed]

5. Di Renzo, M.; Zhou, Z.; George, I.; Becker, K.; Cunningham-Rundles, C. Enhanced apoptosis of T cells in common variable immunodeficiency (CVID): Role of defective CD28 co-stimulation. *Clin. Exp. Immunol.* **2000**, *120*, 503–511. [CrossRef] [PubMed]

6. Giovannetti, A.; Pierdominici, M.; Mazzetta, F.; Marziali, M.; Renzi, C.; Mileo, A.M.; de Felice, M.; Mora, B.; Esposito, A.; Carello, R.; et al. Unravelling the complexity of T cell abnormalities in common variable immunodeficiency. *J. Immunol.* **2007**, *178*, 3932–3943. [CrossRef] [PubMed]

7. Taraldsrud, E.; Fevang, B.; Aukrust, P.; Beiske, K.H.; Floisand, Y.; Froland, S.; Rollag, H.; Olweus, J. Common variable immunodeficiency revisited: Normal generation of naturally occurring dendritic cells that respond to Toll-like receptors 7 and 9. *Clin. Exp. Immunol.* **2014**, *175*, 439–448. [CrossRef] [PubMed]

8. Viallard, J.F.; Camou, F.; Andre, M.; Liferman, F.; Moreau, J.F.; Pellegrin, J.L.; Blanco, P. Altered dendritic cell distribution in patients with common variable immunodeficiency. *Arthritis Res. Ther.* **2005**, *7*, R1052–R1055. [CrossRef] [PubMed]

9. Ochtrop, M.L.; Goldacker, S.; May, A.M.; Rizzi, M.; Draeger, R.; Hauschke, D.; Stehfest, C.; Warnatz, K.; Goebel, H.; Technau-Ihling, K.; et al. T and B lymphocyte abnormalities in bone marrow biopsies of common variable immunodeficiency. *Blood* **2011**, *118*, 309–318. [CrossRef] [PubMed]

10. Conley, M.E.; Notarangelo, L.D.; Etzioni, A. Diagnostic criteria for primary immunodeficiencies. Representing PAGID (Pan-American Group for Immunodeficiency) and ESID (European Society for Immunodeficiencies). *Clin. Immunol.* **1999**, *93*, 190–197. [CrossRef] [PubMed]

11. Chapel, H.; Lucas, M.; Lee, M.; Bjorkander, J.; Webster, D.; Grimbacher, B.; Fieschi, C.; Thon, V.; Abedi, M.R.; Hammarstrom, L. Common variable immunodeficiency disorders: Division into distinct clinical phenotypes. *Blood* **2008**, *112*, 277–286. [CrossRef] [PubMed]

12. Bonilla, F.A.; Barlan, I.; Chapel, H.; Costa-Carvalho, B.T.; Cunningham-Rundles, C.; de la Morena, M.T.; Espinosa-Rosales, F.J.; Hammarstrom, L.; Nonoyama, S.; Quinti, I.; et al. International Consensus Document (ICON): Common Variable Immunodeficiency Disorders. *J. Allergy Clin. Immunol. Pract.* **2016**, *4*, 38–59. [CrossRef] [PubMed]

13. Uzzan, M.; Ko, H.M.; Mehandru, S.; Cunningham-Rundles, C. Gastrointestinal Disorders Associated with Common Variable Immune Deficiency (CVID) and Chronic Granulomatous Disease (CGD). *Curr. Gastroenterol. Rep.* **2016**, *18*, 17. [CrossRef] [PubMed]

14. Cunningham-Rundles, C.; Cooper, D.L.; Duffy, T.P.; Strauchen, J. Lymphomas of mucosal-associated lymphoid tissue in common variable immunodeficiency. *Am. J. Hematol.* **2002**, *69*, 171–178. [CrossRef] [PubMed]

15. Gathmann, B.; Mahlaoui, N.; Gerard, L.; Oksenhendler, E.; Warnatz, K.; Schulze, I.; Kindle, G.; Kuijpers, T.W.; Dutch, W.I.D.; van Beem, R.T.; et al. Clinical picture and treatment of 2212 patients with common variable immunodeficiency. *J. Allergy Clin. Immunol.* **2014**, *134*, 116–126. [CrossRef] [PubMed]

16. Vajdic, C.M.; Mao, L.; van Leeuwen, M.T.; Kirkpatrick, P.; Grulich, A.E.; Riminton, S. Are antibody deficiency disorders associated with a narrower range of cancers than other forms of immunodeficiency? *Blood* **2010**, *116*, 1228–1234. [CrossRef] [PubMed]

17. Kinlen, L.J.; Webster, A.D.; Bird, A.G.; Haile, R.; Peto, J.; Soothill, J.F.; Thompson, R.A. Prospective study of cancer in patients with hypogammaglobulinaemia. *Lancet* **1985**, *1*, 263–266. [CrossRef]

18. Castigli, E.; Wilson, S.A.; Garibyan, L.; Rachid, R.; Bonilla, F.; Schneider, L.; Geha, R.S. TACI is mutant in common variable immunodeficiency and IgA deficiency. *Nat. Genet.* **2005**, *37*, 829–834. [CrossRef] [PubMed]

19. Salzer, U.; Bacchelli, C.; Buckridge, S.; Pan-Hammarstrom, Q.; Jennings, S.; Lougaris, V.; Bergbreiter, A.; Hagena, T.; Birmelin, J.; Plebani, A.; et al. Relevance of biallelic versus monoallelic TNFRSF13B mutations in distinguishing disease-causing from risk-increasing TNFRSF13B variants in antibody deficiency syndromes. *Blood* **2009**, *113*, 1967–1976. [CrossRef] [PubMed]

20. Ng, L.G.; Mackay, C.R.; Mackay, F. The BAFF/APRIL system: Life beyond B lymphocytes. *Mol. Immunol.* **2005**, *42*, 763–772. [CrossRef] [PubMed]

21. Castigli, E.; Scott, S.; Dedeoglu, F.; Bryce, P.; Jabara, H.; Bhan, A.K.; Mizoguchi, E.; Geha, R.S. Impaired IgA class switching in APRIL-deficient mice. *Proc. Natl. Acad. Sci. USA* **2004**, *101*, 3903–3908. [CrossRef] [PubMed]

22. Romberg, N.; Virdee, M.; Chamberlain, N.; Oe, T.; Schickel, J.N.; Perkins, T.; Cantaert, T.; Rachid, R.; Rosengren, S.; Palazzo, R.; et al. TNF receptor superfamily member 13b (TNFRSF13B) hemizygosity reveals transmembrane activator and CAML interactor haploinsufficiency at later stages of B-cell development. *J. Allergy Clin. Immunol.* **2015**, *136*, 1315–1325. [CrossRef] [PubMed]

23. Azizi, G.; Abolhassani, H.; Kiaee, F.; Tavakolinia, N.; Rafiemanesh, H.; Yazdani, R.; Mahdaviani, S.A.; Mohammadikhajehdehi, S.; Tavakol, M.; Ziaee, V.; et al. Autoimmunity and its association with regulatory T cells and B cell subsets in patients with common variable immunodeficiency. *Allergol. Immunopathol.* **2017**. [CrossRef] [PubMed]

24. Pan-Hammarstrom, Q.; Salzer, U.; Du, L.; Bjorkander, J.; Cunningham-Rundles, C.; Nelson, D.L.; Bacchelli, C.; Gaspar, H.B.; Offer, S.; Behrens, T.W.; et al. Reexamining the role of TACI coding variants in common variable immunodeficiency and selective IgA deficiency. *Nat. Genet.* **2007**, *39*, 429–430. [CrossRef] [PubMed]

25. Pieper, K.; Rizzi, M.; Speletas, M.; Smulski, C.R.; Sic, H.; Kraus, H.; Salzer, U.; Fiala, G.J.; Schamel, W.W.; Lougaris, V.; et al. A common single nucleotide polymorphism impairs B-cell activating factor receptor's multimerization, contributing to common variable immunodeficiency. *J. Allergy Clin. Immunol.* **2014**, *133*, 1222–1225. [CrossRef] [PubMed]

26. Schweighoffer, E.; Vanes, L.; Nys, J.; Cantrell, D.; McCleary, S.; Smithers, N.; Tybulewicz, V.L. The BAFF receptor transduces survival signals by co-opting the B cell receptor signaling pathway. *Immunity* **2013**, *38*, 475–488. [CrossRef] [PubMed]

27. Castigli, E.; Wilson, S.A.; Scott, S.; Dedeoglu, F.; Xu, S.; Lam, K.P.; Bram, R.J.; Jabara, H.; Geha, R.S. TACI and BAFF-R mediate isotype switching in B cells. *J. Exp. Med.* **2005**, *201*, 35–39. [CrossRef] [PubMed]

28. Gross, J.A.; Dillon, S.R.; Mudri, S.; Johnston, J.; Littau, A.; Roque, R.; Rixon, M.; Schou, O.; Foley, K.P.; Haugen, H.; et al. TACI-Ig neutralizes molecules critical for B cell development and autoimmune disease. impaired B cell maturation in mice lacking BLyS. *Immunity* **2001**, *15*, 289–302. [CrossRef]

29. Kuijpers, T.W.; Bende, R.J.; Baars, P.A.; Grummels, A.; Derks, I.A.; Dolman, K.M.; Beaumont, T.; Tedder, T.F.; van Noesel, C.J.; Eldering, E.; et al. CD20 deficiency in humans results in impaired T cell-independent antibody responses. *J. Clin. Investig.* **2010**, *120*, 214–222. [CrossRef] [PubMed]

30. Thiel, J.; Kimmig, L.; Salzer, U.; Grudzien, M.; Lebrecht, D.; Hagena, T.; Draeger, R.; Voelxen, N.; Bergbreiter, A.; Jennings, S.; et al. Genetic CD21 deficiency is associated with hypogammaglobulinemia. *J. Allergy Clin. Immunol.* **2012**, *129*, 801–810. [CrossRef] [PubMed]

31. Van Zelm, M.C.; Smet, J.; Adams, B.; Mascart, F.; Schandene, L.; Janssen, F.; Ferster, A.; Kuo, C.C.; Levy, S.; van Dongen, J.J.; et al. CD81 gene defect in humans disrupts CD19 complex formation and leads to antibody deficiency. *J. Clin. Investig.* **2010**, *120*, 1265–1274. [CrossRef] [PubMed]

32. Salzer, U.; Maul-Pavicic, A.; Cunningham-Rundles, C.; Urschel, S.; Belohradsky, B.H.; Litzman, J.; Holm, A.; Franco, J.L.; Plebani, A.; Hammarstrom, L.; et al. ICOS deficiency in patients with common variable immunodeficiency. *Clin. Immunol.* **2004**, *113*, 234–240. [CrossRef] [PubMed]

33. Hutloff, A.; Dittrich, A.M.; Beier, K.C.; Eljaschewitsch, B.; Kraft, R.; Anagnostopoulos, I.; Kroczek, R.A. ICOS is an inducible T-cell co-stimulator structurally and functionally related to CD28. *Nature* **1999**, *397*, 263–266. [CrossRef] [PubMed]

34. Wong, S.C.; Oh, E.; Ng, C.H.; Lam, K.P. Impaired germinal center formation and recall T-cell-dependent immune responses in mice lacking the costimulatory ligand B7-H2. *Blood* **2003**, *102*, 1381–1388. [CrossRef] [PubMed]

35. Offer, S.M.; Pan-Hammarstrom, Q.; Hammarstrom, L.; Harris, R.S. Unique DNA repair gene variations and potential associations with the primary antibody deficiency syndromes IgAD and CVID. *PLoS ONE* **2010**, *5*, e12260. [CrossRef] [PubMed]

36. Tampella, G.; Baronio, M.; Vitali, M.; Soresina, A.; Badolato, R.; Giliani, S.; Plebani, A.; Lougaris, V. Evaluation of CARMA1/CARD11 and Bob1 as candidate genes in common variable immunodeficiency. *J. Investig. Allergol. Clin. Immunol.* **2011**, *21*, 348–353. [PubMed]

37. Orange, J.S.; Glessner, J.T.; Resnick, E.; Sullivan, K.E.; Lucas, M.; Ferry, B.; Kim, C.E.; Hou, C.; Wang, F.; Chiavacci, R.; et al. Genome-wide association identifies diverse causes of common variable immunodeficiency. *J. Allergy Clin. Immunol.* **2011**, *127*, 1360–1367. [CrossRef] [PubMed]

38. Schubert, D.; Bode, C.; Kenefeck, R.; Hou, T.Z.; Wing, J.B.; Kennedy, A.; Bulashevska, A.; Petersen, B.S.; Schaffer, A.A.; Gruning, B.A.; et al. Autosomal dominant immune dysregulation syndrome in humans with CTLA4 mutations. *Nat. Med.* **2014**, *20*, 1410–1416. [CrossRef] [PubMed]

39. Deau, M.C.; Heurtier, L.; Frange, P.; Suarez, F.; Bole-Feysot, C.; Nitschke, P.; Cavazzana, M.; Picard, C.; Durandy, A.; Fischer, A.; et al. A human immunodeficiency caused by mutations in the PIK3R1 gene. *J. Clin. Investig.* **2014**, *124*, 3923–3928. [CrossRef] [PubMed]

40. Chen, K.; Coonrod, E.M.; Kumanovics, A.; Franks, Z.F.; Durtschi, J.D.; Margraf, R.L.; Wu, W.; Heikal, N.M.; Augustine, N.H.; Ridge, P.G.; et al. Germline mutations in NFKB2 implicate the noncanonical NF-κB pathway in the pathogenesis of common variable immunodeficiency. *Am. J. Hum. Genet.* **2013**, *93*, 812–824. [CrossRef] [PubMed]

41. Ombrello, M.J.; Remmers, E.F.; Sun, G.; Freeman, A.F.; Datta, S.; Torabi-Parizi, P.; Subramanian, N.; Bunney, T.D.; Baxendale, R.W.; Martins, M.S.; et al. Cold urticaria, immunodeficiency, and autoimmunity related to PLCG2 deletions. *N. Engl. J. Med.* **2012**, *366*, 330–338. [CrossRef] [PubMed]

42. Lopez-Herrera, G.; Tampella, G.; Pan-Hammarstrom, Q.; Herholz, P.; Trujillo-Vargas, C.M.; Phadwal, K.; Simon, A.K.; Moutschen, M.; Etzioni, A.; Mory, A.; et al. Deleterious mutations in LRBA are associated with a syndrome of immune deficiency and autoimmunity. *Am. J. Hum. Genet.* **2012**, *90*, 986–1001. [CrossRef] [PubMed]

43. Van Montfrans, J.M.; Hoepelman, A.I.; Otto, S.; van Gijn, M.; van de Corput, L.; de Weger, R.A.; Monaco-Shawver, L.; Banerjee, P.P.; Sanders, E.A.; Jol-van der Zijde, C.M.; et al. CD27 deficiency is associated with combined immunodeficiency and persistent symptomatic EBV viremia. *J. Allergy Clin. Immunol.* **2012**, *129*, 787–793. [CrossRef] [PubMed]

44. Mayor, P.C.; Eng, K.H.; Singel, K.L.; Abrams, S.I.; Odunsi, K.; Moysich, K.B.; Fuleihan, R.; Garabedian, E.; Lugar, P.; Ochs, H.D.; et al. Cancer in primary immunodeficiency diseases: Cancer incidence in the United States Immune Deficiency Network Registry. *J. Allergy Clin. Immunol.* **2017**. [CrossRef] [PubMed]

45. Mellemkjaer, L.; Hammarstrom, L.; Andersen, V.; Yuen, J.; Heilmann, C.; Barington, T.; Bjorkander, J.; Olsen, J.H. Cancer risk among patients with IgA deficiency or common variable immunodeficiency and their relatives: A combined Danish and Swedish study. *Clin. Exp. Immunol.* **2002**, *130*, 495–500. [CrossRef] [PubMed]

46. Dhalla, F.; da Silva, S.P.; Lucas, M.; Travis, S.; Chapel, H. Review of gastric cancer risk factors in patients with common variable immunodeficiency disorders, resulting in a proposal for a surveillance programme. *Clin. Exp. Immunol.* **2011**, *165*, 1–7. [CrossRef] [PubMed]

47. IARC *Helicobacter pylori* Working Group. *Helicobacter pylori Eradication as a Strategy for Gastric Cancer Prevention*; IARC Working Group Reports, No. 8; International Agency for Research on Cancer: Lyon, France, 2014. Available online: http://www.iarc.fr/en/publications/pdfs-online/wrk/wrk8/index.php (acccessed on 17 September 2016).

48. Danesh, J. *Helicobacter pylori* infection and gastric cancer: Systematic review of the epidemiological studies. *Aliment. Pharmacol. Ther.* **1999**, *13*, 851–856. [CrossRef] [PubMed]

49. Helicobacter and Cancer Collaborative Group. Gastric cancer and *Helicobacter pylori*: A combined analysis of 12 case control studies nested within prospective cohorts. *Gut* **2001**, *49*, 347–353.

50. Quiding-Jarbrink, M.; Sundstrom, P.; Lundgren, A.; Hansson, M.; Backstrom, M.; Johansson, C.; Enarsson, K.; Hermansson, M.; Johnsson, E.; Svennerholm, A.M. Decreased IgA antibody production in the stomach of gastric adenocarcinoma patients. *Clin. Immunol.* **2009**, *131*, 463–471. [CrossRef] [PubMed]

51. Correa, P.; Piazuelo, M.B. The gastric precancerous cascade. *J. Dig. Dis.* **2012**, *13*, 2–9. [CrossRef] [PubMed]

52. Ajani, J.A.; Lee, J.; Sano, T.; Janjigian, Y.Y.; Fan, D.; Song, S. Gastric adenocarcinoma. *Nat. Rev. Dis. Prim.* **2017**, *3*, 17036. [CrossRef] [PubMed]

53. Wang, L.L.; Yu, X.J.; Zhan, S.H.; Jia, S.J.; Tian, Z.B.; Dong, Q.J. Participation of microbiota in the development of gastric cancer. *World J. Gastroenterol.* **2014**, *20*, 4948–4952. [CrossRef] [PubMed]

54. Xu, L.; Qu, Y.H.; Chu, X.D.; Wang, R.; Nelson, H.H.; Gao, Y.T.; Yuan, J.M. Urinary levels of *N*-nitroso compounds in relation to risk of gastric cancer: Findings from the shanghai cohort study. *PLoS ONE* **2015**, *10*, e0117326. [CrossRef] [PubMed]

55. De Petris, G.; Dhungel, B.M.; Chen, L.; Chang, Y.H. Gastric adenocarcinoma in common variable immunodeficiency: Features of cancer and associated gastritis may be characteristic of the condition. *Int. J. Surg. Pathol.* **2014**, *22*, 600–606. [CrossRef] [PubMed]

56. Coati, I.; Fassan, M.; Farinati, F.; Graham, D.Y.; Genta, R.M.; Rugge, M. Autoimmune gastritis: Pathologist's viewpoint. *World J. Gastroenterol.* **2015**, *21*, 12179–12189. [CrossRef] [PubMed]

57. Kulnigg-Dabsch, S. Autoimmune gastritis. *Wien. Med. Wochenschr.* **2016**, *166*, 424–430. [CrossRef] [PubMed]

58. Bergman, M.P.; Faller, G.; D'Elios, M.M.; Del Prete, G.; Vandenbroucke-Grauls, C.M.J.E.; Appelmelk, B.J. Gastric automminity. In *Helicobacter pylori: Physiology and Genetics*; Mobley, H.L.T., Mendz, G.L., Hazell, S.L., Eds.; ASM Press: Washington, DC, USA, 2001; Chapter 36.

59. Morimoto, Y.; Routes, J.M. Granulomatous disease in common variable immunodeficiency. *Curr. Allergy Asthma Rep.* **2005**, *5*, 370–375. [CrossRef] [PubMed]

60. Daniels, J.A.; Lederman, H.M.; Maitra, A.; Montgomery, E.A. Gastrointestinal tract pathology in patients with common variable immunodeficiency (CVID): A clinicopathologic study and review. *Am. J. Surg. Pathol.* **2007**, *31*, 1800–1812. [CrossRef] [PubMed]

61. Ferlay, J.; Shin, H.R.; Bray, F.; Forman, D.; Mathers, C.; Parkin, D.M. Estimates of worldwide burden of cancer in 2008: GLOBOCAN 2008. *Int. J. Cancer* **2010**, *127*, 2893–2917. [CrossRef] [PubMed]

62. Hamashima, C. Current issues and future perspectives of gastric cancer screening. *World J. Gastroenterol.* **2014**, *20*, 13767–13774. [CrossRef] [PubMed]

63. Calvet, X.; Sanchez-Delgado, J.; Montserrat, A.; Lario, S.; Ramirez-Lazaro, M.J.; Quesada, M.; Casalots, A.; Suarez, D.; Campo, R.; Brullet, E.; et al. Accuracy of diagnostic tests for *Helicobacter pylori*: A reappraisal. *Clin. Infect. Dis.* **2009**, *48*, 1385–1391. [CrossRef] [PubMed]

64. Gisbert, J.P.; Pajares, J.M. Stool antigen test for the diagnosis of *Helicobacter pylori* infection: A systematic review. *Helicobacter* **2004**, *9*, 347–368. [CrossRef] [PubMed]

65. Niv, Y. *H pylori* recurrence after successful eradication. *World J. Gastroenterol.* **2008**, *14*, 1477–1478. [CrossRef] [PubMed]

66. Lee, Y.C.; Chiang, T.H.; Liou, J.M.; Chen, H.H.; Wu, M.S.; Graham, D.Y. Mass Eradication of *Helicobacter pylori* to Prevent Gastric Cancer: Theoretical and Practical Considerations. *Gut Liver* **2016**, *10*, 12–26. [CrossRef] [PubMed]

67. Dinis-Ribeiro, M.; Lopes, C.; da Costa-Pereira, A.; Guilherme, M.; Barbosa, J.; Lomba-Viana, H.; Silva, R.; Moreira-Dias, L. A follow up model for patients with atrophic chronic gastritis and intestinal metaplasia. *J. Clin. Pathol.* **2004**, *57*, 177–182. [CrossRef] [PubMed]

68. Park, S.Y.; Jeon, S.W.; Jung, M.K.; Cho, C.M.; Tak, W.Y.; Kweon, Y.O.; Kim, S.K.; Choi, Y.H. Long-term follow-up study of gastric intraepithelial neoplasias: Progression from low-grade dysplasia to invasive carcinoma. *Eur. J. Gastroenterol. Hepatol.* **2008**, *20*, 966–970. [CrossRef] [PubMed]

69. De Vries, A.C.; Haringsma, J.; Kuipers, E.J. The detection, surveillance and treatment of premalignant gastric lesions related to *Helicobacter pylori* infection. *Helicobacter* **2007**, *12*, 1–15. [CrossRef] [PubMed]

70. Gompels, M.M.; Hodges, E.; Lock, R.J.; Angus, B.; White, H.; Larkin, A.; Chapel, H.M.; Spickett, G.P.; Misbah, S.A.; Smith, J.L.; et al. Lymphoproliferative disease in antibody deficiency: A multi-centre study. *Clin. Exp. Immunol.* **2003**, *134*, 314–320. [CrossRef] [PubMed]

71. Unger, S.; Seidl, M.; Schmitt-Graeff, A.; Bohm, J.; Schrenk, K.; Wehr, C.; Goldacker, S.; Drager, R.; Gartner, B.C.; Fisch, P.; et al. Ill-defined germinal centers and severely reduced plasma cells are histological hallmarks of lymphadenopathy in patients with common variable immunodeficiency. *J. Clin. Immunol.* **2014**, *34*, 615–626. [CrossRef] [PubMed]

72. Wehr, C.; Kivioja, T.; Schmitt, C.; Ferry, B.; Witte, T.; Eren, E.; Vlkova, M.; Hernandez, M.; Detkova, D.; Bos, P.R.; et al. The EUROclass trial: Defining subgroups in common variable immunodeficiency. *Blood* **2008**, *111*, 77–85. [CrossRef] [PubMed]

73. Desar, I.M.; Keuter, M.; Raemaekers, J.M.; Jansen, J.B.; van Krieken, J.H.; van der Meer, J.W. Extranodal marginal zone (MALT) lymphoma in common variable immunodeficiency. *Neth. J. Med.* **2006**, *64*, 136–140. [PubMed]

74. Cunningham-Rundles, C.; Bodian, C. Common variable immunodeficiency: Clinical and immunological features of 248 patients. *Clin. Immunol.* **1999**, *92*, 34–48. [CrossRef] [PubMed]

75. Chapel, H.; Cunningham-Rundles, C. Update in understanding common variable immunodeficiency disorders (CVIDs) and the management of patients with these conditions. *Br. J. Haematol.* **2009**, *145*, 709–727. [CrossRef] [PubMed]

76. Cunningham-Rundles, C.; Lieberman, P.; Hellman, G.; Chaganti, R.S. Non-Hodgkin lymphoma in common variable immunodeficiency. *Am. J. Hematol.* **1991**, *37*, 69–74. [CrossRef] [PubMed]

77. Wotherspoon, A.C.; Ortiz-Hidalgo, C.; Falzon, M.R.; Isaacson, P.G. *Helicobacter pylori*-associated gastritis and primary B-cell gastric lymphoma. *Lancet* **1991**, *338*, 1175–1176. [CrossRef]

78. Gottesman, S.R.; Haas, D.; Ladanyi, M.; Amorosi, E.L. Peripheral T cell lymphoma in a patient with common variable immunodeficiency disease: Case report and literature review. *Leuk. Lymphoma* **1999**, *32*, 589–595. [CrossRef] [PubMed]

79. Jesus, A.A.; Jacob, C.M.; Silva, C.A.; Dorna, M.; Pastorino, A.C.; Carneiro-Sampaio, M. Common variable immunodeficiency associated with hepatosplenic T-cell lymphoma mimicking juvenile systemic lupus erythematosus. *Clin. Dev. Immunol.* **2011**, *2011*, 1–4. [CrossRef] [PubMed]

80. Gammon, B.; Robson, A.; Deonizio, J.; Arkin, L.; Guitart, J. CD8+ granulomatous cutaneous T-cell lymphoma: A potential association with immunodeficiency. *J. Am. Acad. Dermatol.* **2014**, *71*, 555–560. [CrossRef] [PubMed]

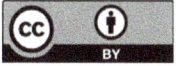

International Journal of
Molecular Sciences

MDPI

Article

Molecular and Pathological Features of Gastric Cancer in Lynch Syndrome and Familial Adenomatous Polyposis

Mara Fornasarig [1,*], Raffaella Magris [1], Valli De Re [2], Ettore Bidoli [3], Vincenzo Canzonieri [4], Stefania Maiero [1], Alessandra Viel [5] and Renato Cannizzaro [1]

[1] SOC di Gastroenterologia Oncologica, Centro di Riferimento Oncologico IRCSS, 33081 Aviano, Italy; raffaella.magris@cro.it (R.M.); smaiero@cro.it (S.M.); rcannizzaro@cro.it (R.C.)
[2] SOSD Immunopatologia e biomarcatori Oncologico, Centro di Riferimento Oncologico IRCSS, 33081 Aviano, Italy; vdere@cro.it
[3] SOC di Epidemiologia, Centro di Riferimento Oncologico IRCSS, 33081 Aviano, Italy; bidolie@cro.it
[4] SOSD di Anatomia Patologica, Centro di Riferimento Oncologico IRCSS, 33081 Aviano, Italy; vcanzonieri@cro.it
[5] SOSD Oncogenetica e Oncogenomica Funzionale, Centro di Riferimento Oncologico IRCSS, 33081 Aviano, Italy; aviel@cro.it
*   Correspondence: mfornasarig@cro.it; Tel.: +39-0434-659436

Received: 26 April 2018; Accepted: 1 June 2018; Published: 6 June 2018

Abstract: Lynch syndrome (LS) and familial adenomatous polyposis (FAP) are autosomal dominant hereditary diseases caused by germline mutations leading to the development of colorectal cancer. Moreover, these mutations result in the development of a spectrum of different tumors, including gastric cancers (GCs). Since the clinical characteristics of GCs associated with LS and FAP are not well known, we investigated clinical and molecular features of GCs occurring in patients with LS and FAP attending our Institution. The Hereditary Tumor Registry was established in 1994 at the Department of Oncologic Gastroenterology, CRO Aviano National Cancer Institute, Italy. It includes 139 patients with LS and 86 patients with FAP. Patients were recruited locally for prospective surveillance. Out of 139 LS patients, 4 developed GC—3 in the presence of helicobacter pylori infection and 1 on the background of autoimmune diseases. All GCs displayed a high microsatellite instability (MSI-H) and loss of related mismatch repair (MMR) protein. One of the FAP patients developed a flat adenoma, displaying low-grade dysplasia at the gastric body, and another poorly differentiated adenocarcinoma with signet ring cells like Krukenberg without HP infection. LS carriers displayed a risk of GC. The recognition of HP infection and autoimmune diseases would indicate those at higher risk for an endoscopic surveillance. Regarding FAP, the data suggested the need of suitable endoscopic surveillance in long survivals with diffuse fundic gland polyps.

Keywords: gastric cancer; lynch syndrome; familial adenomatous polyposis (FAP), helicobacter pylori infection; autoimmune gastritis; fundic gland polyps (FGPs)

---

1. Introduction

Lynch syndrome (LS) and familial adenomatous polyposis (FAP) are the most frequent syndromes in hereditary colorectal cancer (CRC), causing, respectively, 6% and 1% of all CRC. Extracolonic neoplasms are often observed in these syndromes and upper gastrointestinal (GI) malignancies are an important cause of death.

LS is an autosomal dominant disorder caused by germline mutations in one of the mismatch repair (MMR) genes (MSH2, MLH1, MSH6, PMS2) or the EpCAM gene that mainly determines CRC risk. However, these mutations evolve into a spectrum of different extracolonic tumors. Endometrial cancer is the most frequent extracolonic cancer followed by urothelial, small bowel, and gastric cancers (GCs) [1,2]. MSH2, MLH1, and EpCAM carriers display a 46% risk of developing CRC and a 57% risk of endometrial cancer by the age of 75 years. Much lower is the risk for GCs (13%), but it is still higher compared to the 1% risk in the general population. MSH6 carriers instead have a lower risk for CRC (15%), endometrial cancer (46%), and also for GCs (<3%). Tumor tissue of CRC and extracolonic cancers in an LS setting show two peculiar molecular features: microsatellite instability (MSI) that is characterized by length alteration within simple, repeated DNA sequences called microsatellites, and loss of MMR protein expression at immunohistochemical analyses. These two molecular features are useful screening markers to identify patients with LS [3]. Guidelines are mainly focused on CRC prevention, suggesting colonoscopy starting at the age of 20–22 years with a two-year interval for recognition and removal of the precancerous lesions, i.e., adenomatous polyps. There is no consensus for extracolonic cancer prevention and for GCs surveillance [3–5]. GCs in this setting are usually of intestinal type, showing high microsatellite instability (MSI-H) and a loss of relative MMR protein expression. The natural history and pathological transformation pathway are unknown. However, helicobacter pylori (HP) infection represents a predisposing clinical condition to GCs, and its eradication is recommended. Gastric adenomas are rarely observed in LS; however, a recent study reported PGA in 3 patients out of 15 cases of LS GC [6].

FAP is an autosomal dominant hereditary disease caused by germline mutations in the adenomatous polyposis coli (APC) gene with 80–100% penetrance, leading to the development of hundreds to thousands colorectal adenomatous polyps starting in teenage years and CRC at an average age of 39 years. The correlation between genotype and phenotype has been highlighted. The APC gene encodes 2844 aminoacids in 15 exons. The mutation cluster region, located between 1250–1464 codon, is associated with florid and more aggressive colonic polyposis, whereas mutations in 5′ and 3′ regions are related to an attenuated FAP (AFAP) with a lower number of colonic adenomas. Mutations between 140–1309 are linked to papillary thyroid carcinoma and between 1399–1580 to desmoids tumors [7,8]. CRC has been considered an inevitable consequence in the natural history of FAP. Guidelines suggest colonic surveillance starting before teenage and prophylactic colectomy is the recommended treatment for preventing cancer when adenomatous polyposis is not endoscopically manageable or in the presence of adenomas with high-grade dysplasia [5]. Beside CRC, duodenal adenomas and carcinomas and desmoids tumors are the most frequent cause of morbidity and mortality in FAP. Presently, upper gastrointestinal (GI) endoscopy has been included in the surveillance starting at 25 years of age for staging duodenal polyposis, and the intervals are based on the Spigelman score determined by the number and grade of dysplasia of duodenal adenomas. However, GCs have also been reported [9]. Differences in frequency were seen between Western and Eastern countries [10]. A recent paper has described GCs in 0.5% of FAP patients from a US registry [11], while among Japanese FAP patients, the prevalence of GC has been reported to be from 2.8% to 15.5% [12]. The types of gastric lesions associated with GCs in FAP are: fundic gland polyps (FGPs), gastric foveolar-type gastric adenoma, gastric adenoma, and pyloric gland adenoma (PGA) [13]. FGPs are present in more than 60% of FAP patients and they usually display biallelic inactivation of the APC gene often with foci of dysplasia or microadenomatous polyps of the foveolar epithelium [14]. However, malignant progression in FGPs is uncommon and the lifetime risk of GC is reported to be in the range of 0.5–1%. Intestinal-type adenomas are rare (1–2% of gastric polyps) in Western countries compared to Asia (40–50% of gastric polyps) [15]. A strong correlation between gastric adenomas and atrophic gastritis secondary to HP infection has been showed in Japanese FAP patients [12,16]. PGAs have been recently recognized as a new polyp subtype, developing on the mucosa with pyloric metaplasia [17]. They have been found in 6% of FAP patients and high grade dysplasia is seen in 10% of cases. Out of the FAP setting, PGAs have been found in association with autoimmune metaplastic atrophic gastritis [18].

Since the clinical characteristics of GCs associated with LS and FAP are still not well understood, in our study we investigated clinical and molecular features of GCs occurring in these patients attending our Institution.

2. Results

In LS, CRC was the most frequently diagnosed primary cancer (82 patients, 59%), followed by endometrial cancer (55% out of 83 women). Out of 82 patients with CRC, 24 had multiple synchronous lesions with a total of 131 CRCs diagnosed. Mucinous histotype was present in 55.7% (72) of CRCs, and the remaining ones were well or poorly differentiated adenocarcinomas. GC was the fourth most frequently diagnosed extracolonic cancer. Out of 139 patients, 18 (13%) showed HP infection and 4 patients (2.9%) (2 male, 2 female) developed a GC. All GCs displayed MSI-H and the loss of related MMR protein. The four patients with GCs are described as follows. Patient 1 was a 53-year-old man carrying the MLH1 mutation (Table 1, Figure 1) who developed an HP infection negative diffuse-type adenocarcinoma (T2N0) at the fundus (Figure 2a). The tumor displayed the reduction of cytoplasmic expression of E-cadherin (Figure 2b). Four years before diagnosis, he had two PGAs removed at the body with high-grade dysplasia. On that setting, an autoimmune gastritis was diagnosed with already atrophic gastritis and a deficit of acid secretion. Since the reduction of E-cadherin expression in tumor tissue and mutations in the CDH1 gene (codifying for E-cadherin) are strongly associated with diffuse-type adenocarcinoma, we also performed the sequence analysis of germline CDH1 gene. The patient showed common polymorphisms and nonpathogenetic variants (Figure 3). This patient has not developed CRC yet, but he underwent removal of four adenomas with low-grade dysplasia during his colonoscopic surveillance.

Table 1. Molecular and pathological features of gastric cancer and adenoma in Lynch syndrome and FAP.

Mutated Gene	Mutation	Age at Onset	Gender	Histology	Stage
MLH1	c.688G>T p.(Glu230*)	53	M	Diffuse	T2N0
MSH2	c.(?_-68)_(*272_?)del p.(?)	73	F	Intestinal HP+	T2N1
MSH2	c.2334C>A p.(Cys778*)	62	M	Intestinal HP+	T2N0
MSH2	c.(?_-68)_1276+?del p.(?)	40	F	Intestinal HP+	T2N1
APC	c.1863-1866del p. (Thr621fs*8)	54	M	adenoma	
APC	c.1495C>T p.(Arg499*)	72	F	Krukenberg	T3N3

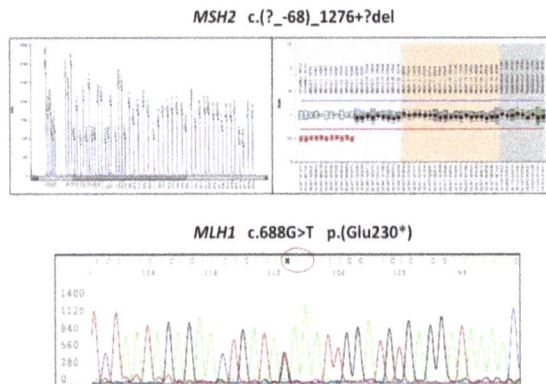

MSH2 c.(?_-68)_1276+?del

MLH1 c.688G>T p.(Glu230*)

Figure 1. Representative mismatch repair gene mutations. **Top** panels: MLPA electropherogram (**left**) and analysis of MLPA data with the Software Coffalyser v.140721.1958 (MRC-Holland, Amsterdam, Holland). (NET (**right**) showing the MSH2 c.(?_-68)_1276+?del variant, corresponding to a large deletion encompassing exons 1–7. **Bottom** panel: Sanger sequencing showing the MLH1 c.688G>T variant producing the truncated p.(Glu230*) protein. The mutated codon (GAA > TAA) is circled in red.

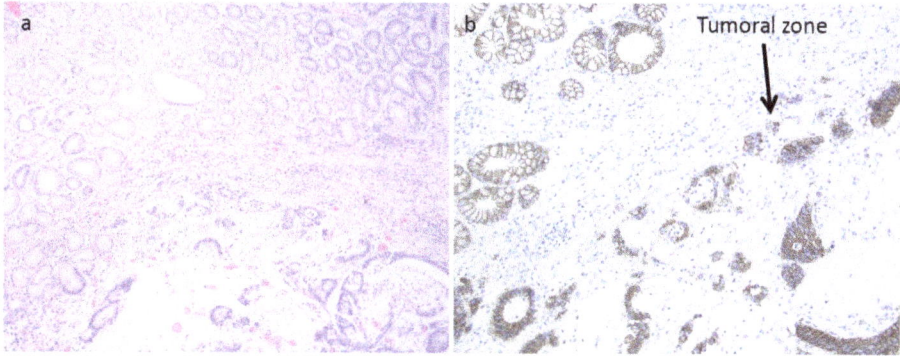

Figure 2. Patient 1: (**a**) Neoplastic cells showing diffuse solid growth and focal vague glandular appearances. H&E staining, original magnification 10×; (**b**) Reduction of E-cadherin expression by immunohistochemical staining, original magnification 20×.

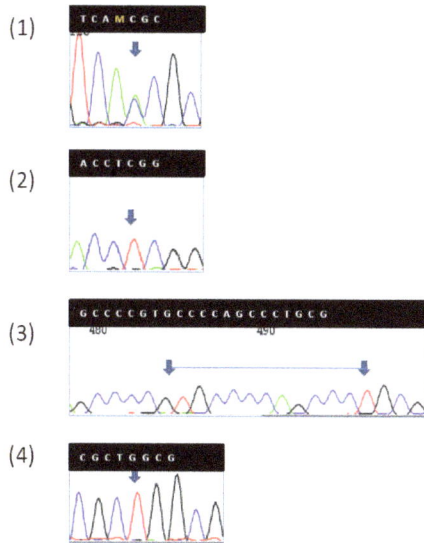

Figure 3. Four germline mutations, one of uncertain significance and three presumably benign were found in the *CDH1* gene. Sequence chromatograms. (**1**) mutation of uncertain significance located in the promoter region of the E-cadherin CDH1 gene (rs16260 C/A); (**2**) mutation located in the intron 1 (rs3743674 T/T); (**3**) insertion located in the intron 1 (rs74406246 ins); (**4**) mutation located in the codon 13 (rs2076 T/T).

Patient 2 (Table 1, Figure 1) was a 73-year-old female carrying an MSH2 mutation with adenocarcinoma moderately differentiated intestinal type at antrum (T2N1) (Figure 4a). She had previous diagnoses of multiple primary cancers (CRC at ascending colon at age 27 years, endometrial cancer at 45 years, CRC at descending colon at 56 years, and urothelial cancer at 65 years). Patient 3 was a 62-year-old male carrying an MSH2 mutation with an adenocarcinoma poorly differentiated intestinal type (T2N0) at corpus (Table 1 and Figure 4b) associated with HP infection. He had already developed multiple CRCs at the ascending colon at age 34 years and at the sigmoid colon at 53 years. Patient 4 was a 40-year-old female carrying an MSH2 mutation with adenocarcinoma intestinal type poorly differentiated at corpus (T2 N1) and HP infection (Table 1 and Figure 4c). A previous CRC at the ascending colon was diagnosed at age 32 years.

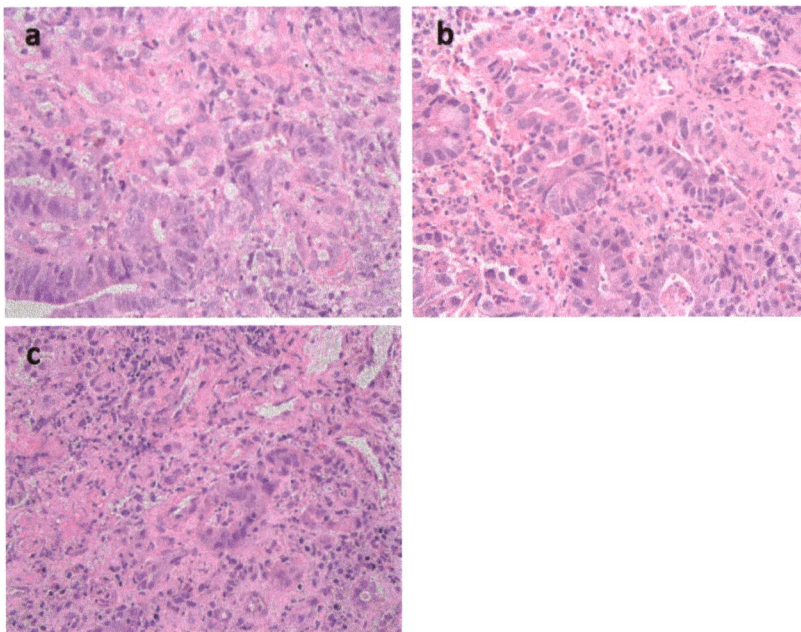

Figure 4. (**a**) Patient 2: moderately differentiated intestinal-type adenocarcinoma; (**b**) Patient 3: moderately differentiated intestinal-type adenocarcinoma; (**c**) Patient 4: moderately and poorly differentiated intestinal-type adenocarcinoma; H&H staining, original magnification 400×.

Out of the 74 FAP patients under surveillance, 64 (94%) were diagnosed with FGPs and 11 (16%) with a diffuse carpeting at fundus and body (Figure 5). After 15 years of prophylactic colectomy, a 54-year-old male developed a flat adenoma displaying low-grade dysplasia at the gastric body about 25 mm in diameter in the presence of diffuse FGPs (Table 1, Figure 6). An adenocarcinoma poorly differentiated with signet ring cells like Krukenberg (T3N+) without HP infection was diagnosed in a 72-year-old female with a previous prophylactic colectomy at age 43 years. She had few FGPs without gastric adenomas and she developed ovary metastasis two years after gastrectomy (Table 1).

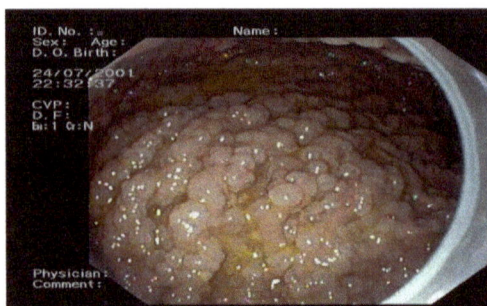

Figure 5. Diffuse fundic gland polyps.

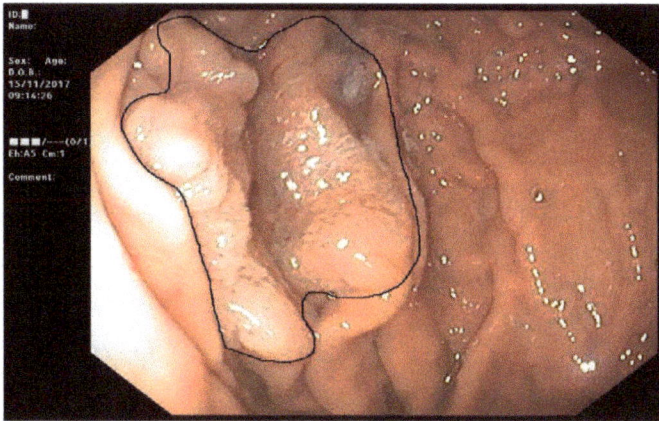

Figure 6. Flat adenoma in fundic gland polyposis.

3. Discussion

This study reports the clinical and molecular features of a small cohort of patients with FAP, LS, and GC who were recorded in the Hereditary Tumor Registry of the Department of Oncologic Gastroenterology at CRO Aviano. The small sample size necessarily implies a limitation of the effectiveness of our report. However, a substantial interesting point comes from our cases since all patients have been genetically characterized, come from the same geographical area, and the surveillance procedures have been performed at our Institution.

Regarding LS, MSI-H and the absence of MMR proteins corresponding to the germline mutation are the molecular features of GCs when they are related to this genetic disease [1,19]. GC has been reported to be one of the most frequent extracolonic malignancies in MSH2 and MLH1 mutation carriers with an estimated lifetime risk up to 13% and a frequency ranging from 1.6% in a Dutch registry to 3.1% in Korea and 10.9% in Finland, with a mean age of 56 years in Western countries and 46 years in Eastern countries [1,2,6]. A correlation with familial GC history had been shown only in Korea. Our regional cancer registry, Friuli Venezia Giulia Cancer Registry, has reported a cumulative lifetime risk of GC of 2.6% for males and 1.2% for women in the general population, which is lower than that estimated for LS patients. The frequency of GC in our cohort was 2.9% in the range of previous reports.

GCs displayed features of LS, such as MSI-H and the lack of MMR protein expression. Our cases had mutations in MLH1 and MSH2, the two genes mainly involved in GC risk [1,20]. The mean age of patients with GC was 57 years, and they did not have a GC family history. Three cases were of the intestinal type and one of the diffuse type. Intestinal GCs are often preceded by chronic atrophic gastritis with intestinal metaplasia and are related to environmental exposures such as diet, smoking, alcohol, and HP infection. In our series, HP infection was observed in all intestinal-type GCs and the diagnosis of cancer was made by upper GI endoscopy in a work up for symptoms. HP infection has been reported in about 20% of GCs in LS [2,6,21]. No differences in the frequency of HP infection were observed between LS carriers and the general population [21]. Diffuse-type GC was already reported in LS, with the highest frequency of 17% [2]. Our case of diffuse-type GC was diagnosed during a follow-up for atrophic gastritis associated with diffuse intestinal metaplasia caused by autoimmune diseases. The patient was positive at antiparietal cell antibodies. Atrophic gastritis was histologically ascertained as was an acid-secretion deficit by pepsinogen I and a low dose of vitamin B12. Two PGAs with high-grade dysplasia were endoscopically removed at the body and diffuse-type cancer was diagnosed four years later. PGAs are a distinct entity, they can derive from deep gastric mucous glands and they are likely accompanied by a background of intestinal metaplasia and autoimmune gastritis. They can evolve into invasive adenocarcinoma displaying pyloric gland differentiation [22]. PGAs were described in 3 out of 15 cases of GCs by Lee [6]. Two cases were diagnosed at the edge of the tumor, and in one case, PGA was removed two years before the GC diagnosis. However, we do not have any information on the association with autoimmune diseases. In autoimmune gastritis inflammatory aggression affects oxytocin glands at the gastric body and fundus leading to atrophia, and parietal cells may be replaced by cells containing mucus, similar to the intestinal ones, i.e., intestinal metaplasia. Atrophic gastritis with intestinal metaplasia is a recognized precancerous condition, usually predisposed to intestinal type adenocarcinoma or to carcinoid tumors in the setting of autoimmune gastritis [23]. GC was diagnosed, although there was a close surveillance of yearly endoscopy since our patient had already developed precancerous lesions as PGAs and he was an LS carrier. Thus, we hypothesized a role of CDH1 in the pathogenesis of GC because the diffuse type is uncommon in autoimmune gastritis; although CDH1 is involved in hereditary diffuse GC, pathogenetic mutations were not found in the molecular analysis. GCs were mainly diagnosed after previous CRCs, and one patient only developed GC as a primary cancer, but we must take into account that he was under colonic surveillance and multiple adenomas were removed. GC guidelines suggest surveillance in countries at higher risk of GC, such as Asian countries, or treatment of HP infection [3–5]. Our GC developed in the two clinical conditions leading to atrophic gastritis: autoimmune gastritis and HP infection. Our results confirmed current guidelines to search for and treat HP infection. Regarding the role of autoimmune gastritis in LS patients, our findings must be confirmed by further research, as it was identified only in one patient in a small cohort.

FAP is a genetic disease with an approximately 100% risk of CRC. Since mortality of CRC has considerably shrunk after the introduction of genetic testing and prophylactic colectomy, surveillance for extracolonic cancer has been suggested [5]. In our cases, metastatic CRCs were diagnosed in 12 patients because they were not aware of their genetic disease; no CRC was diagnosed in the other patients. They started surveillance at the appropriate age and they were treated with prophylactic colectomy or they were still under colonoscopic surveillance. Upper GI endoscopy is recommended for staging duodenal polyposis and the intervals are based on the Spigelman score determined by the number and grade of dysplasia of duodenal adenomas, regardless of gastric polyposis. However, recent data has emerged on GCs developed on the background of FGPs [11]. Unlike Far East populations, GC was uncommon in FAP [10] and our data are in line with previous reports. Actually, our case of GC was not related to FAP; it was a Krukenberg tumor, which is a rare metastatic signet ring cell tumor in the ovary. The stomach is the primary site in the majority of Krukenberg tumor cases, followed by carcinomas of the colon, appendix, and breast. The tumor must display mucin-secreting signet ring cell carcinoma in the dense fibroblastic stroma of the ovary to be defined as a Krukenberg tumor. Instead, another patient developed a large gastric adenoma that was located at the gastric body among diffuse FGPs. This adenoma probably could represent the precancerous lesions on a dysplasia foci or small adenoma on FGP background as reported in [11]. Our cases displayed APC mutations in the same region (between 685–2040 codon) as described by Walton [11]; this finding is, however, controversial because the same correlation was not found with adenomas. Comparing others features reported in GC cases, our patients did not have desmoid tumors or diffuse duodenal adenomas. GC diagnoses in the Japanese FAP cohort differed from British ones as well as our case for multicentric adenocarcinoma foci associated with HP infection and early onset. So far, guidelines on FAP have not accomplished gastric surveillance in patients with diffuse FGPs. Different intervals and new tools such as high-definition and narrow-binding light endoscopes must be considered for detection of small adenomas among diffuse hyperplastic polyposis.

In conclusion, our results confirm the risk of GC in LS carriers and indicate that surveillance programs should include investigation of HP infection. In addition, further studies are still needed the shed light on the role of autoimmune diseases. Regarding FAP, our limited data did not allow us to draw definitive conclusions, but previous reports suggest a suitable endoscopic surveillance for long survivals with diffuse gastric FGPs in Western countries.

4. Materials and Methods

4.1. Patients

One hundred thirty-nine patients with LS and 86 patients with FAP were recorded in the Hereditary Tumor Registry, that was established and approved on the 21th September 1994 by the Institutional Board of CRO-IRCCS, National Cancer Institute of Aviano (PN), Italy. All registered patients or their legal guardian, provided informed written consent. Ethical guidelines for research involving human subjects were respected.

4.1.1. LS Patients

Out of 139 LS patients (83 females, 56 males; mean age 53 years), 33 had mutation in MLH1, 10 in MSH6, and 96 in MSH2. Fifty-seven patients entered surveillance because of asymptomatic mutation carriers and 82 patients were in follow-up after a previous CRC (Figure 7). The average follow-up time was 10.5 years (2–26 years). The surveillance program consisted of colonoscopy starting at age 20 years, repeated every 2 years until the age of 40 years, and annually thereafter. Gynecological surveillance for women started at age 30 years with abdominal ultrasound, with urinary cytology beginning at age 35 years and repeated every 2 years. Upper GI endoscopy was performed according to guidelines only in patients with a family history of GC or because of symptoms until 2005, then the procedure was extended to all carriers staring at age 35, repeated every 3 years. Nowadays, European and American guidelines still give different suggestions [3–5]. Figure 7 describes patient number and types of cancers recorded during the follow-up.

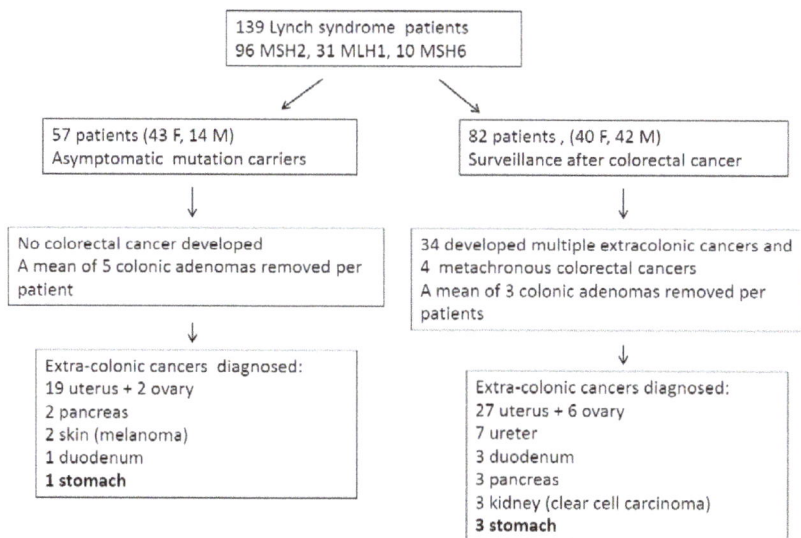

Figure 7. Lynch syndrome patients and cancer registered.

4.1.2. FAP or AFAP Patients

FAP patients (42 female, 44 male; mean age 46.7 years) had mutations identified in the APC gene. Sixty-two patients (32 female, 36 male; mean age 45.6) had mutations between 1250–1464 codon related to more aggressive polyposis and 18 in regions associated with the attenuated form (AFAP) (Figure 8). Upper GI endoscopy was performed according to guidelines starting at age 25 years or at the time of prophylactic colectomy. Twelve patients had a metastatic CRC at FAP diagnosis. Seventy-four patients are still under surveillance (57 with classical FAP and 17 with AFAP) (Figure 2). The average follow-up time was 11.6 years (1–36 years). Forty patients were under surveillance after their prophylactic colectomy and 34 were still in colonoscopic follow-up. FGPs were diagnosed in 64 patients out of 74, with 11 showing a diffuse carpeting of polyps at the fundus and body and 63 displaying a small number of polyps. The endoscopic intervals were determined by the burden and grade of dysplasia of duodenal adenomas classified according to the Spigelman score, varying from every 4 years if no polyps were found to every 3–6 months for diffuse duodenal adenomas or adenomas with high grade dysplasia.

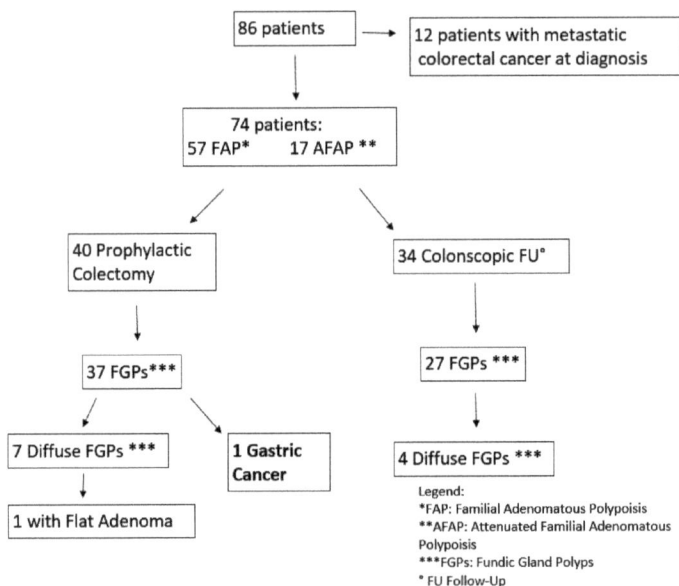

Figure 8. Familial adenomatous polyposis (FAP) patients.

4.2. Histology and HP Infection Status

GCs were classified according to Laurén into intestinal, diffuse, mixed, and indeterminate types, whereas WHO classification identifies five main types, i.e., tubular, papillary, mucinous, signet ring, and mixed carcinomas and a two- or three-tiered differentiation grading. Chronic gastritis, atrophy, intestinal metaplasia, and HP infection were evaluated and graded according to the Sydney classification. HP status was verified by conventional stainings (including H&E and special stains like Giemsa).

4.3. Mutational Analysis

Screening for constitutional point mutations of the three main DNA MMR genes (MSH2, MLH1, and MSH6) and APC gene was carried out on blood DNA by standard procedures of exon-by-exon amplification of the whole genomic region and flanking intron borders, followed by single-strand conformation polymorphism and/or direct bidirectional Sanger sequencing on an AB3130 xl Sequencer (Applied Biosystems/Thermofisher, Foster City, CA, USA) or by next generation sequencing targeting a custom gene panel on a MiSeq platform (Illumina, San Diego, CA, USA). Multiplex-Ligation Dependent Probe Amplification analyses (MLPA, MRC-Holland, Amsterdam, The Netherlands) were also used to detect large gene deletions/duplications.

Screening for mutations of the *CDH1* exons and neighboring intronic sequences was performed using polymerase chain reaction (PCR) with previously described primers and reaction conditions [20]. In short, 15 PCR reactions were performed for a full mutational screening of all 15 exons and splice junctions of the *CDH1* gene. Amplified PCR products were sequenced on the Applied Biosystems 3130 automated sequencer (Applied Biosystems, Foster City, CA, USA) using the Big Dye v3.1 Terminator Cycle Sequencing Kit (Life Technologies, Monza, Italy) and sequence data were aligned and analyzed using CodonCode Aligner software [24].

4.4. Microsatellite analysis

Genomic DNA was obtained from blood and from paraffin-embedded or frozen tissues. Standard MSI analysis was performed on paired tumor–normal tissue DNA samples using the original Bethesda panel of microsatellite markers (*BAT26, BAT25, D2S123, D5S346, D17S250*) or the mononucleotide panel (MSI Analysis System, Promega, WI, USA) including BAT26, BAT25, NR21, NR23, and MONO27. Fluorescent-labeled PCR products were separated by capillary electrophoresis using an ABI3130xl sequencer and evaluated with the GeneMapper software (version number 5, Applied Biosystems/Thermofisher, Foster City, CA). Criteria for definition of MSS and MSI were according to the Bethesda guidelines [25].

4.5. Immunohistochemistry (IHC)

MMR protein: formalin-fixed and paraffin-embedded sections from tumor blocks were stained by an automated method on the Ventana BenchMark Ultra. MLH-1 (M1), MSH2 (G219-1129), MSH6 (44) mouse monoclonal primary antibodies (Roche/Ventana), and PMS2 (EPR3947) rabbit monoclonal antibody (Roche/Ventana) were used to qualitatively identify human DNA MMR proteins. Lesions were considered positive for protein inactivation when a complete absence of nuclear staining was evident in tumor cells with concomitant nuclear staining of adjacent normal epithelial and stromal cells.

E-cadherin: the formalin-fixed, paraffin-embedded tumor block was cut into 4-μm-thick sections for H&E and immunostaining. Immunohistochemistry was performed by using the mouse monoclonal antibody against human E-cadherin (clone 36, Ventana Medical System, Tucson, Arizona). Lesions were considered positive for E-cadherin in the presence of membrane staining.

Author Contributions: M.F. conceived and supervised the whole project, interpreted the results, wrote and prepared the manuscript; R.M. wrote and prepared the manuscript; V.D.R. analyzed CDH1; E.B. provided epidemiologic data on gastric cancer in our region; V.C. performed pathological evaluation and immunohistochemestry; S.M. collected the data; A.V. performed MSI analyses and MMR mutation analyses; R.C. interpreted the results and critically evaluated the manuscript. All authors read and approved the final manuscript for publication.

Conflicts of Interest: The authors declare no conflict of interest.

Abbreviations

AFAP	Attenuated Familial Adenomatous Polyposis
APC	Adenomatous Polyposis Coli
CRC	colorectal Cancer
FAP	Familial Adenomatous Polyposis
FGP	Fundic Gland Polyps
GC	Gastric Cancer
HP	Helicobacter Pylori
IHC	Immunohistochemistry
LS	Lynch Syndrome
MMR	Mismatch repair
MSI-H	High Microsatellite instability
PGA	Pyloric Gland Adenoma
PCR	Polymerase Chain Reaction

References

1. Møller, P.; Seppälä, T.T.; Bernstein, I.; Holinski-Feder, E.; Sala, P.; Evans, D.G.; Lindblom, A.; Macrae, F.; Blanco, I.; Sijmons, R.H.; et al. Cancer risk and survival in path_MMR carriers by gene and gender up to 75 years of age: A report from the Prospective Lynch Syndrome Database. *BMJ Gut* **2017**. [CrossRef] [PubMed]

2. Aarnio, M.; Salovaara, R.; Aaltonen, L.A.; Mecklin, J.P.; Järvinen, H.J. Features of gastric cancer in hereditary non-polyposis colorectal cancer syndrome. *Int. J. Cancer* **1997**, *74*, 551–555. [CrossRef]

3. Vasen, H.F.; Blanco, I.; Aktan-Collan, K.; Gopie, J.P.; Alonso, A.; Aretz, S.; Bernstein, I.; Bertario, L.; Burn, J.; Capella, G.; et al. Revised guidelines for the clinical management of Lynch syndrome (HNPCC): Recommendations by a group of European experts. *BMJ Gut* **2013**, *62*, 812–823. [CrossRef] [PubMed]

4. Giardiello, F.M.; Allen, J.I.; Axilbund, J.E.; Boland, C.R.; Burke, C.A.; Burt, R.W.; Church, J.M.; Dominitz, J.A.; Johnson, D.A.; Kaltenbach, T.; et al. Guidelines on genetic evaluation and management of Lynch syndrome: A consensus statement by the US Multi-society Task Force on colorectal cancer. *Am. J. Gastroenterol.* **2014**, *109*, 1159–1179. [CrossRef] [PubMed]

5. National Comprehensive Cancer Network. *NCCN Clinical Practice Guidelines in Oncology (NCCN Guidelines®) Genetic/Familial High-Risk Assessment*; NCCN.org Version 2017; NCCN: Fort Washington, PA, USA, 2017.

6. Lee, S.E.; Kang, S.Y.; Cho, J.; Lee, B.; Chang, D.K.; Woo, H.; Kim, J.W.; Park, H.Y.; Do, I.G.; Kim, Y.E.; et al. Pyloric gland adenoma in Lynch syndrome. *Am. J. Surg. Pathol.* **2014**, *38*, 784–792. [CrossRef] [PubMed]

7. Goss, K.H.; Groden, J. Biology of the adenomatous polyposis coli tumor suppressor. *J. Clin. Oncol.* **2000**, *18*, 1967–1979. [CrossRef] [PubMed]

8. Groen, E.J.; Roos, A.; Muntinghe, F.L.; Enting, R.H.; de Vries, J.; Kleibeuker, J.H.; Witjes, M.J.; Links, T.P.; van Beek, A.P. Extra-intestinal manifestations of familial adenomatous polyposis. *Ann. Surg. Oncol.* **2008**, *15*, 2439–2450. [CrossRef] [PubMed]

9. Mankaney, G.; Leone, P.; Cruise, M.; LaGuardia, L.; O'Malley, M.; Bhatt, A.; Church, J.; Burke, C.A. Gastric cancer in FAP: A concerning rise in incidence. *Fam. Cancer* **2017**, *16*, 371–376. [CrossRef] [PubMed]

10. Shibata, C.; Ogawa, H.; Miura, K.; Naitoh, T.; Yamauchi, J.; Unno, M. Clinical characteristics of gastric cancer in patients with familial adenomatous polyposis. *Tohoku J. Exp. Med.* **2013**, *229*, 143–146. [CrossRef] [PubMed]

11. Walton, S.J.; Frayling, I.M.; Clark, S.K.; Latchford, A. Gastric tumours in FAP. *Fam. Cancer* **2017**, *16*, 363–369. [CrossRef] [PubMed]

12. Nakamura, K.; Nonaka, S.; Nakajima, T.; Yachida, T.; Abe, S.; Sakamoto, T.; Suzuki, H.; Yoshinaga, S.; Oda, I.; Matsuda, T.; et al. Clinical outcomes of gastric polyps and neoplasms in patients with familial adenomatous polyposis. *Endosc. Int. Open* **2017**, *5*, E137–E145. [CrossRef] [PubMed]

13. Brosens, L.A.; Wood, L.D.; Offerhaus, G.J.; Arnold, C.A.; Lam-Himlin, D.; Giardiello, F.M.; Montgomery, E.A. Pathology and Genetics of Syndromic Gastric Polyps. *Int. J. Surg. Pathol.* **2016**, *24*, 185–199. [CrossRef] [PubMed]

14. Abraham, S.C.; Nobukawa, B.; Giardiello, F.M.; Hamilton, S.R.; Wu, T.T. Fundic gland polyps in familial adenomatous polyposis: Neoplasms with frequent somatic adenomatous polyposis coli gene alterations. *Am. J. Pathol.* **2000**, *157*, 747–754. [CrossRef]

15. Wood, L.D.; Salaria, S.N.; Cruise, M.W.; Giardiello, F.M.; Montgomery, E.A. Upper GI tract lesions in familial adenomatous polyposis (FAP): Enrichment of pyloric gland adenomas and other gastric and duodenal neoplasms. *Am. J. Surg. Pathol.* **2014**, *38*, 389–393. [CrossRef] [PubMed]

16. Matsumoto, T.; Iida, M.; Kobori, Y.; Mizuno, M.; Nakamura, S.; Hizawa, K.; Yao, T. Serrated adenoma in familial adenomatous polyposis: Relation to germline APC gene mutation. *BMJ Gut* **2002**, *50*, 402–404. [CrossRef]

17. Chen, Z.M.; Scudiere, J.R.; Abraham, S.C.; Montgomery, E. Pyloric gland adenoma: An entity distinct from gastric foveolar type adenoma. *Am. J. Surg. Pathol.* **2009**, *33*, 186–193. [CrossRef] [PubMed]

18. Hashimoto, T.; Ogawa, R.; Matsubara, A.; Taniguchi, H.; Sugano, K.; Ushiama, M.; Yoshida, T.; Kanai, Y.; Sekine, S. Familial adenomatous polyposis-associated and sporadic pyloric gland adenomas of the upper gastrointestinal tract share common genetic features. *Histopathology* **2015**, *67*, 689–698. [CrossRef] [PubMed]

19. Gylling, A.; Abdel-Rahman, W.M.; Juhola, M.; Nuorva, K.; Hautala, E.; Järvinen, H.J.; Mecklin, J.P.; Aarnio, M.; Peltomäki, P. Is gastric cancer part of the tumour spectrum of hereditary non-polyposis colorectal cancer? A molecular genetic study. *BMJ Gut* **2007**, *56*, 926–933. [CrossRef] [PubMed]

20. Aarnio, M. Clinico-pathological features and management of cancers in lynch syndrome. *Pathol. Res. Int.* **2012**, *2012*, 350309. [CrossRef] [PubMed]

21. Soer, E.C.; Leicher, L.W.; Langers, A.M.; van de Meeberg, P.C.; van der Wouden, E.J.; Koornstra, J.J.; Bigirwamungu-Bargeman, M.; Vasen, H.F.; de Vos tot Nederveen Cappel, W.H. Equivalent *Helicobacter pylori* infection rates in Lynch syndrome mutation carriers with and without a first-degree relative with gastric cancer. *Int. J. Colorectal Dis.* **2016**, *31*, 693–697. [CrossRef] [PubMed]

22. Hackeng, W.M.; Montgomery, E.A.; Giardiello, F.M.; Singhi, A.D.; Debeljak, M.; Eshleman, J.R.; Vieth, M.; Offerhaus, G.J.; Wood, L.D.; Brosens, L.A. Morphology and genetics of pyloric gland adenomas in familial adenomatous polyposis. *Histopathology* **2017**, *70*, 549–557. [CrossRef] [PubMed]

23. Rustgi, N.; Shroff, S.G.; Katona, B.W. Two Types of Gastric Cancer Caused by the Same Underlying Condition. *Gastroenterology* **2018**, *154*, 1246–1248. [CrossRef] [PubMed]

24. Caggiari, L.; Miolo, G.; Buonadonna, A.; Basile, D.; Santeufemia, D.A.; Cossu, A.; Palmieri, G.; de Zorzi, M.; Fornasarig, M.; Alessandrini, L.; et al. Characterizing Metastatic HER2-Positive Gastric Cancer at the CDH1 Haplotype. *Int. J. Mol. Sci.* **2017**, *19*, 47. [CrossRef] [PubMed]

25. Umar, A. Lynch syndrome (HNPCC) and microsatellite instability. *Dis. Mark.* **2004**, *20*, 179–180. [CrossRef] [PubMed]

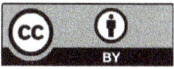

International Journal of
Molecular Sciences

MDPI

Article

Use of Metabolomics as a Complementary Omic Approach to Implement Risk Criteria for First-Degree Relatives of Gastric Cancer Patients

Giuseppe Corona [1,*], Renato Cannizzaro [2], Gianmaria Miolo [3], Laura Caggiari [1], Mariangela De Zorzi [1], Ombretta Repetto [1], Agostino Steffan [1] and Valli De Re [1,*]

[1]   Immunopathology and Cancer Biomarkers Unit, IRCCS-National Cancer Institute, 33081 Aviano, Italy;
      lcaggiari@cro.it (L.C.); mdezorzi@cro.it (M.D.Z.); orepetto@cro.it (O.R.); asteffan@cro.it (A.S.)
[2]   Oncological Gastroenterology Unit, IRCCS-National Cancer Institute, 33081 Aviano, Italy; rcannizzaro@cro.it
[3]   Oncology B Unit, IRCCS-National Cancer Institute, 33081 Aviano, Italy; gmiolo@cro.it
*   Correspondence: giuseppe.corona@cro.it (G.C.); vdere@cro.it (V.D.R.);
      Tel.: +39-043-465-9666 (G.C.); +39-043-465-9672 (V.D.R.); Fax: +39-043-465-9659 (G.C. & V.D.R.)

Received: 25 January 2018; Accepted: 5 March 2018; Published: 7 March 2018

Abstract: A positive family history is a strong and consistently reported risk factor for gastric cancer (GC). So far, it has been demonstrated that serum pepsinogens (PGs), and gastrin 17 (G17) are useful for screening individuals at elevated risk to develop atrophic gastritis but they are suboptimal biomarkers to screen individuals for GC. The main purpose of this study was to investigate serum metabolomic profiles to find additional biomarkers that could be integrated with serum PGs and G17 to improve the diagnosis of GC and the selection of first-degree relatives (FDR) at higher risk of GC development. Serum metabolomic profiles included 188 serum metabolites, covering amino acids, biogenic amines, acylcarnitines, phosphatidylcholines, sphingomyelins and hexoses. Serum metabolomic profiles were performed with tandem mass spectrometry using the Biocrates Absolute*IDQ* p180 kit. The initial cohort (training set) consisted of $n = 49$ GC patients and $n = 37$ FDR. Differential metabolomic signatures among the two groups were investigated by univariate and multivariate partial least square differential analysis. The most significant metabolites were further selected and validated in an independent group of $n = 22$ GC patients and $n = 17$ FDR (validation set). Receiver operating characteristic (ROC) curves were used to evaluate the diagnostic power and the optimal cut-off for each of the discriminant markers. Multivariate analysis was applied to associate the selected serum metabolites, PGs, G17 and risk factors such as age, gender and *Helicobacter pylori* (*H. pylori*) infection with the GC and FDR has been performed and an integrative risk prediction algorithm was developed. In the training set, 40 metabolites mainly belonging to phospholipids and acylcarnitines classes were differentially expressed between GC and FDR. Out of these 40 metabolites, 9 were further confirmed in the validation set. Compared with FDR, GC patients were characterized by lower levels of hydroxylated sphingomyelins (SM(OH)22:1, SM(OH)22:2, SM(OH)24:1) and phosphatidylcholines (PC ae 40:1, PC ae 42:2, PC ae 42:3) and by higher levels of acylcarnitines derivatives (C2, C16, C18:1). The specificity and sensitivity of the integrative risk prediction analysis of metabolites for GC was 73.47% and 83.78% respectively with an area under the curve of the ROC curve of 0.811 that improves to 0.90 when metabolites were integrated with the serum PGs. The predictive risk algorithm composed of the C16, SM(OH)22:1 and PG-II serum levels according to the age of individuals, could be used to stratify FDR at high risk of GC development, and then this can be addressed with diagnostic gastroscopy.

Keywords: gastric cancer; metabolomics; first degree relatives; biomarkers; early diagnosis; pepsinogen

1. Introduction

The GC is the fourth most common cancer and the second leading cause of cancer-related death worldwide [1]. Despite its decline in the last century, GC remains a major public health issue, with approximately 950,000 new cases diagnosed every year worldwide, of whom about 723,000 die from the disease [2]. GC is a genetically and phenotypically heterogeneous disease usually detected at an advanced stage with a median survival below one year.

The marked geographic variation, time trends and the migratory effect on GC incidence suggest that both genetic and environmental factors are implicated in the etiology. Besides the immutable inherent risk factors such as age, gender, race, the presence of *Helicobacter pylori* (*H. pylori*) infection, tobacco and diet are considered the major causes of GC [3]. However, other factors may also influence GC susceptibility. Different studies have reported a GC aggregation within FDR with a risk of two to 10 times higher than that of the general population. With the exclusion of the rare (<1% of GC) hereditary diffuse gastric cancer (HDGC) condition harboring a *CDH1* gene mutation [4], the observed familial clustering of GC cannot, to date, be explain only on genetic bases. The widespread use of upper endoscopy, an invasive but sensitive test for GC diagnosis, is limited by cost, risk complication and discomfort to patients and its use is indicated only for very high risk or symptomatic individuals.

The five-year survival rate continues to be poor (about 25% of cases) for GC, but where early diagnosis of cancer was confined to the inner lining of the stomach wall, a five-year survival rate of 95% can be reached. The problem of late diagnostics is due to a substantial proportion of patients with an asymptomatic or unspecified GC disease. Ideally, the GC disease should be diagnosed at an early stage by surveillance and management of individuals at high risk for GC. So far, extensive screening programs for GC have been introduced with success in high-risk countries such as Japan and South Korea. In Japan, eradication of *H. pylori* has been used as a first prevention strategy [5]; a secondary prevention strategy focuses on the diagnosis of GC in an early stage by using endoscopy. In some cases, the combination of serum pepsinogens (PGs) concentration and the presence of *H. pylori* antibody (ABC method) has been recommended based on the knowledge that PG concentration reflects the grade of gastric atrophy, a precursor condition for GC development [6]. The ABC method has been used for GC mass screening since 2011 in Japan (Nishitokyo Medical Association). However, this method is still debated because of the lack of satisfactory evidence in decreasing the mortality rates of GC [7]. Therefore, the finding of an efficacious non-invasive triage of FDR at increased risk for GC, that should undergo endoscopic examination remains a challenge for GC surveillance, particularly in low GC incidence geographic areas.

Metabolomics has emerged as a fast and efficient method to identify novel cancer biomarkers that gradually become a complementary technique to genomics and proteomics [8,9]. Metabolomics specifically addresses the simultaneous monitoring of hundreds to thousands of small molecules (metabolites < 1 kDa) from bio-fluids and tissue samples. The metabolomic profile is retained to give a biochemical snapshot of the physiopathological conditions of the cells/tissues resulting from the complex interplay between host genetic and environmental factors.

In this study, specific deficiency of serum sphingomyelins, phospholipids and an excess of acylcarnitines lipids were detected in GC as potential risk biomarkers. The integration of serum metabolomic biomarkers with other risk factors such as age and serum PG-II levels enhanced the diagnostic power of the pepsinogen test allowing a risk stratification of FDR for endoscopic GC examination. These results underline the role of the use of the individual's metabolomic trait to complement the FDR screening for precancerous conditions.

2. Results

2.1. Individual Characteristics

Demographic and pathological characteristics of GC patients and FDR in the training and validation sets are reported in Table 1, respectively. The training set comprised 49 GC patients and 37 FDR while the validation set included 22 GC patients and 17 FDR. In both these two sets, age and PG-II level differed significantly ($p < 0.05$) in GC patients and FDR while the other clinical and pathological conditions were superimposable. The odds ratio was 1.12 (95% CI 1.05–1.18) for age, and 1.25 (95% CI 1.10–1.42) for PG-II. The loss of data for histological *H. pylori* infection and GC classification is due to the difficulty of accessing tissue samples collected from the external hospital during routine biopsies for GC diagnosis.

Table 1. GC patients and FDR characteristics in the training set (**a**) and in the validation set (**b**).

(a)			
	GC	**FDR**	p [a]
N	49	37	NS
M/F [b]	27/22	10/27	NS
Age [c]	61 (19–85)	53 (30–69)	0.00009
H. pylori (−) [d,#]	32	25	NS
H. pylori (+) [e,#]	14	10	NS
PG-I (ng/mL) [f]	118.2 (2.7–706.4)	97.2 (3.1–658.4)	NS
PG-II (ng/mL) [g]	17.2 (1.1–104.0)	9.8 (0.2–35.5)	0.0075
G17 (pmol/L) [h]	15.7 (0.9–983.0)	3.7 (0.4–109.8)	NS
Histological GC Type [#]			
Intestinal	17		
Diffuse	11		
Mixed	5		
(b)			
	GC	**FDR**	p [a]
N	22	17	
M/F [b]	12/10	9/8	NS
Age [c]	67 (34–79)	45 (23–78)	0.001
H. pylori (−) [d,#]	12	12	NS
H. pylori (+) [e,#]	4	4	NS
PG-I (ng/mL) [f]	107.5 (3.9–341.2)	87.9 (59.3–112.0)	NS
PG-II (ng/mL) [g]	12.6 (2.8–45.9)	9.0 (4.5–13.8)	0.033
G17 (pmol/L) [h]	3.8 (1.5–500.0)	4.0 (0.5–14.6)	NS
Histological GC Type [#]			
Intestinal	8		
Diffuse	2		
Mixed	1		

[a] Statistical significance of the differences between GC (gastric cancer) and FDR (First-Degree Relatives) evaluated by *t*-test, [b] M: male, F: female, [c] age expressed as median and (range), [d] non infected *H. pylori* patients, [e] infected *H. pylori* patients, [f,g] serum pepsinogen I and II concentration, [h] gastrin 17 serum concentration. [#] data loss is due to no access to tissue samples from the external hospital. NS: not significant.

2.2. Comparison of Serum Metabolomic Profiles of GC and FDR

The serum targeted metabolomic profiles were investigated by tandem mass spectrometry (MS). The MS-targeted approach for serum metabolomic profile analysis adopted in this investigation has the advantage of being highly robust in term of intra- and inter-day precision and accuracy and overall, its application provides absolute quantification of serum metabolites. All these features contribute to making the targeted approach particularly reliable for clinical metabolomic investigations and guarantees a high standard quality among different clinical laboratories. The list of metabolites analyzed by the targeted metabolomics method used in this study is shown in Supplemental Table S1. Metabolomic profile data were analyzed using supervisor partial least squares discrimination analysis (PLS-DA), which explains maximum separation between GC and FDR samples. The result of this multi-parametric approach was summarized in the PLS-DA graph (Figure 1) where each point corresponds to a metabolomic patient profile. The PLS-DA discriminated GC patients and FDR with a classification accuracy of 72% ($R^2 = 0.40$, $Q^2 = 0.20$). Statistical validation of the obtained PLS-DA model was also confirmed with permutation testing ($p < 0.004$). Variable importance in the projection (VIP) of the PLS-DA model indicated that SM(OH)22:1 and SM(OH)22:2 had the higher VIP score (>2.1) (Supplemental Figure S1).

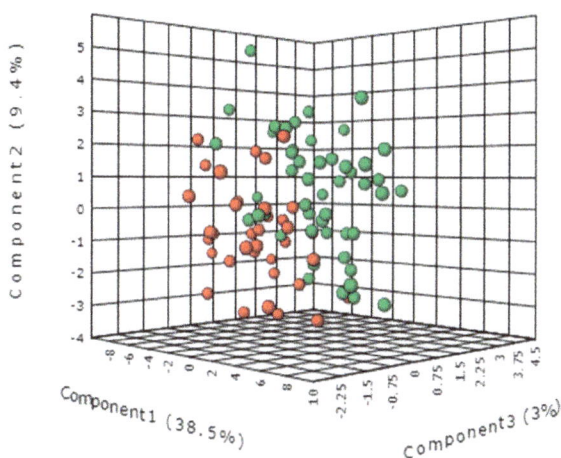

Figure 1. Multivariate partial least squares discrimination analysis (PLS-DA) of serum metabolomic profiles from FDR (red color) and GC patients (green color) in the training set.

2.3. Identification and Selection of the Most Significant Metabolites

From the training data set we selected the most significant metabolites that discriminate GC patients and FDR by both univariate (*t*-test, $p < 0.05$) and multivariate analysis (VIP > 1). Forty metabolites met these criteria and are summarized in Table S2. They include carnitine/acylcarnitines ($n = 7$), aminoacid derivatives ($n = 5$), phosphatidylcholines ($n = 23$) and sphingomyelins ($n = 5$) lipids derivatives. Of these 40 metabolites identified in the training set, nine were further confirmed as differentially expressed in the validation set ($p < 0.05$). They were three hydroxylated sphingomyelins: SM(OH)22:1, SM(OH)22:2, SM(OH)24:1, three acylcarnitines: C2, C16 and C18:1 and three phosphatidylcholine lipids PC ae 40:1, PC ae 42:2 and PC ae 42:3. Figure 2 shows the heat map plot of the concentrations of the validated metabolites that show the main significant change between GC patients and FDR in the training set. Hydroxylated sphingomyelins and phosphatidylcholines lipids showed the highest abundance score in FDR, while acylcarnitine's derivatives presented the lowest abundance score in GC patients. Absolute mean concentration, expressed as serum micromolar concentration, of each validated metabolite in GC patients and FDR are reported in Figure 3. In order to assess the GC's specificity of these nine validated metabolites, every single level of them was compared with those obtained from patients with non-epithelial cancer (i.e., non-Hodgkin lymphoma (NHL), $n = 47$) and with epithelial cancer (i.e., breast cancer, $n = 34$). When compared with FDR, the levels of the acylcarnitine: C2, C16 and, C18:1 were found to be higher in GC as well as in NHL and breast cancer groups. Conversely, the PC derivatives: PC ae 40:1, PC ae 42:2 and PC ae 42:3 as well as the SM derivatives SM(OH)22:1 and SM(OH)22:2 were found to be lower only in the GC patients (Figure S2, Supplemental Data).

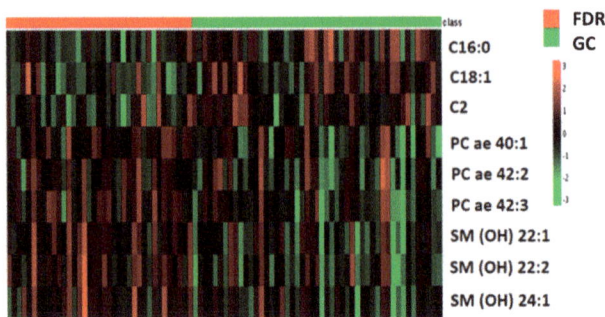

Figure 2. Heat map plot of the differential validated serum metabolites between FDR and GC patients. Data refers to the relative serum concentration level observed in the training set.

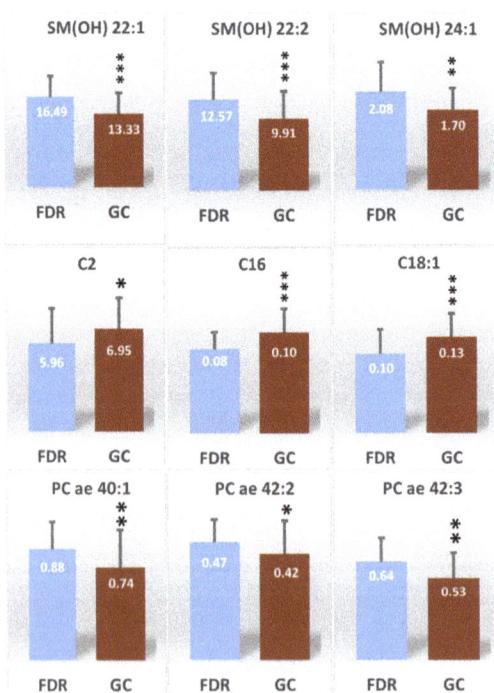

Figure 3. Box plots of the selected and validated differential metabolites (mean ±SD) between FDR and GC patients (training set). For each metabolite the serum concentration mean value is reported inside the box and expressed as μmoles/L. * $p < 0.05$, ** $p < 0.001$, *** $p < 0.0001$.

2.4. Model Performance for Metabolites

In the multifactor logistic regression model containing the nine established metabolites, high C16 and low SM(OH)22:1 metabolites were found to be independent risk factors for GC patients; in the training set the odds ratio (95% CI) were 2.83 (1.66–4.82) and 1.39 (1.19–1.62) for C16 and SM(OH)22:1, respectively. The equation for logistic regression fit was logit(p) = 0.0778 + 44.76 × C16 − 0.26 × SM(OH)22:1. For the training set, the predictive accuracy of the logistic equation measured by ROC curve analysis gave an area under curve (AUC)of 0.81 (95% CI: 0.75–0.89) with a sensitivity of 73.5%

and a specificity of 83.8% (Figure 4a) and an AUC of 0.82 (95% CI: 0.66–0.92) with a sensitivity of 90.9% and a specificity of 59.0% when the same equation was applied to the validation set (Figure 4b).

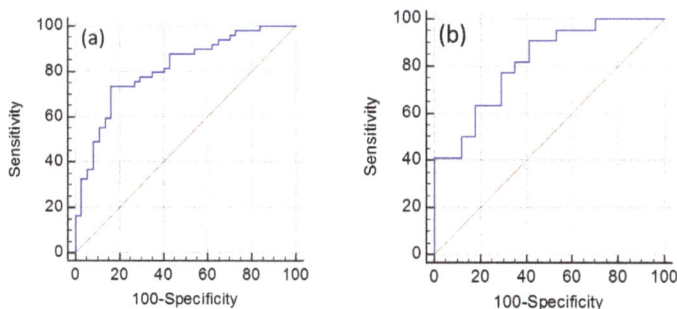

Figure 4. The receiver operating characteristic (ROC) curve plots for the metabolomic model based on C16 and SM(OH)22:1 biomarkers in the training (**a**) and validation set (**b**).

2.5. Effect of H. pylori Infection on Levels of Sphingomyelins and Acylcarnitines

To investigate the effect of *H. pylori* infection on the observed metabolic differences among GC and FDR, all samples were categorized according to the *H. pylori*-infection status and their sphingomyelins or acylcarnitines serum levels. The mean values of the significative sphingomyelins and acylcarnitines metabolites according to *H. pylori* infection status are shown in Figure 5. The main trend in metabolite profile consists in a decrease of SM(OH)22:1 and SM(OH)22:2 levels and an increase of C16 acylcarnitine in both infected and not infected individuals. In addition, a significant decrease of SM(OH)14:1, SM(OH)16:1 and SM(OH)24:1 and an increase in C18:1 acylcarnitine in *H. pylori*-positive GC was observed, while the C2 and C5 acylcarnitines were increased limitedly in negative *H. pylori*-GC.

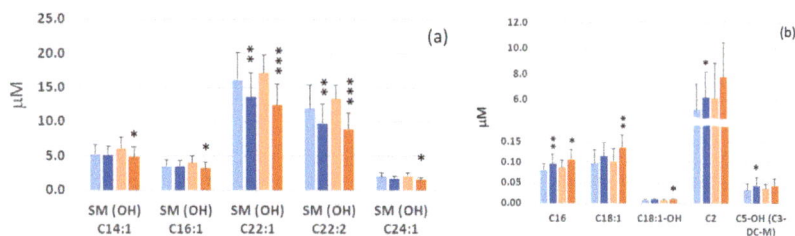

Figure 5. Serum concentrations of significative sphingomyelins phospholipids (**a**) and acylcarnitines derivatives (**b**) in FDR and GC patients according to *H. pylori* infection. Blue and dark-blue columns refer to FDR (*n* = 37) and GC patients (*n* = 44) with negative *H. pylori* infection, respectively. Orange and dark-orange columns refer to FDR (*n* = 14) and GC patients (*n* = 18) with positive *H. pylori* infection, respectively. Statistical comparison performed for FDR vs. GC for both negative and positive *H. pylori* groups by *t*-test: * $p < 0.05$, ** $p < 0.001$, *** $p < 0.0001$.

2.6. Age Effect on the Serum Levels of the SM(OH)22:1 and C16 Metabolites

Since there was a significant difference in the age between FDR and GC patients (median age of 53 vs. 61 for the FDR and GC groups, respectively, $p < 0.001$, Table 1), we further investigated the relationship between the level of metabolites SM(OH)22:1 and C16 and the age of individuals. Considering all the FDR and GC data from both the training and validation sets a significant positive correlation (Spearman's rank test, $p = 0.0076$) was found between the level of C16 metabolite and age (Figure 6a). Conversely, no significant relationship between the SM(OH)22:1 metabolite and age

(Figure 6b) was reported. However, within the single FDR and GC groups, any significant correlation ($p = 0.4609$ and $p = 0.3081$ respectively) was established between the levels of C16 and age.

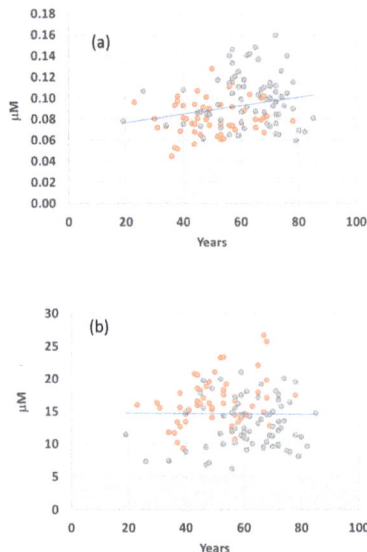

Figure 6. Correlation between C16 (**a**) and SM(OH)22.1 (**b**) serum concentrations and age for FDR (orange) and GC patients (gray). Correlation is performed considering all FDR and GC data. Spearman's rank test < 0.05 is considered significant.

2.7. Integrated Metabolomics Model

Data integration of metabolomics GC signatures with PGs, G17, *H. pylori* infection and individual's clinical data was our ultimate goal. Association of (a) SM(OH)22:1 and (b) C16 metabolites, and (c) serum PG-II level on GC diagnosis was retained in the multivariate model. Although C16 was found related to age when either FDR and GC group were considered separately, it was found independent by age. Therefore, we included both age and C16 as independent covariates in the logistic classification algorithm. The estimated regression coefficients for markers were as follows: 0.0898 for age, 0.0843 for PG-II, 0.283 for SM(OH)22:1 and 0.604 for C16. Thus, the final equation that stratifies FDR at high risk for GC development is computed as follow:

$$Y = -4.97 + 0.0898 \times \text{Age} + 0.0843 \times \text{PG-II} + 0.283 \times \text{SM(OH)22:1} + 0.604 \times \text{C16}$$

In our series, the equation including the metabolites provided a significantly higher capability of detecting GC than that provided by PG-I/PG-II ratio model. The model achieved good discriminatory power (i.e., AUC = 0.857, 95% CI: 0.78–0.91) (Figure 7). Conversely, the analysis performed with the current screening test for GC based on PG-I/PG-II ratio showed a ROC curve with a lower AUC value of 0.765 (95% CI: 0.67–0.84) ($p = 0.0278$) in our series (Figure 7). The prognostic ability of the model was further evaluated by using the optimal cut-off of $Y > 0.063$, as the score from ROC curve analysis was able to better discriminate FDR from GC patients. By using this cut-off, we correctly identified 52 out of the 71 GC patients (73%). Instead, by using a PG-I/PG-II ratio of ≤ 3, which is a commonly used cut-off for GC diagnosis, we correctly identified only nine out of the 71 GC patients (12.7%) (Figure 8). The percentage of false-positive cases by using the $Y > 0.063$ cut-off was nine individuals among the 54 FDR with a high-risk profile, while using the $Y \leq 3$ cut-off for PG-I/PG-II ratio was zero. Individuals identified by the integrated metabolomics/pepsinogen equation have been reported to the gastroenterologist for special attention in the follow-up and, as of now (median follow up of 4 years), they have not developed a GC as confirmed by histological examination of the biopsies. The limited number of FDR (9/54) at higher risk for GC development allows for effective prospective monitoring of these individuals.

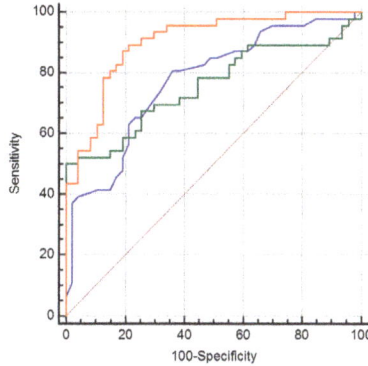

Figure 7. Comparison of ROC curves to test the difference among the areas under 3 dependent ROC curves: patient age (blue), PG-II biomarker (green) and the integrated model including age, PG-II and metabolites (orange).

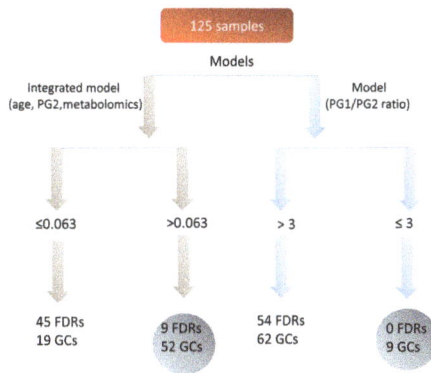

Figure 8. Clinical application of the developed algorithm proposed to identify high risk FDR ($Y = -4.97 + 0.0898$ age $+ 0.0843$ PG-II $+ 0.283$ SM(OH)22:1 $+ 0.604$ C16) compared with the PG-I/PG-II basal model currently in use.

3. Discussion

The prognosis of GC remains poor and its early detection is the key factor to improving survival. Screening and prevention programs offer an opportunity to reduce GC mortality, but only a minority of individuals (<1%) shows an identified germline gene defect (i.e., *CDH1* gene mutation), for which intense surveillance or prophylactic gastrectomy are provided. The identification of high risk individuals without *CDH1* mutations for further endoscopic examination to recognize GC at an early stage remains a key point. Only in Japan, where GC incidence is very high, PG-I/PG-II ratio ≤ 3 was used as a screening of GC risk.

In this study, we explored the potential of a noninvasive screening test for detecting early stage GC in FDR population using a metabolomics tool combined with clinical and pepsinogen tests. Metabolomics is a useful new omic tool to identify specific metabolic dysregulation occurring in GC patients compared with FDR. In our series, the most significant metabolic alterations of GC involve the acylcarnitines, sphingomyelins and phosphatidylcholines pathway. The present study highlighted an integrated model that included sphingomyelin SM(OH)22:1 and acylcarnitine C16 as important risk markers able to identify the large majority of GC (73%). Moreover, among FDR population, a feasible number of high risk individuals (<15%) were identified. These latter FDR have been reported to the gastroenterologist for further endoscopic examination and for special attention follow-up and as of now (median follow-up of 4 years) they have not developed a GC. However, to reach a valid conclusion more time to follow-up is necessary. The integrated model showed a better predictive performance than the PG-I/PG-II ratio test (AUC 0.857 vs. 0.765, respectively). Thus, our data suggested that the herein developed model represents an effective non-invasive test to screen FDR at risk of GC development. The interpretation of findings from this study presents some limitations due to the relatively small sample size and the short time of FDR follow-up as well as potential bias common in retrospective studies.

Despite these limitations, results provided new molecular insights into the metabolism GC's hallmarks. The serum metabolites that were found significantly differentiated between GC and FDR appear specific to GC disease. When the FDR levels were compared with those of patients with non-epithelial cancer such non-Hodgkin lymphoma or epithelial breast cancer (Figure S2, Supplementary Data), the acylcarnitines: C2, C16 and C18:1 and were found increased in all patients with cancer, while, the PC ae 40.1, PC ae 42:2 and PC ae 42:3 as well as the SM(OH)22:1 and SM(OH)22.2 decreased in only the GC group, suggesting that these latter phospholipids derivatives are specific to the GC disease.

Acylcarnitines are the obligate cofactors of mitochondrial fatty acid β-oxidation. The Acyls-CoA derived from fatty acids are unable to penetrate the mitochondrial outer membrane, but by using carnitine palmitoyltransferase activity, the Acyls-CoA are transformed to acylcarnitines, which are then shuttled into the mitochondrial matrix by carnitine-acylcarnitine translocase. Finally, acylcarnitines are converted back to Acyls-CoA by carnitine palmitoyltransferase 2 localized on the inner mitochondrial membrane. Acyls-CoA then enter into the cycle of citric acid to generate NADH and FADH$_2$ to produce ATP along the electron transport chain [10]. An imbalance between the fatty acid uptake and the oxidation due to defects or alterations in mitochondrial respiratory complex activities arises in intracellular concentration of acylcarnitines that may be reflected at the serum level [11]. In our series, C18:1, C18:1(OH) and C16 acylcarnitine levels increased in GC patients according to *H. pylori* infection (Figure 6a), suggesting a positive correlation between these acylcarnitines and the bacterium presence. The oxidative stress is one of the major factors in the development of gastric diseases, while the inflammatory state associated with chronic *H. pylori* infection may increase the risk of GC development due to the continuous exposure to oxidative species. Thus, *H. pylori* infection may partially explain the higher serum level of specific acylcarnitine metabolites shown in our patients. On the other hand, increased acylcarnitines in GC patients may be the consequence of the oxidative stress associated to GC itself or to the higher age of patients since oxidative stress has been reported to increase with aging [12]. Interestingly, we found a positive correlation between C16 acylcarnitine and patient's age (Figure 6). Thus, it is possible that the higher level of C16 carnitine observed in GC patients may be related to both *H. pylori* infection and the age of the patient.

Conversely to acylcarnitines, some phosphatidylcholine derivatives such as PC ae 40.1, PC ae 42:2 and PC ae 42:3 were significantly lower in the serum of GC patients. The lower level of specific serum phospholipids in GC serum could reflect alterations at tumor tissue. A previous metabolomics investigation, performed by a mass spectrometry imaging technique, revealed that GC tissue as compared with normal gastic mucosa may present specific shortages of phosphatidylcholine lipids derivatives i.e., PC 36:4 and PC 34:2 [13,14]. Interestingly, the authors of this study were able to demonstrate that the supplementation of such phosphatidylcholines in the culture medium suppressed the NIH-3T3 transformation by K-Ras as well as the in vitro growth of 4 out of 8 GC cell lines. Moreover, their oral administration was found to also reduce the in vivo growth of GC cells in nude mice without any side effects [13,14]. Overall, these preliminary results underline the importance of the specific serum phospholipids shortage with the GC growth. The lower serum concentrations of other specific phospholipids belonging to the sphingomyelins class observed in this study further reinforce such suggestions.

Sphingomyelins are structural constituents of all cell membranes particularly abundant in the myelin membrane sheaths surrounding axons. Sphingomyelins interact with cholesterol and glycerophospholipids participating in the formation and maintenance of lipid microdomains in the plasma membrane known as lipid rafts. Sphingolipids in lipid rafts modulate many cell processes, such as membrane sorting and trafficking, cell polarization and signal transduction [15]. Through the action of the sphingomyelinase (SMse), the sphingomyelins play a relevant role also in determining the cell fate by hydrolyzing back to ceramide which is an important metabolic intermediate able to induce cellular apoptosis [16]. Thus, sphingolipids have emerged as key effectors in different tumors such as colon cancer, breast cancer, leukemia, esophagus cancer, and brain cancer [17], by controlling various aspects of tumor cell growth and proliferation through ceramide molecules [15]. The specific metabolic signature observed in GC involved a lower serum level of several 2-hydroxylated sphingomyelins (SM(OH)s): SM(OH)22:1, SM(OH)22:2 and SM(OH)24:1 (Figure 3). Collectively, these specific hydroxylated sphingolipids require the action of the cellular fatty acid hydroxylase (FA2H) for their synthesis [18] and like the other sphingomyelins, they can be hydrolyzed to generate 2 hydroxy-ceramide derivatives, which analogously to ceramides have a pro-apoptotic activity [19]. Thus, a shortage of SM(OH)s sphingolipids may contribute to a reduction in cellular ceramide load promoting cell proliferation and tumor survival. Of interest, many cancers, including stomach, pancreas, and colon, show increased nerve density in relation to tumor growth [20]. Nerves infiltrating the GC microenvironment were found to release neurotransmitters to promote tumor growth and reciprocally, tumors secrete neurotrophic factors, that stimulate both nerve outgrowth and cancer cell growth [21]. The lower levels of circulatory sphingomyelins may reflect the increase tumor nerves growth observed in GC. Taken together, these findings suggest further investigations on whether nerve–cancer cell cross-talk involves sphingolipids in GC.

4. Experimental Section

4.1. Participants

Participants were excluded from clinically significant medications, surgery, radiotherapy or chemotherapy for metabolic, liver, kidney diseases or any other cancers. From January 2009 to March 2014, 71 GC patients and 54 FDR were consecutively enrolled at the Oncological Gastroenterology, Centro di Riferimento Oncologico, IRCCS-National Cancer Institute, Aviano, Italy to characterize their serum metabolomic profiles. For all the GC patients diagnosis was confirmed histologically based on tissue specimens. For all FDR individuals, the GC lesion was excluded after gastroscopy and histological examination of the biopsies. Two additional cohorts of patients unrelated to GC patients with a representative non-epithelial (i.e., non-Hodgkin lymphoma; $n = 47$) and epithelial cancer (breast cancer; $n = 34$) were included in the metabolomics investigation as unrelated independent cancer groups. None of GC patients and FDR were treated with proton pump inhibitors. *H. pylori* infection was detected in tissue sections using hematoxylin and eosin and Giemsa stains as previously reported [22]. Serum PG-I, PG-II and G-17 levels were measured as previously reported [22]. Clinical data from GC patients and FDR were collected in a dedicated database in the oncological gastroenterology center. Before enrolling each participant gave informed written consent. The study was approved on December 2008 by the Institutional Review Board (ref no. IRB2008-14).

4.2. Sample Collection

All the study participants were in an overnight fasting state and 5 mL of peripheral venous blood was taken in the morning. The blood was then allowed to clot for 30 min at 37 °C water bath and followed by centrifugation at 3000 rpm for 15 min. Then, the serum supernatant was taken and transferred to a clean tube and stored at −80 °C until further analysis.

4.3. Design of the Study

Based on the diagnosis, participants were randomly divided into 2 sets; the training set included 49 GC patients and 37 FDR and a validation set of 22 GC and 17 FDR. Detailed characteristics of patients are listed in Table 1.

The main steps of the study were: (1) characterization of metabolomic profiles associated with FDR and GC patients, (2) identification and validation of the most important metabolomics GC signatures by using the independent validation sample set, (3) apply multivariate statistical analysis of selected serum metabolites, clinical data and pepsinogen biomarkers to develop an integrated risk model for early stage GC detection, and (4) performance comparison between the model including the metabolites and the model based on PG-I/PG-II risk score.

4.4. Metabolomics Investigation

A high-throughput liquid chromatography-tandem mass spectrometry (LC-MS/MS) platform has been applied to evaluate serum metabolomics profiles. We used the commercial Absolute*IDQ* p180 Kit (Biocrates Life Sciences, Innsbruck, Austria) according to the manufacturer's instructions for the quantification of 188 targeted metabolites covering the following compound classes: amino acids, biogenic amines and polyamines ($n = 40$), acylcarnitines ($n = 40$), di-acyl-phosphatidyl lipids ($n = 92$), sphingolipids ($n = 15$) and hexose ($n = 1$). The complete list of all metabolites investigated is reported in supplemental Table S1. The analytical system consisted of a liquid chromatography Agilent (Agilent, Santa Clara, CA, USA) coupled with an ABI4000 triple quadrupole mass spectrometer (ABsciex, Framingham, MA, USA).

Briefly, 10 µL of serum was loaded onto an inserted filter in a 96-well sandwich plate, which already contained appropriate internal standards, structurally identical but labeled with stable isotopes such as deuterium, ^{13}C, or ^{15}N. The filters were dried under a nitrogen stream, derivatization of amino acids was performed with 5% phenylisothiocyanate (PTC), and filters were dried again. After extraction of metabolites with 500 µL of 5 mM ammonium acetate in methanol, the solution was passed through a filter membrane and diluted with MS running solvent. Final extracts were then analyzed by LC-MS/MS using amino acids and bioactive amines PTC-derivatives the Zorbax SB 100 × 2.1 mm column (Agilent, Santa Clara, CA, USA), and a direct flow injection analysis (FIA-MS/MS) for the analysis of acylcarnitines and phospholipids. Quantification of metabolites was achieved by multiple reaction monitoring, neutral loss and precursor ion scan in positive and negative ion mode. The MS/MS signals were integrated, by using Analyst 1.6.1 (ABsciex, Framingham, MA, USA) and quantified using a calibration curve according to the AS-180 to the manufacturer's instructions. Concentration and validation data were then further processed using the MetIQ software by comparing the results of triplicate analysis of low, medium and high-quality serum controls as an integral part of the analytical.

4.5. Data Processing and Statistical Analysis

Prior to statistical analysis, the serum concentration values of metabolites investigated were set to a log scale and auto-scaled (mean-centered and divided by the standard deviation of each variable). A supervisor multivariate partial least squares discrimination analysis (PLS-DA) was then applied to identify the relevant metabolites that contributed the most significance in differentiating between the GC and FDR groups in the training set. The PLS-DA model was further cross-validated by comparison of the resulting goodness of fit (R^2), predictive ability (Q^2) values, and by internal validation using 1000 permutation tests. A variable importance in projection (VIP) score was applied to rank the patients' metabolites that best distinguished between the GC vs. FDR groups. The relevant metabolites that distinguished the two groups in the training set were selected on the basis of VIP > 1 and by $p < 0.05$ as resulted from the application of univariate *t*-test analysis. The more significant metabolites

Int. J. Mol. Sci. **2018**, *19*, 750

differentially expressed were further validated by the confirmation of significant variable ($p < 0.05$) in the validation set. The ROC curves were constructed to test the diagnostic performance of the more significant metabolomics biomarkers. In a ROC curve, the true positive rate (sensitivity) was plotted against the false positive rate (1-specificity) for different cut-off points of a given parameter. The ROC curve was validated by internal cross-validation and permutation testing. The optimal cut-off was assessed by jointly maximizing sensitivity and specificity. Sensitivity and specificity, computed at the optimal cut-off, were then used for further investigation. All above data processing and the statistical analysis that included ROC analysis were performed using the Metabolanalyst web portals [23]. Correlation between metabolite biomarkers and clinical features was analyzed by the Spearman's rank-order correlation test. Multivariate analysis was used to determine the coefficient value for each of the independent variables and to make the integrated model equation including metabolites, patient age and PG-II biomarker.

5. Conclusions

This exploratory study describes for the first-time serum metabolomic profiles that discriminate GC patients from FDR sharing the same environment and a similar genetic background. As compared with FDR, the GC patients showed specific serum metabolomic signatures characterized by an increase in specific acylcarnitines and a decrease in a distinctive subclass of sphingolipids. The inclusion of such serum metabolomic signatures with patient age and pepsinogen PG-II demonstrated they are a key factor for the development of a model to distinguish FDR from GC patients. Compared with the current PG-I/PG-II screening approach used in Japan, the model proposed showed an improved discrimination between GC patients and the FDR. The current results demonstrate the potential usefulness of the serum metabolomics as a noninvasive tool for the triage of individuals at higher risk of GC development for further endoscopic examination. The feasibility of this approach, as well as the biochemical mechanisms implicated in GC development, remain to be validated and warrant further investigation.

Supplementary Materials: The following are available online at http://www.mdpi.com/1422-0067/19/3/750/s1.

Acknowledgments: The authors would like to thank Leslie Sonnenschein for the English editing and are thankful for the 5 × mille funds from Direzione Scientifica, IRCCS-National Cancer Institute.

Author Contributions: Giuseppe Corona, Renato Cannizzaro and Valli De Re designed the experiments; Giuseppe Corona, Agostino Steffan, Laura Caggiari, Mariangela De Zorzi and Ombretta Repetto contributed to sample analysis, Gianmaria Miolo, Renato Cannizzaro and Valli De Re collected samples and clinical data. Giuseppe Corona, Valli De Re performed data analyses and wrote the manuscript.

Conflicts of Interest: The authors declare no conflict of interest.

References

1. Torre, L.A.; Siegel, R.L.; Ward, E.M.; Jemal, A. Global Cancer Incidence and Mortality Rates and Trends—An Update. *Cancer Epidemiol. Biomarker Prev.* **2016**, *25*, 16–27. [CrossRef] [PubMed]
2. Ferlay, J.; Soerjomataram, I.; Dikshit, R.; Eser, S.; Mathers, C.; Rebelo, M.; Parkin, D.M.; Forman, D.; Bray, F. Cancer incidence and mortality worldwide: Sources, methods and major patterns in GLOBOCAN 2012. *Int. J. Cancer* **2015**, *136*, E359–E386. [CrossRef] [PubMed]
3. Parsonnet, J.; Friedman, G.D.; Vandersteen, D.P.; Chang, Y.; Vogelman, J.H.; Orentreich, N.; Sibley, R.K. *Helicobacter pylori* infection and the risk of gastric carcinoma. *N. Engl. J. Med.* **1991**, *325*, 1127–1131. [CrossRef] [PubMed]
4. Corso, G.; Figueiredo, J.; Biffi, R.; Trentin, C.; Bonanni, B.; Feroce, I.; Serrano, D.; Cassano, E.; Annibale, B.; Melo, S.; et al. E-cadherin germline mutation carriers: Clinical management and genetic implications. *Cancer Metastasis Rev.* **2014**, *33*, 1081–1094. [CrossRef] [PubMed]
5. Asaka, M.; Mabe, K.; Matsushima, R.; Tsuda, M. Helicobacter pylori Eradication to Eliminate Gastric Cancer: The Japanese Strategy. *Gastroenterol. Clin. N. Am.* **2015**, *44*, 639–648. [CrossRef] [PubMed]

6.	Miki, K. Gastric cancer screening by combined assay for serum anti-Helicobacter pylori IgG antibody and serum pepsinogen levels—"ABC method". *Proc. Jpn. Acad. Ser. B Phys. Biol. Sci.* **2011**, *87*, 405–414. [CrossRef] [PubMed]

7.	Yamaguchi, Y.; Nagata, Y.; Hiratsuka, R.; Kawase, Y.; Tominaga, T.; Takeuchi, S.; Sakagami, S.; Ishida, S. Gastric Cancer Screening by Combined Assay for Serum Anti-Helicobacter pylori IgG Antibody and Serum Pepsinogen Levels—The ABC Method. *Digestion* **2016**, *93*, 13–18. [CrossRef] [PubMed]

8.	Corona, G.; Rizzolio, F.; Giordano, A.; Toffoli, G. Pharmaco-metabolomics: An emerging "omics" tool for the personalization of anticancer treatments and identification of new valuable therapeutic targets. *J. Cell Physiol.* **2012**, *227*, 2827–2831. [CrossRef] [PubMed]

9.	Gowda, G.A.; Zhang, S.; Gu, H.; Asiago, V.; Shanaiah, N.; Raftery, D. Metabolomics-based methods for early disease diagnostics. *Expert. Rev. Mol. Diagn.* **2008**, *8*, 617–633. [CrossRef] [PubMed]

10.	Houten, S.M.; Wanders, R.J. A general introduction to the biochemistry of mitochondrial fatty acid beta-oxidation. *J. Inherit. Metab. Dis.* **2010**, *33*, 469–477. [CrossRef] [PubMed]

11.	Noland, R.C.; Koves, T.R.; Seiler, S.E.; Lum, H.; Lust, R.M.; Ilkayeva, O.; Stevens, R.D.; Hegardt, F.G.; Muoio, D.M. Carnitine insufficiency caused by aging and overnutrition compromises mitochondrial performance and metabolic control. *J. Biol. Chem.* **2009**, *284*, 22840–22852. [CrossRef] [PubMed]

12.	Muller, F.L.; Lustgarten, M.S.; Jang, Y.; Richardson, A.; Van, R.H. Trends in oxidative aging theories. *Free Radic. Biol. Med.* **2007**, *43*, 477–503. [CrossRef] [PubMed]

13.	Kurabe, N.; Suzuki, M.; Inoue, Y.; Kahyo, T.; Iwaizumi, M.; Konno, H.; Setou, M.; Sugimura, H. Abstract 394A: Phosphatidylcholine-34:2 and -36:4 have tumor suppressive function for gastric cancer. *Cancer Res.* **2016**, *76* (Suppl. S14), 394A. [CrossRef]

14.	Kurabe, N.; Igarashi, H.; Ohnishi, I.; Tajima, S.; Inoue, Y.; Takahashi, Y.; Setou, M.; Sugimura, H. Visualization of sphingolipids and phospholipids in the fundic gland mucosa of human stomach using imaging mass spectrometry. *World J. Gastrointest. Pathophysiol.* **2016**, *7*, 235–241. [CrossRef] [PubMed]

15.	Breslow, D.K.; Weissman, J.S. Membranes in balance: Mechanisms of sphingolipid homeostasis. *Mol. Cell* **2010**, *40*, 267–279. [CrossRef] [PubMed]

16.	Morad, S.A.; Cabot, M.C. Ceramide-orchestrated signalling in cancer cells. *Nat. Rev. Cancer* **2013**, *13*, 51–65. [CrossRef] [PubMed]

17.	Hendrich, A.B.; Michalak, K. Lipids as a target for drugs modulating multidrug resistance of cancer cells. *Curr. Drug Targets* **2003**, *4*, 23–30. [CrossRef] [PubMed]

18.	Hama, H. Fatty acid 2-Hydroxylation in mammalian sphingolipid biology. *Biochim. Biophys. Acta* **2010**, *1801*, 405–414. [CrossRef] [PubMed]

19.	Kota, V.; Hama, H. 2'-Hydroxy ceramide in membrane homeostasis and cell signaling. *Adv. Biol. Regul.* **2014**, *54*, 223–230. [CrossRef] [PubMed]

20.	Venkatesh, H.; Monje, M. Neuronal Activity in Ontogeny and Oncology. *Trends Cancer* **2017**, *3*, 89–112. [CrossRef] [PubMed]

21.	Hayakawa, Y.; Sakitani, K.; Konishi, M.; Asfaha, S.; Niikura, R.; Tomita, H.; Renz, B.W.; Tailor, Y.; Macchini, M.; Middelhoff, M.; et al. Nerve Growth Factor Promotes Gastric Tumorigenesis through Aberrant Cholinergic Signaling. *Cancer Cell* **2017**, *31*, 21–34. [CrossRef] [PubMed]

22.	De Re, V.; Orzes, E.; Canzonieri, V.; Maiero, S.; Fornasarig, M.; Alessandrini, L.; Cervo, S.; Steffan, A.; Zanette, G.; Mazzon, C.; et al. Pepsinogens to Distinguish Patients With Gastric Intestinal Metaplasia and Helicobacter pylori Infection Among Populations at Risk for Gastric Cancer. *Clin. Transl. Gastroenterol.* **2016**, *7*, e183. [CrossRef] [PubMed]

23.	Xia, J.; Wishart, D.S. Using MetaboAnalyst 3.0 for Comprehensive Metabolomics Data Analysis. *Curr. Protoc. Bioinform.* **2016**, *55*, 14.10.1–14.10.91. [CrossRef]

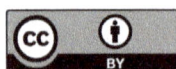

MDPI

St. Alban-Anlage 66

4052 Basel

Switzerland

Tel. +41 61 683 77 34

Fax +41 61 302 89 18

www.mdpi.com

International Journal of Molecular Sciences Editorial Office

E-mail: ijms@mdpi.com

www.mdpi.com/journal/ijms

www.ingramcontent.com/pod-product-compliance
Lightning Source LLC
Chambersburg PA
CBHW051714210326
41597CB00032B/5474